AF773935

Petty's

MUSCULOSKELETAL EXAMINATION and ASSESSMENT

A Handbook for Therapists

SIXTH EDITION

Petty's

MUSCULOSKELETAL EXAMINATION and ASSESSMENT

A Handbook for Therapists

EDITED BY

Dionne Ryder MSc MCSP MMACP FHEA
Visiting Lecturer
School of Health and Social Work
University of Hertfordshire, Hatfield, UK
Private Practitioner
Move and Improve Physiotherapy, St Albans, UK

Kieran Barnard MSc PG Cert BSc (Hons) MCSP MMACP
Advanced Practitioner Physiotherapist
Sussex MSK Partnership, Brighton, UK
Private Practitioner
Flex Physiotherapy, Burgess Hill, UK

FOREWORD BY

Nicola J Petty DPT MSc GradDipPhys FMACP FHEA
Formerly Associate Professor
School of Health Sciences,
University of Brighton, UK

ELSEVIER

First edition 1997
Second edition 2001
Third edition 2006
Fourth edition 2011
Fifth edition 2018
Sixth edition 2024

ISBN: 978-0-323-87471-7

Content Strategist: Andrae Akeh
Content Project Manager: Abdus Salam Mazumder
Design: Margaret M. Reid
Marketing Manager: Deborah Watkins

Printed in Scotland

Last digit is the print number: 9 8 7 6 5 4 3 2 1

CONTENTS

Foreword, vii
Preface, ix
Contributors, xi

1 **Introduction**, 1
Dionne Ryder and Kieran Barnard

2 **Talking the Talk: The Power of Communication**, 3
Lisa Roberts

3 **Subjective Examination/Taking the Patient's History**, 34
Hubert van Griensven and Dionne Ryder

4 **Physical Examination**, 65
Dionne Ryder and Hubert van Griensven

5 **Clinical Reasoning and Assessment: Making Sense of Examination Findings**, 143
Dionne Ryder, Matthew Low, and Neil Langridge

6 **Examination of the Temporomandibular Region**, 173
Helen Cowgill

7 **Examination of the Upper Cervical Region**, 196
Neil Langridge and Gail Forrester Gale

8 **Examination of the Cervicothoracic Region**, 229
Nicola R. Heneghan and Chris Worsfold

9 **Examination of the Thoracic Region**, 257
Nicola R. Heneghan

10 **Examination of Shoulder**, 284
Kevin Hall

11 **Examination of the Elbow Region**, 307
Val Jones

12 **Examination of the Wrist and Hand**, 334
Dionne Ryder

13 **Examination of the Lumbar Region**, 363
Chris Mercer and Amy Kemp

14 **Examination of the Pelvis**, 387
Claire Small

15 **Examination of the Hip Region**, 407
Kieran Barnard and Andrew Kemp

16 **Examination of the Knee Region**, 430
Andrew Kemp and Kieran Barnard

17 **Examination of the Foot and Ankle**, 468
Andrea Moulson

Index, 502

FOREWORD

As a newly qualified physiotherapist in musculoskeletal outpatients, I had 'good' days when patients got better and 'bad' days when patients got worse or did not change, and for a number of years I lived with the discomfort of not really knowing what I was doing. About to give up and leave the profession, the situation was turned around after I completed a year-long musculoskeletal postgraduate course in Melbourne, Australia. Having received such a solid grounding in both the theory and practice of musculoskeletal examination, assessment, treatment and management, it became my passion to pass this knowledge on to others and led to my move into higher education. The challenge I faced was to deliver what I had learnt at postgraduate level in a way that was understandable to an undergraduate student. At the time, some of the concepts and skills were taught on weekend courses and considered to be at postgraduate level, but I saw no reason why undergraduate students could not learn about them. In order to learn about the various concepts, a student would need to have bought more than half a dozen textbooks and so an in-house detailed handbook was written for students, which grew every year. One time when this handbook was on display at a clinical educators' day, a local clinician asked me for a copy for their own personal use. This triggered the decision by myself and Ann Moore to convert the handouts into a textbook, and this was finally achieved when the first edition was published in 1997. I am proud to say that the world-renowned pioneer of musculoskeletal physiotherapy, Geoffrey Maitland, wrote the first foreword of the text. The textbook was well received and further editions followed in 2001, 2006, 2011 and 2018.

To update the fourth edition, and to begin succession planning, I turned from author to editor. I invited well-respected and well-known clinicians and academics to contribute and update each chapter; they did an excellent job in building on the previous edition. Dionne Ryder and Kieran Barnard both made a valuable and significant contribution by writing a number of chapters. During preparation for the fourth edition, I asked Dionne to consider co-editing with me on the fifth edition and I was delighted when she agreed.

I first met Dionne over 20 years ago; we were both teaching Musculoskeletal Physiotherapy in Higher Education Institutions and we were both involved with the Musculoskeletal Association of Chartered Physiotherapists (MACP). Dionne was an ideal editor for the book as she had extensive clinical and educational experience and knew first-hand how to guide the reader in a systematic approach to examination and assessment of the musculoskeletal system. She took the lead in updating the fifth edition and we brought in highly respected clinicians and academics to broaden and deepen the scope of the text, while remaining a systematic step-by-step guide through the examination and assessment process.

During the writing of the fifth edition, I made the decision, with a tinge of sadness, to withdraw completely from any future edition of the book, as my retirement from academia was on the horizon. I asked Dionne and Kieran to co-edit the sixth edition of the book, as well as co-edit the fourth edition of the companion text Petty's Principles of Musculoskeletal Treatment and Management, and I was delighted when they both agreed.

I first got to know Kieran in 2007 as his course leader when he started his MSc Musculoskeletal Physiotherapy at the University of Brighton. During his studies, I remember being impressed by his thoughtful and questioning approach to theoretical issues underpinning practice and his excellence in writing essays. As an Advanced Practitioner and clinical mentor for MSc Musculoskeletal Physiotherapists, Kieran has both clinical and educational expertise which makes him an ideal editor of the book, knowing first-hand what knowledge and skill the reader needs to know to develop clinical expertise.

I have been proud to see this textbook become a core text for many UK undergraduate physiotherapy courses and become well established across the world, with translations into Italian, Spanish, Korean, Japanese, Polish, Turkish, and more recently simplified Chinese and Greek. It has been a very important and significant part of my life for almost 30 years. I feel honoured and delighted to be invited to write the foreword to this sixth edition. The process of writing has allowed me to finally let go of the baton and pass it completely over to Dionne and Kieran in a very tangible and public way. I do so with complete confidence in their stewardship of my work and with my blessing, gift it to them.

Like a bottle of wine, this textbook is getting better with age. The overall structure of the book remains much the same, it continues to offer the reader a step-by-step approach to the subjective and physical examination and assessment of each region of the body. Like previous editions, there is a tremendous amount of information, which has now been updated with more current theory and research evidence all of which is supported by new and updated Tables, Boxes, Figures and Photographs. It is wonderful to see the same contributors from the last edition: Helen Cowgill, Gail Forrester-Gale, Kevin Hall, Andrea Moulson, Lisa Roberts, Hubert van Griensven, Chris Worsfold, and Chris Mercer from the fourth edition, come alongside a number of new well-respected contributors: Nicola Heneghan, Val Jones, Amy Kemp, Andrew Kemp, Neil Langridge, Matthew Low and Claire Small. Their clinical and educational expertise have added further breadth and depth to the text.

Skilled communication is absolutely vital in clinical practice and chapter 2 entitled Talk the Talk: The Power of Communication, has now, quite rightly, been positioned at the start of the book. Throughout this edition, each chapter has new 'knowledge check' boxes with various questions the reader might like to consider to help engage and learn the material, and at the end of each chapter there is a 'review and revise questions' box; both of these could be useful to do individually or in a group. A substantive change has been the addition of case studies into each regional chapter. This is an excellent addition as it helps the reader understand how the examination and assessment process come together for a particular patient.

If the reader is looking for a textbook that gives them a comprehensive, evidence-enhanced step-by-step guide to the examination and assessment of the musculoskeletal system, they need look no further. Developing expertise in this area is quite a challenge, with the requirement to learn hands-on practical skill as well as learning the theory and research that underpins it. This text offers an excellent guide to readers wanting to gain the knowledge and skill in the examination and assessment of the musculoskeletal system.

May you, the reader, be blessed as you seek to develop expertise in the art and science of musculoskeletal examination and assessment.

Dr Nicola J. Petty
Hexham UK

PREFACE

In the new edition of this popular textbook, we have sought to build upon the content conceived and developed by Dr Nicola J Petty over the course of five previous editions. There are seven new contributors joining the existing team, all of whom have significant experience in managing patients with musculoskeletal conditions. There have been developments in the content and structure of the chapters with the inclusion of colour photographs and intext knowledge checks. Each regional chapter concludes with review questions to test the readers' understanding and a case study, allowing the reader to explore how the chapter content informs reasoning of an appropriate patient case.

The contributors have drawn from their own clinical and academic backgrounds to provide a logical and reasoned approach to examination that reflects contemporary practice.

We are grateful, not only for the valuable input each contributor has made to the text, but also for their energy and enthusiasm in completing their chapters under tight timescales and in addition to their busy day-to-day jobs.

Thanks must go to Elsevier and in particular, Poppy Garraway who was instrumental in launching this project and to Abdus Salam Mazumder and Shravan Kumar for their guidance and support throughout the publishing process.

The overall continued aim of the book is to provide a clear and accessible guide to musculoskeletal examination and assessment for pre-registration students. As skilled clinicians we have the opportunity to work closely with patients to facilitate their rehabilitation. This partnership can bring immense satisfaction and reward; however, success is not always easy to achieve with the inherent uncertainty of clinical practice. Each person is a unique blend of physical being, intellect, will, emotion and spirit, living within, and being influenced by, a social and cultural world. Rehabilitation is thus a complex process and requires high levels of clinical expertise. This text aims to provide a comprehensive step-by-step approach to the technical skills and clinical reasoning involved in the examination and assessment of people with musculoskeletal conditions.

Dionne Ryder
Kieran Barnard
Brighton and St Albans 2022

CONTRIBUTORS

The editors would like to acknowledge and offer grateful thanks for the input of all previous editions' contributors, without whom this new edition would not have been possible.

Kieran Barnard, MSc PG Cert BSc (Hons) MCSP MMACP
Advanced Practitioner Physiotherapist
Sussex MSK Partnership, Brighton, UK
Private Practitioner
Flex Physiotherapy, Burgess Hill, UK

Helen Cowgill, BSc(Hons) MCSP MfMACP
Clinical Director of Helen Cowgill Physiotherapy
London, UK
Clinical Lead Physiotherapist
Kings College Hospital NHS Foundation Trust
London, UK

Gail Forrester Gale, MSc PgCert HE SFHEA MCSP MMACP
Associate Dean Enterprise and Income Diversification
Faculty of Health, Education and Society
University of Northampton, Northampton, UK

Kevin Hall, PhD, MSc BSc NIHR Doctoral Fellow MCSP MMACP
Advanced Practice Physiotherapist
Western Sussex Hospitals NHS Foundation Trust
Sussex, UK
Private Practitioner
Kevin Hall Physiotherapy Ltd, Hove, UK

Nicola R. Heneghan, PhD MSc MCSP FMACP
Honorary Senior Lecturer
School of Sport, Exercise and Rehabilitation Sciences
University of Birmingham, Birmingham, UK

Val Jones, MSc Grad Dip Phys MCSP
Clinical Physiotherapy Upper Limb Specialist
Sheffield Shoulder & Elbow Unit
Sheffield Teaching Hospitals NHS Foundation Trust
Sheffield, UK

Amy Kemp, BSc(Hons) PG Dip MCSP MMACP
Advanced Practice Physiotherapist
University Hospitals Sussex NHS Foundation Trust
Worthing, UK

Andrew Kemp, MSc BSc(Hons) MCSP MMACP
Advanced Physiotherapy Practitioner
Research and Audit co-lead and hip and knee pathway lead
HERE
Sussex MSK Partnership, Brighton, UK

Neil Langridge DClinP, MSc BSc(Hons) FCSP FMACP
Director of Clinical and Rehabilitation Services
AECC University College, Bournemouth, UK

Matthew Low, MSc BSc (Hons) MSCPMMACP
Consultant Physiotherapist
University Hospitals Dorset NHS Foundation Trust
Christchurch, UK
Visiting Fellow
Orthopaedic Research Institute
University of Bournemouth, UK

Chris Mercer, MSc PgCert Grad Dip Phys FCSP FMACP
Consultant Physiotherapist
University Hospitals Sussex NHS Foundation Trust
Worthing, UK

Andrea Moulson, MA MSc BSc(Hons) PGCert MCSP MMACP NZRP
Principal Lecturer
School of Health and Social Work
University of Hertfordshire, Hatfield, UK
Clinical Specialist Physiotherapist
The Hillingdon Hospital NHS Foundation Trust
Middlesex, UK

Lisa Roberts, PhD PFHEA FCSP MMACP
Clinical Professor of Musculoskeletal Health
School of Health Sciences
University of Southampton, Southampton, UK
Consultant Physiotherapist
University Hospital Southampton NHS Foundation Trust, Southampton, UK

Dionne Ryder, MSc Grad Dip Phys FHEA MCSP MMACP
Visiting Lecturer
School of Health and Social Work
University of Hertfordshire, Hatfield, UK
Private Practitioner
Move and Improve Physiotherapy, St Albans, UK

Claire Small B, Phty(Hons) M.Phty St PG Cert NMP MCSP FMACP
Chief Clinical Officer, Consultant Physiotherapist
Pure Sports Medicine, London, UK
Honorary Senior Lecturer
Sports & Exercise Medicine
Queen Mary University of London, London, UK

Hubert van Griensven, PhD MSc(Pain) MCSP DipAc FHEA
Institute of Medical and Biomedical Education
St George's, University of London
Cranmer Terrace, London, UK

Chris Worsfold, MSc AFHEA MCSP MMACP
Advanced Musculoskeletal Practitioner
Physiotherapist
The Tonbridge Clinic, Kent, UK

1

Introduction

Dionne Ryder and Kieran Barnard

This text aims to provide guidance to the process of examination and clinical reasoning for patients with musculoskeletal dysfunction.

The text provides a step-by-step approach to the subjective and physical examination of the various regions in the body. Chapter 2 Talking the talk aims to support the reader right through the patient's consultation, highlighting the significance of reflecting on and developing communication skills in order to build strong therapeutic relationships from the outset with our patients.

The next chapter (Chapter 3) on subjective examination provides a general guide to the questions which might be asked, as well as the clinical relevance of questions in developing hypotheses to plan the physical examination. Chapter 4, on the physical examination, provides a guide to performing testing procedures and to understanding the value of the tests. Chapter 5 explores clinical reasoning to make sense of the subjective and physical examination. Thus Chapters 2–5 provide an overview of key principles and as such are considered essential reading setting the scene for regional chapters that follow.

Each regional chapter will follow a similar structure but will seek to identify how these principles are applied to each specific region.

The division of the body into regions is anatomically, biomechanically, functionally and clinically contrived. More realistic regions might, for example, be the cervico-thoracic-shoulder region and the lumbo-pelvic-hip region. One anatomical area may affect another biomechanically; for example, a muscle may span two joints, and nerve involvement may produce symptoms distally as well as at the site of dysfunction. So, while readers are introduced here to the individual regions, they need to maintain an awareness of the broader regional areas that are clinically and functionally relevant for each patient.

Much of the key clinical information is gathered during the subjective examination and often the physical findings simply serve to strengthen the clinical hypothesis generated during the subjective. Careful listening and thoughtful questioning justified through meticulous clinical reasoning during the subjective examination is therefore key (see Chapter 5). Predicting the findings of the physical examination is often a useful way to accelerate the development of a clinician's clinical reasoning skills; however, clinicians must be mindful of the pitfalls of personal bias and understand the value and limitations of the tests they apply.

In terms of physical technique, a word of warning to the novice clinician who may believe what is shown in this text is the only way to do something. What you see in this text is one way of demonstrating an assessment technique favoured by the particular clinician on the particular model at that time. Furthermore, the ability of the photographer to capture the technique will also have affected how the clinician performed it, and of course, the photographs will only be able to capture handling from one angle. Initially, novices have to start somewhere and may want to replicate the techniques shown. Once novices understand what they are trying to achieve with a technique, then they would be wise to consider alternative ways of carrying out the technique, making adaptations for their patients and for themselves. They can determine whether or not their adapted technique is effective and efficient by asking themselves:

- Is it easy and comfortable to perform? The position of the clinician, as well as the position of the patient and plinth height, will all contribute to the ease with which a technique is carried out.
- Is it comfortable for the student model or patient? While learning, it can be helpful for models to imagine they are a patient in pain, so they raise the standard of comfort required and then provide honest and constructive feedback to their partner.
- Does it achieve what it intends to achieve? A technique achieves what it intends to achieve when it is comfortable, accurate, specific, controlled and appropriate, and handling is sensitively adapted to the tissue response. Whenever a technique is being carried out, it is helpful to ask whether you think you are achieving what you are intending to achieve and if not, then adapt your technique. This is not just for novices as they learn techniques; normal everyday clinical practice requires clinicians to adapt their examination procedures to individual patients.

For those learning these examination procedures for the first time, here are some tips on how you might improve your handling which may help make findings from tests more valid and reliable:

- Practise, practise and practise! There is no substitute for plenty of good-quality practice.
- When practising, split the task into bite-sized chunks, building up into a whole. For example, practise hand holds, then application of force, then the hand hold and force on different individuals, then the communication needed with your model, then everything all together on different individuals.
- Imagine what is happening to the tissues when you are carrying out an examination procedure.
- Tell your model very specifically what you want in terms of feedback; model feedback needs to be honest and constructive.
- Verbalize out loud to your model what you are doing.
- When you do a technique, evaluate it and predict the feedback you will receive from your model, so you learn to become independent of your model's feedback.
- Act as a model and feel what is happening.
- Act as an observer: if you can see a good technique and feel a good technique then this can help you to perform a good technique.
- Use a video recording to observe yourself when working with a peer model.
- Imagine yourself doing the examination procedures in your mind in any spare moments.

It is perhaps worth mentioning at the outset that the clinician examining patients with a musculoskeletal condition may not be able to identify a particular structural source of symptoms or ongoing pathological process. In some patients it may be possible—for example, the clinician may suspect a meniscal tear in the knee or a lateral ligament sprain of the ankle. However, in other patients, particularly those for whom symptoms have persisted, the goal of identifying exact pathology is not realistic. All patients whether presenting with acute or persistent musculoskeletal symptoms should be viewed holistically so a person-centred treatment and management approach can be discussed with each person as an individual. The reader is referred to the companion text for further information on the principles of treatment and management of patients with musculoskeletal dysfunction (Barnard & Ryder, 2024).

REFERENCE

Barnard, K., Ryder, D., 2024. Petty's Principles of Musculoskeletal Treatment and Management: A Handbook for Therapists, fourth ed. Elsevier, Edinburgh.

2

Talking the Talk: The Power of Communication

Lisa Roberts

LEARNING OUTCOMES

After studying this chapter, you should be able to:

- Consider the preparations required ahead of a first consultation and how to create a positive first impression.
- Consider the type and style of questions (including TED and Socratic questioning) to use in consultations and the value of using a range of tailored communication approaches.
- Consider the key factors in acquiring, developing and delivering care with empathy, how to manage a patient's distress and listen without judgement to their beliefs and behaviours, without interruption or overlap.
- Consider the sensitivities needed to ask a patient to undress during a physical examination and the different types of touch that can be used in physiotherapy care episodes.
- Identify appropriate language to summarize clinical findings, deliver shared decision-making and person-focused goals, and promote self-management to empower patients and optimize their outcomes and experiences.
- Identify how the key components of the Behaviour Change Wheel can be used in practice and the three steps in offering advice to patients.
- Consider the issues associated with remote consultations compared to traditional, in-person interactions including location, digital challenges and obtaining consent (including the concept of 'material risk').
- Identify the skills needed in closing a consultation and ensure the patient's agenda has been addressed.

CHAPTER CONTENTS

Getting Ready, 4
- Initial Contact, 4
- Preparing Yourself, 5
- Preparing the Environment, 5

Getting Started: Building a Strong Relationship, 6
- Meeting and Greeting, 6
- Additional Companions, 6
- Additional Clinicians, 7
- The Importance of First Impressions, 7

The Main Event, 9
- Opening Questions and Agenda Setting, 9
- Question Styles, 9
- Active Listening, 12
- Empathy, 12

The Content of Physiotherapy Consultations, 13
- Interruptions, 14
- Challenging Conversations, 16
- Documenting Psychological Distress, 17

Person-Focused (or 'Patient-Centered') Care, 18

Remote Consultations, 18
- Clear Signposting, 18
- Additional Concerns About the Technology, 19
- Starting the Call, 19
- Gaining Consent in Remote Consultations, 20
- Looking to the Future, 20

The Physical Examination, 20
- Signposting, 20
- Negotiating Any Need to Undress, 20
- Providing Feedback, 22
- The Power of Touch and Its Role in Communication, 22

Articulating the Assessment Findings and Deciding Together, 23
Perceptions of Diagnosis, 23
Shared Decision-Making, 24
Goal Setting, 26
Changing Behaviour, 26
Motivational Interviewing, 27
Communicating the Treatment Options, 27
Offering Advice, 28
Negotiating an Exit, 29
Acknowledgements, 30
References, 30

Communication is a thread that is woven throughout every clinical interaction. It has been described as the most important aspect of practice that health professionals have to master (Wetherall et al., 1998) and so must be among the most highly developed skills in any clinician's toolkit. The core communication skills that you learn during clinical training will need nurturing and refining throughout your career and, since every patient is unique, each interaction needs to be tailored, as one size does not fit all.

Within healthcare, patient experience (or 'satisfaction') is increasingly used as an indicator of quality (Mazur et al., 2015). It is worth noting, however, that 'satisfaction' is a less-helpful indicator than experience, as it depends upon a patient's expectations (and so could result in disappointment if their expectations are unrealistic, for example expecting a cure for a long-term condition).

Whichever indicator is used, when patients go unheard, the result is 'careless communication, insincere apologies and unclear explanations' (Parliamentary and Health Service Ombudsman, 2012). Furthermore, communication has been cited as the top reason for complaints in the NHS in England (18%) for quarters 3 and 4 in 2020–21, above 'patient care (including nutrition/hydration)' (12.1%) and 'values & behaviours (staff)' (10.6%), which must be addressed (NHS Digital, 2021).

Communication skills form part of a raft of contextual factors (sometimes termed 'nonspecific treatment effects') that have the potential to significantly affect the outcome of a care episode.

Examples of contextual (or 'nonspecific treatment') effects include:

- the relationship between the patient and clinician
- the patient feeling listened to
- the clinician inspiring confidence
- the clinician providing a convincing explanation
- the Hawthorne effect (positive changes in behaviour that occur in individuals when interest is taken in them)
- the physical appearance of the clinician
- the professionalism and behaviour of the clinician
- the environment etc.

Clinicians cannot, and indeed should not, ignore these factors—instead, optimizing them will give the best chance of a good outcome for the patient. And, whilst it may not be possible to achieve an excellent clinical outcome every time, it should always be possible to ensure the patient has a positive experience.

In short, whatever sector you work in, time spent developing your communication skills is essential to maximize the impact of all your other clinical skills.

GETTING READY

Initial Contact

The first contact between a patient and the physiotherapy service is an important marker for what is to follow. Whether the patient has initiated the contact through self-referral, or the clinic made contact by post, telephone, email or text, it is important to think about the appearance and content of this communication, as it informs those all-important first impressions of the service. Asking patients for feedback about their first impressions (once they have got to know the service), can provide key insights for future improvement.

For many patients, seeking healthcare is a significant undertaking and a burden. Patients may have:

- needed to make complex plans to take time off from their usual activities
- had to juggle roles as a carer
- encountered expense and hassle travelling to the clinic, potentially inconveniencing friends or relatives (and impacting their schedules)

- anxieties about what physiotherapy is, and what an initial consultation might involve, ahead of their appointment.

It has been reported that many patients fail to get the best from their consultations because they arrive unprepared, not knowing what the consultation is about, what is likely to happen, and that they will be asked to give an account of their symptoms, concerns and medical history (Caldwell, 2019).

Providing clear information ahead of the consultation can help to minimize these issues and other problems such as non-attendance; patients going to the wrong location; wearing inappropriate clothing; being unable to recall their current medication; not bringing reading glasses etc. Such information needs to be as patient-friendly as possible and is best written by/with the help of people who have used the service and seen it through the lens of a patient or visitor.

When communication is poor and assumptions are made:

> *During the course of our research, one patient with significant back pain told us she physically struggled to her first physiotherapy appointment carrying a huge bag of clothes, because her appointment letter stated, 'please bring some shorts' and she didn't have any. Instead, she 'brought everything else in case', and was so troubled by this single request, she had been lying awake, thinking about it.*

Preparing Yourself

In helping to make a positive first impression, you may wish to make some physical preparations:

Ask yourself:

- *Do I look neat and professional?*
- *Is my clothing clean and well-ironed?*
- *Is my personal hygiene good? (Including avoiding strong-smelling foods before clinic, or strongly scented toiletries when close to patients etc.)*
- *Are my nails short and clean?*
- *Are my hands well-moisturized?*
- *Would I like to be treated by me?!*

In addition to physical preparations, it is essential for clinicians to be aware of their own thought processes if they have received a referral letter ahead of the initial consultation.

Ask yourself: Does it impact your thoughts if you read details like the patient:

- *is currently off sick?*
- *has recurrent symptoms?*
- *is a single parent with a young family?*
- *has sustained a sporting injury?*
- *works as a senior health professional?*
- *has had multiple previous appointments in this service?*
- *has had previous physiotherapy that was reported to be unhelpful?*
- *is involved in ongoing litigation?*

Any of these factors can influence your communication style (positively or negatively, which you may not even be aware of) and so in turn, can impact upon the patient's first impressions of you.

Preparing the Environment

Before inviting a patient into the clinical area, take a minute to check that the area is tidy, that the couch is clean (with fresh paper, if appropriate), and the furniture is arranged appropriately. This is all part of making the patient feel expected, welcome and valued (Fig. 2.1).

Having a clinic room with solid walls rather than curtains can influence the communication that takes place during physiotherapy consultations, as patients may be more guarded if they perceive they can be overheard.

Simple measures like having a radio or music playing could be an option, but in order to avoid copyright infringement in the United Kingdom, it is important to check whether the premises has a 'Performing Right Society (PRS) for Music' license for playing a radio or background music in public, and also a 'Phonographic Performance Ltd (PPL)' license, which collects and distributes money for using recorded music on behalf of record companies and performers. It is possible to purchase a combined license.

KNOWLEDGE CHECK

1. What physical and mental preparations will you make before you go and meet a patient?
2. What can you do in your treatment area to make a positive first impression of the environment?
3. Who do you need to get licenses from if you want to have music or a radio on in your clinic?

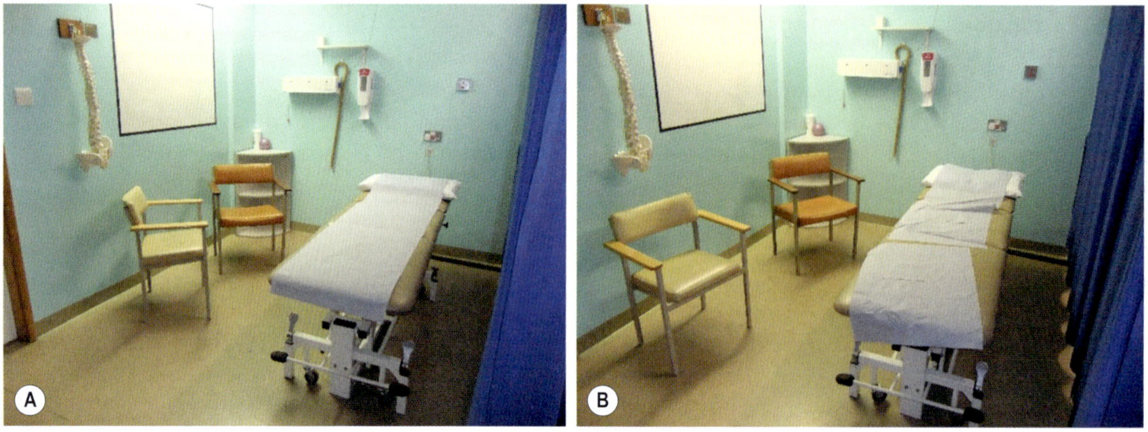

Fig. 2.1 You only have one chance to make a positive first impression (A) – or not (B).

GETTING STARTED: BUILDING A STRONG RELATIONSHIP

Meeting and Greeting

Taking time to smile and welcome patients can go a long way to making them feel at ease, and it should not be underestimated how highly this is valued by patients.

Do you introduce yourself with both your first name and surname? Do you also include your level of experience, such as your job title? In undertaking a needs analysis with patients to develop a leaflet for our department, it was interesting that patients most wanted to know not only the name of their physiotherapist, but also his or her level of experience (Roberts, 2006), or as one patient put it, '*Are they any good?*' This does not necessarily mean using your job title, however as these can be jargonistic.

Whilst there is no universal way to introduce yourself, there are definitely some things to avoid, especially jargon. In many roles in the service sector, it is not necessary to give a job title as the context makes it clear—for example, when someone is booking an appointment for a patient at their reception desk, their role is clear. This may not be so obvious in the case of a physiotherapist working as a first contact practitioner in a health centre, where the patient may not be expecting to see a physiotherapist (depending on the information they have already been given).

However you decide to introduce yourself, it is definitely not helpful to include Agenda for Change bands, as patients are likely to be unaware of what these mean. Table 2.1, includes some examples of things you might like to think about. They are not intended to be scripts, just cues to think about how you introduce yourself to patients.

Additional Companions

If the patient attends with a third party, it is important to greet that person too, check that s/he has actually come with the patient, and that the patient is happy for them to be present in the consultation, rather than waiting outside.

Jamal: Hello—Mrs. Watson?

Mrs. Watson: Yes, hello.

Jamal: My name is Jamal Ferguson, and I'm the physiotherapist who'll be seeing you today. Would you like to come through?

Mrs. Watson gets up to come in, accompanied by a younger woman.

Jamal: And who have you brought with you today?

Mrs. Watson: Oh, this is my daughter, Becky. Can she come in too?

Jamal: Yes that's fine, as long as you're happy for her to come in?

Mrs. Watson: Yes, I'd like that, as I do sometimes get a bit muddled!

TABLE 2.1 Cues on How to Introduce Yourself to Patients

Things to Avoid	Things to Consider
'Hello, my name is Sam Peterson and I'm a band 5 physio'.	*'Hello, my name is Sam Peterson and I'm a physiotherapist'.*
'Hello, my name is Jamie and I'm a physio tec'.	*'Hello, my name is Jamie Smith and I work closely with the physiotherapists and lead the exercise classes'.*
'Hello, my name is Ellie Perkins and I'm a student'.	*'Hello, my name is Ellie Perkins and I'm a final year physiotherapist-in-training'.*
'Hello, my name is Nadia Ahmed and I'm a first contact practitioner'.	*'Hello, my name is Nadia Ahmed and I'm a specialist physiotherapist working with the GPs here, to help with diagnosis'.*

Research indicates that companions attend 16%—25% of primary care encounters and 36%—57% of encounters with patients aged over 60 years (Laidsaar-Powell et al., 2013), and may provide advocacy, as well as practical, informational and emotional support for the patient (Stewart et al., 2021). The companion may be a friend, relative, neighbour or carer, and it is important to know their relationship to the patient, as there may be times in the clinical encounter when the companion adds to the patient's response or even replies to a clinician's turn that was directed to the patient.

When arranging the furniture in the treatment area, your communication will be primarily with the patient; however, you need to think about where the companion will be sitting, as this can influence how involved s/he is/feels in the session.

Additional Clinicians

It may be that the clinician wishes an additional person to be present during a consultation, for example: a student; a colleague completing a peer observation; or someone undertaking work experience etc. It is essential that the clinician explains who this person is, and why the individual wishes to be present.

Where possible, patients should be asked in advance if they are willing for this additional person to be present, so that it is not sprung upon them as they arrive, without much time to think. It is really important that patients are asked in a way that tries to reduce coercion (as far as possible), i.e. in private, and not within sight or ear-shot of the additional person, as the power differential in a clinician-patient relationship already makes it difficult for a patient to decline. Whatever the outcome, it is essential that the patient's wish be respected.

A conversation between the physiotherapist and patient, held in private, away from Helen Michaels, a student physiotherapist in her first year of training who is hoping to be able to sit in and observe the appointment:

Rob: 'Hello, Mr. Stevenson, I'm Rob Johnson, the physiotherapist who phoned last week about this appointment.

Mr. Stevenson: Oh yes, hello.

Rob: You may recall when we spoke, I asked if you would be willing for one of our first-year physiotherapy students to sit in with us today and observe? This is entirely your choice, and it's not a problem if you would rather they didn't.

Mr. Stevenson: No, that's fine. I hope it helps them.

Rob: Thank you, that's really kind. Let's go in, and I'll introduce you to Helen, as she joins us.'

The Importance of First Impressions

As in any interaction, the physiotherapist only has one chance to make a favourable first impression, and it is reported to take only 39 ms for a first impression to be made (Bar et al., 2006) and 'many encounters' to change it (Tongue, 2007).

Handshakes

For some clinicians, using a handshake may feel natural (with some patients), whilst for others, it may not. This is a personal choice, but if used, should be done with sincerity.

According to Emily Post (1940), 'the proper handshake is made briefly: but there should be a feeling of strength and warmth to the clasp, and as in bowing, one should at the same time look into the countenance of the person whose hand one takes'.

A firm handshake accompanied by direct eye contact is generally associated with a more positive first impression, conveying positive individual characteristics, such as openness to experience, extraversion and emotional expressiveness (Katsumi et al., 2017).

Small Talk

Careful thought needs to be given to the use of small talk and social pleasantries. The Cambridge Dictionary (2021) describes small talk as 'conversation about things that are not important, often between people who do not know each other well'. In our research, we found these apparently innocuous phrases turned out to be more important than we perhaps realize:

A physiotherapist accompanied a patient from the waiting room into the clinic and, following an initial introduction, said to a patient *'How are you?'*

> Later the patient confided to the researcher: *'It didn't start off well…when people say to me, "How are you?" I hate it because that is like saying, I don't really care how you are actually, but I'm going to ask out of politeness…. It's one of those statements people should avoid. But you're better off saying, You look crap! You know what I mean? At least you're making a statement!'*
>
> Sincerity is key.

A Good Consultation

Having greeted the patient (and companion) and got into the room, the consultation begins in earnest and has three main purposes (Lipkin et al., 1995), which are to gather information; develop and maintain a therapeutic relationship; communicate information.

The most important determinants of a 'good' consultation have been described by Lærum et al. (2006) as:

1. the patient's perception of being taken seriously
2. giving an understandable explanation of the pain
3. applying patient-centred care
4. reassurance
5. being told what can be done.

Remember: Communication transcends all five of these.

Along with compassion and empathy, rapport has been described as a cornerstone of a positive clinical encounter (Raja et al., 2015). It begins to develop during the initial phase, and taking a history (if done well), resembles a conversation that is paced and directed by both participants (McAllister et al., 2004), rather than an interview or, worse still, an interrogation.

Prosody

It is not only what is said during a clinical encounter that has an impact, but how the spoken word is delivered since communication traditionally incorporates verbal and nonverbal behaviours.

The effectiveness of any verbal message passed on to another person relies on that person's ability to listen, hear and assimilate the message appropriately (Williams, 1997). In addition to the words used, it is not possible to consider verbal communication without looking at the prosodic features that accompany it, including pitch, rhythm, tempo and resonance, as they all influence what is said; for example, nasality (too much air escaping through the nose while talking) is considered likely to create a negative first impression (Candita, 2006).

Nonverbal Behaviours

Meanwhile, nonverbal communication describes all behaviours that convey messages without the use of verbal language (Oliver & Redfern, 1991). There have been attempts in the literature to quantify the relative importance of these behaviours, with estimates of the nonverbal component comprising 55%–97% (Caris-Verhallen et al., 1999), 90% (Hall & Lloyd, 1990) and 93% of the message (Mehrabian, 1971). Although the figures vary, the nonverbal aspects of communication are consistently thought to be more influential than the verbal. Therefore, as Waddell says (2004) when the nonverbal message conflicts with the verbal message, we will probably not believe what is said.

The three most influential factors are reported to be eye contact, smiling and posture (McShane, 1993), alongside other factors such as facial expression and gestures, like a handshake. These have been extensively studied in the field of job interviews:

Eye contact: Researchers concluded that eye contact ranked as one of the top three variables that affected interview ratings (McShane, 1993). It needs to be used with care, however, as constant eye contact can be deemed too intense, while high to moderate levels of contact are considered essential in order to seem engaged and interested (Levine & Feldman, 2002). *[This is particularly important to think about if you are using a laptop or tablet in your clinic, as this can reduce eye contact.]*

Smiling: Levine and Feldman (2002) reported that more time spent smiling (31% vs 16%) was associated with higher scores when interview candidates were rated for their likability. *[In clinical practice, a smile has been deemed even more important than clinical competence—as one patient in our research remarked: 'As long as there's a big smiley face I'm quite happy … a smiley face is more important than clinical skills!']*

Posture: Defined as sitting erect while using hand and facial expressions that are appropriate for the verbal responses that are given, posture is reported to rank just below eye contact in its importance (McShane, 1993). A slouched posture is said to convey an impression of laziness or sloppiness, yet if overdone, sitting completely straight may give the impression of being edgy or overly aggressive, and more frequent posture changes are thought to give better outcomes (Levine & Feldman, 2002). *[It's easier to get into the habit of sitting well as you take a seat at the start of the consultation, as it's one less thing to think about!]*

KNOWLEDGE CHECK

1. How will you introduce yourself to your next new patient?
2. How will you find out the relationship between the patient and the companion s/he arrived with?
3. What steps will you take to gain consent from a patient for a colleague to be present in the clinical encounter with you?
4. How long does it allegedly take for a first impression to be made?
5. What message does your sitting posture convey when you are taking a history from a patient?

THE MAIN EVENT

The early stages of the clinical encounter are when patients present their issues to the clinician. Heritage and Robinson (2006) used the term 'problem presentation' for the stage when patients disclose information about their symptoms. This is reported to be the only time in a healthcare encounter when patients are given the opportunity to describe their condition in their own words and address their own personal agenda (Heritage & Robinson, 2006) and can affect patient's 'satisfaction' (Heritage & Robinson, 2006; Robinson & Heritage, 2006), and adherence to treatment (Zolnierek & Dimatteo, 2009).

Therefore, the physiotherapist's skill in questioning is vital in building a good therapeutic alliance, and according to Miciak et al. (2019), this involves establishing a meaningful connection, in which patients and clinicians feel seen, heard and appreciated. It is integral to the therapeutic relationship (Miciak et al., 2019; McCabe et al., 2021) and like any skill, requires practice.

Opening Questions and Agenda Setting

Communication within physiotherapy is underexplored, and little attention has been given to how 'best' to open clinical encounters. To study this phenomenon, our team audio-recorded 42 initial consultations and 17 first follow-up encounters between qualified physiotherapists and patients with back pain in an adult musculoskeletal, primary care outpatient setting (Chester et al., 2014).

We identified 11 different opening questions in the initial consultations (Table 2.2) and seven in the follow-up visits (Table 2.3). We then used these findings to determine clinicians' preferences in a national survey, posted on the four most relevant professional networks (sports medicine, orthopaedics, massage and soft-tissue therapy, and pain management) of the national, interactive Chartered Society of Physiotherapy (iCSP) website, to canvass opinion more widely.

The preferred 'key clinical question' for an initial encounter among the 43 physiotherapists who responded was: *'Do you want to just tell me a little bit about your [problem presentation] first of all?'*

For follow-up encounters: *'How have you been since I last saw you?'* Although the survey response in this study was small, this topic generated much discussion among clinicians on their preferences for opening patient encounters and building a strong therapeutic relationship.

Question Styles

Developing skills in questioning is fundamental to clinical practice. It is important to keep questions short and simple, ensuring they only address one issue at a

TABLE 2.2 Preferred Phrasing of the Key Clinical Question in Initial Back Pain Consultations

Rank	Score	Phrase
1st	83	*Do you want to just tell me a little bit about [problem presentation, e.g. knee, back] first of all?*
2nd	77	*I've had this referral through. Tell me what's happened.*
3rd	71	*The referral says you've got [problem presentation]; is this correct?*
4th	65	*How can I help you today?*
5th	57	*What we'll do today is just have a bit of a chat about [problem presentation], I believe it is. All right?*
6th	45	*It's your [problem presentation] that you're here for, is it?*
7th	35	*What problem are you having at the moment?*
8th	30	*Do you want to tell me your story?*
9th	29	*Do you want to start off by telling me whereabouts you're getting your pain at the moment?*
10th	28	*I know a little bit from the GP; when did this start?*
11th	17	*How long have you had [problem presentation] for?*

Chester et al. (2014).

TABLE 2.3 Preferred Phrasing of the Key Clinical Question in a Follow-Up Back Pain Encounters

Rank	Score	Phrase
1st	158	*How have you been since I last saw you?*
2nd	131	*How did you get on with the [treatment, e.g. exercises, hydro, injection, massage]?*
3rd	82	*How have you been feeling from a [problem presentation, e.g. knee, back] point of view?*
4th	71	*How are you getting on?*
5th	54	*How have you been?*
6th	18	*Are the [problem presentation] symptoms ongoing?*
7th	12	*What was the take-home message that you got from me last time?*

Chester et al. (2014).

time. Asking closed questions, for example, '*Have you got another appointment booked?*' is likely to result in a short, focused answer to this yes/no interrogative. Meanwhile, open questions such as, '*How is your knee pain affecting you?*' will invite patients to give a fuller account and can be particularly helpful in establishing the impact of the symptoms on their lives.

There is a hybrid form of open-focused questions where the question style is open, but the scope is directed towards a particular topic. This can reduce the number of questions asked and the need for probes—e.g. Asking '*How do your shoulder symptoms affect you getting washed and dressed?*' is preferable to asking '*Does your shoulder affect you getting washed and dressed?*' and then having to follow up with further probing questions to find out how.

'TED' Questions

These questions involve 'tell', 'explain' or 'describe' stems and can encourage patients to share their experiences and provide insights that can be used to help plan treatment goals.

Examples of TED questions:

- *Can you tell me how your neck pain started?*
- *Can you explain how these symptoms are affecting your life at the moment?*
- *Can you describe the feeling in your leg?*
- *Can you describe to me how your back pain varies throughout the day?*
- *Can you tell me what you think is the most important thing for us to focus on in this session?*

Socratic Questions

Named after the philosopher Socrates, this style of questioning uses open-ended questions that are concise, focused and designed to encourage reflection. They are frequently used in cognitive behavioural therapy and also in education and coaching circles and can be particularly useful when discussing the patient's assumptions, values and beliefs. Paul and Elder (2016) identified six types of Socratic questions. Table 2.4 includes some examples of how they may be applied in a physiotherapy consultation.

Sensitive Questioning

Patients often worry when seeing a health professional that they will be judged about aspects of their life, such as their lack of exercise; the choice to smoke; weight; dietary habits; or other lifestyle choices/circumstances.

TABLE 2.4 Socratic Questions That Encourage Reflection in a Physiotherapy Consultation

Question Type	Examples
Clarification	• *What do you think is the most important issue here?*
Assumption-probing	• *What makes you think that?*
Probing reasoning and evidence	• *Can you give me an example?*
Perspectives and viewpoints	• *Can you think of any ways to change this?*
Implications and consequences	• *How does this affect you/your life?*
Questioning the question	• *What do you think was important about that question?*

These worries can be heightened by contextual ('nonspecific') factors such as the clinician's appearance—for example, sitting in front of a physiotherapist, who may be wearing what the patient perceives as a gym kit (sports top, trainers etc.), may result in a patient giving a socially desirable answer about his/her activity levels.

Through carefully crafted questions, you can help patients feel comfortable to give an honest account of their life, whilst minimizing perceptions of judgement:

Physio: After everything that's happened, it must have been a real challenge to get going again and even think about going out?

Patient: Yes, it's really hard.

Physio: Can you tell me a bit more about that? If I can understand what it's really like for you now, it'll help when we think about some goals that you might want to achieve.

Questions That Involve Handing Over Control

It can be particularly helpful during the clinical interview, to ask questions that are designed to specifically hand over control to the patient:

Handing over control to the patient:

- *'You know your body better than anyone; what do you think is happening in your back?'*

At the end of the clinical interview:

- *'Before we go on to have a look at your foot, is there anything else that we haven't talked about that you think is important and want to raise?'*

Handing over control in this way shifts the balance of power to the patient, as the clinician is not presupposing a specific angle or problem, or displaying prior knowledge of the patient's problem, in what Heritage (2012) calls a less knowledgeable (K−) epistemic status. This can reveal some interesting and important beliefs; for example, if a patient has concerns that the label of 'degeneration' in his/her spine means he/she thinks his/her spine is crumbling, this will be a useful starting point to discuss he/her beliefs, in readiness for any decisions about possible treatment options. It is useful to explore these beliefs and what or who has influenced them, especially as many patients now search the internet before seeking healthcare.

Specifically giving control to the patient at the end of the clinical interview can provide another opportunity to ensure his/her agenda is met. This recognizes the issues may be multifactorial, as evidenced by the EPaC

(Elicitation of Patient Concerns) study in the United Kingdom, where an analysis of 185 primary care in-person video-recordings with GPs revealed an average of 2.1 concerns were raised per 10-minute appointment (Stuart et al., 2019).

Seeking any additional issues at this point in the consultation may help prevent 'door-knob concerns', where the patient is metaphorically on their way out with their hand on the door knob, and an additional concern surfaces, often the most important one (Finset, 2016), or they leave with unmet needs. In primary care, unvoiced health concerns have been associated with worsening symptoms, increased anxiety, additional visits and increased burden and costs (time and resources) both for patients and the service (Heritage et al., 2007; Stuart et al., 2019).

> **KNOWLEDGE CHECK**
> 1. How will you phrase your key clinical question for a new patient presenting with a history of elbow pain?
> 2. How will you phrase your key clinical question when a patient returns for their first follow-up appointment after you previously assessed his/her neck?
> 3. Can you provide three examples of TED questions that you could use when taking a history from a patient with a hand injury?
> 4. Can you give one example of a Socratic question that will probe the patient's assumption that walking will increase his/her ankle pain?
> 5. How will you hand over control to the patient at the end of the clinical interview?

Active Listening

Sacks et al. (1974) maintain that people take turns talking by following a set of conventional rules that assign speaker time and direction, and any deviation could indicate a person's attempt to display power, status or influence.

Practical guides to clinical communication skills concur with Sacks' model, and the two most important skills have been identified as the ability to allow the patient to speak without interruption and the ability truly to hear what the patient is trying to say (Jackson, 2006).

It is important to note that the letters in 'listen' also spell 'silent' (Fig 2.2). As well as knowing what to say, a key skill for the physiotherapist to master is to know when to be silent and, as in the title of the book by

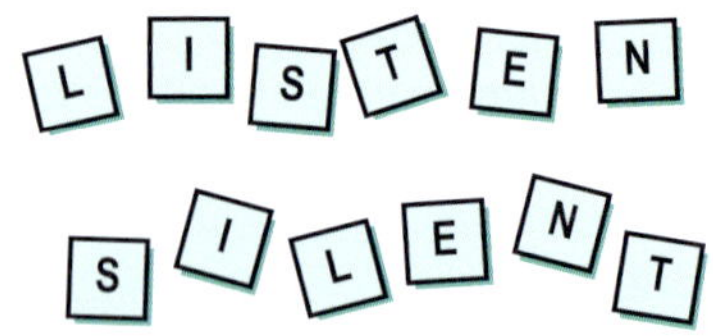

Fig. 2.2 'Listen' also spells 'silent'.

Cathy Jackson, to *Shut up and Listen!* (Jackson, 2006). Even short pauses can be very empowering for patients and provide them with an opportunity to bring up an issue that is important to them.

Audio-recording consultations, with patients' permission, can be a really useful learning tool to help clinicians explore whether there are any periods of silence in the consultation and, if so, what follows from the patient: is it a question; a more affective account of his/her symptoms (e.g. how they feel)? This may then reveal an expression of a deeper worry or concern.

Empathy

Empathy is difficult to define and is considered in healthcare to be an understanding and communication of another person's situation (Shapiro, 2008). Cox et al. (2012) define it as the 'ability to understand and identify with the feelings or emotional states of others… comprising both affective and cognitive aspects', which Misch and Peloquin (2005) describe as 'having empathy' and 'showing empathy' respectively.

It is not clear when or how clinicians successfully acquire a high level of empathic skills. When Millie Allen, in our group, conducted three focus groups with 11 qualified and six student physiotherapists to explore this issue, the majority of clinicians considered empathy to be an innate characteristic (Allen & Roberts, 2017):

> *In our research, one senior clinician said when discussing empathy: 'It's not something that you can just go on a course and learn, accept that it is something that will probably get better and better over time … accept that it is there as something to be developed as part of your practice.'*

From the focus group findings, we created a model to highlight the specific factors that participants identified that may affect the acquisition, development and delivery of empathy during a clinical encounter (Fig. 2.3). This highlights the complexity of this enigma:

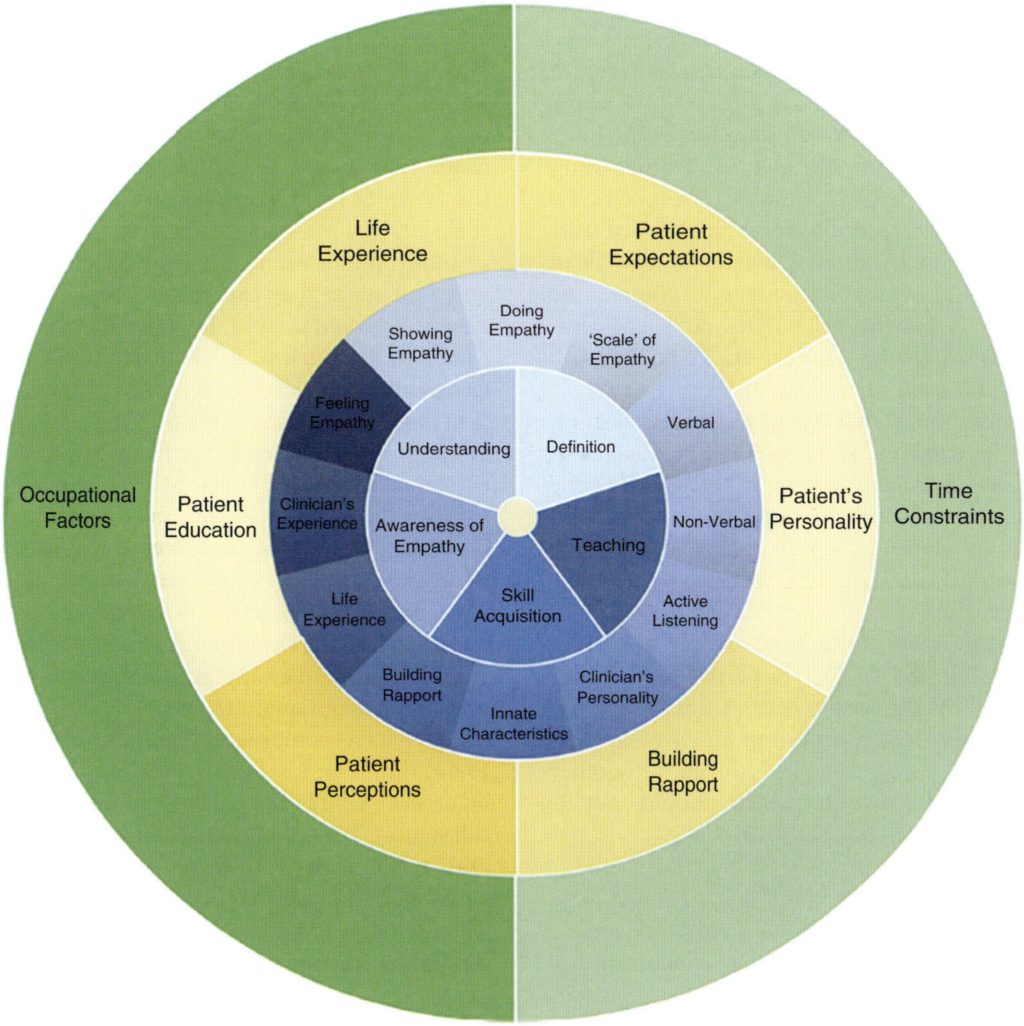

Fig. 2.3 Model of acquiring, developing and delivering empathy within clinical practice. (Allen & Roberts, 2017.)

Empathy remains a much-coveted, holy grail of communication, that is both highly valued and worthy of future research, especially as the best approach to acquiring and enhancing empathic communication skills remains unclear.

In our study, participants were in agreement that it is possible to develop empathic communication skills but disagreed as to whether empathy can be directly taught or not. They considered the optimal time to develop empathic communication skills was while working in a clinical setting, where they can be directly applied in practice, and suggested emphasis should be placed on the continued development of empathic communication skills throughout a clinician's career.

THE CONTENT OF PHYSIOTHERAPY CONSULTATIONS

Compared to medicine, there has been less work undertaken to identify communication practices within physiotherapy, and in particular, examining associations between communication practice and outcomes (Parry, 2008).

In our early research, we undertook a cross-sectional, observational study to measure the verbal communication taking place between clinicians and 25 patients with back pain in a UK primary care setting (Roberts et al., 2013). The mean duration of the initial consultations was 38 minutes and 59 seconds (range 26 minutes 21 seconds to 53 minutes 16 seconds). The content of the audio-recordings was categorized using the Medical Communications Behavior System (Wolraich et al., 1982), which categorizes 13 clinician behaviours and 7 patient behaviours, and has three miscellaneous categories (shown in Table 2.5 with added examples from our research).

Our results showed that the physiotherapists spoke more than the patients (49.5% vs 33.1%, respectively), with the most prevalent categories of speech being 'history/background probes' and 'content remarks' respectively, as clinicians asked questions about patients' symptoms, and patients discussed how these affected their lives.

Both groups spent little time overtly discussing emotions (1.4% and 0.9%, respectively). Analysis further highlighted the prominence of 'advice' given in the initial consultation, constituting 12.5% of the total time, establishing it as a key player in the physiotherapist's treatment repertoire, which should not be underestimated (Roberts et al., 2013).

Interruptions

In this work mapping the verbal content of physiotherapy consultations, we noted that concurrent talk was more prevalent among experienced clinicians compared with less-experienced practitioners (7.6% vs 2.6%, respectively) and interruptions were common (Roberts et al., 2013).

Further analysis of the 25 initial consultations demonstrated that physiotherapists interrupted patients answering the key opening question about their back pain in 60% of cases. This is not unique to physiotherapy: Marvel et al. (1999) found, in a sample of 264 consultations with primary care family physicians in the United States, that 45.5% of patients were interrupted (or 'redirected') while giving their 'statement of concerns' and this was associated with fewer concerns mentioned by patients, late-arising concerns and missed opportunities to gather important patient data. On average, patients were given 23.1 seconds to itemize their concerns before interruption from the physician (Marvel et al., 1999).

Langewitz et al. (2002) reported that patients will take, on average, 92 seconds to explain their problem in an outpatient setting if they are not interrupted. Studies have shown, however, that 25%–76% of patients are interrupted by physicians before they finish talking, and the mean talking time is reduced to only 12–23 seconds (Beckman & Frankel, 1984; Marvel et al., 1999; Rhodes et al., 2001).

Interruptions are not restricted to the problem presentation stage; they can occur at any time during the clinical encounter, and be by either the patient or clinician (Beckman & Frankel, 1984). Such interruptions may lead to delays in patients expressing their concerns (Irish & Hall, 1995) and the clinician missing opportunities to gather relevant information (Beckman & Frankel, 1984; Marvel et al., 1999).

Two different types of 'interruptions' have been identified by Kitzinger (2008), 'overlaps' and 'interruptions' although at present, these definitions are not universal and, in practice, the terms are often applied interchangeably (Drummond, 1989; Kitzinger, 2008). Table 2.6 lists two examples from our research, with the overlap/interruption underlined.

Our data set comprised 975 minutes of data made up of 15,489 turns (7659 by patients; 7647 by clinicians; and 183 by others, such as the patients' spouse or other clinical colleagues). We found that clinicians were 7 times more likely to interrupt than patients (284 and 39 respectively); however, overlaps were 1.5 times more prevalent among patients ($n = 582$), compared to clinicians ($n = 385$) (Roberts & Burrow, 2018) (Fig. 2.4).

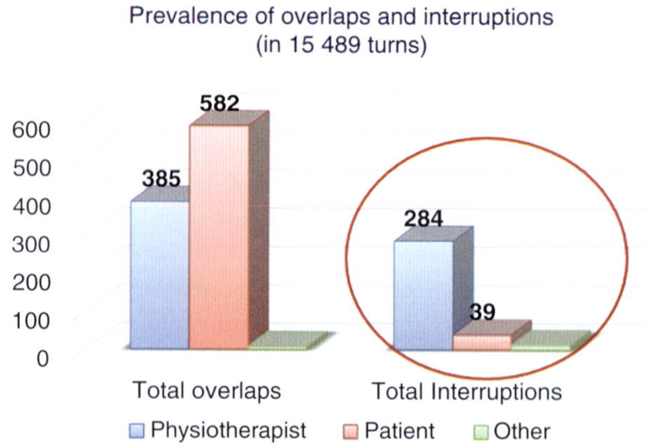

Fig. 2.4 Prevalence of overlaps and interruptions (25 initial back pain consultations). (Roberts & Burrow, 2018.)

TABLE 2.5 Examples of the Categories in the Medical Communications Behavior System (MCBS)

	Category	Includes	Example from Research
Physiotherapist	Content behaviours	History/background probes	*'And did you have the back discomfort at the time or was it purely just the leg pain?'* (patient 5: line 33)
		Checks for understanding information	*'When you were told about you having the sort of wear and tear and the arthritis ... was it explained to you exactly what is going on?'* (patient 1: line 412)
		Advice/suggestion	*'If you bring your leg up towards your chest for me and just hug the knee, can you feel that sort of stretching out the back here?'* (patient 5: line 781)
		Restatement	*'Just to go back to when it started, you said it started to get worse about a year ago?'* (patient 7: line 54)
		Clarification	(Following a patient's description of her recurring symptoms): *'So it [the back pain] was sort of episodic?'* (patient 4: line 37)
	Affective behaviours	Emotional probes	*'How would you feel about ... me referring you to one of the community rehabilitation teams, who can come out and see you in your home ... and see if there's anything that we can do to help you?'* (patient 9: line 385)
		Reassurance/support	*'So the fact that you can control it [the back pain] quite well—not to worry at the moment'* (patient 1: line 477)
		Reflection of feelings	Patient: *'I'm just concerned it might be arthritis going into my back ...'* Therapist: *'Right. That's what you, how you're thinking?'* (patient 1: line 776)
		Encourages/acknowledges	*'I know what you mean'* (patient 1: line 547)
	Negative behaviours	Disapproval	*'Tsk. OK. OK. So, I'm still trying to ascertain when the right hip pain came on'* (patient 20: line 116)
		Disruptions	(Knock at the door) *'Oh sorry, do you mind if I just quickly answer that?'* (patient 2: line 1011)
		Jargon	*'I'm going to teach you an exercise ... which is to work on your transversus abdominis, which is a deep, core stabilizing muscle, OK?'* (patient 4: line 605)
Patient	Content behaviours	Content questions	(Responding to an answer on a health questionnaire to the question *'Do you have diabetes?'*): *'Did I tick that by mistake?'* (patient 10: line 81)

Continued

TABLE 2.5 **Examples of the Categories in the Medical Communications Behavior System (MCBS)—cont'd**

Category	Includes	Example from Research
	Content remarks	*'Oh well, I crouched down to get the bag from under my bed and you know, something went'* (patient 3: line 39)
	Checks for understanding	*'What I'm gathering is, I have to re-strengthen the muscles that have become … like an elastic band. They've gone really thin? Huh?* (patient 2: line 1306)
Affective behaviours	Encourages	*'I would say that was spot on'* (patient 14: line 90)
	Emotional expressions	*'I think it's the old situation of, I've hurt myself, I'm a bit scared and I don't really want to do anything again, yeah'* (patient 2: line 585)
Negative behaviours	Disapproval	Therapist: *'It's too hot outside?'* *Patient: 'Well, it is when you've got to walk round in circles in this hospital'* (patient 7: line 5)
	Disruptions	e.g. Knock on the door from another clinician enquiring whether the room contains a particular piece of equipment
Miscellaneous categories	Social amenities	*'Come on in and have a seat. Right. Did you catch my name?'* (patient 6: line 4)
	Silence	
	Unclassifiable	e.g. When the physiotherapist and patient talk over each other

Wolraich et al. (1982).

The main functions for interruptions by clinicians and patients were to 'seek' or 'give' additional information respectively. A trend was noted that female physiotherapists were three times more likely to interrupt than male clinicians and overall, the prevalence of interruptions in same-sex consultations was twice as likely as in mixed-sex encounters; however, the small sample size precluded secondary analyses.

This work highlights the importance for physiotherapists to be aware of the extent to which they interrupt or overlap their talk with patients, and the impact this has on an interaction.

KNOWLEDGE CHECK

1. What is the difference between an overlap and an interruption?
2. How long will patients take on average in an outpatient setting to explain their problem, if they are not interrupted?

Challenging Conversations

Sometimes it can be difficult to discuss social and emotional issues with patients. Indeed, it has been reported that doctors have been reluctant to inquire about

TABLE 2.6 Overlap and Interruption

Overlaps	Defined as: an error in projecting where a speaker is planning to end his or her turn (Kitzinger, 2008). Here is an example where the physio interrupts to seek clarification: Patient: *I did try those heat pads that you can put, that you can buy...* Physio: *Ah the ones that you can stick on?* Patient: *...yeah, and they were no good.* Physio: *No good. OK.*
Interruptions	Defined as: a start-up at a point in a speaker's talk where it cannot possibly be completed (Kitzinger, 2008). Physio: *Are, are you on any medication?* Patient: *I am, just for depression. That's...* 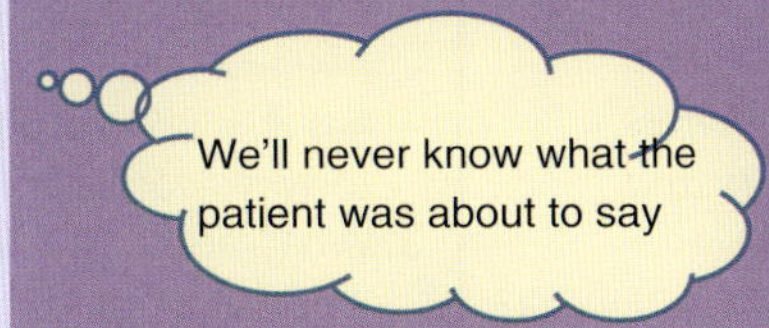 Physio: *Do you know what it's called, that one?* Patient: *It's um, um Fluoxetine.*

the social and emotional impact of patients' problems for fear it will increase the patients' distress, take up too much time and threaten their own emotional survival. Consequently, they respond to emotional cues with strategies to block further disclosure:

Strategies used by doctors to block further disclosure:

- offering advice and reassurance before the main problems have been identified
- explaining away distress as normal
- attending to physical aspects only
- switching topic
- or 'jollying' patients along. (Maguire & Pitceathly, 2002)

It is important for physiotherapists to be aware of times when they are tempted to (or indeed do) use such strategies and the consequences.

Another source of challenging conversation can be when a patient becomes upset during a clinical encounter. It is essential to have a box of tissues to hand that the patient can readily access, without needing to ask, should the need arise.

Sharing such moments can be a powerful component in a therapeutic relationship, as the patient conveys emotional distress and, although the clinician may feel quite helpless and not know what to say, sometimes words are not necessary, and just being there and listening is a source of comfort.

If given time and space to cry, patients will stop at their own pace. Ensuring privacy is important, and it might help to use phrases like, 'I'm sorry this is difficult', or 'please take your time', which gives them some space, whilst acknowledging their distress.

However difficult the situation, it is important to resist any urges to ask the patient to stop crying, or for clinicians to display their own embarrassment or awkwardness. This is a time when it can be really helpful to relinquish control and let the patient lead. It can be an opportunity to find out more about the patient's coping skills and what has helped in the past—knowledge that can be useful to help the patient think about facing the difficulties that lie ahead. Looking back on the consultation, the patient is unlikely to remember whether you asked about an aspect of their past medical history, but they will be very aware of how they felt and how you responded when they were at a low ebb.

Even the most experienced clinicians can feel really challenged when patients become angry or distressed, and it is important to seek support and debrief with colleagues to help process the experience and further develop your healthy coping skills for the future.

Documenting Psychological Distress

When documenting difficult encounters, it is essential to avoid labelling patients with judgmental phrases like 'yellow flaggy', 'heart-sink', displaying 'psychological overlay' or 'supra-tentorial'. This has damaging consequences for the patient, for your credibility and for the profession.

Feeding back to referring medical colleagues about the care episode provides an opportunity to demonstrate the professional, sensitive and thorough communication skills that physiotherapists can deliver.

An example of explaining findings in a professional, nonjudgmental way:

> *The patient presented with causal beliefs that his pain was the direct result of the lifting incident at work, with subsequent loss of personal control, negative treatment beliefs and significant consequences (including loss of earnings, potential job security and inability to return to his twice-weekly football).*

PERSON-FOCUSED (OR 'PATIENT-CENTERED') CARE

In developing person-focused (often termed 'patient-centred') care, clinicians are advised to attend not only to the disease but to patients' experience of symptoms, the impact of the condition and what really matters to them (Pollock, 2001; Walseth et al., 2011).

Patient-centred care is characterized by regarding the patient-as-person, a biopsychosocial perspective, sharing power and responsibility, and therapeutic alliance (Paul-Savoie et al., 2018). In such an approach, establishing meaningful connections, shared decision-making, self-management support, and patient-centred communication are essential components, and the key elements are summarized in Fig. 2.5 (Hutting et al., 2021).

A clinical interview provides an excellent opportunity to deliver person-focused care. This includes creating an adequate conversational space to elicit the patient's agenda (i.e. understanding, impact of pain, concerns, needs and goals) and helps ensure s/he feels listened to and heard.

An approach to focusing on the person when treating patients with musculoskeletal pain and disability has been outlined (Caneiro et al., 2019) and includes screening for biopsychosocial factors and health comorbidities; embracing patient-centred communication; providing health education using active learning approaches; coaching patients towards active self-management; and addressing comorbid health factors (when appropriate).

Skills in delivering person-focused care are key to promoting and optimizing health across the life-course and ensuring the patient has the best outcome and experience possible. Therefore time spent developing these skills to a high level is essential.

KNOWLEDGE CHECK

1. What strategies can you use in a consultation where the patient becomes upset?
2. How would you document that during the clinical interview, the patient said he did not think physiotherapy would help for his recurrent back pain as he has a 'slipped disc and trapped nerve, and so can't go to work' for the foreseeable future?
3. What are the key elements in person-focused (or 'patient-centred') care?

REMOTE CONSULTATIONS

As society becomes more digitalized, there is a strong drive in healthcare to support alternatives to traditional in-person interactions, including remote consultations by telephone and virtual platforms. This agenda was highlighted in the service transformations that took place in physiotherapy services at the onset of the COVID-19 pandemic.

Whilst many key communication skills are transferable from traditional to remote consultations, there is an even greater emphasis on verbal communication skills and prosody during these interactions.

Clear Signposting

It is important to provide clear information ahead of the appointment for patients that it is a *health consultation* and they may wish to take the call somewhere private (and not while at a supermarket, while out walking with friends, while driving, at work, or undertaking home improvements etc., as we experienced in our service at the start of the pandemic!).

Many patients do not realize they may be asked to perform certain tasks, or if it is a video call, they may be asked to de-robe as part of the examination, as they would in a face-to-face interaction and so again, clear signposting is paramount.

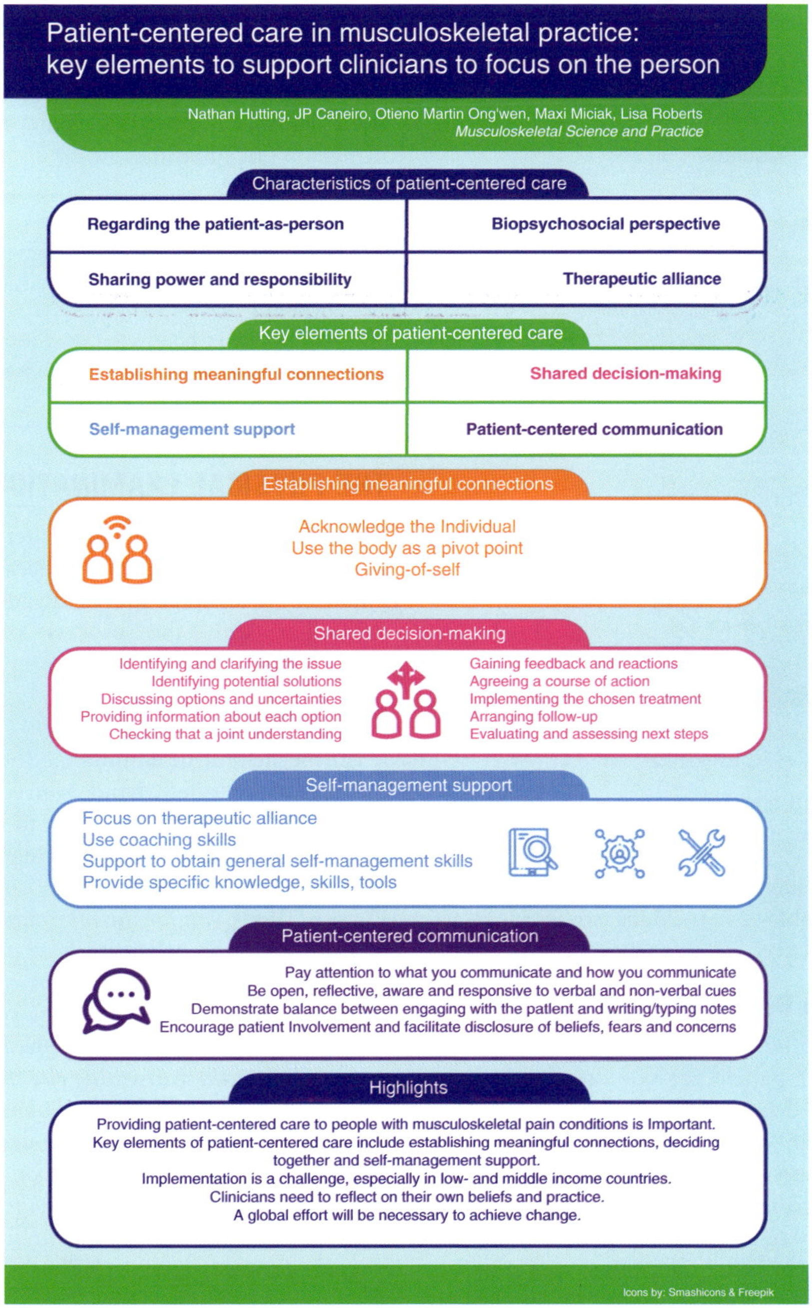

Fig. 2.5 Key elements of patient-centred care in musculoskeletal practice. (Hutting et al., 2021.)

Additional Concerns About the Technology

There are additional challenges, for example, patients (and clinicians) may be anxious about the technology which may result in a degree of 'digital fumbling' at the start of the call (Roberts & Osborn-Jenkins, 2021).

Starting the Call

In an earlier masterclass, we explored the preparation and delivery of remote consultations and highlighted the importance of the opening sequence of the call (Roberts & Osborn-Jenkins, 2021). Fig. 2.6 summarizes

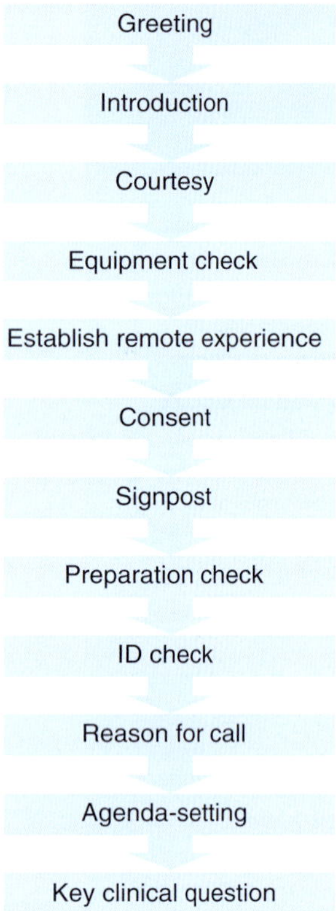

Fig. 2.6 Stages for starting a remote consultation. (Roberts & Osborn-Jenkins, 2021.)

the 12 stages we identified of starting a remote consultation and Table 2.7 includes some ideas to consider in your practice.

Gaining Consent in Remote Consultations

With remote consultations, as it is the clinician who has made the call and the patient has not attended in person, there is not the degree of implied consent that is afforded to traditional consultations.

In Table 2.7 in turn 14, the clinician seeks express consent (when the patient explicitly indicates his/her agreement) for a remote consultation. It is also important to gain express consent if any other staff may be involved in the call, for example, a student on clinical placement, again ensuring the patient is asked before anyone else joins the call and while minimizing coercion.

Looking to the Future

In scaling-up and optimizing digital health services, the differences in communication between remote and in-person consultations must be recognized. There is an urgent need for undergraduate training and continuing professional development to include some reflection on the differences in the communication skills required in remote consultations compared with in-person consultations.

> **KNOWLEDGE CHECK**
> 1. What information does the patient need in advance to ensure they are taking the call in an appropriate location?
> 2. How will you open your next remote consultation?
> 3. How will you gain express consent to go ahead with the consultation?

THE PHYSICAL EXAMINATION

Having completed the clinical interview, the next stage is (usually) to undertake a physical examination. It is important to signpost this clearly, as the patient may be unfamiliar with the process of a physiotherapy consultation.

Signposting

It can be helpful to summarize the key findings from the clinical interview, hand over control to ensure the patient has had the opportunity to raise the things that matter most to them, and then signpost the next stage of the consultation:

Physio: *'Thank you for the information you've given me. It's been really helpful to hear about your back and leg pain, how it affects your sleep, the challenges you're facing at work and how you've stopped taking the Ibuprofen due to its side effects on your gut. Before we go on, is there anything else that you would like to raise that we haven't talked about?*

Patient: *No, I think they're the main things.*

Physio: *Fine. What would be good would be to have a look at how you move, what things you can do and what you find more difficult, to help make a plan going forward. Is that OK?'*

Negotiating Any Need to Undress

It is important for physiotherapists to remember that patients may feel considerable unease at having to get undressed. Simple measures, like leaving the cubicle while the patient undresses and providing a towel/cover nearby to preserve the patient's dignity can all help in this respect.

TABLE 2.7 Starting a Remote Call

Turn	Speaker		Feature
1	Patient:	*Hello?*	
2	Physio:	*Hello. Please can I speak with Mr. Stuart Evans?*	Greeting: *In the form of a request, using both the patient's forename and surname to help identify the intended recipient*
3	Patient:	*Speaking.*	
4	Physio:	*My name's Katie Clifton. I'm a senior physiotherapist at the Woodgate Health Centre.*	Introduction: *The clinician introduces herself with her forename, surname and a simplified job title*
5	Patient:	*Oh yes, hello, I was expecting a call.*	
6	Physio:	*Is now a good time?*	Courtesy: *Check to see if it is convenient for the patient to take the call at this time and identify any time restrictions*
7	Patient:	*Yes, it's fine.*	
8	Physio:	*Can I just check that you can hear* me OK?*	Equipment check: *This is an opportunity for both parties to adjust their lighting, screen angles etc.* *It is usually easier for the clinician to initiate contact if there is a loss of connection.*
9	Patient:	*Yep*	
10	Physio:	*And just in case we lose connection for any reason, which rarely happens, is it OK to call you back straight away on this number?*	
11	Patient:	*Yes, that's OK.*	
12	Physio:	*Good. So, is this the first time you've had a physiotherapy consultation by phone?*	Establish experience: *Useful to orient the clinician to the amount of explanation and signposting that may be required*
13	Patient:	*Yes*	
14	Physio:	*Well, the content will be similar to as if we were in the health centre, and just to let you know, all your information is treated confidentially and stored securely, as normal. Are you happy to go ahead with this by phone?* *One thing that is different, you might well hear me tapping my keyboard as I'll be making some notes as we go, to capture important things you're saying.* *So, is there anything you need to get before we start (e.g. pen and paper)?*	Reassure: *The clinician reassures the patient that the consultation will be thorough, and the data will be secure.* Consent: *Express consent is gained for a virtual consultation.* Signpost: *When people hear typing, they commonly assume the caller is otherwise engaged / not listening. Signposting can help build the relationship and feedback to a patient that what they are saying is important.*
15	Patient:	*No, I'm good to go.*	Preparation check: *Could also include list of medications, or invite a companion to join*
16	Physio:	*That's good. I just need to check a couple of details to confirm I have the correct records open: Please could you tell me your date of birth?*	ID check: *The clinician uses 2 pieces of data to confirm she is speaking to the intended recipient. This must be done before any health information is given about the reason for the call to prevent a data breach.*
17	Patient:	*[patient gives details]*	
18	Physio:	*and the first line of your address?*	
19	Patient:	*[patient replies]*	

Continued

TABLE 2.7 Starting a Remote Call—cont'd

Turn	Speaker		Feature
20	Physio:	*Thank you. Right, I've seen from the referral that you've been having some problems with your left knee which I'd like to ask you about. Please do let me know if there's anything in particular you want to cover today. [Pause]*	Orient to reason for call [K+] and agenda setting: *The clinician chooses to display prior knowledge of the patient's symptoms and preparation for the call. The agenda setting helps tailor the consultation to the patient's needs and align with their expectations.*
21	Patient:	*OK. Will do*	
22	Physio:	*So to start with, can you tell me about the problem you're having with your knee?*	Key clinical question: *Inviting the patient to talk about their presenting condition*

Roberts and Osborn-Jenkins (2021).

The physiotherapist's communication skills can go a long way to smoothing what might be a potentially difficult situation here. For example, explaining to a patient why it is necessary to ask him/her to remove an item of clothing is only courteous. It is important to think about the wording of such a question and avoid potentially patronizing phrases such as, 'Please could you take off your shirt for me'. In this poorly constructed turn, it is unclear if the clinician is asking the patient to remove an item of clothing or instructing them, and whether they have any choice in the matter.

In negotiating any need to undress, it is important to clearly explain why it is necessary and to be culturally aware. Here are some ideas (that are not intended to be a script, but as something to help you reflect on the wording you use).

- *Would you be willing to remove your top, just so that I can see more clearly how your shoulder is moving?*
- *In order to check out your knee and see how it moves, it would be really helpful to actually see the joint. Do you have any shorts with you? [Patient says no]. OK, not a problem, we can work around it. Would you be able to either take your trousers off or if you prefer, you can roll them right up if they'll go?*
- *To help us find out what's causing this, I need to have a closer look at your hip. Some of the movements can become restricted by your trousers and so would you be willing to remove them just for this part of the assessment? [Patient agrees]. Great. I'll step outside and give you a moment to get ready and here's a towel to put across you, to keep you covered. I'll just be outside – please let me know when you're ready, and if you could lie on the couch on your back, that would be good.*

Providing Feedback

The physiotherapist can help allay some concerns when observing, by explaining what s/he is looking for. Providing some feedback and simply explaining that s/he is looking at the shape of the person's spine, for example, comparing the muscle formations on the right and left side and looking for any signs of muscle wasting or spasm etc, not only shows respect for the patient, it can also lessen the chance of dissatisfaction with the consultation.

Examples exist where patients have formally complained about clinicians 'making' them get undressed and staring at them, which they found 'humiliating'. In our research about expectations, when we asked patients about what they were hoping would happen at their first appointment, one patient (who had previously attended physiotherapy) replied, *'not asking you to do things that make you look absolutely ridiculous like take too many clothes off and stand/walk around like it'*.

The Power of Touch and Its Role in Communication

Touch is considered a core element of therapeutic practice in many health disciplines and can be very powerful on a physical, psychological and emotional level.

It can have several different functions for the physiotherapist, including:

- *'instrumental touch'*—(such as executing a special test or treatment technique)
- *'demonstration'*—(for example when a therapist applies touch to show how to modify an activity or perform an exercise)

- *'affective touch'*—making tactile contact with the patient, for example when offering an empathic response. (Roberts & Bucksey, 2007).

Before touching the patient, it is helpful to explain why you wish to undertake a test, what it will involve and specifically gain the patient's permission:

Physio: 'I'd like to do a test that looks at how well the nerves glide and slide in your arm. This would involve placing one of my hands lightly on your fingers while placing the other hand on your shoulder to keep it still. It shouldn't be uncomfortable at all. Is this OK?

Patient: Yes, that's fine.

Physio: Please let me know if you get any symptoms anywhere in the neck or arm as we go. You're in charge—please say if you'd like to stop at any time.'

Touch, in the form of palpation, can also help identify areas of discomfort and pain and can have an important therapeutic effect, as the patient feels the physiotherapist is 'on the spot' and understands the problem.

Equally, if hands-on assessment or treatment is not being undertaken or offered, it is important to carefully communicate this to the patient, as they may have come with an expectation of a tactile experience (or treatment). Expectation can play a significant role in the contextual ('nonspecific treatment') effects, which can therefore impact the outcome and the patient's experience.

KNOWLEDGE CHECK

1. How will you signpost that you have finished the clinical interview and are moving to the physical examination in your next assessment?
2. How will you ask a patient to remove their shirt for you to examine their thoracic spine?
3. How will you signpost testing myotomes in a physical examination?

ARTICULATING THE ASSESSMENT FINDINGS AND DECIDING TOGETHER

Perceptions of Diagnosis

One of the most challenging aspects of a clinical consultation is to explain the findings from the examination to the patient and set-up the discussions about further investigations or potential treatment options.

When the going gets tough, it is common for clinicians to regress to using jargon and making assumptions about the patient's level of knowledge and understanding. The only way to be clear about the patient's understanding of his/her symptoms is to ask them, which is why a question like: '*You know your body better than anyone; what do you think is happening?*' is an excellent place to start.

Following the examination, patients essentially want to know:

- what is causing the problem?
- what can be done about it?
- how quickly/will it resolve?

They want a simple strapline of what is wrong so that when a family member, friend or work colleague asks how they got on at their appointment, they can legitimize their symptoms and give a short account of what is going on.

Unfortunately, clinicians can increase patients' fears and anxieties through their explanations, when using words like 'chronic', 'degeneration', 'wear and tear' etc. Among the most-commonly used, unhelpful words are given in Table 2.8.

It is little wonder then if a clinician tries to minimize concerns by saying, '*Your chronic back pain is caused by mild degeneration and a small amount of wear and tear to the spine*', the patient becomes fearful, as s/he may hear instead: '*The situation is dire, your*

TABLE 2.8 Examples of Words That Can Be Misunderstood and Provoke Fear

What the Clinician Says	What the Patient Hears	Possible Alternatives
• Chronic—(i.e. Meaning it has lasted more than 3 months)	• It's dire (as this is how 'chronic' can be used in everyday language)	• Persistent
• Degeneration	• My spine is crumbling	• Age-related changes
• Wear and tear	• Some tissues are tearing	• Age-related changes (normal ageing process, akin to skin wrinkles/grey hair etc.)

spine is crumbling and is physically weakening by structures that are tearing'. Ouch! This can then make conversations about keeping active much more challenging.

Shared Decision-Making

Having reached a clinical diagnosis and communicated the findings, the next stage is the process of deciding together about appropriate treatment. Shared decision-making is described as both a philosophy and a process whereby clinicians engage patients as partners, to make choices about care based on clinical evidence and patients' informed preferences (Coulter & Collins, 2011). At present, a universally agreed definition is lacking, and a systematic review cited 161 definitions using 31 concepts (most commonly 'patient preferences' and 'options') (Makoul & Clayman, 2006).

The principal components of shared decision-making have been identified (Table 2.9) (Elwyn & Charles, 2009):

Observational studies have shown shared decision-making is rarely implemented in practice. Our team set about measuring the prevalence of shared decision-making in 80 clinical encounters involving physiotherapists and patients with back pain (Jones et al., 2014), using the 12-item OPTION scale (Elwyn & Charles, 2009). Although initially devised to rate general practice consultations, the scale contains generic phasing 'applicable to any clinical setting' (Elwyn & Charles, 2009). It measures the overall shared decision-making, scoring the clinician-initiated behaviour from an observer's perspective.

The tool rates 12 behavioural concepts on an ordinal scale, ranging from 0: 'the behaviour is not observed', to 4: 'the behaviour is observed and executed to a high standard'. Scores are summed and scaled to give an overall percentage, and the higher the score, the greater the shared decision-making competency attained, with 60% generally accepted to correlate with the lowest meaningful competency level (Elwyn & Charles, 2009). Reliability of the OPTION tool has been demonstrated, with the interrater intraclass correlation coefficient (0.62), kappa scores for interrater agreement (0.71), Cronbach's alpha (0.79) and intrarater test-retest reliability (0.66) all above acceptable thresholds (Elwyn & Charles, 2009).

In our study, observing consultations involving patients with back pain and physiotherapists in a primary care setting, there were 42 initial consultations (allocated 45 minutes) and 38 follow-up appointments (allocated 30 minutes). Care episodes ranged from one to six appointments per patient, giving a total of 80 consultations. The overall mean OPTION score was 24% (range 10.4%—43.8%), with 23.6% and 24.5% for the initial and follow-up consultations respectively. Table 2.10 shows the mean score for the individual scale items, including minimum and maximum ranges and score distributions (Jones et al., 2014).

The modal score for 10 out of 12 items in the OPTION scale was 1 out of a possible 4, which indicates the clinicians consistently demonstrated only a 'minimal' attempt to perform these behaviours. The exceptions were 'exploring the patient's concerns', which was consistently 'not observed' and therefore scored 0, and 'expressing the need to review the decision', which scored 2, indicating clinicians regularly achieved the 'baseline skill level'. No shared decision-making behaviour was consistently performed to a 'good' or 'high' standard (Jones et al., 2014).

Providing patients with a list of options was the only behaviour that was exhibited by every clinician across all observed encounters ($n = 80$), but in nearly three-quarters (73.8%) of consultations, this was only done to a 'perfunctory' level. In only 1.3% of consultations, the option to defer treatment ($n = 2$) or take no action ($n = 1$) was provided—evidence that physiotherapists rarely considered doing nothing a viable option in this cohort of patients reporting back pain (Jones et al., 2014).

These findings concur with other clinical contexts and healthcare professions. In another physiotherapy study using the OPTION scale, Dierckx et al. (2013) analyzed 210 Flemish encounters from 13 self-employed clinicians and reported a mean score of 5.2% (range 0%—31%), considerably lower than the mean of 24% identified in this UK study. More broadly, Couët et al. (2015) conducted a systematic review of 2489 consultations across 29 international studies, involving general practitioners, cardiologists, psychiatrists, oncologists, dietitians and nurses, treating a variety of medical conditions (most frequently cancer, diabetes and depression) and identified a mean OPTION score of 23% (9%—37%).

In the current climate, it is vital that clinicians involve patients appropriately in decisions affecting

TABLE 2.9 The Core Components of Shared Decision-Making

- Identifying and clarifying the issue
- Identifying potential solutions
- Discussing options and uncertainties
- Providing information about the potential benefits, harms and uncertainties of each option
- Checking that patients and professionals have a joint understanding
- Gaining feedback and reactions
- Agreeing on a course of action
- Implementing the chosen treatment
- Arranging follow-up
- Evaluating outcomes and assessing the next steps

Elwyn and Charles (2009).

TABLE 2.10 Shared Decision-Making in Consultations Between Physiotherapists and Patients With Low-Back Pain

Item	Shared Decision-Making Behaviour	Mean Score (min–max)	0 (%)	1 (%)	2 (%)	3 (%)	4 (%)
1	The clinician draws attention to an identified problem as one that requires a decision-making process	0.7 (0–3)	48.8	33.8	16.3	1.3	0.0
2	The clinician states that there is more than one way to deal with the identified problem	0.8 (0–3)	41.3	36.3	21.3	1.3	0.0
3	The clinician assesses patient's preferred approach to receiving information to assist decision-making	0.6 (0–3)	58.8	27.5	10.0	3.8	0.0
4	The clinician lists 'options', which can include the choice of 'no action'	1.4 (1–3)	0.0	73.8	25.0	1.3	3.8
5	The clinician explains the pros and cons of options to the patient	0.8 (0–3)	42.5	38.8	15.0	3.8	0.0
6	The clinician explores the patient's expectations (or ideas) about how the problem(s) are to be managed	1.0 (0–4)	41.3	27.5	22.5	6.3	2.5
7	The clinician explores the patient's concerns (fears) about how problem(s) are to be managed	0.3 (0–2)	77.5	17.5	5.0	0.0	0.0
8	The clinician checks that the patient has understood the information	1.3 (0–3)	17.5	36.3	43.8	2.5	0.0

Continued

TABLE 2.10 **Shared Decision-Making in Consultations Between Physiotherapists and Patients With Low-Back Pain—cont'd**

Item	Shared Decision-Making Behaviour	Mean Score (min–max)	0 (%)	1 (%)	2 (%)	3 (%)	4 (%)
9	The clinician offers the patient explicit opportunities to ask questions during decision-making process	1.2 (0–2)	18.8	46.3	35.0	0.0	0.0
10	The clinician elicits the patient's preferred level of involvement in decision-making	0.7 (0–3)	58.8	16.3	22.5	2.5	0.0
11	The clinician indicates the need for a decision-making (or deferring) stage	1.2 (0–3)	7.5	70.0	20.0	2.5	0.0
12	The clinician indicates the need to review the decision (or deferment)	1.7 (0–4)	5.0	42.5	31.3	18.8	2.5

Key (Elwyn & Charles, 2009)
0 = The behaviour is not observed.
1 = A minimal attempt is made to exhibit the behaviour.
2 = The clinician asks the patient about his or her preferred way of receiving information to assist decision.
3 = The behaviour is exhibited to a good standard.
4 = The behaviour is observed and executed to a high standard.

Jones et al. (2014).

their healthcare to ensure it is person-focused and optimizes any contextual/nonspecific treatment effects. This will enhance patients' experience and is likely to reduce the potential for complaints and litigation.

Our findings showed that shared decision-making was underdeveloped in these back pain consultations and this aspect of practice would be a good area for physiotherapists to invest time in, to develop their skills further.

Goal Setting

Clinicians can enhance their shared decision-making abilities through self-awareness and adopting a goal-oriented approach. Empirical work by Vermunt et al. (2018) resulted in a 3-level model for goal setting: (1) symptom- or disease-specific goals (to obtain relief from symptoms); (2) functional goals; and (3) fundamental goals (drawing on a person's values, hopes and priorities in life).

Vermunt et al. (2018) recommend setting goals at all three levels, *starting* with fundamental goals. These drive the discussions about function and symptom-specific goals and ensure that decisions are genuinely made together.

Changing Behaviour

Implementing evidence-based practice and public health agendas depends on successful behaviour change interventions (Michie et al., 2011), which are common to physiotherapy practice. A plethora of theories and frameworks exist, including the Behaviour Change Wheel, which was developed from 19 frameworks, incorporating capability, opportunity, motivation and behaviour. It comprises:

- *physical capability*, which can be achieved through physical skill development or potentially through enabling interventions such as medication, surgery or prostheses

- *psychological capability*, which can be achieved through imparting knowledge or understanding, training emotional, cognitive and/or behavioural skills or through enabling interventions such as medication
- *reflective motivation*, which can be achieved through increasing knowledge and understanding, eliciting positive (or negative) feelings about behavioural target
- *automatic motivation*, which can be achieved through associative learning that elicits positive (or negative) feelings and impulses and counter-impulses relating to the behavioural target, habit formation or direct influences on automatic motivational processes (e.g. via medication)
- *physical and social opportunity*, which can be achieved through environmental change (Michie et al., 2011).

The Behaviour Change Wheel starts with the question: 'What conditions internal to individuals and in their social and physical environment need to be in place for a specified behavioural target to be achieved?' This comprehensive approach is highly pertinent to physiotherapy (Fig. 2.7), and time spent studying behaviour change at the undergraduate and postgraduate level cannot be recommended highly enough.

Motivational Interviewing

Motivational interviewing is a collaborative, goal-oriented style of communication with particular attention to the language of change and has become popular within physiotherapy. It is designed to strengthen the personal commitment to a specific goal by eliciting and exploring the patient's own reasons for change, within an atmosphere of acceptance and compassion (Miller & Rollnick, 2013).

With this approach, the physiotherapist uses active listening and communication skills to elicit the patient's own positive reasons for change, with the aim of avoiding confrontation or resistance to behaviour change, which can be particularly helpful when encouraging patients to make difficult lifestyle changes such as taking more exercise or reducing their alcohol intake. This approach can help clinicians to provide patients with the tools they need for self-management and to be able to change his/her behaviour

Communicating the Treatment Options

Gaining Consent for Treatment

Appropriately and adequately gaining consent is vital in providing safe, patient-centred, collaborative care. There is a legal, ethical and clinical necessity to gain an informed consent from the patient, and that is the case whether s/he is physically present with you or on the telephone or a remote platform.

When information about an intervention is disclosed, it needs to include the 'material' risks, benefits and alternatives of the treatment and information about the likely impact of not accepting any treatment at all. In a landmark case in 2015 (Montgomery *v.* Lanarkshire Health Board), there is a move from the 'reasonable clinician' to the 'reasonable patient', and it is essential for all clinicians to be familiar with this case.

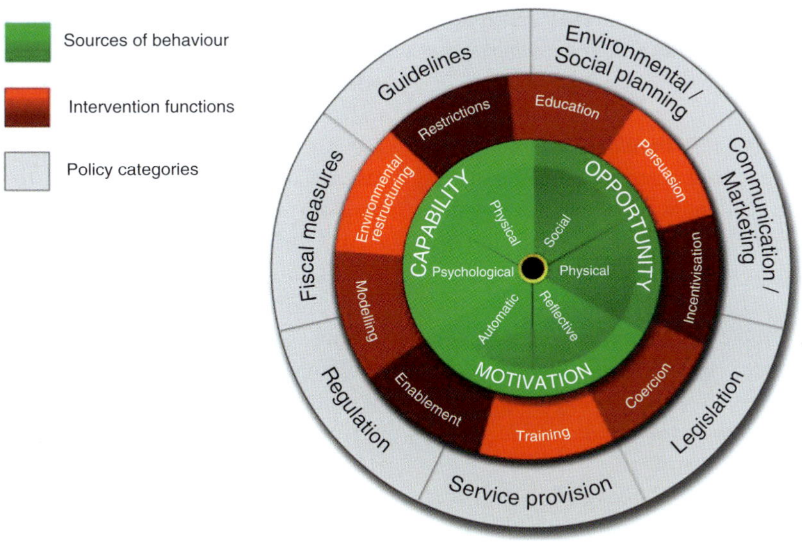

Fig. 2.7 The Behaviour Change Wheel. (From Michie et al., 2011.)

The test of materiality is:

> *...whether, in the circumstances of the particular case, a reasonable person in the patient's position would be likely to attach significance to the risk, or the doctor is, or should reasonably be aware, that the particular patient would be likely to attach significance to it.*
>
> ***Montgomery* v. *Lanarkshire Health Board***

In a therapeutic environment, there may be an assumption that because a patient has attended, s/he has consented to receive treatment; however, this is not the case. Therefore after an assessment, it is the clinician's responsibility to communicate the diagnosis clearly, so the patient is able to understand the nature of the condition and the options available.

In understanding this, the patient should have options for treatment (including self-management), watchful waiting (with the potential to start treatment later if required), or the option of not receiving any treatment (as it is their choice). These discussions should include any benefits or potential risks/consequences, and this discussion must be accurately documented. Here is an example of how this might happen in practice:

Physio: OK. So, from what you've told me, and the assessment we've just done, the main problem is the stiffness in your shoulder and how difficult it's making everyday tasks like washing your hair and doing up your bra.

Patient: Yes, and putting washing on the line.

Physio: Absolutely. Well, there are several treatment options. Let's go through these and then see where you would like to start.

Patient: OK

Physio: The best way to get this shoulder moving is for you to do some exercises and activities at home every day that I can show you now, to stretch the tissue where it's got stiff, and help you get better movement. It's also really important to strengthen the muscles, and I can show you ways to help with this too.

We can also do a couple of sessions of manual (or 'hands-on') treatment, which would involve coming here for the session and me applying some techniques called mobilizations, alongside your home stretching and strengthening exercises.

It's up to you whether you would like to start with the exercises to see how you get on first, or whether you want to have the manual therapy alongside? I know you've got a lot on at the moment and my estimate is that it'd probably be 1-2 sessions. The mobilizations are likely to improve your range quicker but won't help with the strength—that's really down to the exercises. There is a chance you may have a bit of discomfort in the shoulder after the manual treatment, but this is likely to be mild and short-lasting—to be honest, it will feel as if the arm has had a bit of a work-out!

Of course, all of this is your choice. If you don't want to do any exercises or hands-on treatment, my honest opinion is that your shoulder is likely to remain stiff, and I don't know whether or not it would eventually resolve by itself.

What are your thoughts about what you would like to happen next?

Best-practice models propose that the consent process is voluntary, patients consent freely and in a noncoercive environment and that patients have the capacity to make decisions, whilst having the opportunity to ask questions (Goldfarb et al., 2012).

Offering Advice

As we saw in our research, 'advice' given in the initial consultation constituted 12.5% of the duration (Roberts et al., 2013), and it is a cornerstone of physiotherapy practice.

Using the 'Ask-Offer-Ask' approach, based on the Ask-Tell-Ask framework (Barnett, 2001), can help build a two-way conversation with the patient to share health information (Roberts & Osborn-Jenkins, 2021). The first 'ask' establishes what information and strategies the patient is aware of and provides patients with an opportunity to raise their own ideas and enables the advice to be tailored. This collaboration strengthens self-efficacy (i.e. an individual's belief that they can do a particular task/behaviour) and is reported to have positive effects on pain and physical activity engagement (Degerstedt et al., 2020), while also providing an opportunity to address any unhelpful beliefs that the patient may have.

Focusing on 'offering' advice, rather than 'giving' or 'telling', is likely to be better received by the patient, avoiding psychological reactance, a term used to describe the feelings and thoughts that occur when a person perceives there are threats to his/her freedom (Dorrance Hall, 2019).

The second 'ask' empowers patients to reflect on their understanding and consider any barriers they can identify with the advice:

1st ask: '*Can you tell me about any ways you are aware of that can help manage your leg pain and swelling and if there's anything in particular you'd like to know?*'

Offer: '*Would you like me to suggest some other ideas that might help you manage the swelling?*'

2nd ask: '*Can you tell me how you might be able to fit this in with your day, and if you think there will be any difficulties in giving this a try?*'

Skills in offering advice and reassurance are integral to enabling people to self-manage their symptoms. In an observational study, we found physiotherapists used advice to reassure patients, to encourage, explain and prepare (Osborn-Jenkins & Roberts, 2021) (Fig. 2.8).

From this research, we concluded it is particularly important for all clinicians to develop a high level of skill in offering advice to avoid ambiguous, contradictory or unhelpful messages that may evoke fear or increase disability. Again, training and sharing ideas in offering advice constitute excellent opportunities for continuing professional development.

NEGOTIATING AN EXIT

Soliciting whether the patient has any other concerns near the end of the consultation is a commonly used strategy, and Robinson and Heritage (2016) showed

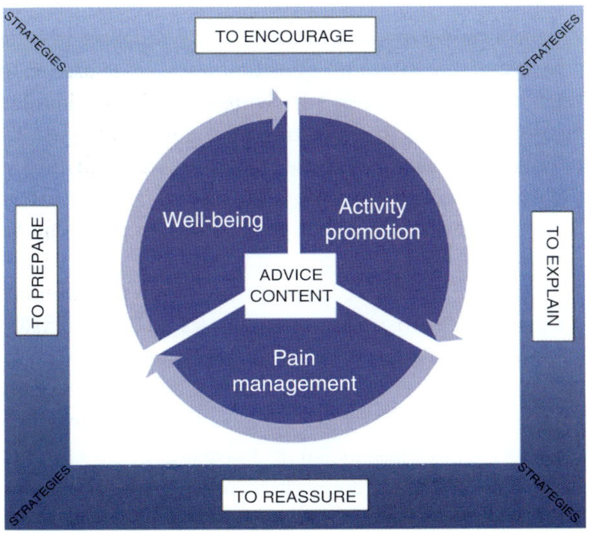

Fig. 2.8 Model of content and contextual categories in the advice given to patients with low back pain. (Osborn-Jenkins & Roberts, 2021.)

in the United States that this was understood by patients to bring the appointment to a close.

Research has found that if the question is phrased '*Is there anything else I can help you with?*' the '*anything else*' can impede patients from raising additional concerns, as this is polarized to prefer a 'no response' (Heritage et al., 2007). If the '*anything else*' is replaced with '*something else*', it becomes positively polarized and favours a 'yes' response (Heritage et al., 2007). It's worth trying out!

It has also been found that using 'concern-seeking' questions to elicit patients' agendas ('*Do you have other concerns?*') resulted in patients being more likely to volunteer a new health concern than if 'question-seeking' questions were used ('*Do you have other questions?*'), (Robinson et al., 2016).

Other forms of closing sequences may include providing some written materials or providing a closing offer to send some online resources, exercise apps etc.

Leaving a positive final impression of the consultation is vitally important. Silverman et al. (1998) have proposed four main skills that contribute to a satisfactory ending of the consultation:

1. summarizing the session
2. contracting with the patient about what happens next
3. providing a safety net of what to do if the plan is not working, when and how to seek help
4. final checks that the patient is comfortable with the plan and has the opportunity to ask questions or discuss any other items.

In negotiating an exit, is important to listen out for any subtle displays of dissatisfaction and address these before the consultation ends. In a study looking at how callers convey their satisfaction with calls to a cancer helpline, Woods et al. (2015) described patients downgrading their appreciation with phrases like '*alright then*' or '*thank you anyway*' using flat, unenthusiastic prosody, suggesting the patients' expectations have not (yet) been fulfilled.

If all has gone to plan, patients should be leaving the consultation with a clear understanding of their clinical diagnosis and any further investigations or potential treatment options. Most importantly, they should have had a positive experience with physiotherapy. The clinician should also have experienced a positive interaction and been able to optimize the nonspecific treatment effects, to maximize the outcome of the care episode.

KNOWLEDGE CHECK

1. How will you explain to a patient with osteoarthritis that the x-ray of his/her knee showed moderate degenerative changes?
2. How many of the 12 shared decision-making behaviours do you routinely include when discussing findings at the end of an initial assessment?
3. Can you name the six domains in the inner ring of the Behaviour Change Wheel?
4. Can you explain the material risk to a patient of a treatment involving physiological joint mobilization?
5. How could you start a conversation in which you think you will be advising a patient about how to improve his/her sleep patterns?
6. How will you negotiate an exit if a patient says '*Well, thank you anyway*'?

Acknowledgements

The author wishes to acknowledge the work of the research team, in particular: Dr Neil Langridge, Lisa Osborn-Jenkins, Sally Bucksey, Chris Whittle, Lucy Jones, Emily Chester, Natalie Robinson, Faye Burrow, Millie Allen, Lucy Brindle, Simon Stewart and the patients and staff in the United Kingdom who have generously given their time, shared their knowledge and made this research program possible.

REVIEW AND REVISE QUESTIONS

1. Think about a recent initial consultation that you have completed. Did it go well? Can you list any contributing factors as to why you think it went well, relating to:
   (a) the patient
   (b) you
   (c) the patient's problem presentation
   (d) the environment
   (e) anything else?
2. Think about a recent initial consultation that has not gone quite so well. Can you list any contributing factors as to why this might be, related to:
   (a) the patient
   (b) you
   (c) the patient's problem presentation
   (d) the environment
   (e) anything else?

   What has given you the impression that this encounter could have gone better? At what point in the consultation did you get this impression? What can you learn from this?

3. In thinking about a recent consultation, what (if any) topics did you cover with the patient before you sat down at the start of the assessment (e.g. walking through to the clinic room)? What topics did you cover before asking about the patient's problem presentation? How did you phrase the specific opening question about the patient's problem presentation? Do you always use a similar form of words to this when taking a history?
4. With the patient's consent, try audio recording a clinical consultation. How frequently do you interrupt patients, and what effect does this appear to have had?
5. Using the audio recording, how many of the 12 shared decision-making behaviours in the OPTION tool can you identify in your practice?

REFERENCES

Allen, M.V., Roberts, L.C., 2017. Perceived acquisition, development and delivery of empathy in musculoskeletal physiotherapy encounters. J. Commun. Healthc. 10, 304–312. https://doi.org/10.1080/17538068.2017.1366000.

Bar, M., Neta, M., Linz, H., 2006. Very first impressions. Emotion 6, 269–278.

Barnett, P.B., 2001. Rapport and the hospitalist. Am. J. Med. 111 (9B), 31S–35S. https://doi.org/10.1016/s0002-9343(01)00967-6.

Beckman, H.B., Frankel, R.M., 1984. The effect of physician behaviour on the collection of data. Ann. Intern. Med. 101, 692–696.

Caldwell, G., 2019. The process of clinical consultation is crucial to patient outcomes and safety: 10 quality indicators. Clin. Med. 19 (6), 503–506.

Cambridge Dictionary, 2021. Available: https://dictionary.cambridge.org/dictionary/english/small-talk (accessed 29 August 2021.

Candita, J.E., 2006. More than just a good cv: Creating a favourable first impression in job interviews. PhD Thesis, college of law and business school of management. The University of Western, Sydney.

Caneiro, J.P., Roos, E.M., Barton, C.J., O'Sullivan, K., Kent, P., Lin, I., et al., 2019. It is time to move beyond "body region silos" to manage musculoskeletal pain: five actions to change clinical practice. Br. J. Sports Med. 54, 438–439. https://doi.org/10.1136/bjsports-2018-100488.

Caris-Verhallen, W., Kerkstra, A., Bensing, J.M., 1999. Nonverbal behavior in nurse-elderly patient communication. J. Adv. Nurs. 29, 808–818.

Chester, E.C., Robinson, N.C., Roberts, L.C., 2014. Opening clinical encounters in an adult musculoskeletal setting. Man. Ther. 19, 306–310.

Couët, N., Desroches, S., Robitaille, H., Vaillancourt, H., Leblanc, A., Turcotte, S., et al., 2015. Assessments of the extent to which health-care providers involve patients in decision making: a systematic review of studies using the OPTION instrument. Health Expect. 18, 542–561.

Coulter, A., Collins, A., 2011. Making shared decision-making a reality. No decision about me, without me. The king's fund. Available online at: http://www.kingsfund.org.uk/.

Cox, C., Uddin, L., Di Martino, A., Castellanos, F.X., Milham, M.P., Kelly, C., 2012. The balance between feeling and knowing: affective and cognitive empathy are reflected in the brain's intrinsic functional dynamics. Soc. Cogn. Affect. Neurosci. 7, 727–737.

Degerstedt, Å., Alinaghizadeh, H., Thorstensson, C., Olsson, C.B., 2020. High self-efficacy – a predictor of reduced pain and higher levels of physical activity among patients with osteoarthritis: an observational study. BMC Musculoskelet. Disord. 21, 380. https://doi.org/10.1186/s12891-020-03407-x.

Dierckx, K., Deveugele, M., Roosen, P., Devisch, I., 2013. Implementation of shared decision making in physical therapy: observed level of involvement and patient preference. Phys. Ther. 93, 1321–1330.

Dorrance Hall, E., 2019. Why we hate people telling us what to do. https://www.psychologytoday.com/gb/blog/conscious-communication/201906/why-we-hate-people-telling-us-what-do. Accessed 06 August 2021.

Drummond, K., 1989. A backward glance at interruptions. Western J. Speech Commun. 53, 150–166.

Elwyn, G.M., Charles, C., 2009. Shared decision-making: the principles and the competencies. In: Edwards, A., Elwyn, G. (Eds.), Evidence-Based Patient Choice. Oxford University Press, Oxford, pp. 118–143.

Emily Post, E., 1940. Etiquette; 'The blue book of social usage'. Funk & Wagnalls, New York, p. 23.

Finset, A., 2016. When patients have more than one concern. Patient Educ. Couns. 99 (5), 671. https://doi.org/10.1016/j.pec.2016.03.016.

Goldfarb, E., Fromson, J.A., Gorrindo, T., Birnbaum, R.J., 2012. Enhancing informed consent best practices: gaining patient, family and provider perspectives using reverse simulation. J. Med. Ethics 38, 546–551.

Hall, T., Lloyd, C., 1990. Nonverbal communication in a health care setting. Br. J. Occup. Ther. 53, 383–387.

Heritage, J., 2012. Epistemics in action: action formation and territories of knowledge. Res. Lang. Soc. Interact. 45, 1–29.

Heritage, J., Robinson, J.D., 2006. The structure of patients' presenting concerns: physicians' opening questions. Health Commun. 19, 89–102.

Heritage, J., Robinson, J.D., Elliott, M.N., Beckett, M., Wilkes, M., 2007. Reducing patients' unmet concerns in primary care: the difference one word can make. J. Gen. Intern. Med. 22 (10), 1429–1433. https://doi.org/10.1007/s11606-007-0279-0.

Hutting, N., Caneiro', J.P., Ong'wen, O.M., Miciak, M., Roberts, L., 2021. Patient-centered care in musculoskeletal practice: key elements to support clinicians to focus on the person. Musculoskelet. Sci. Pract. 57, 102434. https://doi.org/10.1016/j.msksp.2021.102434.

Irish, J.T., Hall, J.A., 1995. Interruptive patterns in medical visits: the effects of role, status and gender. Soc. Sci. Med. 41, 873–881.

Jackson, C., 2006. Shut up and listen! A brief guide to clinical communication skills. Dundee University Press, Dundee, p. 1.

Jones, L.E., Roberts, L.C., Little, P.S., Mullee, M.A., Cleland, J.A., Cooper, C., 2014. Shared decision-making in back pain consultations: an illusion or reality? Eur. Spine J. 23 (Suppl. 1), S13–S19.

Katsumi, Y., Kim, S., Sung, K., Dolcos, F., Dolcos, S., 2017. When nonverbal greetings "make it or break it": the role of ethnicity and gender in the effect of handshake on social appraisals. J. Nonverbal Behav. 41, 345–365.

Kitzinger, C., 2008. Conversation analysis: technical matters for gender research. In: Harrington, K., Litosseliti, L., Sauntson, H., et al. (Eds.), Gender and Language Research Methodologies. Palgrave Macmillan, Hampshire, pp. 119–138.

Lærum, E., Indahl, A., Sture Skouen, J., 2006. What is 'the good back consultation'? A combined qualitative and quantitative study of chronic low back pain patients' interaction with and perceptions of consultations with specialists. J. Rehabil. Med. 38, 255–262.

Laidsaar-Powell, R.C., Butow, P.N., Bu, S., Charles, C., Gafni, A., Lam, W.W., et al., 2013. Physician-patient-companion communication and decision-making: a systematic review of triadic medical consultations. Patient Educ. Couns. 91, 3–13. https://doi.org/10.1016/j.pec.2012.11.007.

Langewitz, W., Denz, M., Keller, A., Charles, C., Gafni, A., Lam, W.W.T., et al., 2002. Spontaneous talking time at start of consultation in outpatient clinic: cohort study. Br. Med. J. 325, 682–683.

Levine, S.P., Feldman, R.S., 2002. Women and men's nonverbal behaviour and self-monitoring in a job interview setting. Appl. H R M Res. 7 (1), 1–14.

Lipkin, M., Putnam, S.M., Lazare, A., 1995. The medical interview: clinical care, education and research. Springer, New York.

Maguire, P., Pitceathly, C., 2002. Key communication skills and how to acquire them. Br. Med. J. 325, 697–700.

Makoul, G., Clayman, M.L., 2006. An integrative model of shared decision making in medical encounters. Patient Educ. Couns. 60, 301–312.

Marvel, M.K., Epstein, R.M., Flowers, K., Beckman, H.B., 1999. Soliciting the patient's agenda: have we improved? J. Am. Med. Assoc. 281, 283–287.

Mazur, M., McEvoy, S., Schmidt, M.H., Bisson, E.F., 2015. High self-assessment of disability and the surgeon's recommendation against surgical intervention may negatively impact satisfaction scores in patients with spinal disorders. J. Neurosurg. Spine 22, 666–671.

McAllister, M., Matarasso, B., Dixon, B., Shepperd, C., 2004. Conversation starters: re-examining and reconstructing first encounters within the therapeutic relationship. J. Psychiatr. Ment. Health Nurs. 11, 575–582.

McCabe, E., Miciak, M., Roduta, R.M., Sun, H., Kleiner, M.J., Holt, C.J., et al., 2021. Development of the physiotherapy therapeutic relationship measure. Eur. J. Physiother. 1–10. https://doi.org/10.1080/21679169.2020.1868572.

McShane, T.D., 1993. Effects of nonverbal cues and verbal first impressions in unstructured and situational interview settings. Appl. H R M Res. 4 (2), 137–150.

Mehrabian, A., 1971. Silent Messages. Wadsworth, Belmont, CA.

Michie, S., van Stralen, M.M., West, R., 2011. The behaviour change wheel: a new method for characterising and designing behaviour change interventions. Implement. Sci. 6, 42.

Miciak, M., Mayan, M., Brown, C., Joyce, A.S., Gross, D.P., et al., 2019. A framework for establishing connections in physiotherapy practice. Physiother. Theory Pract. 35, 40–56. https://doi.org/10.1080/09593985.2018.1434707.

Miller, W.R., Rollnick, S., 2013. Motivational interviewing. helping people change, third ed. Guilford Press, New York.

Misch, D., Peloquin, S., 2005. Developing empathy through confluent education. J. Phys. Ther. Educ. 19, 41–51.

Montgomery (Appellant) v Lanarkshire Health Board (Respondent), 2015. UKSC 11, on appeal from [2013] CSIH 3; [2010] CSIH 104.

NHS Digital, 2021. Data on written complaints in the NHS – 2020–21. Available at: https://digital.nhs.uk/data-and-information/publications/statistical/data-on-written-complaints-in-the-nhs/2020-21-quarter-3-and-quarter-4. accessed 31 August 2021.

Oliver, S., Redfern, S., 1991. Interpersonal communication between nurses and elderly patients: refinement of an observational schedule. J. Adv. Nurs. 16, 30–38.

Osborn-Jenkins, L., Roberts, L., 2021. The advice given by physiotherapists to people with back pain in primary care. Musculoskelet. Sci. Pract. 55, 102403.

Parliamentary and Health Service Ombudsman, 2012. Listening and learning: the ombudsman's review of complaint handling by the NHS in England 2011–12. The Stationery Office, London, p. 7.

Parry, R., 2008. Are interventions to enhance communication performance in allied health professionals effective, and how should they be delivered? Direct and indirect evidence. Patient Educ. Couns. 73, 186–195.

Paul, R., Elder, L., 2016. The thinker's guide to the art of socratic questioning. The Foundation for Critical Thinking. Rowman & Littlefield, Lanham, Maryland.

Paul-Savoie, E., Bourgault, P., Potvin, S., Gosselin, E., Lafrenaye, S., 2018. The impact of pain invisibility on patient-centered care and empathetic attitude in chronic pain management. Pain Res, Manag, pp. 1–8. https://doi.org/10.1155/2018/6375713.

Pollock, K., 2001. 'I've not asked him, you see, and he's not said': understanding lay explanatory models of illness is a prerequisite for concordant consultation. Int. J. Pharm. Pract. 9, 105–117.

Raja, S., Hasnain, M., Vadakumchery, T., Hamad, J., Shah, R., Hoersch, M., 2015. Identifying elements of patient-centered care in underserved populations: a qualitative study of patient perspectives. PLoS One 10, e0126708.

Rhodes, D.R., McFarland, K.F., Finch, W.H., Johnson, A.O., 2001. Speaking and interruptions during primary care office visits. Fam. Med. 33, 528–532.

Roberts, L., 2006. First impressions: an information leaflet for patients attending a musculoskeletal out-patient department. Physiotherapy 92, 179–186.

Roberts, L., Bucksey, S., 2007. Communicating with patients: what happens in practice? Phys. Ther. 87 (5), 586–594.

Roberts, L., Whittle, C., Cleland, J., Wald, M., 2013. Measuring verbal communication in initial physical therapy encounters. Phys. Ther. 93, 479–491.

Roberts, L.C., Burrow, F.A., 2018. Interruption and rapport disruption: measuring the prevalence and nature of verbal 'interruptions' during back pain consultations. J. Commun. Healthc. 11, 95–105. https://doi.org/10.1080/17538068.2018.1449289.

Roberts, L., Osborn-Jenkins, L., 2021. Delivering remote consultations: talking the talk. Musculoskelet. Sci. Pract. 52, 102275. https://doi.org/10.1016/j.msksp.2020.102275.

Robinson, J.D., Heritage, J., 2006. Physicians' opening questions and patients' satisfaction. Patient Educ. Couns. 60, 279–285.

Robinson, J.D., Heritage, J., 2016. How patients understand physicians' solicitations of additional concerns: implications for up-front agenda setting in primary care. Health Commun. 31 (4), 434–444. https://doi.org/10.1080/10410236.2014.960060.

Robinson, J.D., Tate, A., Heritage, J., 2016. Agenda-setting revisited: when and how do primary-care physicians solicit patients' additional concerns? Patient Educ. Couns. 99 (5), 718–723. https://doi.org/10.1016/j.pec.2015.12.009.

Sacks, H., Schegloff, E.A., Jefferson, G., 1974. A simplest systematics for the organization of turn-taking for conversation. Language 50, 696–735.

Shapiro, J., 2008. Walking a mile in their patients' shoes: empathy and othering in medical students' education. Philos. Ethics Humanit. Med. 3 (1), 1–11.

Silverman, J., Kurtz, S., Draper, J., 1998. Skills for communicating with patients. Radcliffe Medical Press, Oxford, p. 10.

Stewart, S.J., Roberts, L., Brindle, L., 2021. Romantic partner involvement during oncology consultations: a narrative review of qualitative and quantitative studies. Patient Educ. Couns. 104 (1), 64–74. https://doi.org/10.1016/j.pec.2020.08.018.

Stuart, B., Leydon, G., Woods, C., Gennery, E., Elsey, C., Summers, R., et al., 2019. The elicitation and management of multiple health concerns in GP consultations. Patient Educ. Couns. 102 (4), 687–693. https://doi.org/10.1016/j.pec.2018.11.009.

Tongue, S., 2007. Every day brings a first impression. Nurs. Stand. 22, 62.

Vermunt, N.P., Harmsen, M., Elwyn, G., Westert, G.P., Burgers, J.S., Olde Rikkert, M.G., et al., 2018. A three-goal model for patients with multimorbidity: a qualitative approach. Health Expect. 21, 528–538. https://doi.org/10.1111/hex.12647.

Waddell, G., 2004. The back pain revolution, second ed. Churchill Livingstone, Edinburgh, p. 243.

Walseth, L.T., Abildsnes, E., Schei, E., 2011. Lifestyle, health and the ethics of good living: health behaviour counselling in general practice. Patient Educ. Couns. 83, 180–184.

Wetherall, D., Silverman, J., Kurtz, S., et al., 1998. Skills for communicating with patients. Radcliffe Medical Press, Oxford vii.

Williams, D., 1997. Communication skills in practice, a practical guide for health professionals. Jessica Kinglsey, London, pp. 1–27.

Wolraich, M., Albanese, M., Reiter-Thayer, S., Barratt, W., 1982. Factors affecting physician communication and parent–physician dialogues. J. Med. Educ. 52, 621–625.

Woods, C.J., Drew, P., Leydon, G.M., 2015. Closing calls to a cancer helpline: expressions of caller satisfaction. Patient Educ. Couns. 98 (8), 943–953. https://doi.org/10.1016/j.pec.2015.04.015.

Zolnierek, K.B., Dimatteo, M.R., 2009. Physician communication and patient adherence to treatment: a meta-analysis. Med. Care 47, 832–834.

3

Subjective Examination/Taking the Patient's History

Hubert van Griensven and Dionne Ryder

LEARNING OUTCOMES

After studying this chapter, you should be able to:

- Identify the importance of the subjective examination in understanding the patient and their presentation.
- Complete a body chart with an appreciation of the relevance of each aspect.
- Explain the concepts of irritability and severity and how judgements of each can be made using subjective data.
- Discuss the importance of a range of screening questions to assess for serious conditions and existing comorbidities.
- Explore the significance of collecting details of the patient's history in understanding the present complaint.
- Understand how subjective data is used to plan the physical examination.

CHAPTER CONTENTS

Introduction, 34
Subjective Examination/Taking the Patient's History, 35
The Patient's Context and Their Perspective on Their Experience, 36
Body Chart, 37
Impact on Function, 44
Aggravating and Easing Factors, 45
Severity and Irritability of Symptoms, 46
Twenty-Four-Hour Behaviour of Symptoms, 47
Stage of the Condition, 47
Risk Factors for Chronicity and Poor Treatment Outcome, 48
Screening/Special Questions, 49
Radiographs, Medical Imaging and Tests, 55
Past Medical History, 55
Family History, 56
History of the Present Condition, 56
Planning the Physical Examination, 56
Appendix 3.1 Physical Examination Planning Sheet (Short Version), 58
Appendix 3.2 Clinical Reasoning Form Using Hypothesis Categories, 59
References, 61

INTRODUCTION

This chapter covers the general principles of the subjective examination. Through discussion with the patient, the clinician seeks to understand what has brought the patient to the clinic. To fully understand the patient, the clinician must consider all factors that may impact on a person's health (Fig. 3.1) (World Health Organization (WHO), 2001).

Throughout the subjective examination the clinician is continuously reasoning, seeking to understand possible

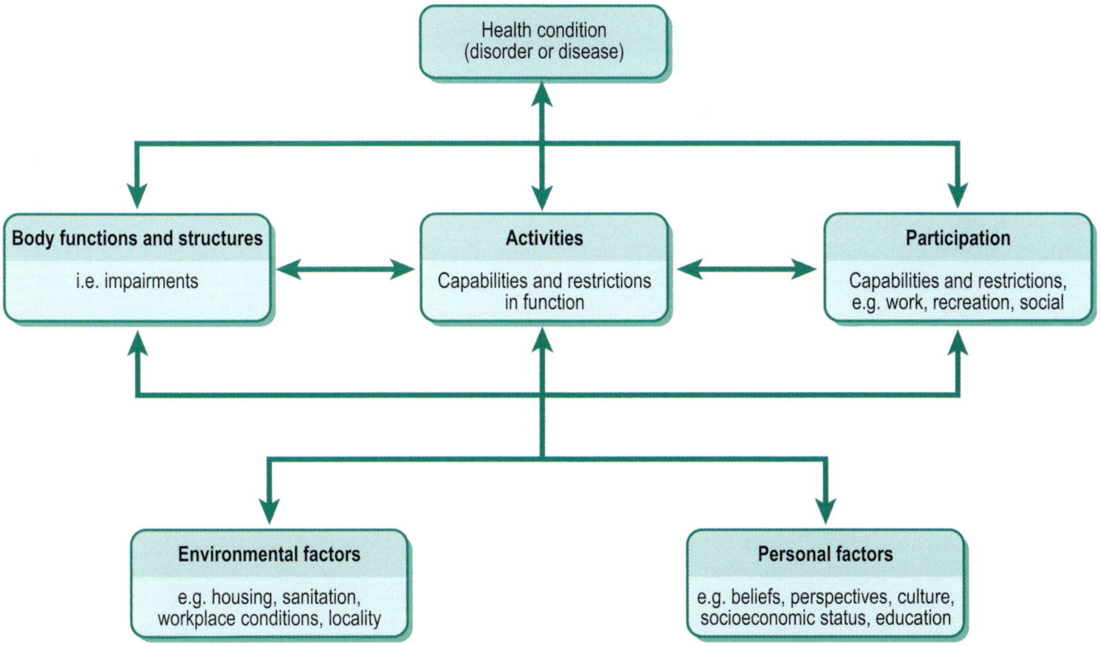

Fig. 3.1 Framework of Health and Disability. (Source: World Health Organisation. (2001). International classification of functioning, disability and health. Geneva: World Health Organisation. http://www.who.int/classifications/icf/en/)

causes of the patient's presenting symptoms, and considering contributing physical and psychosocial factors, so that appropriate management options can be offered.

Clinical reasoning has been described as:

> *A reflective process of clinical enquiry and analysis, carried out by a health professional in collaboration with the patient. The aim is to understand the patient and their clinical problems in their context, in order guide examination, treatment and management of the patient.*
>
> ***Jones & Rivett, 2019***

Research has identified that clinicians often use a number of clinical reasoning approaches, which can be broadly divided into those with a diagnostic focus such as hypothetico-deductive reasoning (Rivett & Higgs, 1997), pattern recognition (Barrows & Feltovich, 1987) and those utilizing interactive processes, such as narrative or collaborative reasoning (Edwards et al., 2004a). Expert clinicians demonstrate greater flexibility in their ability to switch between reasoning strategies compared with novice clinicians (Jones, 1995; Edwards et al., 2004b; Jones & Rivett, 2004; Jones et al., 2008). Hypothesis categories which reflect the ICF framework of Functioning Disability and Health have been proposed to assist in the organization of knowledge and reasoning throughout the subjective and physical examination (WHO, 2001) (Box 3.1). More detailed information on clinical reasoning is provided in Chapter 5.

SUBJECTIVE EXAMINATION/TAKING THE PATIENT'S HISTORY

The quality of the information gained in the subjective examination is dependent on the communication and clinical reasoning skills of the clinician. The information in the subjective examination is key, with experts spending twice as long as novices, in gathering this information (Doody & McAteer, 2002). For further details, please refer to Chapter 2.

This chapter aims to provide an overview of the questions often asked to enable clinicians to obtain relevant information on which to base a person-centred, physical examination. It outlines a very

BOX 3.1 Hypothesis Categories Framework

Activity capability/restriction: what activities the patient is able and unable to do (e.g. walking, lifting, sitting)

Participant capability/restriction: the patient's ability/inability to be involved in life situations, i.e. work, family and leisure activities

Patients' perspectives on their experience and social influences: an important category in its own right as it must be acknowledged that patients' perceptions will have a significant impact on their presentation and response to treatment

Pathobiological mechanisms: the state of the structures or tissues thought to be producing the patient's symptoms in relation to tissue pathology, ongoing tissue damage, the stage of the healing process and the pain mechanisms involved

Physical impairments and associated structure/tissue sources: the target tissue from where symptoms may be coming, in conjunction with the resulting impairment. Sole identification of specific tissues is often difficult, and management directed to the resulting impairment whilst hypothesizing the pathological processes involved is most effective

Contributing factors to the development and maintenance of the problem: these may be environmental, psychosocial, behavioural, physical or heredity factors. Environmental factors may include a patient's workstation or work environment, home situation. Psychosocial factors may include the patient's belief that pain or exercise 'will do harm' resulting in fear avoidant behaviours, or misunderstanding the nature of the problem resulting in catastrophization. Behavioural factors may include what patients do at work or at home, their level of physical activity, such as they may lead a very sedentary lifestyle. Physical contributing factors include elements such as reduced range of movement and muscle weakness. Heredity factors play a part in the development of some musculoskeletal conditions, such as ankylosing spondylitis and osteoarthritis (Solomon et al., 2001)

Precautions/contraindications to physical examination and treatment: this includes the severity and irritability of the patient's symptoms, response to screening questions and the underlying nature of the problem

Management strategy and treatment plan: will be based on reasoning of the subjective data and in agreement through discussion with the patient

Prognosis: this can be affected by factors such as the stage and extent of the injury as well as the patient's expectation, personality and lifestyle. Psychosocial (yellow flags) risk factors, patient's perceived stress at work (blue flags) and work conditions, including employment and sickness policy as well as type and amount of work (black flags), are considered to influence the outcome of treatment strongly. Orange flags indicate mental health disorders which will need to be managed appropriately by trained professionals (Main & Spanswick, 2000; Jones & Rivett, 2004)

From Jones and Rivett (2019).

detailed subjective examination, which the clinician must tailor to the individual patient. The clinician must ask themselves: What is it I want to know and how will the information influence my reasoning? The aim of the subjective examination is to obtain sufficient information for the clinician to clinically reason and plan a safe, person-specific and efficient physical examination, which seeks to confirm or refute initial hypotheses on the causes of the patients' presenting symptoms.

The most important findings in the subjective examination are highlighted in the clinicians' notes with asterisks (*) for easy reference. They can be used to evaluate management interventions.

A summary of the subjective examination is shown in Table 3.1.

The Patient's Context and Their Perspective on Their Experience

Establishing the patient's personal views and expectations is a useful way to open the subjective examination. The clinician invites the patient to explain in their own words why they are seeking help. 'Can you tell me about…' (Gask & Usherwood, 2002). Insight into the patient's perspective can help the clinician to frame the examination within a person-centred context (Goodrich & Cornwell, 2008):

- It makes it clear that the clinician is interested in the patient as a person and helps to build rapport between clinician and patient.
- It identifies whether the reason for referral stated in the referral letter corresponds with the patient's reason for attending.

TABLE 3.1 Summary of Subjective Examination

	Key Information
The patient's context and their perspective on their experience	Patient's expectations, beliefs, goals—identifying their perspective—impact on their quality of life Age, details of their lifestyle—home and work situations, dependents and leisure activities, level of physical activity
Body chart	Details of current symptoms, description, distribution, quality, intensity, abnormal sensations, relationship of symptoms
Behaviour of symptoms	Impact on daily activities, aggravating factors, easing factors, coping strategies, assessment of severity and irritability of the condition, behaviour of symptoms over 24 h, stage of the condition. Risk factors for chronicity
Medical screening questions and family history	General health, weight change—gain or loss, medication incl. steroids, anticoagulants, other existing conditions (e.g. diabetes, thyroid dysfunction, cardiovascular risk factors, neurological screening for spinal cord or cauda equina symptoms, details of recent imaging, blood tests, family history—cancer, coronary heart disease, osteoporosis, rheumatoid arthritis)
Past medical history	Relevant medical history (e.g. hospital admissions, previous episodes, effect of previous treatment if any)
History of present condition	History of each symptomatic area—how and when symptoms began, stage of the condition—how symptoms have behaved over time

Based on Nicholas et al. (2016).

- It identifies what is important to the patient and to what extent the patient's symptoms are problematic for them in their lives. A deep appreciation of their experience is essential for a collaborative and person-centred approach which has been shown to increase treatment adherence, outcomes and patient satisfaction.
- It identifies how the patient views their problem and so can assist in identifying what their expectations and goals are of attending physiotherapy. For example, a patient may be seeking a reassuring explanation of their symptoms and not wish to have treatment.

In order to understand the patient fully, it is important that their presenting symptoms are viewed within the context of the patient's social and work environment. This may help to explain the onset progression or reasons for the persistence of the patient's problem.

In order to identify to what extent the patient's symptoms are problematic to them, the clinician may use brief screening questions such as the following (Aroll et al., 2003; Barker et al., 2014):

- In the past month, has your pain been bad enough to stop you from doing many of your day-to-day activities? This provides an impression of the pain's impact on function, as well as activities such as work, leisure and social interaction. It also provides initial insight into the patient's interpretation of, and response to, the pain.
- In the past month, has your pain been bad enough to make you feel worried or low in mood? This provides initial information about the impact of the pain on the patient's mental and emotional wellbeing.

The answers to these questions can guide the therapist's explanation, reassurance and rehabilitation approach at a later stage.

Body Chart

A body chart (Fig. 3.2) is an example of a visual representation of the area and type of symptoms the patient is experiencing. The clinician uses this information to inform their reasoning and guide further questioning.

Area of Current Symptoms

The clinician is advised to map out the area of the symptoms precisely. Although the most common symptom of musculoskeletal dysfunction is pain, it must not be assumed to be the only presenting

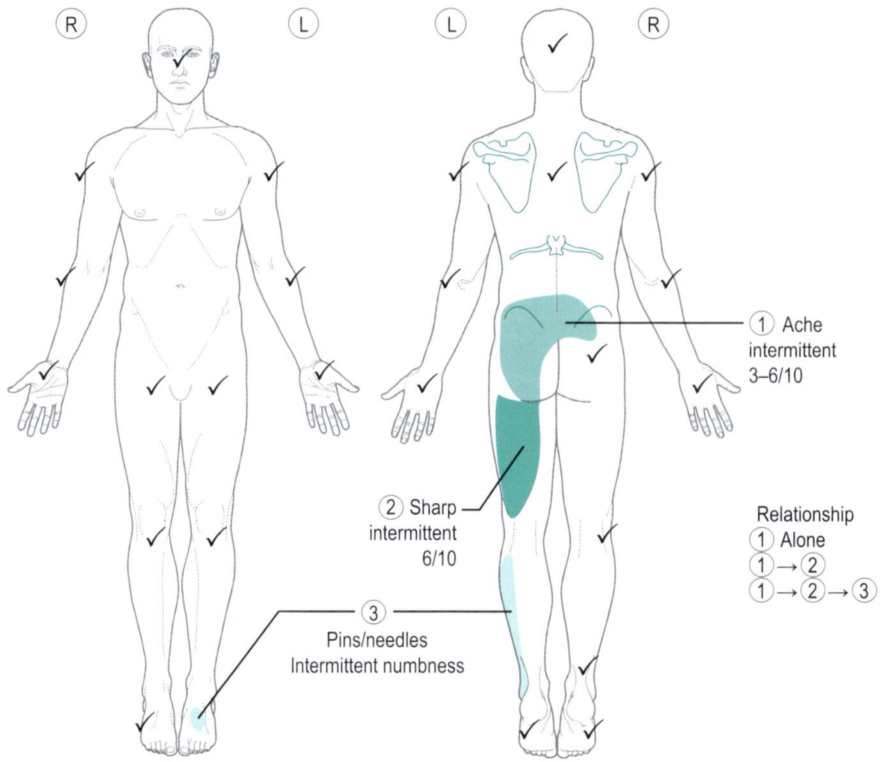

Fig. 3.2 A Body Chart. (Redrawn from Grieve 1991, with permission.)

symptom. Patients often report a range of other symptoms, e.g. crepitus, clicking or locking. It is important to use the words chosen by the patient to identify their symptoms, e.g. an ache or a catch, in order to represent the patient's experience accurately.

It is useful to ask the patient where they feel the symptoms are coming from: 'If you had to put your finger on one spot where you feel it is coming from, where would you put it?' This can help to pinpoint the source of the symptoms although careful reasoning is needed in interpreting this information. It may be an area of pain referral since symptoms can be felt in one area but emanate from elsewhere. For example, pain felt in the elbow may be produced locally or may be due to pathology in the cervical spine, the shoulder or the radial nerve (see section on referred pain below).

Asking the patient to identify which symptom troubles them most (if more than one area) can help to focus the examination and prioritize treatment. It is also important to remember that the patient may describe only the worst symptom, but lesser or different symptoms may be highly relevant to the understanding of the patient's condition. For example, referred symptoms into the limbs may originate in spinal segments.

Areas Relevant to the Region Being Examined

All other relevant areas are checked for the presence of any symptoms and any unaffected areas are marked with ticks (✓) on the body chart.

Pain: The Most Common Presenting Symptom

The International Association for the Study of Pain (IASP) defines pain as:

An unpleasant sensory and emotional experience associated with, or resembling that associated with, actual or potential tissue damage (www.iasp-pain.org).

The IASP also notes that pain is always a personal experience that is influenced to varying degrees by biological, psychological, and social factors. It is different for every individual. It is difficult to estimate the extent of another person's psychological and

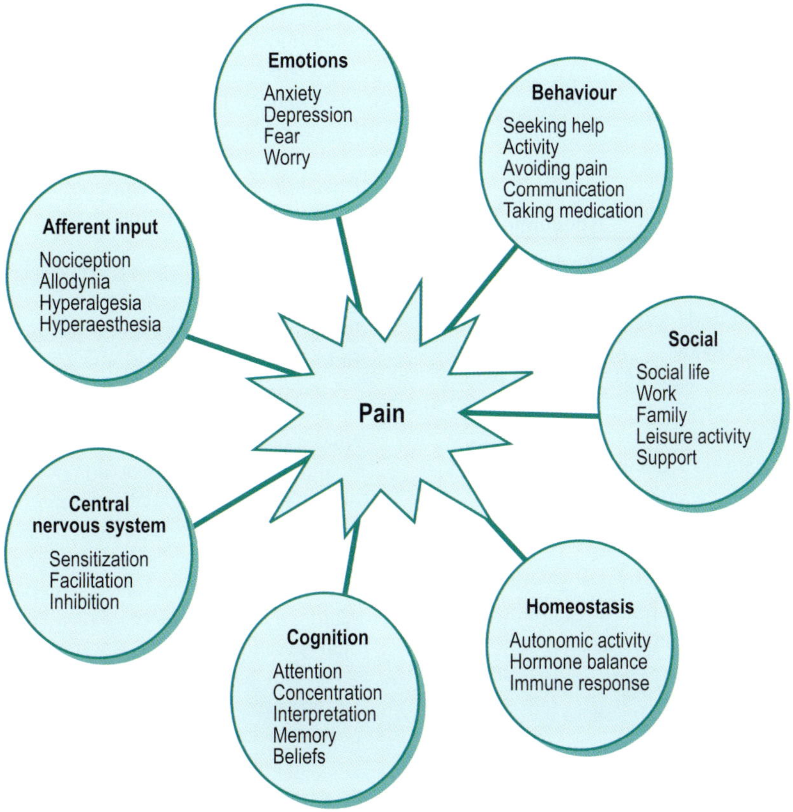

Fig. 3.3 Dimensions of Pain.

emotional experience of pain. A person's report of an experience as pain should therefore be respected; if something is painful to the patient, then the clinician must accept that. The definition highlights the complexity of pain and makes it clear that pain always has an emotional aspect. It also demonstrates that pain does not require tissue damage, even if it is experienced as such by the patient. Pain may be widespread or focal. It may or may not follow an anatomical distribution. Pain has many dimensions, as shown in Fig. 3.3.

Quality of the Pain

The clinician asks the patient: 'How would you describe your pain?' The adjectives the patient uses to describe their pain may be of an emotional rather than a physical nature, such as torturous, miserable or terrifying, which may provide insight into the way the patient experiences their pain. Descriptions of the pain such as burning, sharp or stabbing can assist identification of the physiological mechanism involved. This, along with the location and behaviour of symptoms, may assist in determining the structures at fault (Box 3.2). An understanding of the neurobiological mechanisms responsible for pain can help to formulate a treatment approach specifically targeting these mechanisms (Woolf, 2004). Peripheral origins of pain can be either nociceptive or neuropathic, and pain may be enhanced by nociplastic changes. Patients may use emotive descriptors of their pain that provide an impression of how they experience it subjectively. Further information can be found in Barnard and Ryder (2024), Chapter 10.

Pain intensity. Pain intensity can be measured using numerical or visual analogue rating scales (Hinnant, 1994). These are outlined in Fig. 3.4.

To complete a numerical rating scale (NRS), the patient is asked to indicate the number which best describes the intensity of their pain. Typically, the

BOX 3.2 Pain Characteristics

Nociceptive Pain

Pain that arises from actual or threatened damage to non-neural tissue and is due to the activation of nociceptors (www.iasp-pain.org). This is different from neuropathic pain, see below. Nociceptive pain can be the consequence of tissue damage or mechanical, inflammatory and ischaemic influences.

Characterized by:

Mechanical	Inflammatory	Ischaemic
Localized intermittent pain Predictable consistent response to mechanical stimuli e.g. stretch, compression or movement No/less pain on waking but (more) pain on rising Usually mild to moderate severity Responds to simple painkillers and non-steroidal anti-inflammatory drugs (NSAIDs)	Constant/ varying pain Worsened rapidly by movement Latent pain Night pain and pain on waking High irritability and severity Movements limited by pain Responds to non-steroidal anti-inflammatory drugs (NSAIDs)	Usually intermittent Predictable pattern • Aggravated by sustained postures and/ or repetitive activities • Eased by change of position or by cessation of a repetitive activity

Reference: van Griensven (2013).

Peripheral Neuropathic Pain

Pain caused by a lesion or disease of the peripheral somatosensory nervous system (www.iasp-pain.org). Somatosensory refers to information about the body per se including visceral organs, rather than information from the world external to the body. The mere presence of certain symptoms or signs suggestive of neuropathy (e.g. touch-evoked pain) does not justify the use of the term *neuropathic* (ibid.). Please note that neuropathic pain may also be due to a lesion or disease in the central nervous system (for instance, after a spinal cord lesion or stroke), in which case it is called *central* neuropathic pain.

May manifest as:

Neuro-anatomical distribution, i.e. along a spinal segment or peripheral/cranial nerve pathway/course

Typical descriptions include burning, sharp, shooting and electric shocklike, although neuropathic pain can manifest in many different ways

Allodynia (pain provoked by stimuli that are normally innocuous), paraesthesia (abnormal sensation such as tingling or pins & needles), dysaesthesia (painful paraesthesia), hypoaesthesia, hyperaesthesia and possibly a mixture of these

Provoked by nerve stretch, nerve compression (Phalen's test) or nerve palpation (Tinel's test)

Possible associated hypoaesthesia or analgesia (partial or complete sensory loss), muscle weakness and autonomic changes

Poor response to simple analgesia and anti-inflammatory medication

Response to passive treatment varies

References: Cook, van Griensven & Jesson (in press), Finnerup et al. (2016).

Nociplastic Pain

Pain that arises from altered nociception despite no clear evidence of actual or threatened tissue damage causing the activation of peripheral nociceptors or evidence of disease or lesion of the somatosensory system causing the pain (www.iasp-pain.org). In other words, a patient may have pain as a consequence of a change in function of the somatosensory nervous system, with no findings indicating a nociceptive or neuropathic origin of the pain. It is possible for a pain to have both a nociceptive and a nociplastic component (ibid.) (i.e. the pain may have a clear origin in the tissues, but an altered function of the somatosensory nervous system changes the way the pain is experienced).

Enhanced pain sensitivity and pain perception in an individual may be due to neurophysiological mechanisms. They are not an indication of psychological overlay and must be interpreted with caution.

One of the mechanisms that may underlie nociplastic changes is called *central sensitization*. It is defined as an increased responsiveness of nociceptive neurons in the central nervous system to their normal or subthreshold afferent input (www.iasp-pain.org). Central sensitization cannot be measured in people but allodynia and hyperalgesia to some sensory tests may suggest that it is present—see (van Griensven et al., 2020) for an overview.

May manifest as:

Hyperalgesia (increased sensitivity to painful stimuli)

Allodynia (pain in response to innocuous stimuli)

Inconsistent response to stimuli and tests

Patients having difficulty in locating and describing their pain

The pain seems to have 'a mind of its own'

Widespread, nonanatomical distribution

Simple analgesics may be ineffective

Unpredictable or failed response to passive treatments

References: Woolf (2012), van Griensven et al. (2020).

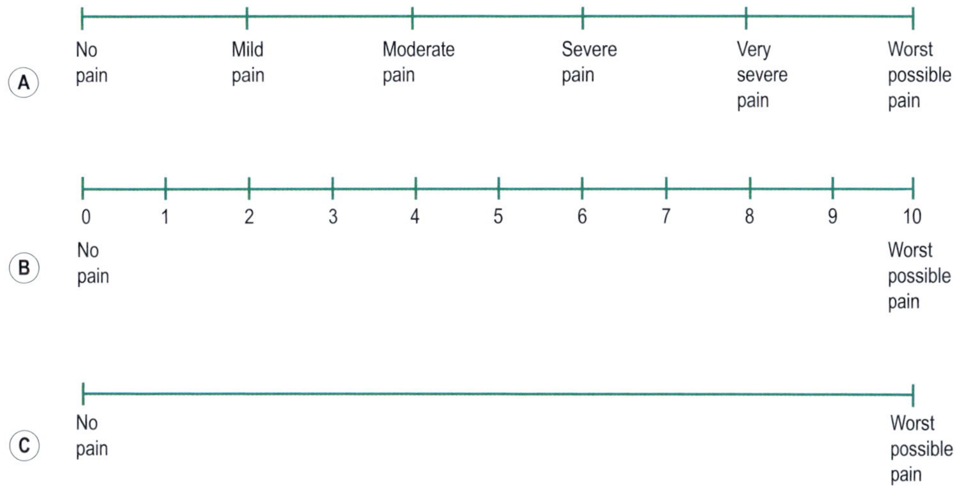

Fig. 3.4 Pain Intensity Rating Scales. (A) Simple descriptive pain rating scale. (B) 1–10 numerical pain intensity scale. (C) Visual Analogue Scale. (From Hinnant 1994. © Williams and Wilkins.)

numbers are presented on an 11-point NRS ranging from 0 to 10. The anchor on the left is 0, representing an absence of pain, while 10 on the right represents the worst imaginable pain. For the Visual Analogue Scale (VAS), the patient is asked to mark on a 100 mm line the point that best represents the intensity of their pain, with descriptors at either end. The line has no marks, numbers or words between the two anchors. The VAS score is the distance in mm of the mark from 0. The requirements of a line that is exactly 100 mm long and measurement in millimetres make an NRS more practical for clinical use. Finally, some scales use words (from *no pain* to *worst possible pain*) or emojis (from smiling to very sad).

The clinician has to be clear and consistent when the patient is asked to fill in a pain score, specifically if a comparison is to be made at a later date. For example, it must be clear whether the patient is asked about their pain on the day, on average, or at its worst. Some clinicians ask the patient to score their pain at its best as well as its worst to establish a range. A set of pain rating scales developed by the British Pain Society asks the patient to score their pain on the day, but also on average over the past week (https://www.britishpainsociety.org/british-pain-society-publications/pain-scales-in-multiple-languages/). The set also includes scales for distress associated with the pain (on the day and on average), the level of interference with activities and the effectiveness of previous treatment.

Pain scales are not interchangeable (i.e. someone who marks their pain at 80 mm on a VAS will not necessarily give the pain a description of 8 out of 10 on the NRS). Pain intensity scores can be repeated several times a day, over the course of a treatment or as part of a pain diary. This can be done to construct a pain profile from which the behaviour of the patient's pain, or the effectiveness of a treatment for pain, can be judged. There is however recognition that measuring a range of different domains to include condition-specific function, general health status, work disability, patient satisfaction as well as pain is important in evaluating interventions in patients with persistent problems (Chiarotto et al., 2016; van Griensven & Strong, in press).

Referred pain. Pain which is felt distant to the tissue in which it originates is known as referred pain. The more proximal the source of the pain, the more extensive is the possible area of referral. For example, the zygapophyseal joints in the lumbar spine can refer symptoms to the leg and foot (Mooney & Robertson, 1976), the hip joint typically refers symptoms no further than the knee, while the joints of the foot tend to produce local symptoms only. Referred pain is thought to be the consequence of the convergence of sensory neurones onto a common secondary neurone in the spinal cord (Bogduk, 2009). Fig. 3.5 illustrates how afferents from for instance viscera or deep somatic structures converge on a secondary neurone in the dorsal horn, which normally responds mainly to nociceptive input from cutaneous regions (McMahon, 1997; Arendt-Nielsen et al., 2000).

Spinal structures such as facet joints, ligaments and discs can also produce somatically referred pain (Bogduk, 2009). This type of pain is distinct from radicular pain, which results from sensitization of the nerve root

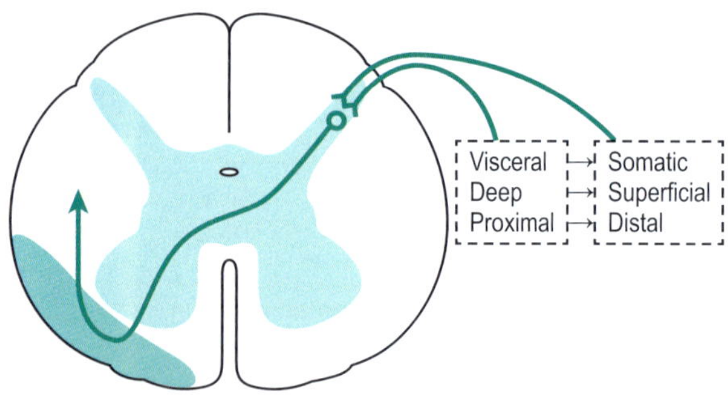

Fig 3.5 Dorsal Horn Pathways Underlying Referred Pain. Primary neurones from different tissues synapse with a single secondary neurone. Input from the more commonly stimulated neurone (box on the right) is either shared with, or facilitated by, the input from the less commonly stimulated neurone (box on the left) (McMahon, 1997). The arrows between the boxes indicate the direction of pain referral. (From Lindsay et al. 1997, with permission.)

and has a lancinating quality (ibid). Detailed questioning about the nature of the pain and neurological symptoms, followed by a detailed examination, is essential to distinguish between these types of spinal pain.

Visceral pain may also be referred to muscles and skin, thus generating somatic pain and sensitization (Cervero & Laird, 2004). Areas of referred symptoms from the viscera are shown in Fig. 3.6 (Lindsay et al., 1997). Pain from viscera is notoriously diffuse and poorly localized (Al-Chaer & Traub, 2002).

Pain is most likely to be referred to tissues innervated by the same segments, as pain is 'projected' from the viscera to the area supplied by corresponding somatic afferent fibres (see Fig. 3.7). In addition, the uterus is capable of referring symptoms to regions innervated by both T10–L2 and S2–S5 (van Cranenburgh, 1989). Symptoms referred from the viscera can sometimes be distinguished from those originating in the musculoskeletal system when they are not aggravated by activity or relieved by rest, but this is not always the case. The clinician needs to be aware that symptoms can be referred from the spine and trunk to the periphery, from the periphery to more peripheral regions (e.g. hip to knee or shoulder to elbow), and from the viscera to the spine and trunk.

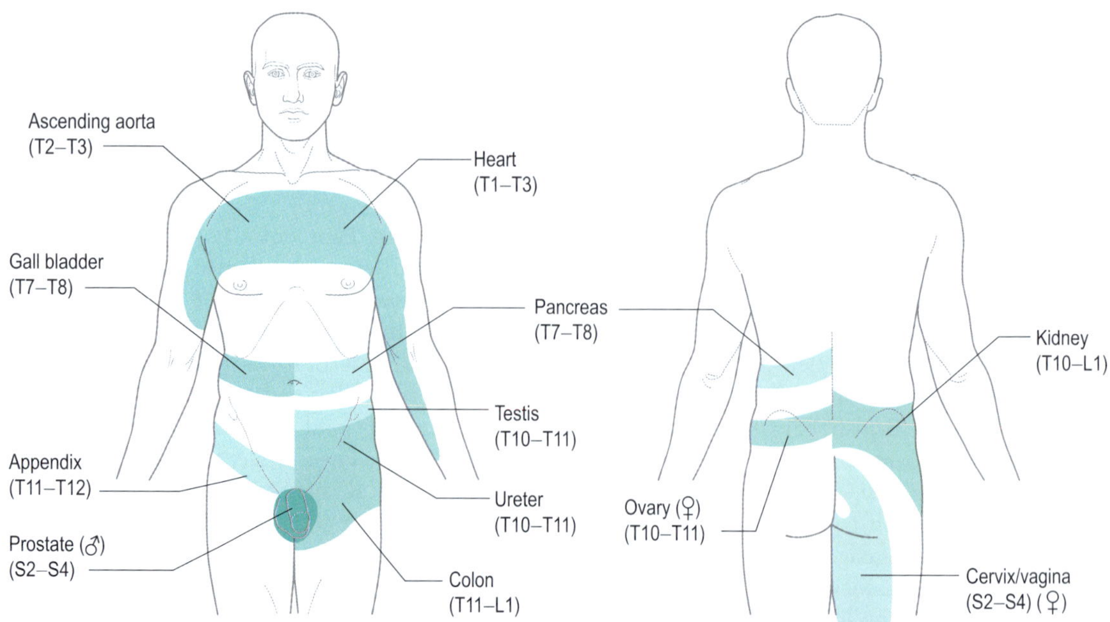

Fig. 3.6 Sites of Referred Pain From the Viscera.

Body chart 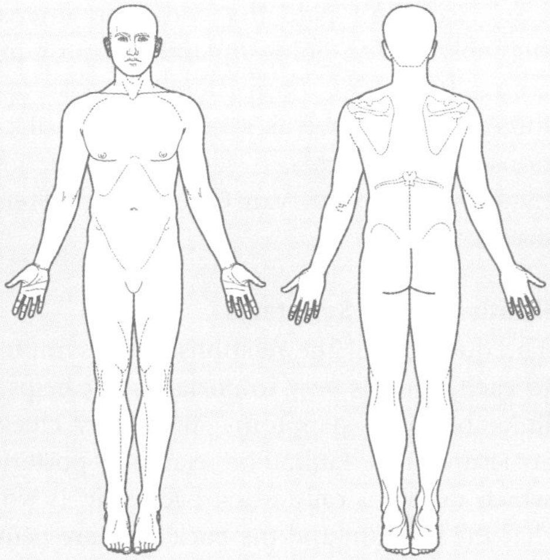 Relationship of symptoms	Name Age Date Patient's perspective / Social history Patient expectations Capabilities / Restrictions HPC Improving Static Worsening FH General health Weight
Intensity of pain 0 1 2 3 4 5 6 7 8 9 10	Special questions Medication X-ray/scan/investigations
Aggravating factors	24-hour behaviour Night / On waking a.m. Midday p.m.
Easing factors	Primary hypothesis/alternative hypotheses
Severity Irritability High/moderate/low Yes No	Plan for physical examination **Must** **Should** **Could**

Fig. 3.7 Subjective Examination Chart.

Another potential source of referred musculoskeletal pain is an *active trigger point*, described as an exquisitely tender spot in discrete bands of tight muscle that produce local and referred pain (Bron & Dommerholt, 2012). Although trigger points were originally described as potentially arising in any soft tissue (Travell & Simons, 1983), they are now seen as associated with muscle overuse, overactivity or trauma (Dommerholt, 2011; Bron & Dommerholt, 2012). For trigger points and their characteristic area of referral see (Donnelly et al., 2013).

Abnormal sensations. Areas of abnormal sensation are mapped out on the body chart.

Abnormal sensations include paraesthesia (abnormal sensation), anaesthesia (complete loss of sensation), hypoaesthesia (reduced nonpainful sensation), hyperaesthesia (heightened nonpainful stimulation) and allodynia (pain provoked by stimuli that are normally nonpainful). Paraesthesia includes sensations of tingling, pins and needles, swelling, tight bands around part of the body and water trickling over the skin. When painful, it is known as dysaesthesia. Detailed descriptions and definitions can be found at www.iasp-pain.org.

The sensory changes listed above can be generated anywhere along a peripheral or cranial nerve, including nerve root, spinal cord or brain. A common cause for loss of sensation is nerve compression (e.g. when part of the brachial plexus is compressed by a cervical rib or when a median nerve compression results in carpal tunnel syndrome). Knowledge of the cutaneous distribution of nerve roots (dermatomes), brachial and lumbosacral plexuses, and peripheral nerves enables the clinician to distinguish between the sensory loss from a root lesion and a peripheral nerve lesion. Cutaneous innervation areas and dermatomes are shown in Chapter 4 (see Figs 4.12–4.15).

Constant or Intermittent Symptoms

The word 'constant' is used here to mean symptoms that are felt unremittingly for 24 hours a day; any relief of symptoms even for a few minutes would mean that the symptoms were intermittent. Some patients describe their pain as constant until asked whether they are ever without pain. The frequency of intermittent symptoms is important as there may be wide variations, from symptoms being felt once a month to once an hour. Specific details are useful at this stage so that progress can be clearly monitored at subsequent treatment sessions. Constant pain that does not vary is characteristic of serious pathology (e.g. neoplastic disease). Constant pain that varies in intensity may be suggestive of on-going inflammatory or infective processes. Pain with a consistent response to mechanical forces, for instance as a consequence of certain positions or movements, is suggestive of a nociceptive or tissue-based origin (van Griensven & Trendafilova, in press).

Relationship of Symptoms

The question of the relationship of symptomatic areas to each other is very important as it helps to establish links between symptoms and gives clues about the structure(s) at fault. For example, posterior leg pain which develops only when back pain is worse suggests that the leg pain and the back pain are being produced by the same structure.

This completes the information that can be documented on the body chart. An example of a completed body chart is shown in Fig. 3.3

KNOWLEDGE CHECK

1. Why do we ask patients to describe their pain?
2. How can pain intensity be quantified, and why is this useful?
3. What is referred pain?
4. Why is a report of constant pain of potential concern?

Impact on Function

The clinician asks how the symptoms affect the patient's daily function including activities such as sitting, standing, walking, running, washing, driving and lifting, which may impact on their ability to participate in work, family life and leisure activities.

The impact of functional impairment can be measured using a range of patient-reported outcome measures (PROMS). Some are generic (e.g. the Patient Specific Functional Scale), whilst others are region or disease specific (e.g. Roland Morris Questionnaire or Oswestry Disability Index). Outcome measures provide baseline measures which can be used to evaluate the impact of future interventions. The selection of measures must take into account a range of considerations such as suitability for a particular patient as well as reliability and validity (Kyte et al., 2015).

Aggravating and Easing Factors

Aggravating and easing information helps the clinician to hypothesize the likely underlying reasons for the patient's symptoms (e.g. the structure(s) at fault). It also helps to judge the severity (S) and irritability (I) of the patient's symptoms so the clinician can begin to plan the physical examination.

Further questioning can also establish the patient's response to their pain and the impact of their coping strategies. This provides insight into the relative contribution of personal factors within the framework of functioning, health and disability (WHO, 2001).

Aggravating Factors

For each symptomatic area, the clinician asks the patient if they are able to identify what aggravates or reproduces their symptoms. The clinician uses this information to analyse the aggravating movement or position and to hypothesize what structures may be causing symptoms. For example, the clinician would expect theoretically known aggravating factors for suspected hip and knee problems such as squatting and going up and down stairs. If the patient is unable to identify an aggravating factor, this increases the clinician's index of suspicion that the problem may not have a musculoskeletal origin.

Detailed information (Box 3.3) helps identify functional restrictions, and the most notable are highlighted on the patient's clinical records with asterisks (*), to be explored in the physical examination. They can be used as reassessment markers to evaluate treatment interventions.

Easing Factors

These are movements or positions that ease the patient's symptoms. As with the aggravating factors, the exact movement or position and the time it takes to ease each symptom are established. This information helps the clinician judge irritability and therefore how difficult or easy it may be to relieve the patient's symptoms during the physical examination. Symptoms that are readily eased by changes in movement or position may respond to treatment quickly. The clinician analyses in detail the easing movement or position to hypothesize which structures are causing the symptoms. The effect of the easing of one symptom on the other symptoms is established, as this helps to identify whether there is a relationship between symptoms.

BOX 3.3 Examples of Questions to Establish Irritability, Severity and Relationship of Symptoms.

How quickly are the patient's symptoms reproduced?	The time it takes to bring on the symptoms (or make them worse) indicates how irritable the symptoms are and so how difficult or easy it may be to reproduce the patient's symptoms in the physical examination. For example, knee symptoms that are felt after a 90-minute football match will be harder to reproduce in the clinic than symptoms provoked by climbing a single flight of stairs.
Is the patient able to maintain a position or movement?	If symptoms are too severe the patient may report having to stop a particular activity. For example, a patient reporting symptoms along the course of the median nerve may be severely limited in typing due to the mechanosensitivity of the nerve tissue.
What happens to other symptoms when this symptom is produced or made worse?	This information helps to confirm the relationship between the symptoms. If different symptoms are aggravated by the same position or movement, it suggests that the symptoms are being produced by the same source or structure(s).

Coping Strategies

Having established aggravating and easing factors, the clinician must identify whether and how the patient is using these to manage their condition. For example, they may have changed or abandoned activities in response to their symptoms. The clinician must judge whether this accommodation is likely to be helpful or not. Short-term reduction or avoidance of some activities can be an effective strategy to overcome an injury and is therefore known as *adaptive*. Finding ways to continue functioning in the presence of pain can also be adaptive. On the other hand, avoiding most activities over a long period of time may be *maladaptive*: it may avoid pain but also leads to a decline in fitness and functional ability, possibly interfering with social activities, work and leisure. Maladaptive coping strategies can contribute to and perpetuate the patient's problem and compromise treatment (Harding & Williams, 1995; Shorland, 1998; Main et al., 2008). Unhelpful coping strategies may include:

- Activity avoidance—leading to disuse, lack of fitness, reduced strength and flexibility. This strategy may reduce participation in leisure activities and work with additional social and financial consequences.
- Underactivity/overactivity cycles: activity avoidance on days with pain, followed by excessive activity on other days. Reduced activity tolerance due to disuse on 'bad' days leads to tissue overload on 'good' days. Over time there may be a gradual increase in pain and a decrease in activity.
- Long-term use of medication may lead to side effects such as constipation, indigestion and drowsiness. While medication may help to control symptoms, its side effects are likely to build up over time and interfere with general function and recovery. Moreover, the patient may become drug dependent.
- Visiting a range of therapists and specialists in the pursuit of a diagnosis or cure (Butler & Moseley, 2003).
- An unwillingness to take control but persisting with passive and unhelpful coping strategies.

Severity and Irritability of Symptoms

The clinician must reason whether the patient's symptoms are severe and/or irritable so that the physical examination can be carried out in a way that avoids unnecessary exacerbation of the patient's symptoms.

Severity of the Symptoms

The severity of the symptoms is the degree to which symptoms restrict or stop movement and/or function and is related to the intensity of the symptoms (Banks & Hengeveld, 2014). For example, the clinician asks a patient with shoulder pain 'When you are reaching up for something from the kitchen cupboard and you feel the sharp pain in your shoulder can you continue to reach or do you have to stop?' Symptoms are defined as severe if a movement at a certain point in range provokes symptoms so intense that the movement must be ceased immediately.

If symptoms are severe, the patient will not tolerate structures being tested more extensively, such as the application of overpressures, repeated or combined movements. For these patients, movements must be performed up to or just short of the first onset of symptoms. On the other hand, when symptoms are of low severity the patient will be able to tolerate more extensive testing (Banks & Hengeveld, 2014). Severity is often expressed by clinicians as a subjective descriptive measure in terms of being of mild, moderate or high severity.

Irritability of the Symptoms

Irritability is a combination of the amount of provocation required to produce a symptom, its severity and how long it takes for it to ease (Banks & Hengeveld, 2014).

For example, when a movement produces or increases pain which continues to be present for a period of time, then the symptom(s) are considered to be irritable. Any pain lasting more than a few seconds requires a pause between tests to allow symptoms to return to their resting level. If the symptom disappears as soon as the movement is stopped, then the symptom is considered to be nonirritable.

The clinician might ask: 'When you are reaching up for something from the kitchen cupboard and you get the sharp pain in your shoulder and you stop. What happens to your pain?' If the pain eases immediately, the pain is considered to be nonirritable and physical testing can be more extensive (e.g. selected movements could be sustained) repeated etc. If the symptoms take minutes to disappear then the symptoms are irritable, so the clinician uses their reasoning to justify a limited physical examination to avoid making the patient's symptoms worse and to identify pain-easing strategies.

Occasionally latent irritability may occur, for example, if symptoms are neurogenic in origin, where a movement or position may induce symptoms that are delayed by some minutes.

Patient's symptoms often present as a combination requiring careful reasoning. They may be nonsevere but irritable, severe but nonirritable, or both severe and irritable, for example.

Twenty-Four-Hour Behaviour of Symptoms

Night Symptoms

Quality of sleep is integral to a person's wellbeing. Sleep quality and quantity have been linked to the risk of persistent pain (Finan et al., 2013; Afolalu et al., 2018). An understanding of a patient's sleep pattern can be explored.

- Does the patient have difficulty getting to sleep because of the symptom(s)? Lying down reduces compressive forces on weight-bearing joints so may ease symptoms provoked by upright postures.
  - How many hours of sleep do they get each night?
  - Which positions are most comfortable and uncomfortable for the patient? The clinician can analyse these positions to inform their reasoning.
  - How many and what type of pillows are used by the patient? How are they placed? This information may be relevant for patients with cervical spine pain because the pillows may create excessively flexed or side-flexed cervical spine resting positions.
  - Does the patient use a firm or soft mattress, and has it recently been changed? Alteration in sleeping posture caused by a new mattress is sometimes sufficient to provoke spinal symptoms.
  - Is the patient woken by symptoms and, if so, which symptoms? Are they associated with movement (e.g. turning over in bed or position?)
  - To what extent do the symptoms disturb the patient at night?
    - How many times in any one night is the patient woken?
    - How many nights in the past week was the patient woken?
    - What does the patient do when woken? For example, can the patient reposition or do they have to get up? If they get up what do they do? Do they take pain relief? Sit/lie on the sofa?
    - Can the patient get back to sleep?
    - How long does it take to get back to sleep?

It is useful to be as specific as possible so that this information can be used to judge severity, irritability and a possible contribution of a lack of sleep to the pain. The information can guide treatment priorities and provide a baseline to evaluate response to treatment.

Morning Symptoms

What are the patient's symptoms in the morning on waking before movement? Do they wake feeling refreshed and rested in the morning? When the patient gets up, what happens to their symptoms? Prolonged morning pain and stiffness that improves minimally with movement may be suggestive of an inflammatory process such as rheumatoid arthritis (Magee & Manske, 2021). Minimal or absent pain with stiffness in the morning is associated with degenerative conditions such as osteoarthrosis or cervical spondylosis (Huskisson et al., 1979; Rao et al., 2007).

Evening Symptoms

Symptoms at the end of the day may depend on the patient's daily activity levels. Symptoms aggravated by movement and eased by rest generally indicate a mechanical problem of the musculoskeletal system. Symptoms that increase with activity may be due to repeated mechanical stress, an inflammatory process or a degenerative process.

KNOWLEDGE CHECK

1. Explain the value of asking patients about activities that provoke their symptoms.
2. How would you explain the terms adaptive and maladaptive?
3. Can you give examples of unhelpful strategies patients may adopt in response to their symptoms?

Stage of the Condition

Knowing whether the symptoms are getting better, getting worse or remaining unchanged gives an indication of the stage of the condition and helps the clinician to clinically reason a prognosis. Symptoms that are deteriorating tend to take longer to respond to treatment than symptoms that are resolving. It is important to understand the natural history of the condition under consideration (van Griensven, 2005).

Risk Factors for Chronicity and Poor Treatment Outcome

In the first weeks or months, certain aspects of a patient's presentation may suggest that they have an increased chance that their acute or subacute pain will become persistent (see Table 3.2). These are known as *risk factors* for chronicity and poor treatment outcome. In back pain, psychological and social risk factors have been referred to as *psychosocial yellow flags* (Kendall et al., 1997; Waddell, 2004). A list of yellow and other flags is provided in Table 3.2 Risk factors and yellow flags draw the clinician's attention to the possibility of chronicity, but they are not to be confused with diagnoses or absolute predictors of a patient's recovery (Mallen et al., 2007). The clinician is therefore advised to verify whether a patient's risk factors may or may not be relevant to them. It is equally important not to give up on a patient on the basis of risk factors, but to address the issues that may prevent them from making a full recovery.

Systematic reviews have identified risk factors in patients with musculoskeletal pain (Artus et al., 2017). The following findings may predict poor recovery or poor response to treatment:

Pain-related risk factors
- High pain intensity
- Widespread pain
- Pain of long duration

Psychological risk factors
- Somatization (physical symptoms caused by mental and emotional problems)
- Anxiety
- Depression

Social risk factors
- A high level of functional disability

There is evidence that the use of pain medication and a patient's level of education are not risk factors.

Questionnaires may help to identify the risk level of patients, such as the STarT Back for back pain (https://startback.hfac.keele.ac.uk/) and the short form of the Örebro Musculoskeletal Pain Screening Questionnaire (ÖMPSQ-short) for patients with low back pain (Simula et al., 2020).

If a patient is thought to be at risk of developing persistent pain, it is important to make every effort to optimize pain control. This may include advice, physiotherapy intervention and liaising with the GP or physician regarding prescription medication.

TABLE 3.2 Types of Flags

Flag	Nature	Example
Red	Symptoms suggestive of serious pathology e.g. cauda equina, fracture, tumour	Severe unintended weight loss, progressive neurological symptoms
Orange	Psychopathology	Clinical depression, personality disorder
Yellow	Psychological reaction to symptoms	Unhelpful beliefs regarding nature of the pain, belief that pain must be avoided, worry anxiety
Blue	Perceptions about effect of work on pain or health	Belief that work will cause further injury, belief that manager is not supportive
Black	Obstacles to recovery beyond patient and clinician—contextual factors such as socioeconomic status, access to healthcare	Work that cannot be adapted, lack of return to work options, overly solicitous family members

Based on Linton et al. (2011), Waddell (2004), Main and George (2011), Nicholas et al. (2016).

Screening/Special Questions

Screening questions must always be asked in order to identify existing conditions and co-morbidities which may be contraindications or precautions to physical examination and/or treatment Table 3.3. The clinician needs to clinically reason regarding the pathology that may be underlying the patient's condition and screen for any features of their presentation that suggests a nonmusculoskeletal origin, such as visceral or systemic conditions or indicators of more serious pathology (Deyo et al., 1992; Goodman et al., 2018).

Signs and symptoms suggestive of serious spinal pathology such as tumours, infection, fracture or cord/cauda equina compression are referred to as *red flags*. Table 3.4 It is important to realize that the presence of a single red flag does not necessarily suggest the presence of a serious pathology but needs to be reasoned within the context of the whole person. The International Federation of Orthopaedic Manipulative Physical Therapists (IFOMPT) endorsed framework supports clinical reasoning for red flags (Finucane et al., 2020) (see Chapter 11, Barnard & Ryder, 2024).

TABLE 3.3 Examples of Precautions/Contraindications to Physical Testing and Treatment

Aspects of Subjective Examination	Subjective Information	Possible Cause/Implication for Examination and/or Treatment
Body chart	Constant unremitting pain	Malignancy, systemic, inflammatory cause will require minimal physical screening and referral onward for further investigation
	Symptoms in the upper limb below the acromion or symptoms in the lower limb below the gluteal crease	Possible nerve root compression. Carry out appropriate neurological integrity tests in physical examination
	Widespread sensory changes and/or weakness in upper or lower limb	Compression on more than one nerve root, metabolic (e.g. diabetes, vitamin B_{12}), systemic (e.g. rheumatoid arthritis)
Aggravating factors	Symptoms severe and/or irritable	Care in treatment to avoid unnecessary provocation or exacerbation
Special questions	Feeling unwell	Systemic or metabolic disease
	General health: • history of malignant disease, in remission	Would not exclude manual testing and treatment
	• active malignant disease if associated with present symptoms	Symptoms do not fit a typical MSK presentation.
	• active malignant disease not associated with present symptoms	Would require reasoning of location of the disease and impact of disease process and possible treatment impact on overall tissue health
	• hysterectomy	Increased risk of osteoporosis
	Recent unexplained weight loss	Malignancy, systemic
	Diagnosis of bone disease (e.g. osteoporosis, Paget's brittle bone)	Bone may be abnormal and/or weakened
	Diagnosis of rheumatoid arthritis or other inflammatory joint disease	Avoid strong direct force to bone, especially the ribs Avoid accessory and physiological movements to upper cervical spine and care with other joints

Continued

TABLE 3.3 Examples of Precautions/Contraindications to Physical Testing and Treatment—cont'd

Aspects of Subjective Examination	Subjective Information	Possible Cause/Implication for Examination and/or Treatment
	Diagnosis of infective arthritis	In active stage immobilization is treatment of choice
	Diagnosis of spondylolysis or spondylolisthesis	Avoid strong direct pressure to the subluxed vertebral level
	Systemic steroids	Osteoporosis, poor skin condition requires careful handling, avoid tape
	Anticoagulant therapy	Increased time for blood to clot. Soft tissues may bruise easily
	Human immunodeficiency virus (HIV)	Check medication and possible side effects
	Pregnancy	Ligament laxity, may want to avoid strong forces
	Diabetes	Delayed healing, peripheral neuropathies
	Bilateral hand/feet pins and needles and/or numbness	Spinal cord compression, peripheral neuropathy
	Difficulty walking	Spinal cord compression, peripheral neuropathy, upper motor neurone lesion
	Disturbance of bladder and/or bowel function	Cauda equina syndrome
	Perineum (saddle)	Cauda equina syndrome
	Anaesthesia/paraesthesia	
	For patients with cervicothoracic symptoms: dizziness, altered vision, nausea, ataxia, drop attacks, altered facial sensation, difficulty speaking, difficulty swallowing, sympathoplegia, hemianaesthesia, hemiplegia	Cervical artery dysfunction, upper cervical instability, disease of the inner ear
	Heart or respiratory disease	May preclude some treatment positions
	Oral contraception	Increased possibility of thrombosis—may avoid strong techniques to cervical spine
	History of smoking	Circulatory problems—increased possibility of thrombosis
Recent history	Trauma	Possible undetected fracture, e.g. scaphoid

It is important for clinicians to be aware of the non-linear course of diseases such as cancer. There are three identified stages: the *subclinical stage* where there are pathological changes in the absence of signs and symptoms, the *prodromal stage* characterized by vague nonspecific symptoms with few signs and the *clinical stage* more easily identifiable because there are signs and symptoms. The clinician needs to be constantly alert as early stages of serious conditions can manifest as musculoskeletal conditions and monitoring is an ongoing process (Greenhalgh & Selfe, 2010).

In addition to red flags, clinicians need to be aware of possible red herrings, i.e. misattribution of symptoms by the patient or clinicians leading to reasoning errors (Greenhalgh & Selfe, 2004).

TABLE 3.4 Hierarchical List of Red Flags

>50 years+	<10 and >51 years	Age 11–19	Loss of mobility, trips, falls and problems with stairs
Hx of Cancer+	Medical Hx Ca, TB, HIV, or IV drug use, osteoporosis	Weight loss 5%–10% of BW (3–6 months)	'Bothersome legs'
Unexplained weight loss +	Weight loss >10% of BW (3–6 months)	Constant progressive pain	Weight loss <5% of BW (3–6 months)
Failure to improve after 1/12 of conservative treatment	Severe night pain	Bandlike pain	Smoking
	Loss of sphincter tone and S4	Abdominal pain and changed bowel habit	Systemically unwell trauma bilateral pins and needle
	Bladder and bowel symptoms	Inability to lie supine	Previous failed treatment Thoracic pain
	+ve extensor plantar response	Spasm and disturbed gait	Headache Marked articular stiffness

BW, Body weight; *HIV,* human immunodeficiency virus; *IV,* intravenous; *TB,* tuberculosis.
Reference: Greenhalgh and Selfe (2010).

General Health

The clinician should explore lifestyle choices with the patient (e.g. diet, smoking, alcohol intake, use of recreational drugs, levels of physical activity). Feelings of stress, anxiety or depression can also affect health. Feeling unwell or tired is common with systemic, metabolic or malignant disease (Greenhalgh & Selfe, 2010).

Weight Loss

Has the patient had any change in their weight? If the patient reports weight loss it is important to establish if this was planned. If not, can they explain it, for instance through a change in physical activity or their diet or have they been feeling unwell? Have their symptoms impacted on their appetite? How much have they lost and over what period of time? The clinician needs to be alert especially if the patient reports having lost 5%–10% of their body weight over a period of 3–6 months as this level of loss may be indicative of malignancy or systemic diseases such as tuberculosis (TB) or human immunodeficiency virus (HIV) (Finucane et al., 2020). Weight gain may result in increased load through musculoskeletal structures or may be associated with a reduction in physical activity.

Cardiovascular Disease

Does the patient have a history of cardiovascular disease (e.g. hypertension, angina, myocardial infarction or stroke?) How is their condition managed (e.g. medication and monitoring?) A pacemaker will be a contraindication to certain electrotherapy modalities (Watson T www.electrotherapy.org).

Altered hemodynamics is a red flag, as vascular pathologies such as deep vein thrombosis have pain as an initial feature. Subjectively patients may report exercise-induced nondermatomal pain which is described as pulsing or throbbing. Clinicians will therefore need to consider whether the symptoms reported are linked to the risk factors for that patient e.g. sedentary lifestyle, history of smoking, history, smoking or high BMI, which raise suspicion of an underlying vascular pathology. Family history of cardiovascular disease is relevant for example Abdominal Aortic Aneurysm can present as non-mechanical back pain (van Wyngaarden et al., 2014).

Respiratory Disease

Does the patient have a condition which affects their breathing (e.g. asthma)? If so, how is it managed and do they take medication (e.g. an inhaler)? Medications prescribed for long-term respiratory conditions include steroids, which can affect bone health leading to osteoporosis. In addition, patients with breathing problems may present with reduced exercise tolerance and be unable to lie supine or prone due to breathlessness.

Epilepsy

Is the patient epileptic? If so, what type of seizures does s/he have? Are they medicated? Is their condition well controlled? When was their last seizure? Are there any specific triggers? Side effects of anticonvulsant medication include an impact on mood and an increased risk of osteoporosis (Arora et al., 2016).

Thyroid Disease

Does the patient have a history of thyroid disease? Is their thyroid under or overactive? How well is it managed? Thyroid dysfunction is associated with a higher incidence of musculoskeletal conditions such as adhesive capsulitis, Dupuytren's contracture, trigger finger and carpal tunnel syndrome (Cakir et al., 2003).

Diabetes Mellitus

Is the patient diabetic? If so, is it type 1 or 2? How long since their diagnosis? How is their diabetes managed? How well-controlled is the condition? Patients with diabetes can present with a range of musculoskeletal conditions such as carpal tunnel syndrome, adhesive capsulitis and peripheral neuropathy (Greenhalgh & Selfe, 2010). Healing of tissues is likely to be slower in the presence of this disease, which impacts on prognosis (Brem & Tomic-Canic, 2007).

Cancer

It is important to ask specifically about a history of cancer. A history of a first-degree relative (e.g. parent) or sibling may be relevant, as some cancers have a strong family history (e.g. breast cancer which tends to metastasize to bone along with prostate, kidney, lung and thyroid) (Greenhalgh & Selfe, 2010; Finucane et al., 2020). A history of a malignant disease which is in remission does not contraindicate physical examination or treatment, although presenting symptoms must be confirmed as musculoskeletal in origin. If, on the other hand, there is active malignancy, the primary aim of the physical examination will be to clarify whether the presenting symptoms may be caused by the malignancy or whether there is a separate musculoskeletal disorder. Symptoms thought to be associated with malignancy will require onward referral.

Tuberculosis

With the incidence of TB on the rise, particularly in deprived socioeconomic groups (Bhatti et al., 1995), clinicians must be alert and ask about symptoms such as night sweats, weight loss and fatigue. Most extra-pulmonary TB presents in the spine T10–L1 and patients in the early stages may well present with back ache. A previous history should also be noted as TB can remain dormant for 30–40 years.

Human Immunodeficiency Virus

HIV is an acquired disease affecting the immune system leaving infected patients vulnerable to serious illnesses however they can remain asymptomatic for up to 10 years. The skeletal system is affected in 1%–2% of patients who are HIV negative and 60% of patients who are HIV positive (Greenhalgh & Selfe, 2010). HIV is a neurotrophic virus causing demyelination of the central and peripheral nervous system tissues from the early stages of infection. This can result in patients presenting with myelopathies affecting the spinal and/or painful sensory peripheral neuropathies producing symptoms in the patient's hands or feet (Goodman et al., 2018).

Inflammatory Arthritis

Has the patient been diagnosed with inflammatory arthropathy? Is the patient presenting with symptoms of a inflammatory disease such as rheumatoid arthritis or spondylarthritis? Is there a family history of Rheumatoid Arthirits (RA), spondyloarthritis or psoriasis? Do they have associated extra-articular inflammatory conditions such as inflammatory bowel disease, uveitis, or psoriasis of nails or skin? (MacMillan et al., 2021). Symptoms vary between individuals but usually, patients report an insidious onset which may be associated with feelings of malaise, fever, poor appetite, weight loss and fatigue. Have they had recent gastro-intestinal or genito-urinary infections as these can trigger reactive arthritis. They may well have been referred with diffuse musculoskeletal pain and on questioning report spontaneous swelling of joints, especially of the hands and feet, and inflammation of tendon attachments to bone. Early morning stiffness that lasts longer than 30 minutes is relevant in suspecting inflammatory diseases (McCrum, 2019). If an inflammatory arthropathy is suspected, the patient needs referral onward to rheumatology for further investigations. In patients with existing RA, care needs to be taken in the physical examination because of possible joint erosion and chronic synovitis, especially affecting ligamentous stability of the upper cervical spine. Bone health may also be compromised due to steroidal medication.

Osteoporosis

The clinician will need to ask patients if they have been diagnosed with osteoporosis as this would be a precaution to physical testing. Osteoporosis is the most prevalent of the metabolic bone diseases, the incidence of which increases in postmenopausal women over 50. Questions about menstrual cycles and menopause can offer insights into hormonal influences on bone health. Secondary osteoporosis is also seen in patients with endocrine and metabolic disorders such as hyperthyroidism or inflammatory conditions (e.g. RA or Crohn's disease) (Greenhalgh & Selfe, 2019). Osteoporosis can also be a side effect of long-term use of certain medications such as steroids and anticonvulsants (Finucane et al., 2020). Lifestyle factors with increased risk of insufficiency fractures have been identified as smoking more than 20 cigarettes daily, and consumption of more than 3 units of alcohol a day. Asking about nutritional health is relevant as restrictive diets or a history of eating disorders will impact on bone health. Clinicians need to take a detailed history to identify risk factors to inform reasoning and refer on if there are concerns (e.g. patients may present with episodic acute thoracic/high lumbar pain associated with compression fractures) (Goodman et al., 2018).

Neurological Symptoms

Has the patient experienced any neural symptoms such as tingling, pins and needles, pain, weakness or hypersensitivity? The clinician must clinically reason whether symptoms are likely to originate from the central nervous system (CNS) or the peripheral nervous system. For spinal conditions, gathering the following information will assist with reasoning:

Has the patient experienced symptoms suggestive of spinal cord compression (i.e. compression of the spinal cord that runs from the foramen magnum to L2)? This can occur at any spinal level but is most common in the cervical spine, often as a result of spinal stenosis causing cervical myelopathy. Typical symptoms (e.g. pain, neck stiffness, paresthesia, weakness, clumsiness, disequilibrium, difficulty with bladder control and decreased mobility) and signs (e.g. decreased cervical range of motion, sensory abnormalities, weakness, spasticity and gait disturbance) become more obvious as the disease progresses (Salvi et al., 2006). These symptoms are an indication for neurological integrity tests in the physical examination. Metastatic disease may also be a cause of cord compression, with severe pain often described as bandlike around the trunk as a significant presenting feature in addition to neurological changes in the legs. Symptoms of spinal cord compression require urgent onward referral for an emergency magnetic resonance imaging (MRI) scan (Greenhalgh & Selfe, 2010; Finucane et al., 2020; Greenhalgh et al., 2020).

Clinicians screen patients for cauda equina syndrome (CES), usually caused by a prolapsed intervertebral disc or metastatic disease. Compression of the conus medullaris at the level of L1–2 produces sensory and motor neural problems, the most significant of which is irreversible bladder and bowel dysfunction (Greenhalgh & Selfe, 2010). Patients may be embarrassed answering questions about bladder, bowel and sexual dysfunction, so the clinician must explain why this information is important. Using appropriate language patients are asked if they have noticed changes in bladder or bowel sphincter disturbance which could include retention, loss of control (incontinence), hesitancy, urgency or a sense of incomplete evacuation. Does the patient have any loss of sensation (hypoaesthesia) around their anus, perineum or genitals when using toilet paper? Have they experienced changes in sexual function (e.g. loss of sensation or inability to achieve an erection)? These symptoms must be clinically reasoned in the light of any associated back pain as well as co-existing conditions and medications (such as amitriptyline) which may provide an alternative explanation for changes in bladder or bowel function. CES is relatively rare but if suspected is defined as a surgical emergency, with early surgical spinal decompression producing the most successful outcomes. Clinicians need to remain vigilant, safety-net patients deemed at risk and have a pathway protocol in place so that patients can be managed quickly and appropriately (Greenhalgh et al., 2020; Finucane et al., 2020) (see Chapter 9, Barnard & Ryder, 2024)

Cervical Artery Dysfunction

Patients who present with neck pain and headaches should be screened for cervical artery dysfunction (CAD). Questions seek detailed information about a history of possible exposure to trauma or infection (Thomas, 2016) and any symptoms indicating ischaemia such as visual disturbance, changes in hearing, taste, swallowing or speech difficulties, balance or gait disturbance, limb weakness or paraesthesia. A clinical pattern may emerge from the subjective history that does not fit a typical musculoskeletal pattern. The clinician must reason all risk factors such as cardiovascular health, hypertension, high cholesterol or family history of stroke, in order to recognize elements of a clinical pattern which may indicate a vascular cause. For further information, the reader is directed to (Rushton et al., 2020) and Chapter 8 (Barnard & Ryder, 2024).

Neuropathic Pain Symptoms

Neuropathic pain is pain caused by a lesion or disease of the somatosensory nervous system (www.iasp-pain.org). If the clinician suspects that their patient's pain may be of a neuropathic nature, validated neuropathic screening tools may be helpful. These tools enable the clinician to score the patient's signs and symptoms in a systematic way. Commonly used screening tools are the Leeds Assessment of Neuropathic Symptoms and Signs (LANSS), the Neuropathic Pain Questionnaire (NPQ), Douleur Neuropathique en 4(DN4), painDETECT and ID-Pain (Bennett et al., 2007). LANSS and DN4 include a few simple physical tests such as brush allodynia and pin prick threshold.

Hypermobility Spectrum Disorder

Joint hypermobility-related disorders affecting connective tissue can range from asymptomatic generalized joint laxity to symptomatic hypermobility which has been defined as hypermobility spectrum disorder (HSD) and hypermobile Ehlers-Danlos syndrome (hEDS). Has the patient been diagnosed with HSD or hEDS? Patients with HSD/hEDS may present with widespread diffuse pain, whilst also reporting a range of symptoms such as fatigue and visceral problems and may have a history of recurrent musculoskeletal conditions (Russek et al., 2019). If hEDS is suspected, five simple questions can help to contribute to the identification of this syndrome (Hakim & Grahame, 2003):

1. Can you now (or could you ever) place your hands flat on the floor without bending your knees?
2. Can you now (or could you ever) bend your thumb to touch your forearm?
3. As a child, did you amuse your friends by contorting your body into strange shapes or could you do the splits?
4. As a child or teenager, did your kneecap or shoulder dislocate on more than one occasion?
5. Do you consider yourself 'double-jointed'?

These questions are included within the diagnostic criteria developed to improve subjective screening, physical examination and appropriate manage for this group of patients (Russek et al., 2019).

KNOWLEDGE CHECK

1. Give examples of red flags for serious spinal pathology.
2. What screening questions are relevant to ask to establish risk factors for cardiovascular disease?
3. What are the symptoms of cervical myelopathy?
4. How would you screen for cauda equina syndrome?

Drug Therapy

A series of questions about medication can inform the clinical reasoning process.

1. Has the patient been on long-term medication/steroids? High doses of corticosteroids for a long period of time can weaken the skin and cause osteoporosis. In this case, the patient requires careful handling and avoidance of the use of tape so that the skin is not damaged. Owing to the raised likelihood of osteoporosis, strong direct forces on the bones are inadvisable.
2. Long-term use of medication may lead to side effects such as constipation, indigestion and drowsiness as well as perhaps causing the patient to become drug dependent. This may interfere with their general function and hinder their recovery.
3. Has the patient been taking anticoagulants? If so, care is needed in the physical examination and treatment in order to avoid trauma to tissues and consequent bleeding.
4. Medication use can provide information about the pathological process and may affect treatment. For example, the efficacy of anti-inflammatory medication suggest the presence or absence of inflammation. The WHO three-step analgesic ladder recommends suitable analgesia based on the level and underlying mechanism of a patient's pain. For a comprehensive account of pain pharmacology, the reader is directed to Smith and Muralidharan (in press). Care may be needed if the patient attends for assessment/treatment soon after taking painkillers, as the pain may be temporarily masked. The clinician also needs to be aware of any side effects of the drugs. The clinician must continue to monitor medication use and be prepared to discuss a patient's medication with medical colleagues.
5. Have all of the patient's drugs been prescribed or is the patient self-medicating with (additional) over-the-counter preparations? Does the patient take illicit drugs such as cannabis?
6. Has the medication helped? For example, a positive response to anti-inflammatory medication is suggestive of an inflammatory process, while a lack of response suggests other origins of and/or influences on the patient's symptoms.

Radiographs, Medical Imaging and Tests

Has the patient been x-rayed or had other medical tests? If so, what did they reveal, and what does the patient understand about what they have been told? Plain radiographs are useful to diagnose fractures, arthritis and serious bone pathologies such as infection, osteoporosis or tumours. Imaging can provide useful information, but the findings must always be correlated with the patient's clinical presentation. This is particularly true for spinal radiographs, which may reveal normal age-related degenerative changes of the spine that do not necessarily correlate with the patient's symptoms (Brinjikji et al., 2015). There is evidence that imaging results can negatively affect the patient's sense of well-being (Sharma et al., 2020). Imaging reports can contribute to persistent pain if patients are not provided with the context of normal epidemiological data (McCullough et al., 2012). For this reason, routine spinal radiographs are no longer considered indicated for non-traumatic spinal pain (NICE, 2016).

Other imaging techniques include computed tomography (CT), MRI, myelography, discography, bone scanning and arthrography. The results of these tests can help to determine the nature of the patient's condition but must be requested only based on sound reasoning and clinically indication. Further details of these tests and their diagnostic value can be found in Goodman et al. (2018).

Has the patient had other investigations such as blood tests? A full blood count (FBC) will provide information on number of red and white blood cells and platelets. This is a useful initial screening test because results outside normal ranges could indicate a number of conditions. It can be followed up with more specific tests such as erythrocyte sedimentation rate (ESR) a useful indicator of serious pathology for example malignant myelomas and TB. C-reactive protein (CRP) is commonly tested to detect inflammatory diseases and infections. Further information on clinical interpretation of blood tests (Basten, 2019).

Past Medical History

The following information is obtained from the patient and/or medical notes:

Details of any medical history such as major or longstanding illnesses, accidents or surgery that are relevant to the patient's condition.

Family History

The clinician asks about any relevant family history that may indicate a patient's predisposition for a condition. An understanding of the family history may also help to explain a patient's perceptions of their problem.

History of the Present Condition

Details of the onset of the patient's presenting condition is often discussed earlier in the initial examination, but it is useful to revisit again once the clinician has more information about the patient's symptoms. For each symptomatic area, the clinician ascertains:

- Whether there was a known or unknown cause that provoked the onset of the symptom (e.g. trauma or change in lifestyle that may have triggered symptoms).
- Whether there was a sudden or slow onset of symptoms.
- The relationship of symptoms. The clinician asks when each symptom began in relation to others. If, for example, their low back pain started 5 weeks ago and increased a week ago when the posterior thigh pain developed, it would suggest that the back and thigh pain are associated. If there was no change in the back pain when the thigh pain began, the symptoms may not be related and different structures may be producing the two pain areas.
- How long symptoms have been present.
- Whether the patient has sought any treatment already and, if so, what type of treatment and to what effect.
- History of any previous symptoms (e.g. the number and duration of previous episodes) when they occurred, possible causes, and whether the patient fully recovered between episodes. If there have been no previous episodes, has the patient experienced other symptoms such as stiffness which may have been a precursor to the development of pain?
- Whether the patient had treatment previously. If so, what type? What was the outcome of any past treatments for the same or a similar problem? Past treatment records, if available, may be obtained for further information. A previously successful treatment modality may be successful again; however, possible reasons for a recurrence should be discussed.
- Whether the patient feels their symptoms are getting better, worse or staying the same.
- What the patient believes is the cause of their symptoms and what they think will help them to recover.

Planning the Physical Examination

When all information has been collected, the subjective examination is complete. A summary of this first part of the patient examination can be found in Fig. 3.7.

It is useful at this stage for the clinician to reconfirm the patient's understanding of their main complaint, and to offer them the opportunity to add anything they have not raised so far, before explaining the purpose and plan for the physical examination. For ease of reference, important subjective findings are highlighted with asterisks (*), specifically one or more functional restrictions. These can be re-examined at subsequent sessions to evaluate treatment interventions.

Refer to Appendix 3.1 for a short planning form to assist in focusing the physical examination prompting the following questions:

Are there any contraindications to a physical examination that need to be explored further, such as red flags (e.g. cord compression)? Are there any precautions to elements of the physical examination such as recent fracture, trauma, steroid therapy or rheumatoid arthritis?

Clinically reasoning throughout the subjective examination using the distribution of symptoms, pain mechanisms, the behaviour of symptoms and the history of onset, the clinician needs to decide on structures that could be the cause of the patient's symptoms. The clinician needs a prioritized list of working hypotheses based on the most likely causes of the patient's symptoms. These may include the structures in the symptomatic area (e.g. joints, muscles, nerves and fascia, as well as the regions which may refer pain into the area). Potential origins of pain referral need to be examined as a possible cause of symptoms (e.g. for upper limb pain: cervical spine, thoracic spine, shoulder and wrist and hand). In complex cases it is not always possible to examine fully at the first attendance so, using clinical reasoning skills, the clinician will need to prioritize and justify what *must* be examined in the first assessment session, and what *should* or *could* be followed up at subsequent sessions.

What are the pain mechanisms driving the patient's symptoms, and what does it mean for the clinician's understanding of the problem and subsequent management decisions? For example, pain associated with repetitive activities is suggestive of inflammatory or neurogenic nociception. This would justify an early assessment of activities and advice to the patient to pace activities. The patient's acceptance and willingness to be an active participant in management will depend on his or her perspective and subsequent behavioural response to the symptoms. For example, if a patient is demonstrating fear-avoidance behaviours, the clinician's ability to explain and educate the patient will be pivotal to achieving a successful outcome.

Once the clinician has decided on the tests to include in the physical examination, the next consideration will be how the physical tests need to be carried out. Are symptoms severe and/or irritable? Will it be easy or hard to reproduce each symptom? If symptoms are severe, physical tests may be carried out to just before the onset of symptom production or just to the onset of symptom production; further stressing of tissues (i.e. overpressures, will not be carried out). If symptoms are irritable, physical tests may be examined to just before symptom production or just to the onset of provocation, with fewer physical tests being examined to allow for rest periods between tests. In cases of low severity and irritability, will it be necessary to use combined movements or repetitive movements to reproduce the patient's symptoms?

A clinical reasoning form based on the hypothesis categories framework (see Box 3.1) suggested by Jones and Rivett (2004) can be useful to help guide a clinician's clinical reasoning (Appendix 3.2).

REVIEW AND REVISE QUESTIONS

1. How would you identify irritability and severity, and why is it useful to establish?
2. What is allodynia?
3. What are the risk factors for osteoporosis that you could screen for in the subjective history?
4. What are red herrings?
5. What questions do we ask about diabetes mellitus and why?
6. What questions do we ask about a patient's medications and why?
7. What can plain radiographs detect?

APPENDIX 3.1 PHYSICAL EXAMINATION PLANNING SHEET (SHORT VERSION)

Physical examination planning sheet (short version)

Contraindications	

Precautions	

Symptom	1		2		3	
	Y	N	Y	N	Y	N
Severity						
Irritability						

Symptom	1	2	3
To stop short of P1 symptom reproduction (P1)			
To partial reproduction			
To full reproduction			

Pain mechanisms

Input mechanism		Processing mechanism	Output mechanism
Nociceptive symptoms	Neuropathic symptoms	Nociplastic pain e.g. central sensitization	Behaviour, motor function, thoughts beliefs cognition, autonomic nervous system

To test	→	Expected findings
Must Neuro integrity Y ○ N ○	→	
Should	→	
Could	→	

APPENDIX 3.2 CLINICAL REASONING FORM USING HYPOTHESIS CATEGORIES

Clinical reasoning form using hypothesis categories (Jones and Rivett 2004)

1. Activity and participation capabilities / restrictions

Activity capability	Restriction
Participation capability	Restriction

2. Patients perspectives on their experience.
Examples:
- Their understanding
- Their feelings
- Their coping strategies
- Attitude to self-management and physical activity
- Their beliefs/what does this experience mean to them
- Their expectations
- Their goals

3. Pathobiological mechanisms

3.1 Tissue sources / tissue healing e.g. at what stage of the inflammatory healing process would you judge the principal disorder to be?

3.2 Pain mechanisms.
List the subjective evidence which supports each specific mechanism of symptoms.

Input mechanism		Processing mechanism	Output mechanism
Nociceptive symptoms	Neuropathic symptoms	Nociplastic changes	Behaviour, motor function, thoughts beliefs cognition, autonomic nervous system

Reflect on this pie chart the proportional involvement of the pain mechanisms

Nociceptive
Peripheral neuropathic
Nociplastic changes
Autonomic nervous system

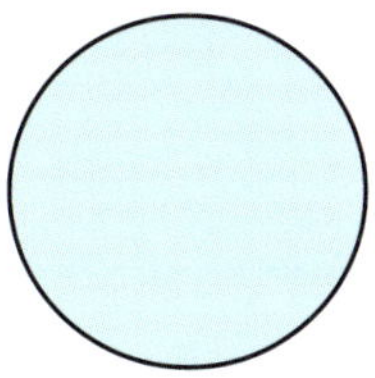

4. The sources of the symptoms
List in order of likelihood the possible structures at fault for each area / component of symptoms.

Tissue sources	Symptom 1:	Symptom 2:	Symptom 3:	Symptom 4:
Local				
Referred				
Neurogenic				
Vascular				
Visceral				

5. Contributing factors
Examples:
- Physical
- Environmental
- Psychosocial
- Health related

6. History of symptoms
Onset / physical impairment / stage / implications for physical examination.

7a. List for each area of symptoms

	Aggravating activity	Time to aggravate	Stops the activity	Easing the activity	Time to ease	Irritability Y/N	Severity Y/N
Symptoms 1 (P_a)							
Symptoms 2 (P_a)							

8. Give an indication of the proportion of inflammatory to mechanical components in this patient's pain presentation, together with the clinical features that support or negate your hypothesis.

Mechanical -- Inflammatory

Justification	Justification

9. Health considerations, precautions and contraindications to physical examination and management.

9.1 Does the patient have any health, red flag or precaution to limit your physical examination?
Consider the following in relation to red flags?

9.2 Will reproduction of symptoms easy or difficult to reproduce? **How vigorously would you examine this patient for each area of symptoms?**

Symptom	Short of P^1	To P^1 only	25% reproduction of pain	Full reproduction of pain
P_1				
P_2				
P_3				

9.3 Will a neurological integrity examination be necessary? Y N

Justify your decision:

10. Indicate your primary (working) hypothesis (H1) regarding the cause of the patient's complaint and identify evidence to support this decision. Identify alternative hypotheses including evidence.

Primary hypothesis (H1)	Alternative H	Alternative H	Alternative H	Alternative H
Evidence:				

To test	→	Expected findings
Must Neuro integrity Y ○ N ○	→	
Should	→	
Could	→	

REFERENCES

Afolalu, E.F., Ramlee, F., Tang, N., 2018. Effects of sleep changes on pain-related health outcomes in the general population: a systematic review of longitudinal studies with exploratory meta-analysis. Sleep Med. Rev. 39, 82–97.

Al-Chaer, E., Traub, R., 2002. Biological basis of visceral pain: recent developments. Pain 96 (3), 221–225.

Arendt-Nielsen, L., Laursen, R., Drewes, A., 2000. Referred pain as an indicator for neural plasticity. In: Sandkühler, J., Bromm, B., Gebhart, G. (Eds.), Nervous System Plasticity and Chronic Pain. Elsevier, Amsterdam, pp. 344–356.

Aroll, B., Khin, N., Kerse, N., 2003. Screening for depression in primary care with two verbally asked questions: cross sectional study. Br. Med. J. 327, 1144–1146.

Arora, E., Singh, H., Gupta, Y.K., 2016. Impact of antiepileptic drugs on bone health: need monitoring, treatment and prevention strategies. J. Fam. Med. Prim. Care 5, 248–253.

Artus, M., Campbell, P., Mallen, C., Dunn, K., Van Der Windt, D., 2017. Generic prognostic factors for musculoskeletal pain in primary care: a systematic review. BMJ Open. 7, e012901.

Banks, K., Hengeveld, E., 2014. The Maitland Concept as a clinical practice framework for neuromusculoskeletal disorders. In: Hengeveld, E., Banks, K. (Eds.), Maitland's Vertebral Manipulation. Churchill Livingstone, Edinburgh. Chapter 1.

Barker, C., Taylor, A., Johnson, M., 2014. Problematic pain — redefining how we view pain? Br. J. Pain 8 (1), 9–15.

Barnard, K., Ryder, D., (2024). Principles of Musculoskeletal Treatment and Management: A Guide for Therapists, fourth ed. Churchill Livingstone, Edinburgh.

Barrows, H.S., Feltovich, P., 1987. The clinical reasoning process. Med. Educ. 21, 86–91.

Basten, G., 2019. Blood Results in Clinical Practice: A Practical Guide to Interpreting Blood Test Results, second ed. M&K Publishing.

Bennett, M., et al., 2007. Using screening tools to identify neuropathic pain. Pain 127, 199–203.

Bhatti, N., Law, M.R., Morris, J.K., Halliday, R., Moore-Gillon, J., 1995. Increasing incidence of tuberculosis in England and Wales: a study of the likely causes. Br. Med. J. 310, 967–969.

Bogduk, N., 2009. On the definitions and physiology of back pain, referred pain, and radicular pain. Pain. 147 (1–3), 17–19.

Brem, H., Tomic-Canic, M., 2007. Cellular and molecular basis of wound healing in diabetes. J. Clin. Invest. 117, 1219–1222.

Bron, C., Dommerholt, J., 2012. Etiology of myofascial trigger points. Curr. Pain Headache Rep. 16, 439–444.

Brinjikji, W., Luetmer, P., Comstock, B., Bresnahan, B., Chen, L., Deyo, R., et al., 2015. Systematic literature review of imaging features of spinal degeneration in asymptomatic populations. Am. J. Neuroradiol 36, 811–816.

Butler, D., Moseley, L., 2003. Explain Pain. Neuro Orthopaedic Institute, Adelaide.

Cakir, M., Samanci, N., Balci, N., Balci, M.K., 2003. Musculoskeletal manifestations in patients with thyroid disease. Clin. Endocrinol. 59, 162–167.

Cervero, F., Laird, J., 2004. Referred visceral hyperalgesia: from sensations to molecular mechanisms. In: Brune, K., Handwerker, H. (Eds.), Hyperalgesia: Molecular Mechanisms and Clinical Implications. IASP Press, Seattle, pp. 229–250.

Chiarotto, A., Terwee, C., Ostelo, R., 2016. Choosing the right outcome measurement instruments for patients with low back pain. Best Pract. Res. Clin. Rheumatol. 30, 1003–1020.

Cook, N., van Griensven, H., Jesson, T. (in press) Neuropathic pain and complex regional pain syndrome. In: van Griensven & Strong Pain – A textbook for health professionals, third ed. Elsevier, Edinburgh.

Deyo, R.A., Rainville, J., Kent, D.L., 1992. What can the history and physical examination tell us about low back pain. J. Am. Med. Assoc. 268, 760–765.

Dommerholt, J., 2011. Dry needling – peripheral and central considerations. J. Man. Manip. Ther. 19 (4), 223–237.

Donnelly, J., Fernández -De-Las-Peñas, C., Finnegan, M., Freeman, J., 2013. Travell, Simons and Simons' Myofascial Pain and Dysfunction: The Trigger Point Manual. Lippincott Williams & Wilkins, Philadelphia.

Doody, C., McAteer, M., 2002. Clinical reasoning of expert and novice physiotherapists in an outpatient orthopaedic setting. Physiotherapy. 88, 258–268.

Edwards, I., Jones, M., Carr, J., Braunack-Mayer, A., Jensen, G.M., 2004b. Clinical reasoning strategies in physical therapy. Phys. Ther. 84, 312–330.

Edwards, I., Jones, M., Hillier, S., 2006. The interpretation of experience and its relationship to body movement: a clinical reasoning perspective. Man. Ther. 11, 2–10.

Edwards, I., Jones, M., Higgs, J., Trede, F., Jensen, G., 2004a. What is collaborative reasoning? Adv. Physiother. 6(2), 70-83.

Finan, P., Goodin, B., Smith, M., 2013. The association of sleep and pain: An update and a path forward. J. Pain 14 (12), 1539–1552.

Finnerup, N., Haroutiunian, S., Kamerman, P., Baron, R., Bennett, D., Bouhassira, D., et al., 2016. Neuropathic pain: an updated grading system for research and clinical practice. Pain 157, 1599–1606.

Finucane, L., Downie, A., Mercer, C., Greenhalgh, S., Boissonnault, W., Pool Goudzwaard, A., et al., May 2020. International framework for red flags for potential serious spinal pathologies. J. Orthop. Sports Phys. Ther. 50 (7), 350–372. https://doi.org/10.2519/jospt.2020.9971. Epub 21.

Gask, L., Usherwood, T., 2002. ABC of psychological medicine. The consultation. Br. Med. J. 324, 1567–1569.

Goodman, C., Heick, J., Lazaro, R., 2018. Differential diagnosis for physical therapists. Screening for Referral, sixth ed. Elsevier, St Louis.

Goodrich, J., Cornwell, J., 2008. Seeing the Person in the Patient. The Point of Care Review. The King's Fund, London.

Greenhalgh, S., Finucane, L., Mercer, C., Selfe, J., 2020. Safety netting in the face of uncertainty. Musculoskel. Sci. Pract. 48, 102179.

Greenhalgh, S., Selfe, J., 2004. Margaret a tragic case of spinal Red Flags and Red Herrings. Physiotherapy. 90, 73–76.

Greenhalgh, S., Selfe, J., 2010. Red Flags II: A Guide to Identifying Serious Pathology of the Spine. Elsevier, Edinburgh.

Greenhalgh S., Selfe J. 2019 Red flags and blue lights. mangaing serious spinal pathology Elsevier Edinburgh

Grieve, G.P., 1991. Mobilisation of the Spine, fifth ed. Churchill Livingstone, Edinburgh.

Hakim, A., Grahame, R., 2003. A simple questionnaire to detect hypermobility; and adjunct to the assessment of patients with diffuse musculoskeletal pain. Int. J. Clin. Pract. 57, 163–166.

Harding, V., Williams, A.C., de, C., 1995. Extending physiotherapy skills using a psychological approach: cognitive-behavioural management of chronic pain. Physiotherapy 81, 681–688.

Hinnant, D.W., 1994. Psychological evaluation and testing. In: Tollison, C.D. (Ed.), Handbook of Pain Management, second ed. Williams & Wilkins, Baltimore.

Huskisson, E.C., Dieppe, P.A., Tucker, A.K., Cannell, L.B., 1979. Another look at osteoarthritis. Ann. Rheum. Dis 38, 423–428.

Jones, M.A., 1995. Clinical reasoning and pain. Man. Ther. 1, 17–24.

Jones, M., Jensen, G., Edwards, I., 2008. Clinical reasoning in physiotherapy. In: Higgs, J., Jones, M.A., Loftus, S. (Eds.), Clinical Reasoning in the Health Professions, third ed. Butterworth Heinemann/Elsevier, Amsterdam, pp. 245–256.

Jones, M.A., Rivett, D.A., 2004. Clinical reasoning for manual therapists. Butterworth-Heinemann, Edinburgh.

Jones, M.A., Rivett, D.A., 2019. Clinical reasoning in musculoskeletal practice. Elsevier, Edinburgh.

Kendall, N., Linton, S., Main, C., 1997. Guide to Assessing Psychosocial Yellow Flags in Acute Low Back Pain. Accident Rehabilitation and Compensation Insurance Corporation and National Advisory Committee on Health and Disability. Wellington, NZ.

Kyte, D., Calvert, M., Van de Wees, P.J., Ten Hove, R., Tolan, S., Hill, J.C., 2015. An introduction to patient reported outcome measures PROMS in physiotherapy. Physiotherapy. 101 (12), 119–125.

Lindsay, K.W., Bone, I., Callander, R., 1997. Neurology and Neurosurgery Illustrated, third ed. Churchill Livingstone, Edinburgh.

Linton, S., Shaw, W., 2011. Impact of psychological factors in the experience of pain. Phys. Ther. 91, 700–711.

MacMillan, A., Corser, A., Clark, Z., McCrum, C., Gaffney, K., 2021. Masterclass: axial spondyloarthritis for osteopaths and manual therapists. Int. J. Osteopath. Med. 41, 45–46.

Magee, D., Manske, R., 2021. Orthopedic Physical Assessment, seventh ed. Saunders Elsevier, St. Louis.

Main, C.J., George, S.Z., 2011. Psychologically informed practice for management of low back pain: future directions in practice and research. Phys. Ther 91, 820–824.

Main, C.J., Spanswick, C.C., 2000. Pain Management: An Interdisciplinary Approach. Churchill Livingstone, Edinburgh.

Main, C., Sullivan, M., Watson, P., 2008. Pain Management. Practical Applications of the Biopsychosocial Perspective in Clinical and Occupational Settings, second ed. Churchill Livingstone, Edinburgh.

Mallen, C., Peat, G., Thomas, E., Dunn, K., Croft, P., 2007. Prognostic factors for musculoskeletal pain in primary care: a systematic review. Br. J. Gen. Pract. 57, 655–661.

McCrum, C., 2019. When to suspect spondyloarthritis: a core skill in musculoskeletal clinical practice. Musculoskelet. Sci. Pract. 44, 1–3.

McCullough, B.J., Johnson, G.R., Martin, B.I., Jarvik, J.G., 2012. Lumbar MR imaging and reporting epidemiology: do epidemiologic data in reports affect clinical management? Radiology. 262 (3), 941–946.

McMahon, S., 1997. Are there fundamental differences in the peripheral mechanisms of visceral and somatic pain? Behav. Brain Sci. 20, 381–391.

Mooney, V., Robertson, J., 1976. The facet syndrome. Clin. Orthop. Relat. Res. 115, 149–156.

NICE. 2016 Low back pain and sciatica in over 16s: assessment and management.

Nicholas, M., Linton, S., Watson, P., Main, C., 2016. Early identification and management of psychosocial risk factors ('Yellow Flags') in patients with low back pain: a reappraisal. Phys. Ther. 91, 737–753.

Rao, R., Currier, B., Todd, A., 2007. Degenerative cervical spondylosis pathogenesis and management. JBJS Am. 89, 1360–1378.

Rivett, D.A., Higgs, J., 1997. Hypothesis generation in the clinical reasoning behavior of manual therapists. J. Phys. Ther. Educ. 11, 40–45.

Rushton, A., Rivett, D., Carlesso, L., Flynn, T., Hing, W., Kerry, R., 2014. International framework for examination of the cervical region for potential cervical arterial dysfunction prior to orthopaedic manual therapy intervention. Man. Ther. 9 (3), 222–228.

Russek, L.N., Stott, P., Simmonds, J., 2019. Recognizing and effectively managing hypermobility-related conditions. Phys Ther. 99, 1189–1200.

Salvi, F., Jones, J., Weigert, B., 2006. The assessment of cervical myelopathy. Spine J. 6 (6), S182–S189.

Sharma, S., Traeger, A.C., Reed, B., Hamilton, M., O'Connor, D.A., Hoffmann, T.C., et al., 2020. Clinician and patient beliefs about diagnostic imaging for low back pain: a systematic qualitative evidence synthesis. BMJ Open 10. e037820. https://doi.org/10.1136/bmjopen-2020-037820.

Shorland, S., 1998. Management of chronic pain following whiplash injuries. In: Gifford, L. (Ed.), Falmouth 115–134. Topical Issues in Pain. Neuro-Orthopaedic Institute UK.

Simula, A., Ruokolainen, O., Oura, P., Lausmaa, M., Holopainene, R., Paukkunen, M., et al., 2020. Association of STarT Back Tool and the short form of the Örebro Musculoskeletal Pain Screening Questionnaire with multidimensional risk factors. Nat. Sci. Rep. 10 (1), 11.

Smith M.T. & Muralidharan (in press) Pain pharmacology and the pharmacological management of pain. In: van Griensven H. & Strong J. Pain – A textbook for health professionals, third ed. Elsevier, Edinburgh.

Solomon, L., Warwick, D., Nayagam, S., 2001. Apley's System of Orthopaedics and Fractures, eighth ed. Arnold, London.

Thomas, L., 2016. Cervical arterial dissection: an overview and implications for manipulative therapy practice. Man. Ther. 21, 2–9.

Travell, J., Simons, D., 1983. Myofascial Pain and Dysfunction: The Trigger Point Manual. Williams & Wilkins, Baltimore.

van Cranenburgh, B., 1989. Inleiding in de toegepaste neurowetenschappen, deel 1, Neurofilosofie (Introduction to Applied Neuroscience, Part 1, Neurophysiology) third. In: Uitgeversmaatschappij de Tijdstroom. Lochum.

van Griensven, H. Trendafilova, T. (in press). Neurophysiology of pain. In: van Griensven, H., Strong, J. (Eds.), Pain. A Textbook for Health Professionals, third ed. Churchill Livingstone, Edinburgh.

van Griensven, H., 2005. Pain in Practice – Theory and Treatment Strategies for Manual Therapists. Elsevier, Edinburgh.

van Griensven, H. 2013. Neurophysiology of pain. In: van Griensven, H., Strong, J., Unruh, A. Pain – A textbook for health professionals, second Ed. Elsevier, Edinburgh.

van Griensven, H., Schmid, A., Trendafilova, T., Low, M., 2020. Central sensitization in musculoskeletal pain: lost in translation? J. Orthop. Sports Phys. Ther. 50, 592–596.

van Griensven H. & Strong J. (in press). Pain – A textbook for health professionals, third ed. Elsevier, Edinburgh.

van Wyngaarden, J., Ross, M., Hando, B., 2014. Abdominal aortic aneurysm in a patient with low back pain. J. Orthop. Sports Phys. Ther. 44 (7), 501–507.

Waddell, G., 2004. The Back Pain Revolution, second ed. Churchill Livingstone, Edinburgh.

Watson, T., www.electrotherapy.org.

Woolf, C., 2004. Pain: moving from symptom control toward mechanism specific pharmacologic management. Ann. Intern. Med. 140, 441–451.

Woolf, C., 2012. Central sensitisation: implications for the diagnosis and treatment of pain. Pain. 152 (3), S2–S15.

World Health Organization (WHO), 2001. International Classification of Functioning. Disability and Health. World Health Organization, Geneva. http://www.who.int/classifications/icf/en/.

4

Physical Examination

Dionne Ryder and Hubert van Griensven

LEARNING OUTCOMES

After studying this chapter, you should be able to:

- Identify the key components of the physical examination.
- Discuss how the selection of physical tests is justified from the subjective examination.
- Identify the clinical reasoning required in interpreting physical examination findings.
- Discuss the limitations of the physical examination in confirming a structural diagnosis.

CHAPTER CONTENTS

Introduction, 65
Interpretation of Tests, 66
Physical Examination Step by Step, 67
Observation, 67
Functional Ability/Physical Performance Tests, 72
Active Physiological Movements, 72
Modifications of Active Movements, 75
Joint Integrity Tests, 78
Passive Physiological Movements, 78
Muscle Tests, 78
Sensorimotor/Neurological Tests, 89
Other Neurological Tests, 126
Palpation, 126
Accessory Movements, 126
Movement Diagrams, 129
Completion of the Physical Examination, 133
References, 139

INTRODUCTION

The physical examination should not be the indiscriminate application of routine tests. Following on from the subjective examination the clinician should have already identified a 'must, should and could' plan, tailored to the individual patient and based on a primary hypothesis. Clinicians use their clinical reasoning to select and adapt the order of testing according to the patient and their presenting condition. This chapter will cover the principles of physical examination. More specific regional examination procedures are described in the relevant chapters.

Physical testing should be selective and justified through clinical reasoning, with the aim of collecting evidence to rule in or rule out hypotheses. This way the physical examination is based on the findings of the subjective examination and the clinician considers whether a specific musculoskeletal problem or a broader dysfunction is likely to be the main barrier to recovery. A relatively recent onset, a clear mechanism of injury, and consistent symptom behaviour and location of symptoms suggestive of specific physical structures, favour an approach based on *ruling in*, i.e. the clinician focuses on establishing the tissues at fault and contributing factors.

On the other hand, if the problem is widespread, long-standing, or has had a significant influence on the patient's overall well-being and function, an approach of *ruling out* is advocated. For this type of presentation, it may not be meaningful to attempt to find a tissue at fault. Not only may persistence and dysfunction have led to a wider range of tissues or systems involved, but a specific tissue diagnosis may also not be helpful because the main barriers to recovery are likely to be of a different nature. For example, feeling depressed or having become very deconditioned may prevent a person from recovering. These problems may be more significant than a specific musculoskeletal injury. The clinician therefore attempts to rule out the presence of specific diagnoses suggested by the subjective examination, to ensure that there is no need to target specific tissues.

The aims of the physical examination can be summarized as follows:

- To determine whether specific structure(s) and/or factor(s) are responsible for producing or maintaining the patient's symptoms.
- To assess whether and how function has been affected.
- To explore the influence of behavioural aspects on the patient's condition and presentation.

INTERPRETATION OF TESTS

Several factors should be considered in interpreting the findings of physical tests. If symptoms are reproduced, aggravated or eased, then there may be an assumption that the test has somehow affected the structures at fault or the physiological mechanisms involved. No test stresses individual structures in isolation—each affects a number of tissues, both locally and at a distance. For example, knee flexion will affect the tibiofemoral and patellofemoral intraarticular and periarticular joint structures, surrounding soft tissues and nerves, as well as the hip, spine and ankle.

If an abnormality is detected in a structure which could theoretically refer symptoms to the symptomatic area, then that structure should be considered a potential source of the symptoms and examined. The potential origin of the referred pain must be tested and confirmed through the reproduction of symptoms.

The term *objective* is sometimes applied to the physical examination. It suggests that this part of the examination is not prejudiced and that the tests are valid and reliable, producing robust results. However, this is misleading as most tests rely on the skill of the clinician to observe, move and palpate, and are always subject to interpretation.

When interpreting the findings of physical tests, it is important to consider their sensitivity and specificity values. These values indicate how likely a positive or negative test will rule in or rule out a suspected diagnosis. For example, the *sensitivity* of the Lachman's test to detect tears of the anterior cruciate ligament is the proportion of people with an ACL tear who will test positive, i.e. it is the ability of the test to detect the condition. However, some people without a tear may also have a positive response. The *specificity* of the Lachman's test is its ability to correctly rule out those without an ACL tear (true negative rate). Sensitivity and specificity relate to the tests and not the prevalence of the condition within a given population.

Predictive values can be more valuable than specificity and sensitivity because they predict the likelihood of a positive or negative result within a particular population, e.g. people playing a contact sport such as rugby are more likely to sustain an ACL tear than tennis players.

Likelihood ratios (LRs) summarize the diagnostic accuracy by combining sensitivity and specificity information. An LR greater than 1 indicates the likelihood that a pathology is present, while less than 1 indicates absence of the pathology, with values closer to 0 making absence of the pathology highly likely. LR+ is the likelihood of ruling in the pathology when the test is positive, while LR− is the likelihood of ruling it out when the test is negative. An LR+ greater than 2 and LR− less than 0.5 suggests that a test's result is more accurate (Valdes & LaStayo, 2013).

The clinician needs to take these factors into account when clinically reasoning a patient's presentation based on the findings of the physical examination. The clinician should collate and clinically reason all information obtained from the subjective and physical examination in order to make sense of the patient's overall presentation, i.e. 'making features fit' (Hengeveld & Banks, 2014). If features are not consistent or not fitting a recognized musculoskeletal pattern, the clinician must question why that might be. They must keep an open mind to avoid bias, thinking logically throughout the physical examination, reflecting in action by using a process of continuous assessment or reasoning. Jumping to conclusions based on the findings of just one or two tests is likely to result in errors and misattribution of symptoms, leading to misguided management decisions and poor outcomes.

TABLE 4.1 Summary of the Physical Examination

Observation	Informal and formal observation of posture, muscle bulk and tone, soft tissues, gait, function and patient's response.
Active physiological movement	Active movements. With selective adaptions such as repeated, sustained, in functional/combined positions.
Passive physiological movement	Passive movements. With selective adaptions such as repeated, sustained, in functional/combined positions. Passive physiological accessory movement. Passive physiological intervertebral movement.
Joint integrity tests	For example, knee adduction (varus) and abduction (valgus) stress tests.
Muscle tests	Strength, control, length, isometric contraction.
Nerve tests	Neurological integrity, neurosensitivity tests including response to load and nerve palpation.
Special tests	Vascular, soft tissue.
Palpation	Superficial and deep soft tissues, bone, joint, ligament, muscle, tendon and nerve.
Joint tests	Accessory movements to test available glides in a range of directions: anterior/posterior, medial/lateral, caudad/cephalad.

Key findings of the physical examination, which form patient-specific reassessment markers to evaluate interventions, are marked with an asterisk (*) (Hengeveld & Banks, 2014).

For an overview of the physical examination see Table 4.1.

PHYSICAL EXAMINATION STEP BY STEP

Observation

Initial Observation

The clinician's observation of the patient begins from the moment they first meet. How is the patient moving? A reluctance to move may suggest how the patient is affected both physically and as a person. Does the patient appear to be in pain? During the subjective examination, is the patient comfortable or constantly shifting position? This informal observation may well be as informative as the formal assessment, as a patient may not adopt their usual posture when examined formally. The clinician can also observe whether the patient is using aids (prescribed or nonprescribed) such as collars, sticks and corsets and whether they are being used appropriately.

Informal and formal observation can give the clinician initial cues:

1. The pathology, for example, local inflammations, e.g. olecranon bursitis produces a localized swelling over the olecranon process.
2. Factors that may contribute to the patient's problem. If a muscle appears wasted on observation, the clinician needs to judge the relevance of this observation to the patient's presenting symptoms and to test a possible relationship with symptom production.

There is also an opportunity to collaboratively reason with the patient through on-going dialogue to gain their perspective. Using questions such as 'How does that feel?' 'What do you make of that?' strengthens continued collaboration and data collection.

The clinician should note whether the patient is demonstrating signs of illness behaviour, i.e. altered behaviour in response to pain, injury or illness. For example, is a patient bracing or breath holding prior to moving? This may suggest illness behaviour, which may be appropriate or adaptive in an acute situation, but may also be maladaptive when maintained over time and have become a driver of symptoms. If the clinician suspects altered behaviour in response to pain may be contributing to the patient's pain experience, then changing the context can be useful. For example, strategies such as breathing out on movement to reduce bracing.

Formal Observation

Observation of posture. It should be remembered that the posture a patient adopts reflects a multitude of factors, not only an indication of musculoskeletal and neural tissue sensitivity/capacity but also the patient's behavioural response to their symptoms which may be protective, influenced by emotions and their body image.

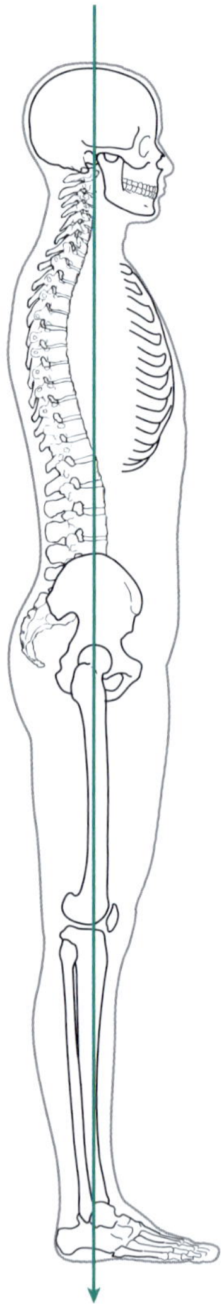

Fig. 4.1 Ideal alignment. (From Kendall et al. 1993 © Williams and Wilkins.)

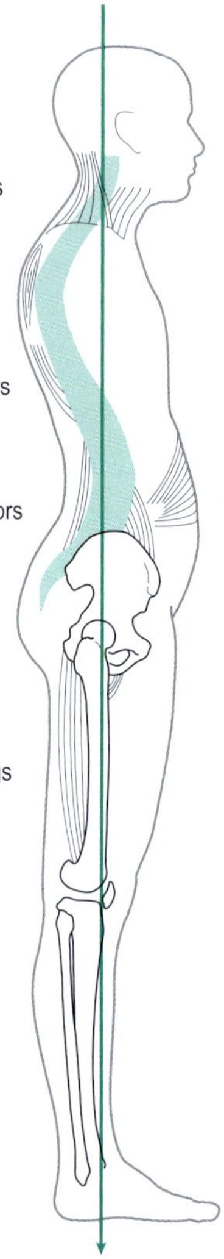

Fig. 4.2 Kyphosis–lordosis posture. (After Kendall et al. 1993 © Williams & Wilkins.)

The clinician observes posture by examining anterior, lateral and posterior views of the patient noting relevant deformities, e.g. scoliosis that may need referring onward for monitoring.

Ideal alignment is described as a posture that is considered the most efficient (Kendall et al., 2010) (Fig. 4.1). Additionally, Kendall et al. (2010) described a number of postural types such as kyphosis–lordotic, sway and flat back postures (Figs. 4.2–4.4); however, there is an acceptance that normal variation exists, and there is no strong evidence to support a link with 'correct' posture and a patient's presenting symptoms (Slater et al., 2019).

Clinically reasoning the relevance of a patient's posture is vital to establish whether it may be a driver for their presenting symptoms. Assumptions must not be made as there is no ideal posture and attempts to uniformly change/correct posture without assessing its contribution to a patient's symptoms will be ineffective and potentially instil unhelpful beliefs.

Observations may include noticing skin creases at various spinal levels indicating possible regions of 'give'

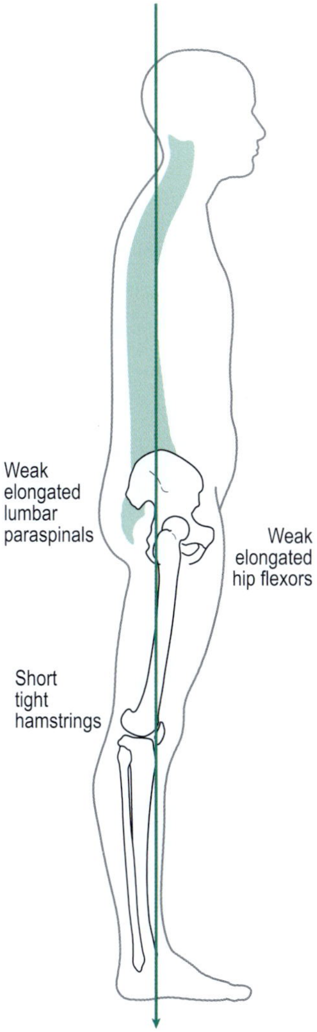

Fig. 4.3 Flat-back posture. (After Kendall et al. 1993 © Williams & Wilkins.)

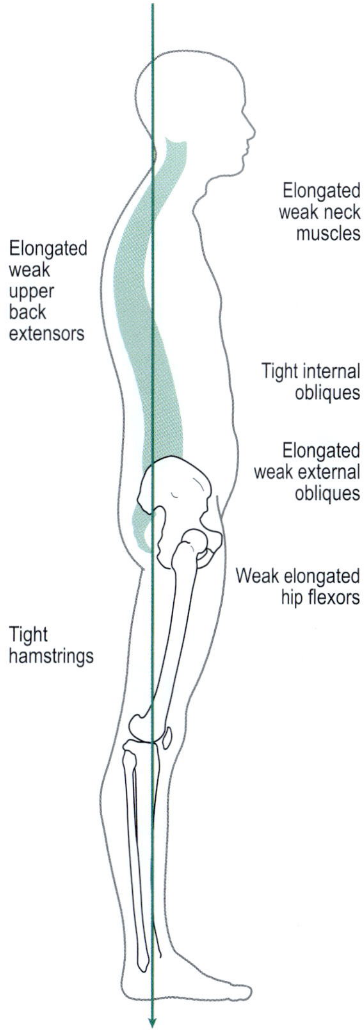

Fig. 4.4 Sway-back posture. (After Kendall et al. 1993 © Williams & Wilkins.)

or excessive mobility. An example would be a crease at the mid-cervical spine indicating a focus of movement at that level; if the patient has reported neck pain this observation could be tested by altering trunk and neck postures to assess pain response. If relevant this finding could be followed up later on in the examination when assessing active movement, passive accessory intervertebral movement (PAIVM) and passive physiological intervertebral movement (PPIVM), to confirm or refute a hypothesis of hypermobility at this level as a contributor to the patient's neck pain.

The clinician may also decide to observe the patient in sustained postures and during habitual/repetitive movement where these are relevant to the problem. Sustained postures and habitual movements are thought to play a role in the development of dysfunction (Sahrmann, 2002).

If a patient reports persistent low back pain when sitting, an assessment in this position is most relevant. If the patient is observed to hold a very upright posture with their pelvis in anterior pelvic tilt, and lumbar spine extended then the clinician will need to assess this position to identify whether it is contributing to the patient's ongoing pain (Fig. 4.5A). If a more relaxed posture results in a reduction in the patient's back pain (Fig. 4.5B), this suggests a link between the posture and

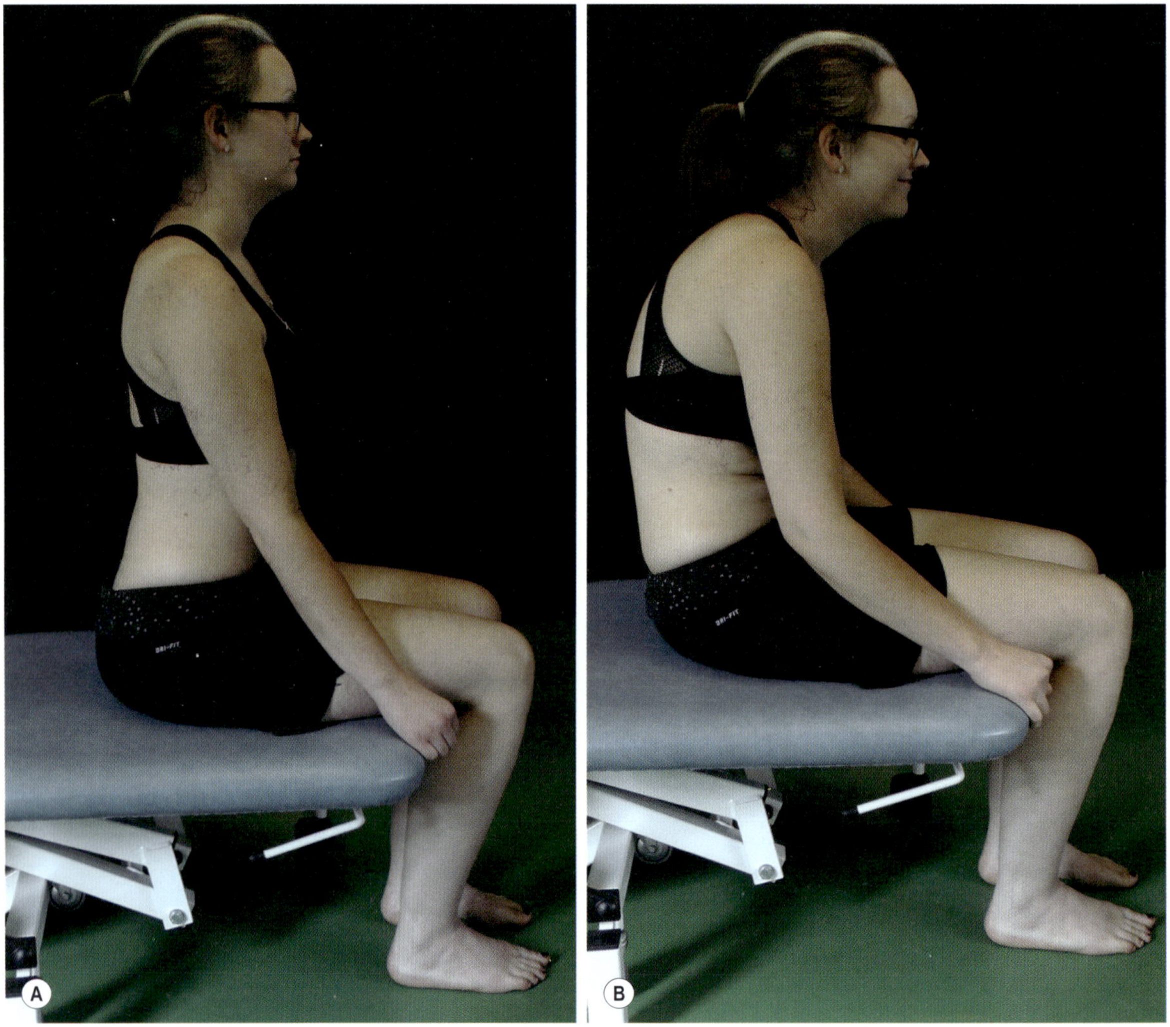

Fig. 4.5 The effect of spinal posture. (A) Patient adopts an upright posture with lumbar extension and anterior pelvic tilt (B) In posterior pelvic tilt the lumbar spine is in flexion.

symptoms and a postural driver can be 'ruled in'. If there is no change in symptoms, then posture as a driver is less likely. This level of individual assessment has been demonstrated to improve outcomes in some patients with persistent low back pain (Wernli et al., 2020).

An example of a habitual movement pattern may be a patient with lumbar spine pain who has pain when bending forwards. The patient is observed to bend predominantly at the lumbar spine, perhaps due to limitation in hamstring length or hip flexibility (Fig. 4.6A). Controlling this lumbar spine 'give' on flexion and encouraging more flexion through the hips may reduce symptoms (Fig. 4.6B). On the other hand, the patient may brace before they move, anticipating pain and demonstrate greater trunk extensor muscle activity on forward flexion. Encouraging the patient to breath out, relax and bend may reduce symptoms. Alternatively assessing trunk flexion in sitting changes the context and reduces the level of threat which may improve pain-free range of movement.

Observation of muscle form. The clinician observes the shape, bulk and tone of the patient's muscles, comparing the left and right sides. It must be remembered that handedness, type, level and frequency of

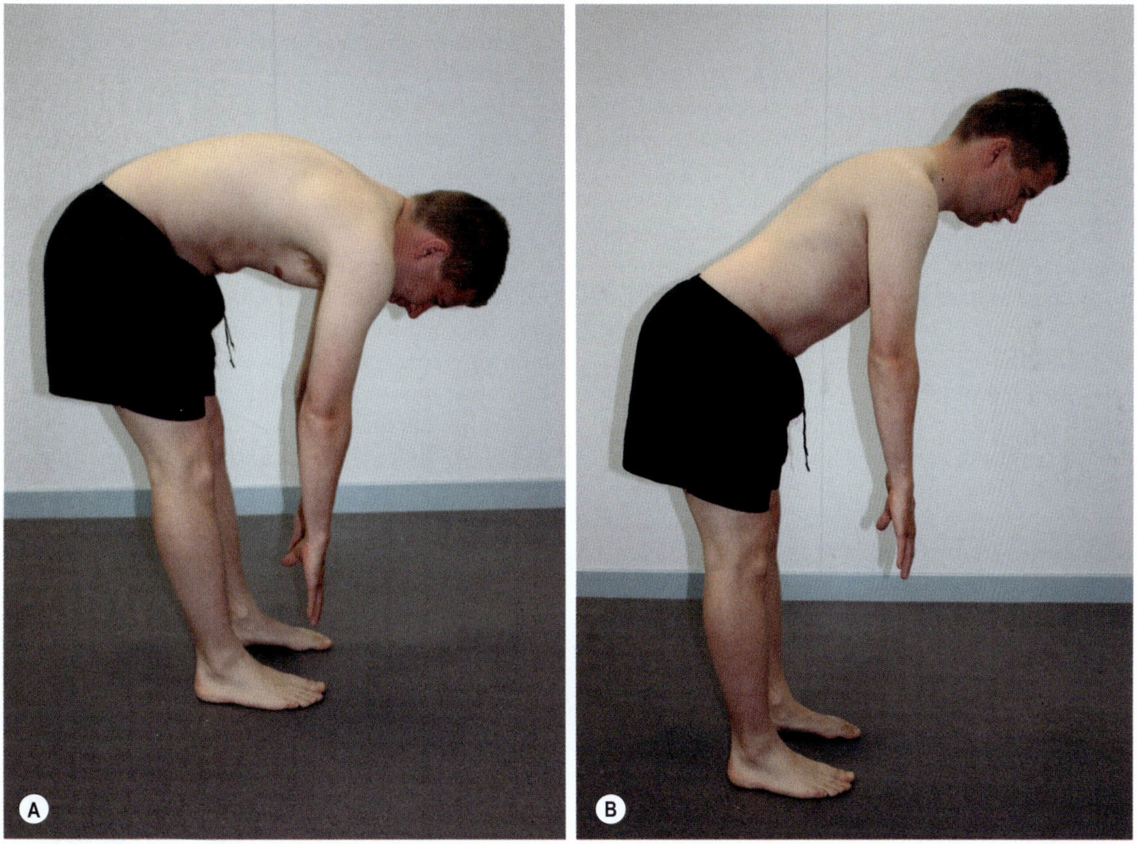

Fig. 4.6 On bending forwards the patient may bend predominantly at the lumbar spine (A) or at the hips (B).

physical activity, including certain activities such as rowing or playing the guitar, may produce asymmetries in muscle bulk.

Observation of soft tissues. Soft tissues local to the patient's symptoms and more generally can be observed, noting the colour and texture of the skin, the presence of scars, abnormal skin creases, swelling of the soft tissues and effusion of the joints. Skin creases may reflect a change in normal biomechanics. Skin colour and texture may suggest the state of the circulation (a bluish tinge suggesting cyanosis or bruising, and redness suggesting inflammation), sympathetic changes such as increased sweating or piloerection and the presence of other diseases. For example, complex regional pain syndrome 1 (CRPS 1) may result in excessive hair growth, red, blue or shiny skin that has lost its elasticity and nails which have become brittle and ridged. Scars may indicate injury or previous surgery; they will be red if recent and white and avascular if old.

Functional ability may be tested in the observation to examine specific activities such as gait, stair climbing, reaching and sit to stand.

Observation of gait. Gait assessment is often applicable for patients with spinal and lower-limb problems. Ideally, the patient wears shorts and is assessed without socks or shoes. The clinician observes the patient's gait from the front, behind and the side, looking at the trunk, pelvis, hips, knees, ankles and feet through both swing and stance phases of the gait cycle. A detailed description of systematic gait observation can be found in Magee and Manske (2021). Videoing and software applications may enhance this observation process. Accelerometers and cameras in smartphones and smart watches can also be useful.

Common abnormalities of gait include the following:

1. An antalgic gait due to pain in the pelvis, hip, knee or foot is characterized by a shortened stance phase of the affected limb, resulting in a

shortened swing phase and step length on the unaffected leg.

2. An arthrogenic gait, resulting from stiffness or deformity of the hip or knee, is characterized by exaggerated plantarflexion of the opposite ankle and circumduction of the stiff leg to clear the toes.
3. A gluteus maximus gait, is a result of the weakness of this muscle. The patient produces a posterior thoracic movement to maintain hip extension during the stance phase.
4. Weakness of the gluteus medius muscle can present with two compensatory strategies. The patient may display an excessive lateral movement of the trunk towards the affected limb during the stance phase of the gait cycle, to keep the patient's centre of gravity over the affected limb ('compensated' Trendelenburg). Alternatively, the contralateral hip may 'drop' due to gluteus medius weakness on the affected limb during the loading/stance phase (positive Trendelenburg sign).
5. A drop-foot gait is due to the weakness of the ankle and foot dorsiflexors, caused by muscle or neural system dysfunction. The patient compensates by lifting their knee higher on the affected side so that their toes clear the ground. Due to a lack of dorsiflexor control at heel strike, there is an audible foot slap.

Functional Ability/Physical Performance Tests

The effects of musculoskeletal problems on global function can be assessed using standardized and validated physical performance tests. This also provides functional outcome measures that can be used to evaluate progress. The outcomes of the tests reflect a combination of factors such as pain, strength, flexibility, fitness and respiratory/cardiovascular function. For an overview see (Harding et al., 1994; Galindo, 2005).

Commonly used outcome measures include:

- Walking tests. The patient walks at their own pace up to a predetermined maximum period, for instance, 5 or 10 minutes. Time, distance and rests are recorded.
- Shuttle walking test (Singh et al., 1992). The patient walks up and down a 10 m track in increasingly short time intervals. Time and distance are recorded.
- Stand-up tests. Involve repeated standing up and sitting down with hands folded across the chest, over a predetermined period or a maximum number of repetitions.
- Stair climbing tests. The patient ascends and descends a standard set of stairs for a predetermined period.
- Functional reach test (Duncan et al., 1990). The patient reaches forward along a horizontal ruler at shoulder level, without stepping out or losing balance. The distance reached without falling is recorded.

Further assessment of function can be achieved with validated questionnaires. Questionnaires may be specific to a pathology or localized body region, but the following cover broad regions and conditions:

- Upper limb: QuickDASH (Institute for Work and Health, 2006)
- Lower limb: Lower Extremity Functional Score (LEFS) (Binkley et al., 1999)
- Low back: Roland Morris Disability Questionnaire (RMDQ) or Oswestry Disability Questionnaire (ODQ) (Roland & Fairbank, 2000)
- Neck: Neck Disability Index (NDI) (Sterling & Rebbeck, 2005).

KNOWLEDGE CHECKS

1. What may suggest illness behaviour in how a patient presents in the clinic?
2. How can an assessment of functional ability contribute to clinical reasoning in a patient case?
3. What is the value of using outcome measures?

Active Physiological Movements

An active physiological movement is defined as a movement that can be performed actively by the patient. Examples include active flexion, extension, abduction, adduction and medial and lateral rotation. These movements test joint range and integrity, muscular and nervous system control, as well as the patient's willingness to move. It is worth mentioning that the range of movement is influenced by factors such as age, gender, occupation, time of day, temperature, emotional status, effort, medication, injury and disease, and that there are wide variations in the range of movement between individuals (Gerhardt, 1992). The clinician determines what is normal for the patient, e.g. by comparing both sides as some patients may have asymptomatic generalized joint laxity.

If patients present with symptoms suggestive of symptomatic joint hypermobility, then there are diagnostic criteria that would rule in hypermobility spectrum disorder (HSD) and Ehlers-Danlos syndrome (hEDS) (Russek et al., 2019). The Beighton 9-point score can be used to assess whether a patient has hypermobility at specific joints (Beighton et al., 1973):

- Ability to put hands flat on the floor when standing with straight knees (1 point).
- Ability to hyperextend elbows (1 point per side).
- Ability to hyperextend knees (1 point per side).
- Ability to passively touch forearm with thumb (1 point per side).
- Ability to passively extend the little finger beyond 90 degrees (1 point per side).

The relevance of the score will depend on the person's age. A score of 6/9 for children, 5/9 for adolescents and 4/9 for those over 50 would indicate hypermobility. This score is combined with an additional point for a positive response to two out of five questions about historical hypermobility. In addition, diagnostic criteria also include a range of additional features related to body-wide systems, e.g. cardiovascular alongside symptoms such as fatigue (Russek et al., 2019).

Standard Active Testing

The choice, order and extent of active movement testing are guided by the severity and irritability of the patient's presenting symptoms, as well as the clinician's working hypotheses of the underlying cause of symptoms.

The aims of assessing active physiological movements are to:

- Determine the pattern, quality, range and pain response for each movement.
- Reproduce all or some of the patient's symptoms—the movements that produce symptoms are analysed and guide reasoning for further testing.
- Identify factors that may have predisposed to, or arisen from, the patient's presentation.
- Establish markers (asterisks*) to evaluate treatment.

The following information can be noted during active movements:

1. Quality of movement
2. Range of movement. Joint range can be measured clinically using a goniometer, tape measure or visual estimation. Readers are directed to other texts on details of joint measurement (Norkin & White, 2016).
3. Symptom reproduction, e.g. pain (local and referred).
4. The occurrence of muscle spasms during the movement.

Active movement is considered normal if there is painless, full range of movement. The procedure for testing active physiological movement is as follows:

- Resting symptoms should be established prior to each movement so that the effect of the movement on the symptoms can be clearly ascertained.
- The active physiological movement is carried out and the quality of movement is observed, noting the smoothness and control of the movement, any deviation from a normal movement pattern and the muscle activity involved.
- Next, altered movement patterns can be corrected to assess whether this changes symptoms. If symptoms do not change on movement correction, the altered movement pattern is not relevant to the patient's problem (Van Dillen et al., 2009).
- Both quality and range of movement can be tested further by modifying the patient's posture during active movements (Sueki et al., 2013). For example, active shoulder movement can be retested with the clinician systematically modifying thoracic, scapular and humeral positions in order to identify possible drivers of symptoms. Modification is regarded as relevant if it produces a 30% improvement in symptoms, and with a consistent response to repeated movement (Lewis, 2009).
- Active physiological movements test not only the function of joints but also of muscles and nerves. This interrelationship is well explained by the *movement system balance theory* (Sahrmann, 2002). This theory suggests that there is an ideal mode of movement system function and that any deviation from this mode is less efficient and increases the load on components of the system (Comerford & Mottram, 2013).

Ideal movement system function depends on:

- The maintenance of precise movement of rotating parts, i.e. the instantaneous axis of rotation (IAR) should follow a normal path. The pivot point about which the joint moves constantly changes during physiological movements and its location at any instant is referred to as the IAR. The shape of joint surfaces and the mobility and length of soft-tissue structures (skin, ligament, tendon, muscle and nerves) are all thought to affect the position of the IAR (Sahrmann, 2002).

- Normal muscle length. As mentioned, muscles can become shortened or lengthened and this will affect the quality and range of movement.
- Normal motor control, i.e. the precise and coordinated action of muscles.
- Normal relative stiffness of contractile and noncontractile tissue.
- Normal kinetics, i.e. normal movement function of joints proximal and distal to the area under consideration.

Therefore a movement dysfunction may be due to several factors, such as shortened tissue, muscle weakness or pain (Sahrmann, 2002).

The behaviour of the pain (both local and referred) throughout the joint range is recorded. The clinician asks the patient to indicate where in the range of movement pain is first felt or increased and then how this pain is affected by further movement. The clinician can ask the patient to rate the intensity of pain as discussed in Chapter 3. The behaviour of pain through the range can be documented using a movement diagram, which is described later in this chapter.

Muscle spasm observed during movement is noted. Muscle spasm is an involuntary contraction of muscle as a result of nerve irritation or secondary to injury of structures, such as bone, joint or muscle. It occurs in order to prevent movement and further injury.

Overpressure

Overpressure can be applied at the end of a physiological range. If the patient's symptoms allow, i.e. are nonsevere, the clinician applies a passive force to take the movement to or towards the end of its range. In this situation overpressure could be classified as a passive movement; however, normal convention includes overpressure within active movement testing. If the resistance to movement felt by the clinician on applying overpressure is considered to be normal and symptoms are not reproduced, then the joint is considered cleared as a contributor to the patient's symptoms (Hengeveld & Banks, 2014).

Overpressure needs to be carried out carefully if it is to give accurate information. The following guidelines may help the clinician:

1. The patient needs to be comfortable suitably supported and prepared.
2. The clinician needs to be in a comfortable position, i.e. the couch adjusted to the correct height.
3. For accurate/efficient direction of the overpressure force, for larger joints the clinician's body may need to be positioned in line with the direction of the force.
4. The force is applied slowly and smoothly to the end of the available range while communicating with the patient throughout.
5. At the end of the available range, the clinician may apply small oscillatory movements to feel the resistance at a point in the range (Hengeveld & Banks, 2014).

There are a variety of ways of applying overpressure. The choice will depend on factors such as the health, age and size of the patient, the joint being tested and the size of the clinician. While applying overpressure, the clinician will:

- Feel the quality of the movement.
- Note the range of further movement.
- Feel the resistance through the latter part of the range and at the end of the range.
- Note any pain (local and referred) on overpressure.
- Feel for the presence of any muscle spasm throughout the range.

Some clinicians do not add overpressure if the movement is limited by pain. In situations where severity and irritability are high, this is correct. However, the clinician cannot be certain that the movement is limited by pain, so they can explore further when irritability and severity are low. That said, it can be informative to apply overpressure in the presence of pain: it can cause the pain to ease, stay the same or get worse. This information can help the clinician to clinically reason the movement limitation and to select a treatment dose. For example, when the pain eases or stays the same on overpressure, a more provocative movement may be chosen next. This would not be done if the pain had increased. When applying an overpressure to a movement limited by pain, it is vital to apply the force extremely slowly and carefully, thereby only minimally increasing the patient's pain.

Normal movement should be pain-free, smooth and resistance-free until the later stages of the range, when resistance will gradually increase until it limits further movement. Less than optimal quality of movement could be demonstrated by the patient's facial expression, e.g. excessive grimacing due to excessive effort or pain, by limb trembling due to muscle weakness or by compensatory movements elsewhere.

Movement can be limited by one or more factors, such as articular surface contact, limit of ligamentous, muscle or tendon extensibility, and apposition of soft tissue. Each of these factors will give a different quality of resistance. For example, wrist flexion and extension are limited by increasing tension in the surrounding ligaments and muscles; knee flexion is limited by soft-tissue apposition of the calf and thigh muscles; elbow extension is limited by bony apposition. Thus each movement for each joint has a different end-feel. The quality of this resistance felt at the end of the range has been categorized by Cyriax (1982) and Kaltenborn (2002), as shown in Table 4.2.

The resistance is considered abnormal if a joint does not have its characteristic end-feel, e.g. if knee flexion has a hard end-feel, or if the resistance is felt too early or too late within the normal range of movement. Additionally, Cyriax describes three abnormal end-feels: empty, springy and muscle spasm (Table 4.3).

Modifications of Active Movements

Further modification of the active range of movement can be gained in a number of ways (Box 4.1), as described below.

Combined Movements

Combined movement is movement in one plane combined with movement in at least one other plane. For example, lumbar flexion may be combined with lateral flexion or wrist extension with radial deviation. Reasons for combining movements in this way include:

- To gain further information about a movement dysfunction.
- To explore a functional activity which involves combined movement in a number of planes.
- To increase the load on the underlying tissues, particularly the joint.

TABLE 4.3 Abnormal Joint End-Feels

Cyriax	Kaltenborn	Description
Empty feel	Empty	No resistance offered due to severe pain secondary to serious pathology such as fractures, active inflammatory processes and neoplasm
Springy block		A rebound feel at end range, e.g. with a torn meniscus blocking knee extension
Spasm		Sudden end-feel due to muscle spasm

Abnormality is also recognized if a joint does not have its characteristic end-feel or if the resistance is felt too early or too late in what is considered the normal range.
Cyriax (1982) and Kaltenborn (2002).

BOX 4.1 Modifications to the Examination of Active Physiological Movements

- Overpressure
- Combined movements
- Repeated movements
- Speed of movement
- Compression or distraction
- Sustained movements
- Injuring movements
- Differentiation tests
- Functional ability

TABLE 4.2 Normal End-Feels

Cyriax	Kaltenborn	Description
Soft-tissue approximation	Soft-tissue approximation or soft-tissue stretch	Soft end-feel, e.g. knee flexion or ankle dorsiflexion
Capsular feel	Firm soft-tissue stretch	Fairly hard halt to movement, e.g. shoulder, elbow or hip rotation due to capsular or ligamentous stretching
Bone to bone	Hard	Abrupt halt to the movement, e.g. elbow extension

Cyriax (1982) and Kaltenborn (2002).

Following examination of the active movements and various combined movements, the patient can be categorized into one of three patterns (Edwards, 1999):

1. Regular stretch pattern. This occurs when the symptoms are produced on the opposite side from that to which movement is directed. An example is a patient with left-sided neck pain which is reproduced on cervical flexion, right lateral flexion and right rotation, with all other movements full and pain-free. The term *stretch* is used here to describe the general stretch of spinal structures reproducing the patient's symptoms.
2. Regular compression pattern. This occurs when the symptoms are reproduced on the side to which the movement is directed. If left-sided neck pain is reproduced on cervical extension, left lateral flexion and left rotation, while all other movements are full and pain-free, the patient is said to have a regular compression pattern. The term *compression* is used to describe the general compression of spinal structures. A recording of the findings of combined movements of the lumbar spine for a patient with left-sided low back pain is illustrated in Fig. 4.7.
3. Irregular pattern. Patients who do not clearly fit into a regular stretch or compression pattern are categorized as having an irregular pattern. In this case, symptoms are provoked by a mixture of stretching and compressing movements.

The information from combined movements, along with the severity and irritability, can help to confirm or refute a primary hypothesis. The clinician can use this information to inform further testing by positioning the patient to either increase or decrease the stretching or compressing effect. For example, accessory movements can be carried out with the spine at the limit of a physiological movement or in a position of maximum comfort.

To verify further whether a joint is a source of the patient's symptoms, accessory movements may be carried out (explained later in this chapter). The use of

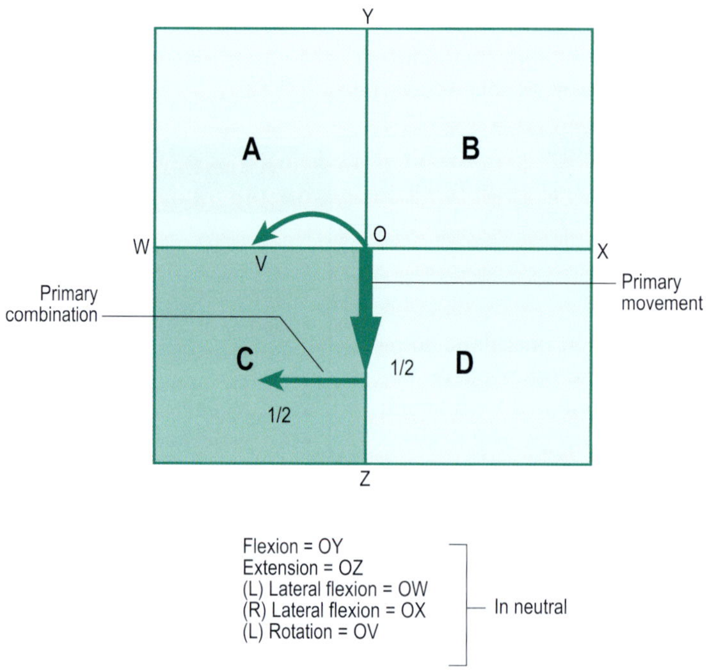

Fig. 4.7 Recording combined movements. Movements can be quickly and easily recorded using this box. It assumes that the clinician is standing behind the patient so that (A) and (B) refer to anterior, and (C) and (D) to posterior parts of the body; (A) and (C) are left side and (B) and (D) are right side. The box depicts the following information: left rotation is limited to half range; extension and left lateral flexion in extension range are half normal range. The symptoms are in the left posterior part of the body (represented by the shading). (From Edwards 1999, with permission.)

combined movements and accessory movements together may be referred to as *joint clearing tests*, or *screening tests*. Normally, if strong end-of-range combined movements and accessory movements do not reproduce the patient's symptoms and reassessment asterisks remain the same, then the joint is not considered to be a source of the patient's symptoms, i.e. it has been screened. If symptoms are produced or there is reduced range of movement, the joint cannot be considered cleared and may require further examination. Combined movements to clear a joint are generally considered more stressful physiological movements. Suggestions for different joints are provided in Table 4.4.

TABLE 4.4 Joint Clearing Tests

Joint	Physiological Movement
Temporomandibular joint	Open/close jaw, side-to-side movement, protraction/retraction
Cervical spine	Quadrants (flexion and extension)
Thoracic spine	Rotation and quadrants (flexion and extension)
Lumbar spine	Flexion and quadrants (flexion and extension)
Sacroiliac joint	Anterior and posterior gapping
Shoulder girdle	Elevation, depression, protraction and retraction
Shoulder joint	Flexion and hand behind back
Acromioclavicular joint	All movements (particularly horizontal flexion)
Sternoclavicular joint	All movements
Elbow joint	All movements
Wrist joint	Flexion/extension and radial/ulnar deviation
Thumb	Extension carpometacarpal and thumb opposition
Fingers	Flexion at interphalangeal joints and grip
Hip joint	Squat and hip quadrant
Knee joint	All movements
Patellofemoral joint	Medial/lateral glide and cephalad/caudad glide
Ankle joint	Plantarflexion/dorsiflexion and inversion/eversion

Repeated Movements

Repeating a movement several times may alter the quality and range of the movement. There may be a gradual increase in range with repeated movements because of the effects of hysteresis on the collagen-containing tissues such as joint capsules, ligaments, muscles and nerves (Threlkeld, 1992). If a patient with a Colles fracture who has recently come out of plaster was to move their wrist into flexion repeatedly, the range of movement would probably increase. Examining repeated movements may also demonstrate muscle fatigue or altered quality of movement, and symptoms may increase or decrease. Repeated movements are an integral part of the McKenzie method of mechanical diagnosis and therapy of the spine (May & Clare, 2015).

Speed of Movement

Movements can be carried out at different speeds and symptoms are noted. Increasing the speed of movement may be necessary in order to replicate the patient's functional restriction and reproduce their symptoms. For example, a footballer with knee pain may only feel symptoms when running fast and symptoms may only be reproduced in clinic with quick movements of the knee. One of the reasons why the speed of movement can alter symptoms is that the rate of loading of viscoelastic tissues affects their extensibility and stiffness (Threlkeld, 1992).

Sustained Movements

A movement can be held within or at the end of the range, and the effects on symptoms are noted. This approach may be very valuable in assessing patients who have reported that their symptoms are aggravated by sustained postures. In this position the soft-tissue structures are being stretched, so they lengthen due to tissue creep thought to be due to redistribution of water content within the tissue (Threlkeld, 1992). Range of movement would therefore increase in normal tissue and providing the load matched the tissues capacity, range would be restored on the release of load/stretch. Pathological tissues may be sensitized and will behave differently if the load exceeds their capacity due to healing/reorganization.

Injuring Movement

The movement related to the injury can be tested. This may be necessary when symptoms have not been reproduced by the movements described above or if the patient has transient symptoms.

Differentiation Tests

These tests are useful to distinguish between two structures suspected to be a source of the symptoms. A position that provokes symptoms is held constant and then a movement that increases or decreases the stress on one of the structures is added. The effect on symptoms is noted. For example, in the straight leg raise (SLR) test, hip flexion with knee extension can be held constant, creating tension on the sciatic nerve as well as the hip extensor muscles (particularly hamstrings). Cervical flexion is then added. This increases the tension on the sciatic nerve without altering the length of the hip extensors. This can help to differentiate between nerve and muscle structures.

Joint Integrity Tests

These are specific tests to determine the stability of a joint, for example, Lachman's test for an anterior cruciate knee injury at the knee. In acute presentations, integrity tests may be carried out early in the examination, as instability will influence, and may contraindicate, further testing. Sides will be compared to identify the normal range for individual patients. Specific tests are described in the relevant regional chapters.

Passive Physiological Movements

Passive movements allow the clinician to identify the full available joint range which is normally greater than can be achieved actively by the patient. The available passive range varies between individual patients. As considered in the discussion of overpressures, the clinician will feel for the quality of movement, resistance through the range, symptom reproduction and end feel. The clinician must interpret the findings of the active and passive examinations together.

A comparison of the response of symptoms to the active and passive movements can help to clinically reason whether the structure at fault is contractile or not. If the lesion is of noncontractile or inert tissue, such as a ligament, then active and passive movements will be painful and/or restricted in the same direction. For instance, if the anterior joint capsule of the proximal interphalangeal joint of the index finger is shortened, there will be pain and/or restriction of finger extension, whether this movement is carried out actively or passively. If the lesion is in contractile tissue (i.e. muscle), then active and passive movements are painful and/or restricted in opposite directions: when the muscle contracts or when it is being stretched. For example, a muscle lesion in the anterior fibres of the deltoid will be painful on active flexion of the shoulder joint and on passive extension of the shoulder.

Compression or distraction of a joint's articular surfaces can be added during the movement. If the lesion is intraarticular then the symptoms are often made worse by compression and eased by distraction (Magee & Manske, 2021).

While active physiological movements of the spine are an accumulation of movement at a number of vertebral segments, passive movements are used to localize movements. Spinal passive movement is assessed segmentally using PPIVMs. To do this, the clinician feels the movement of adjacent spinous processes, articular pillars or transverse processes during physiological movements. An overview of how to perform PPIVMS is given in each relevant chapter and a full description can be found in Hengeveld & Banks (2014). A quick and easy method of recording PPIVMs is shown in Fig. 4.8. This method can also be used to record active movements.

KNOWLEDGE CHECK

1. Give examples of active physiological movements at the hip joint.
2. How can you modify active movements, and why might you choose to do this?
3. Explain the difference between active and passive movement testing.

Muscle Tests

The effect of muscle dysfunction can impact the whole musculoskeletal system. Dysfunction in muscle will impact on joints and nerves and vice versa as they are dependent on each other for normal function. The selection of muscle tests will depend on the clinician's working hypothesis. Is the dysfunction as a result of trauma/pathology within the muscle system such as a

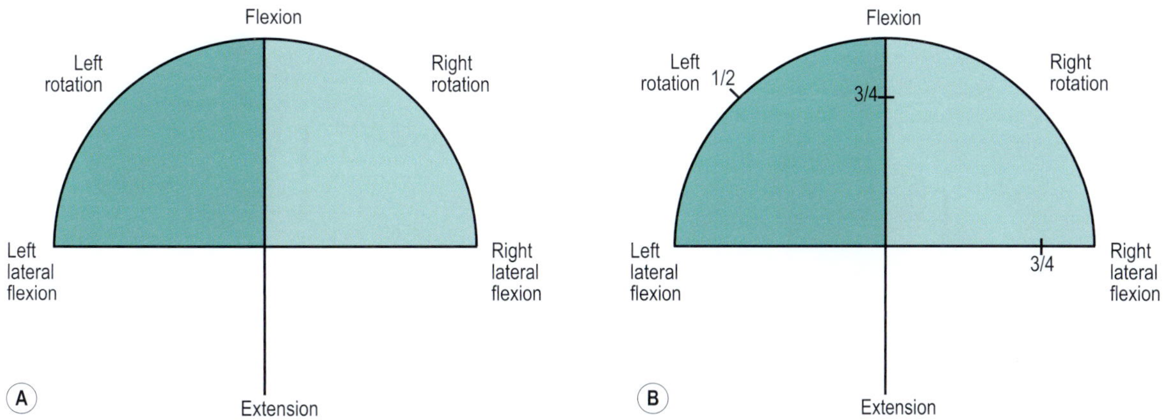

Fig. 4.8 (A) Recording passive physiological intervertebral movements (PPIVMs). (B) Example of a completed PPIVM recording for a segmental level. Interpretation: there is three-quarters range of flexion and right lateral flexion and one-half range of left rotation. There is no restriction of extension.

muscle strain or tendinopathy? Is there muscle inhibition due to pain from joint pathology? Ligamentous instability will result in reduced mechanoreceptor feedback which will alter muscle activity. Is there a neural component, e.g. nerve root lesion? The reader is directed to Chapter 4, Barnard and Ryder (2024).

Comerford and Mottram (2013) suggest that optimal muscle function requires muscles to be able to:

- Concentrically shorten to produce movement—*mobility function.*
- Isometrically hold positions and postures—*postural control function.*
- Eccentrically lengthen—stability function.
- Provide proprioceptive feedback to the central nervous system for on-going coordination and regulation.

Due to their anatomy and physiology, some muscles are more efficient in terms of a mobility function, while others are better suited to a stability function.

A classification system first applied to the lumbar spine by Bergmark (1989) was further refined by Comerford and Mottram (2001). Muscles are grouped under three broad headings: local stabilizer, global stabilizer and global mobilizer. Generally speaking, *local stabilizer muscles* maintain a low, continuous activation in all joint positions, regardless of the direction of joint motion. They tend to become inhibited in the presence of pain. Examples include the vastus medialis obliquus and deep neck flexors. *Global stabilizers* are activated on specific directions of joint movement, providing eccentric control and rotatory movement. When dysfunctional, they tend to become long and weak. Examples include gluteus medius, superficial multifidus, and internal and external obliques. *Global mobilizers* produce direction-specific movement, particularly concentric movement. When dysfunctional, they tend to become short and overactive. Examples include hamstrings and sternocleidomastoids (Comerford & Mottram, 2013). Further characteristics of each classification are given in Table 4.5.

- It is important to remember that individual muscles do not function in isolation and are dependent on a balance between agonists and antagonists, as well as other local and distant muscle groups.

There is a close functional relationship between agonist and antagonist muscles. Activation of the agonist is associated with reciprocal inhibition of the antagonist. This means that overactivity of a muscle is associated with inhibition of the antagonist group, which may in turn become weak. This produces what is known as *muscle imbalance*, i.e. a disruption of the coordinated interplay of muscles. Muscle imbalance can occur when a muscle becomes shortened and alters the position IAR of the joint. This change will result in the antagonist muscle being elongated and weak. Postural positions have been shown to influence trunk muscle activation patterns and altered muscle patterns have been linked to lumbopelvic pain (Dankaerts et al., 2006). For example, in a patient with a kypholordotic posture, the erector spinae muscles will be overactive,

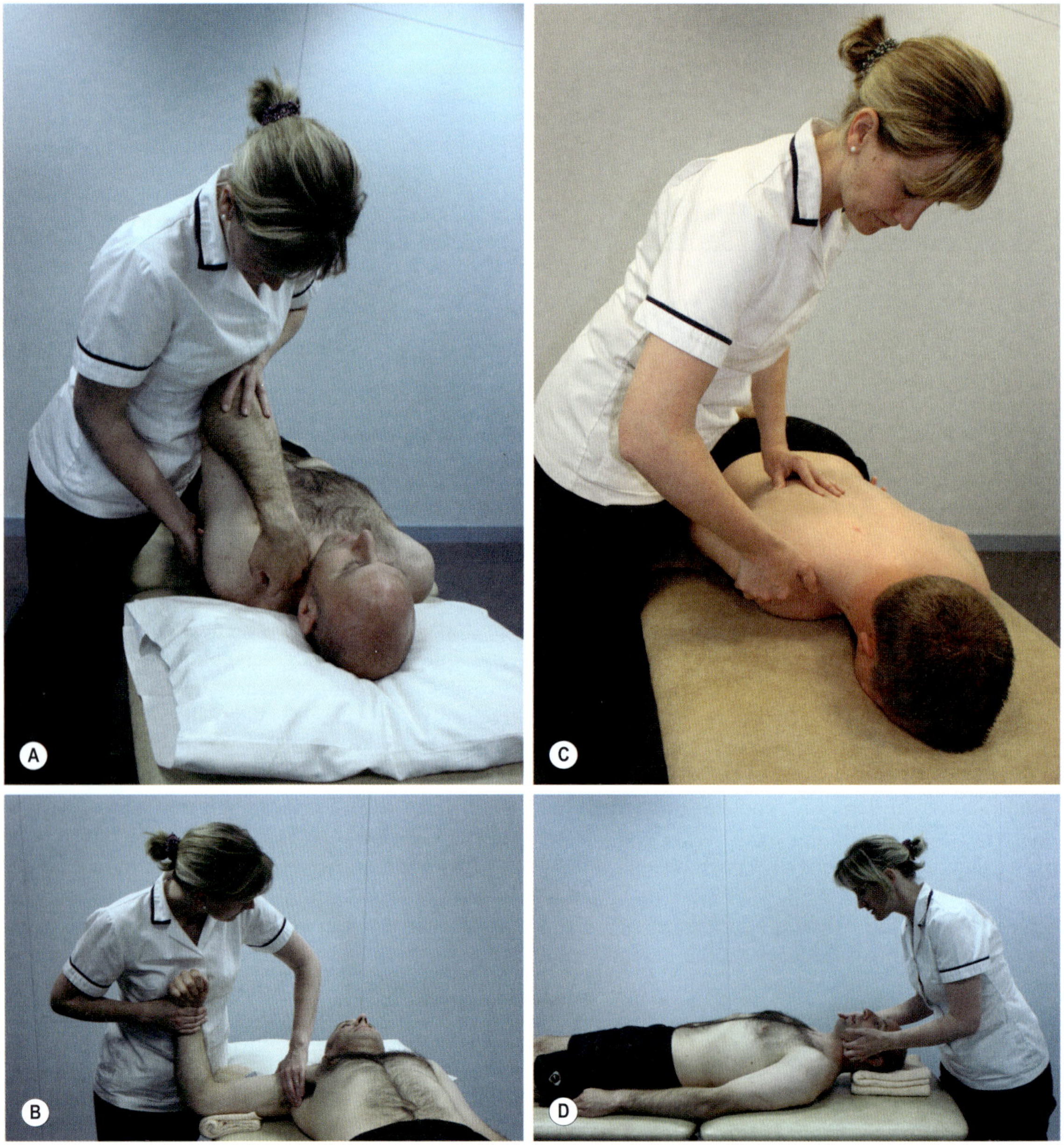

Fig. 4.9 Testing the strength of individual muscles prone to become weak (Cole et al., 1988; Janda, 1994; Jull & Janda, 1987). (A) Serratus anterior. The patient lies supine with the shoulder flexed to 90 degrees and the elbow in full flexion. Resistance is applied to shoulder girdle protraction. (B) Subscapularis. In supine with the shoulder in 90 degrees abduction and the elbow flexed to 90 degrees. A towel is placed underneath the upper arm so that the humerus is in the scapular plane. The clinician gently resists medial rotation of the upper arm. The subscapularis tendon can be palpated in the axilla, just anterior to the posterior border. There should be no scapular movement or alteration in the abduction position. (C) Lower fibres of trapezius. In prone lying with the arm by the side and the glenohumeral joint placed in medial rotation, the clinician passively moves the coracoid process away from the plinth such that the head of the humerus and body of scapula lie horizontal. Poor recruitment of lower fibres of trapezius would be suspected from an inability to hold this position without substitution by other muscles such as levator scapulae, rhomboid major and minor or latissimus dorsi. (D) Deep cervical flexors. The patient lies supine with the cervical spine in a neutral position and is asked to tuck the chin in. If there is poor recruitment the sternocleidomastoid initiates the movement.

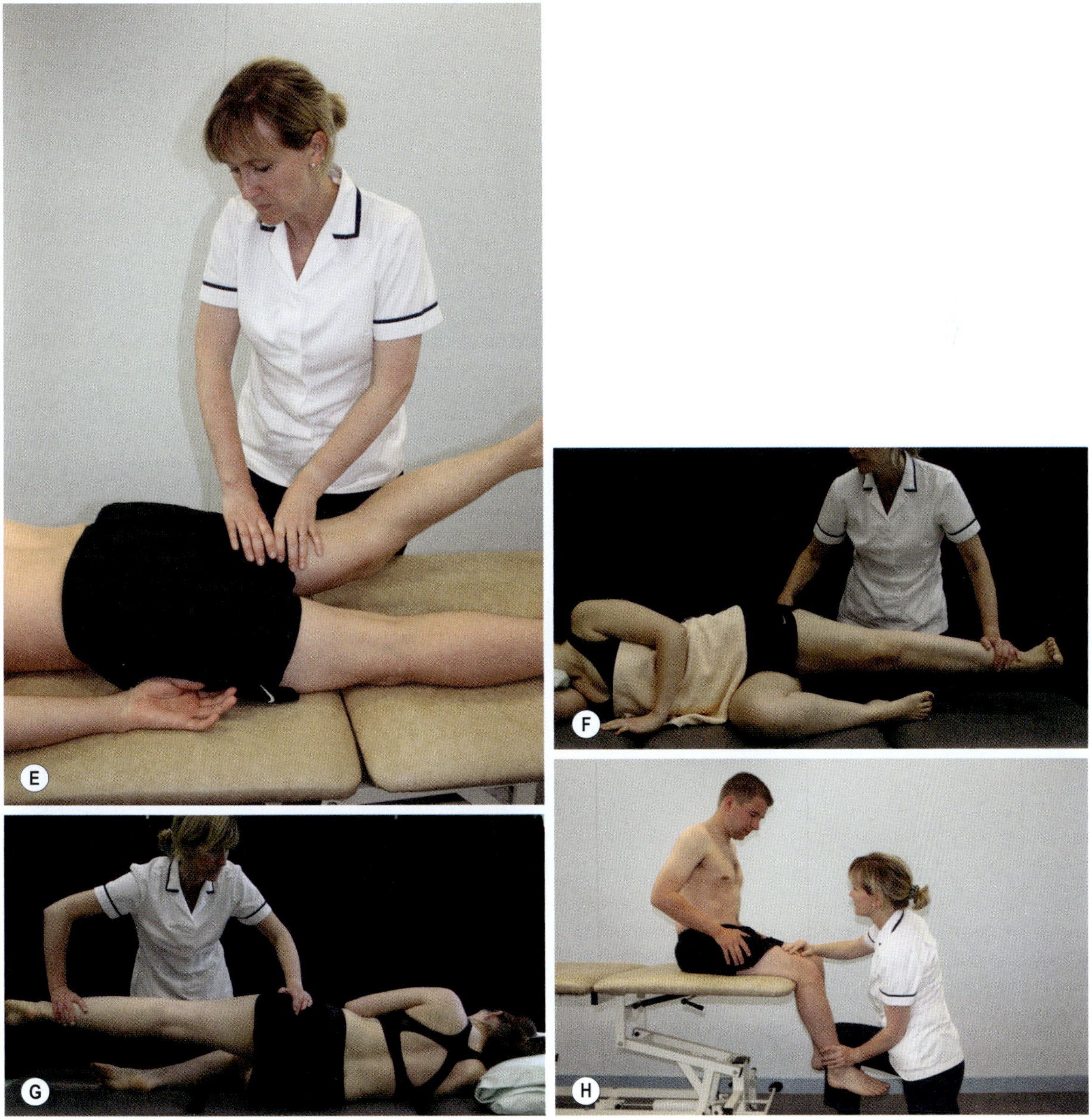

Fig. 4.9, cont'd (E) Gluteus maximus. The clinician resists hip extension. A normal pattern would be hamstring and gluteus maximus acting as prime movers and the erector spinae stabilizing the lumbar spine and pelvis. Contraction of gluteus maximus is delayed when it is weak. Alternatively, the therapist can passively extend the hip into an inner-range position and ask the patient to hold this position isometrically (Jull & Richardson, 1994). (F) Posterior gluteus medius. The patient is asked to abduct the uppermost leg actively with the hip in extension and slight lateral rotation. Resistance can be added by the clinician. Use of hip flexors to produce the movement may indicate a weakness in the lateral pelvic muscles. Other substitution movements include lateral flexion of the trunk or backward rotation of the pelvis. Inner-range weakness is tested by passively abducting the hip; if the range is greater than the active abduction movement, this indicates inner-range weakness. (G) Gluteus minimus. The clinician resists abduction of the hip. (H) Vastus lateralis, medialis and intermedius. The clinician resists knee extension.

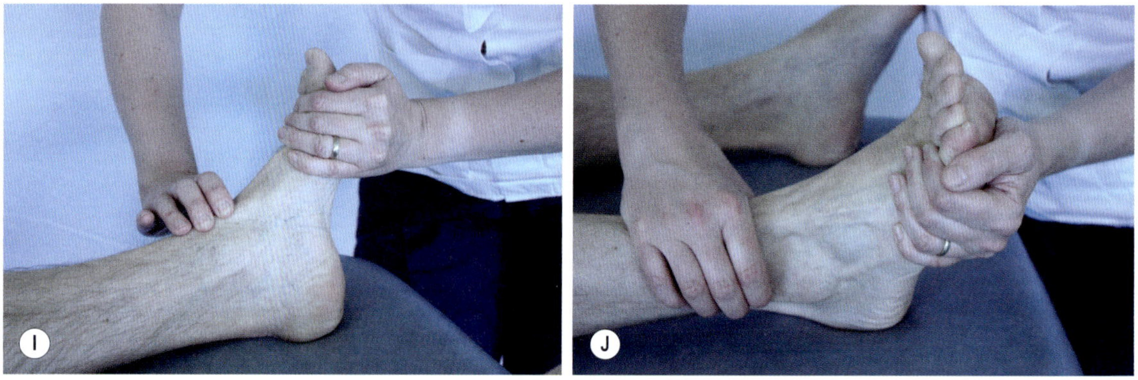

Fig. 4.9, cont'd (I) Tibialis anterior. The clinician resists ankle dorsiflexion and inversion. (J) Peroneus longus and brevis. The clinician resists ankle eversion.

TABLE 4.5 Common Muscle Patterns/Reaction of Muscles to Stress

Muscles Prone to Become Tight	Muscles Prone to Become Weak
Masseter, temporalis, digastric and suboccipital muscles, levator scapulae, rhomboid major and minor, upper trapezius, sternocleidomastoid, pectoralis major and minor scalenes, flexors of the upper limb, erector spinae (particularly thoracolumbar and cervical parts), quadratus lumborum, piriformis, tensor fasciae latae, rectus femoris, hamstrings, short hip adductors, tibialis posterior, gastrocnemius	Serratus anterior, middle and lower fibres of trapezius, deep neck flexors, mylohyoid, subscapularis, extensors of upper limb, gluteus maximus, medius and minimus, deep lumbar multifidus, iliopsoas, vastus medialis and lateralis, tibialis anterior and peronei

Jull and Janda (1987), Janda (1994), and Comerford and Mottram (2013).

resulting in an elongated and underactive rectus abdominis. Muscle imbalance can also occur as a result of reflex inhibition of muscle and weakness in the presence of pain and/or injury. To assess whether movement dysfunction is a contributor to the patient's symptoms the clinician could seek to alter the movement pattern through verbal or handling cues, or positioning, and note the symptom response.

Muscle testing must involve examination of the strength and length of both agonist and antagonist muscle groups.

The following tests are commonly used to assess muscle function: muscle strength, muscle control, muscle length and isometric muscle tests. Region-specific tests can be found in the relevant chapters.

Muscle Strength

Strength is usually tested manually with an isotonic contraction through the available range of movement and graded according to the Medical Research Council (MRC) scale (Medical Research Council, 1976) shown in Table 4.6.

TABLE 4.6 Grades of Muscle Strength

Grade	Muscle Activity
0	No contraction
1	Flicker or trace of contraction
2	Active movement, with gravity eliminated
3	Active movement against gravity
4	Active movement against gravity and resistance
5	Normal strength

Medical Research Council, 1976. Aids to the Investigation of Peripheral Nerve Injuries. HMSO, London. Reproduced with kind permission of the Medical Research Council.

Muscle strength will depend on the age, gender, build and usual level of physical activity of the patient. Details of muscle tests can be found in Kendall et al. (2010).

Some muscles are thought to be prone to inhibition and weakness, see Table 4.7 (Jull & Janda, 1987; Janda, 1994, 2002; Comerford & Mottram, 2001).

They are characterized by hypotonia, decreased strength and delayed activation, with atrophy over a prolonged period of time (Janda, 1993). Sahrmann (2002) suggests that these muscles tend to lengthen if resting in an elongated position as a result of poor posture.

As a consequence, examination of the strength of these muscles, in particular, is recommended. Methods of manual muscle strength testing are shown in Fig. 4.9. Digital dynamometers are increasingly used to measure strength in clinic settings to provide more objective data on performance.

Muscle Control

Muscle control is tested by observing the recruitment and coordination of muscles during active movements. Some of these movements will have already been analysed in functional and active movement examination,

TABLE 4.7 Classification of Muscle Function Roles in Terms of Function, Characteristics and Dysfunction

Local Stabilizer	Global Stabilizer	Global Mobilizer
Examples		
Transversus abdominis	Internal and external obliques	Rectus abdominis
Deep lumbar multifidus	Superficial multifidus	Iliocostalis
Psoas major (posterior fasciculi)	Spinalis	Hamstrings
Vastus medialis oblique	Gluteus medius	Latissimus dorsi
Middle and lower trapezius	Serratus anterior	Levator scapulae
Deep cervical flexors	Longus colli (oblique fibres)	Scalenus anterior, medius and posterior
Function and Characteristics		
Increases muscle stiffness to control segmental movement	Generates force to control range of movement	Generates torque to produce movement
Controls the neutral joint position. Contraction does not produce change in length and so does not produce movement. Proprioceptive function: information on joint position, range and rate of movement	Controls particularly the inner and outer ranges of movement. Tends to contract eccentrically for low-load deceleration of momentum and for rotational control	Produces joint movement, especially movements in the sagittal plane. Tends to contract concentrically. Absorbs shock
Activity is independent of direction of movement	Activity is direction-dependent	Activity is direction-dependent
Continuous activation throughout movement	Noncontinuous activity	Noncontinuous activity
Dysfunction		
Reduced muscle stiffness, loss of joint neutral position (segmental control). Delayed timing and recruitment	Poor control of inner and outer ranges of movement, poor eccentric control and rotation dissociation. Inner- and outer-range weakness of muscle	Muscle spasm. Loss of muscle length (shortened), limiting accessory and/or physiological range of movement
Becomes inhibited	Reduced low-threshold tonic recruitment	Overactive low-threshold, low-load recruitment
Local inhibition	Global imbalance	Global imbalance
Loss of segmental control	Increased length and inhibited stabilizing muscles result in underpull at a motion segment	Shortened and overactive mobilizing muscles result in overpull at a motion segment

but other specific tests are carried out here. Relative strength is assessed by observing the pattern of muscle recruitment, the quality of movement and palpation of muscle activity in various positions. It should be noted that this relies on the observational and palpatory skills of the clinician; for a detailed description of palpation, the reader is directed to Muscolino (2016). An important term within the concept of muscle control is recruitment (or activation), which refers to the timed onset of muscle activity. For a more in-depth description of this concept the reader is directed to Sahrmann (2002), and Comerford and Mottram (2013).

Muscle Length

Testing of muscle length is particularly important for muscles that tend to become tight and thus lose their extensibility (Comerford & Mottram, 2013) (see Table 4.7). These muscles are characterized by hypertonia, increased strength and faster activation time (Janda, 1993). Methods of testing the length of individual muscles are outlined in Fig. 4.10.

There are two important comments to make regarding muscle length tests. First, although these tests are described according to individual muscles, a number of muscles will be tested simultaneously. This is important when interpreting a test: it cannot be assumed when testing the upper trapezius muscle that it is only this muscle that is reduced in length. For example, levator scapulae and the scalene muscles may also be shortened, thus contributing to the reduced movement. Second, Fig. 4.10 shows some of the many muscle length tests; the choice of tests must be specific

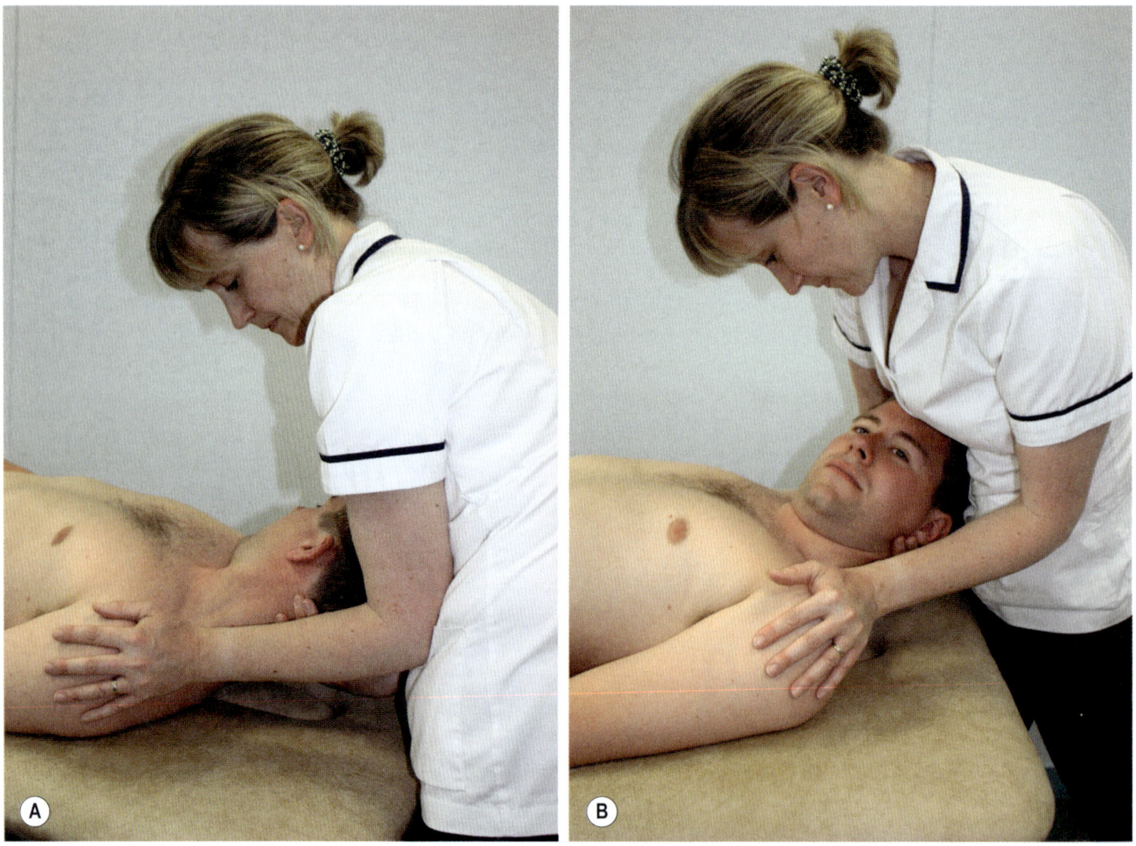

Fig. 4.10 Testing the length of individual muscles prone to becoming short (Jull & Janda, 1987; Cole et al., 1988; Janda, 1994; Kendall et al., 2010). (A) Levator scapulae. A passive stretch is applied by contralateral lateral flexion and rotation with flexion of the neck and shoulder girdle depression. Restricted range of movement and tenderness on palpation over the insertion of levator scapulae indicate tightness of the muscle. (B) Upper trapezius. A passive stretch is applied by passive contralateral lateral flexion, ipsilateral rotation and flexion of the neck with shoulder girdle depression. Restricted range of movement indicates tightness of the muscle.

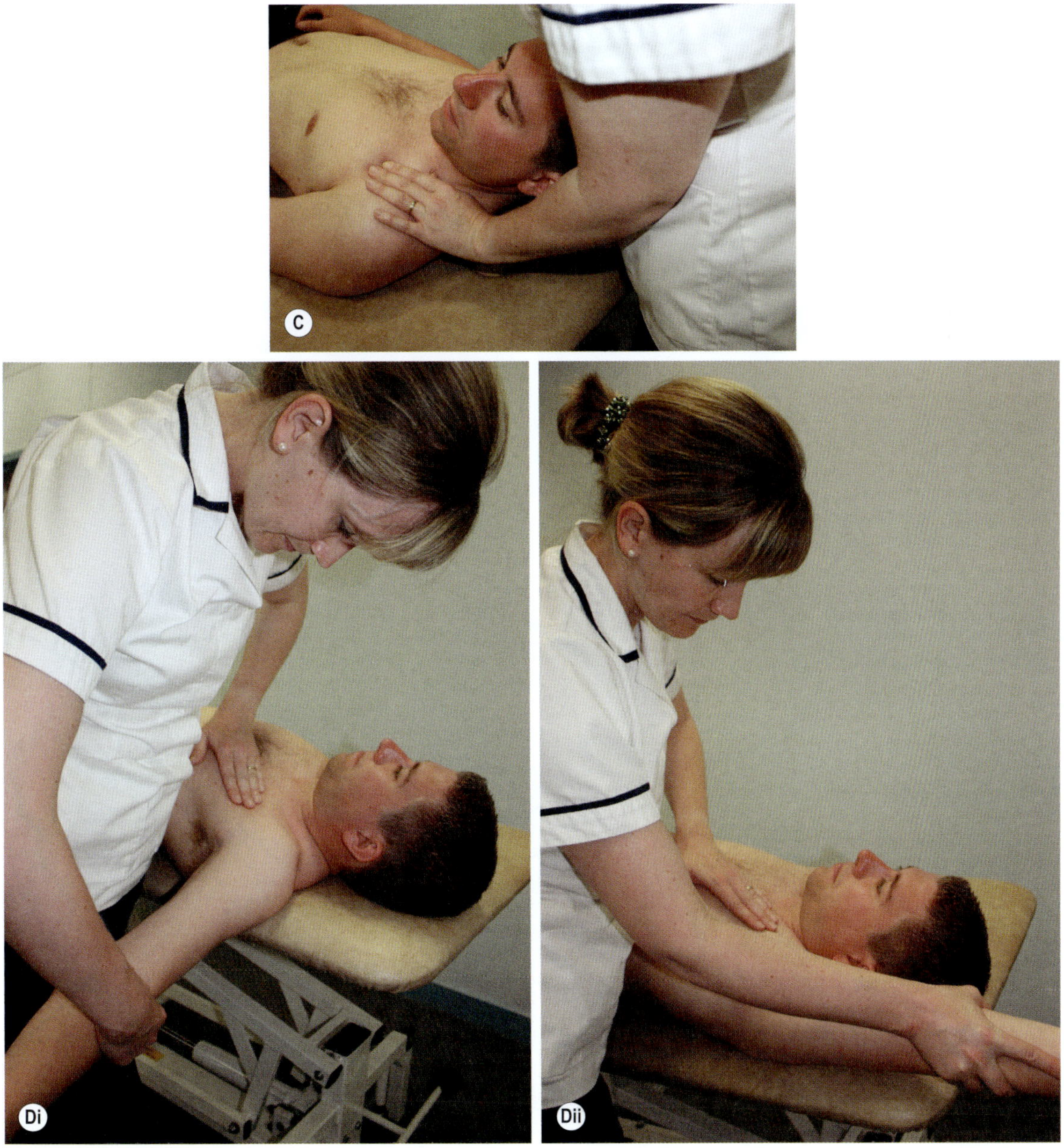

Fig. 4.10, cont'd (C) Sternocleidomastoid. The clinician tucks the chin in and then laterally flexes the head away and rotates towards the side of testing. The clavicle is stabilized with the other hand. (D) Pectoralis major. (i) Clavicular fibres—the clinician stabilizes the trunk and abducts the shoulder to 90 degrees. Passive overpressure of horizontal extension will be limited in range and the tendon becomes taut if there is tightness of this muscle. (ii) Sternocostal fibres—the clinician elevates the shoulder fully. Restricted range of movement and the tendon becoming taut indicate tightness of this muscle.

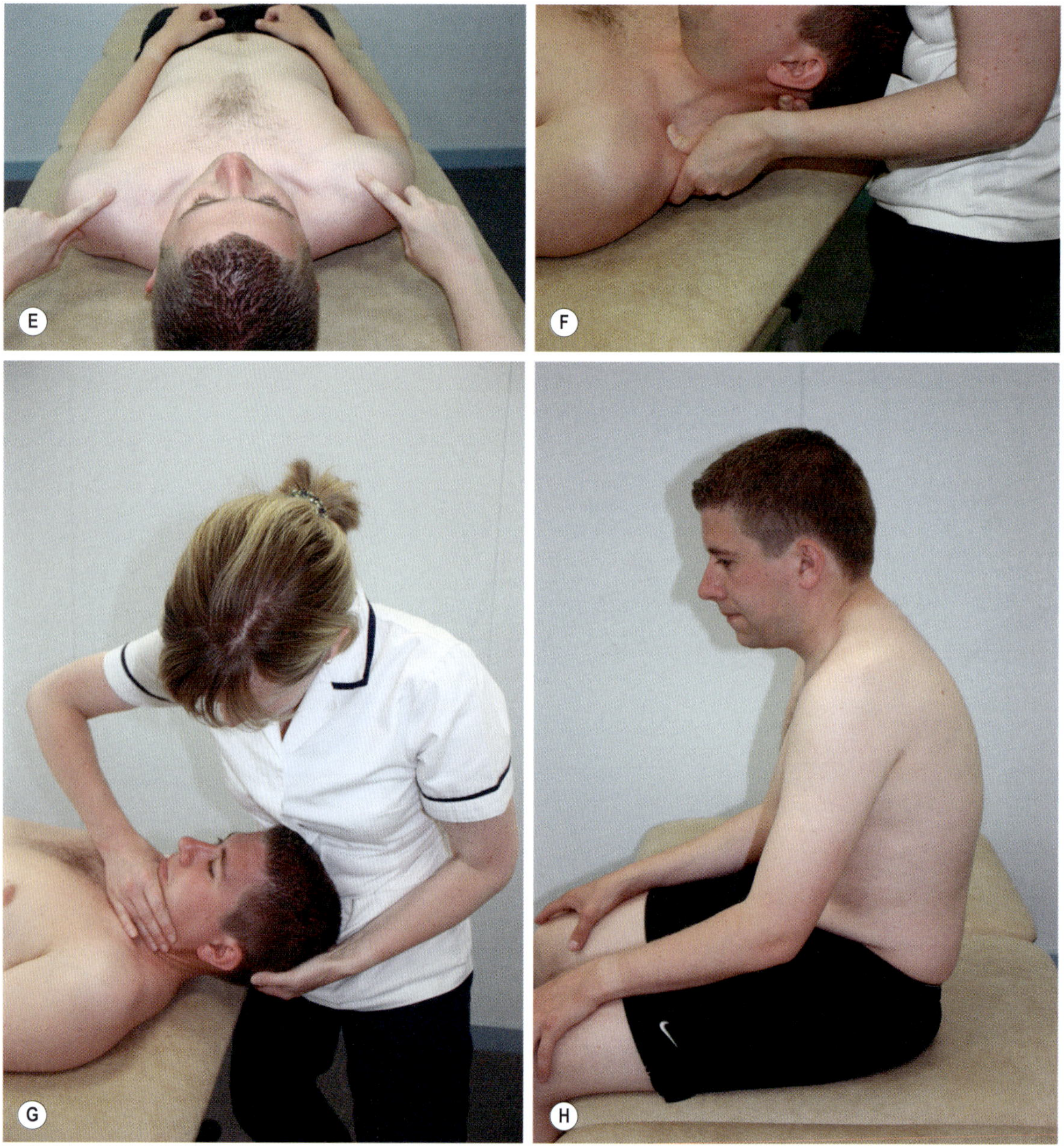

Fig. 4.10, cont'd (E) Pectoralis minor. With the patient in supine and arm by the side, the coracoid is found to be pulled anteriorly and inferiorly if there is a contracture of this muscle. In addition, the posterior edge of the acromion may rest further from the plinth on the affected side. (F) Scalenes. Fixing first and second ribs, the clinician laterally flexes the patient's head away and rotates towards the side of testing for anterior scalene; contralateral lateral flexion tests the middle fibres; contralateral rotation and lateral flexion test the posterior scalene muscle. (G) Deep occipital muscles. The right hand passively flexes the upper cervical spine while palpating the deep occipital muscles with the left hand. Tightness on palpation indicates tightness of these muscles. (H) Erector spinae. The patient slumps the shoulders towards the groin. Lack of flattening of the lumbar lordosis may indicate tightness.

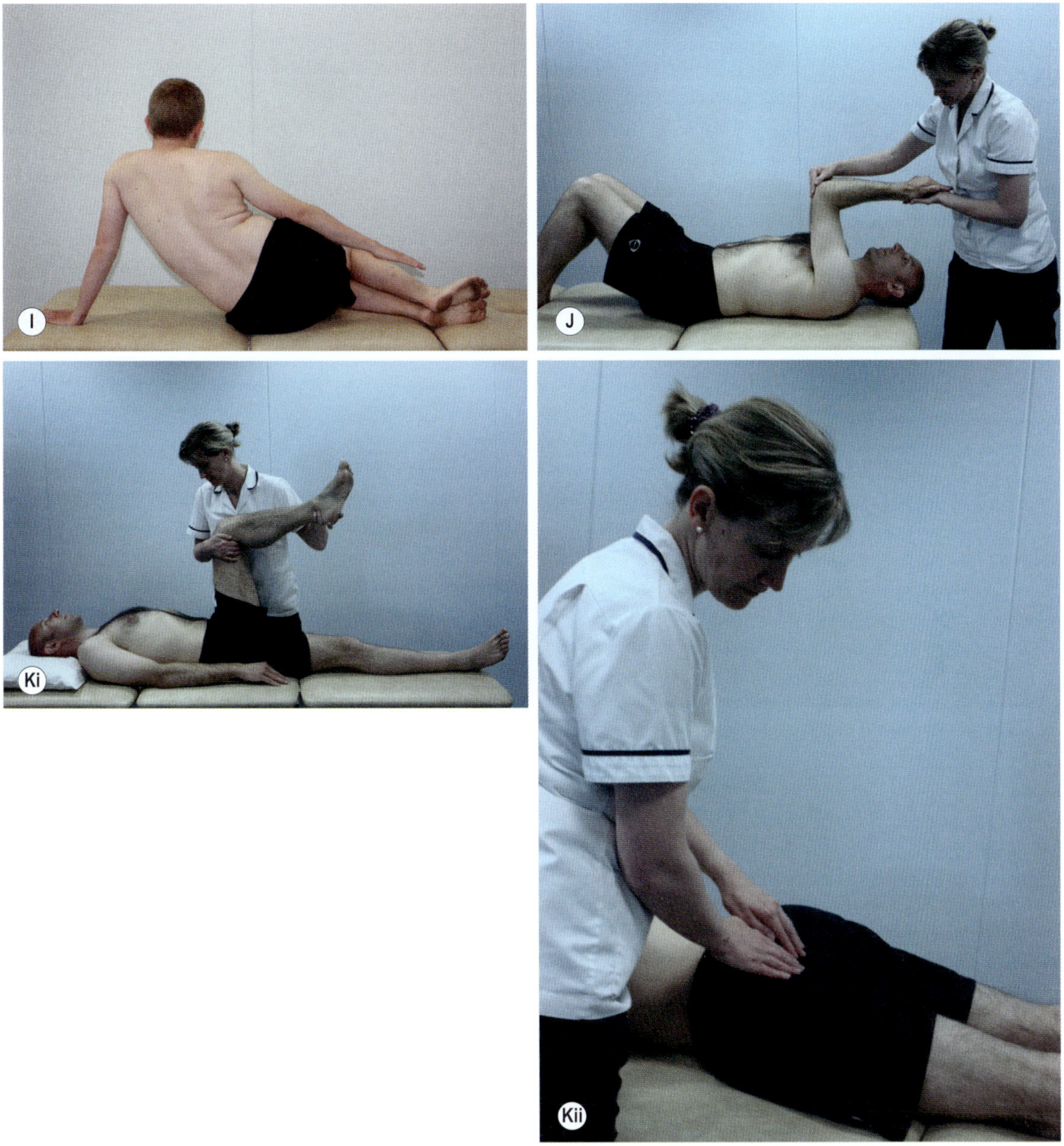

Fig. 4.10, cont'd (I) Quadratus lumborum. The patient pushes up sideways as far as possible without movement of the pelvis. Limited range of movement, lack of curvature in the lumbar spine and/or abnormal tension on palpation (just above the iliac crest and lateral to erector spinae) indicate tightness of the muscle. (J) Latissimus dorsi. With the patient in crook-lying with the lumbar spine flat against the plinth and the gleno-humeral joints laterally rotated, the patient is asked to elevate the arms through flexion. Shortness of latissimus dorsi is evidenced by an inability to maintain the lumbar spine in against the plinth and/or inability to elevate the arms fully. (K) Piriformis. (i) The clinician passively flexes the hip to 90 degrees, adducts it and then adds lateral rotation to the hip, feeling the resistance to the limit of the movement. There should be around 45 degrees of lateral rotation. (ii) Piriformis can be palpated if it is tight by applying deep pressure at the point at which an imaginary line between the iliac crest and ischial tuberosity crosses a line between the posterior superior iliac spine and the greater trochanter.

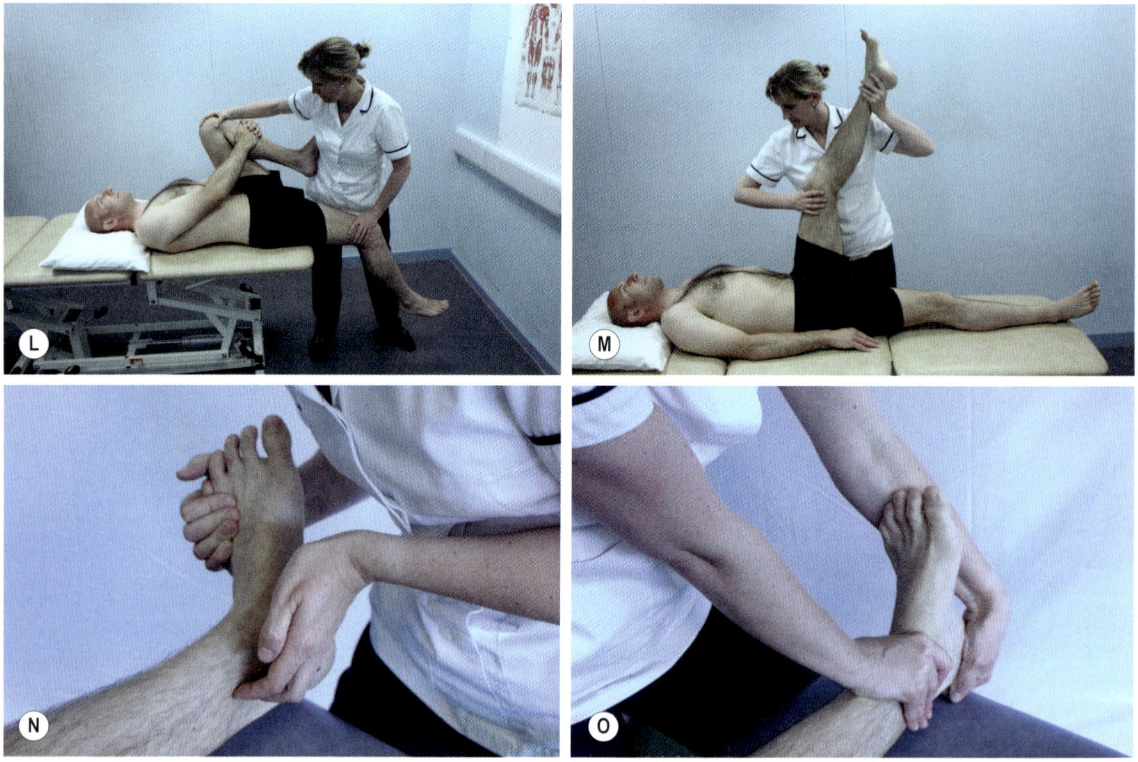

Fig. 4.10, cont'd (L) Iliopsoas, rectus femoris and tensor fasciae latae. The left leg is stabilized against the clinician's side. The free leg will be flexed at the hip if there is tightness of iliopsoas. An extended knee indicates tight rectus femoris. Abduction of the hip, lateral deviation of the patella and a well-defined groove on the lateral aspect of the thigh indicate tight tensor fasciae latae and iliotibial band. Overpressure to each of these movements, including hip abduction for the short adductors, will confirm any tightness of these muscles. (M) Hamstrings. With the patient lying supine, the clinician passively flexes the hip to 90 degrees and then the knee is passively extended. (N) Tibialis posterior. The clinician dorsiflexes the ankle joint and everts the forefoot. Limited range of movement indicates tightness of the muscle. (O) Gastrocnemius and soleus. Gastrocnemius length can be tested by the range of ankle dorsiflexion with the knee extended and then flexed. If the range increases when the knee is flexed, this indicates tightness of gastrocnemius.

to the individual patient and justified using reasoning. For example, to test the length of the hamstring muscles fully, the clinician may investigate a number of different components such as hip flexion with additional adduction/abduction and/or medial/lateral rotation. Similarly, for levator scapulae, the clinician may examine varying degrees of cervical flexion, contralateral lateral flexion and contralateral rotation, while varying the order of the movements. For further information on fully investigating muscle length, the reader is directed to Muscolino (2016).

Muscle length is tested by the clinician stabilizing one end of the muscle, and then slowly and smoothly moving the body part to stretch the muscle from the other end. The following information is noted:

- Quality of movement.
- Range of movement.
- The presence of resistance through the range of movement and at the end of the range of movement: the quality of the resistance may identify whether muscle, joint or neural tissues are limiting the movement.
- Pain behaviour (local and referred) through the range.

Reduced muscle length, i.e. muscle shortness or tightness, occurs when the muscle cannot be stretched to its normal length. This may occur as a result of compensatory changes between agonist and antagonist muscles, so the clinician is required to reason muscle length findings within a context of movement analysis.

Isometric Muscle Testing

This may help to differentiate symptoms arising from contractile rather than inert tissues. The joint is put into a resting position (so that the inert structures are relaxed), and the patient is asked to hold this position against the resistance of the clinician. The clinician observes the quality of the muscle contraction to hold this position. The patient may, for example, be unable to prevent the joint from moving, adopt compensatory substitution strategies or hold with excessive muscle activity; any of these responses suggest neuromuscular dysfunction. If symptoms are reproduced on isometric contraction, it can be reasoned that symptoms are coming from the muscle, although it must be remembered that there will also be shearing and compression of inert structures such as joints. If a more thorough examination of muscle function is justified, isometric strength can be tested at various points in the physiological range.

Cyriax (1982) describes six possible responses to isometric muscle testing:

1. Strong and painless—normal
2. Strong and painful—suggests minor lesion of muscle or tendon, e.g. lateral epicondylalgia
3. Weak and painless—complete rupture of muscle or tendon or disorder of the nervous system
4. Weak and painful—suggests gross lesion, e.g. fracture of patella
5. All movements painful—suggests peripheral and/or sensory sensitization.
6. Painful on repetition—suggests intermittent claudication.

The clinician must bear in mind that pain is a subjective experience, while effort is a behaviour influenced by other factors such as fear related to effort and pain.

> **KNOWLEDGE CHECK**
> 1. What is required for muscle function to be optimal?
> 2. What factors will influence an individual's muscle strength?
> 3. How is muscle strength graded and documented?

Sensorimotor/Neurological Tests

Inclusion of sensorimotor assessment must be clinically reasoned, based on the patient's presenting symptoms. Symptoms such as weakness, numbness or pain with neuropathic characteristics will raise the index of suspicion of a neural source, especially when felt along the course of a nerve. Symptoms suggestive of upper motor neuron (UMN) lesions, e.g. bilateral distribution of symptoms, should prompt the clinician to include additional tests of the CNS. The findings of a sensorimotor assessment will assist in confirming or ruling out a neural source of symptoms and allow for screening of suspected red flags such as cord compression and differentiation between UMN and lower motor neuron (LMN) lesions. This helps to guide appropriate management.

Sensorimotor/neurological examination includes:

- Neurological integrity: testing the ability of the nervous system to conduct action potentials:
  - Sensory perception
  - Coordination
  - Tone
  - Muscle power
  - Reflexes
- Neural sensitivity
  - Neurodynamic tests (the response of the nervous system to load/movement)
  - Neural palpation

Integrity of the Nervous System

The most common condition affecting the peripheral nervous system is entrapment neuropathy. Over the last decade, there has been increased understanding of the underlying pathophysiological mechanisms of symptoms (Schmid et al., 2013; Schmid, 2015; Schmid et al., 2020). For further details see Chapter 6, Barnard and Ryder (2024).

Compression of peripheral nerves can cause a reduction or abolition of signal conduction. Depending on the type(s) of neurone that is affected by the compression, possible effects are:

- Reduced sensation (sensory neurons or afferents).
- Reduced muscle activation (motor neurons or efferents).
- Reflex changes, either increased or decreased. Reflexes involve sensory neurons, motor neurones and the spinal cord.

- Altered skin colour, sweating and piloerection (sympathetic neurons).
- Paraesthesia (sensory neurons).

Increased neural sensitivity, such as hyperaesthesia, hyperalgesia and allodynia, is suggestive of sensitization rather than compression. Sensitization may affect the peripheral nerve (e.g. as a consequence of inflammation or infection) or the central nervous system.

In order to examine the integrity of peripheral nerves, three tests are carried out: skin sensation, muscle strength and deep tendon reflexes. If a nerve root lesion is suspected, the tests carried out are referred to as dermatomal (area of skin supplied by one nerve root), myotomal (group of muscles supplied by one nerve root) and reflexal.

Sensory changes. Reduced sensation may be due to compression or a lesion of the sensory nerves anywhere from terminal branches in the receptor organ, e.g. from joints or skin to spinal nerve root and central nervous system (Fig. 4.11).

Knowledge of the cutaneous distribution of nerve roots (dermatomes) and peripheral nerves enables the clinician to distinguish whether a sensory loss may be due to a lesion of a nerve root or a peripheral nerve. The cutaneous nerve distribution and dermatomes are shown in Figs. 4.12–4.15.

It must be remembered however that there is a great deal of variability from person to person, as well as an overlap between the cutaneous supply of peripheral nerves (Walton, 1989) and dermatome areas (Downs & LaPorte, 2011). Bones may have segmental innervation patterns called sclerotomes, but the evidence for these is extremely poor (Inman & Saunders, 1944; Ivanusic, 2007).

To test sensation, the patient should be in a relaxed and supported position with their skin exposed. The

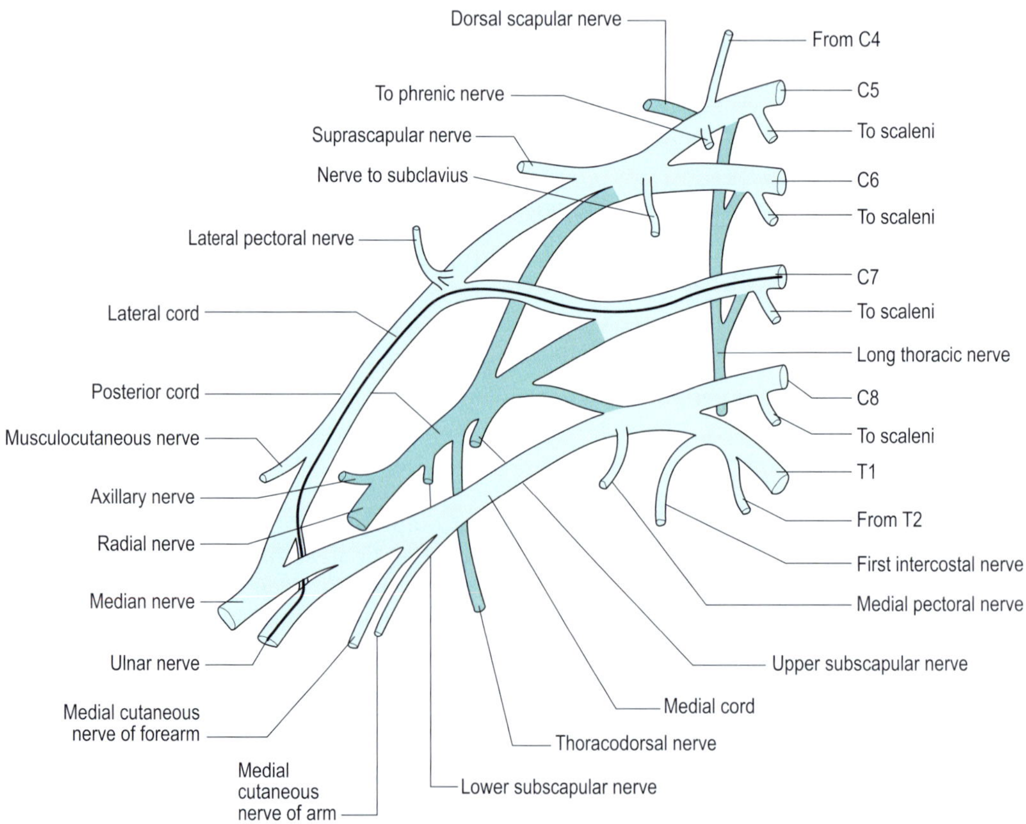

Fig. 4.11 A plan of the brachial plexus showing the nerve roots and the formation of the peripheral nerves. (From Williams et al. 1995, with permission.)

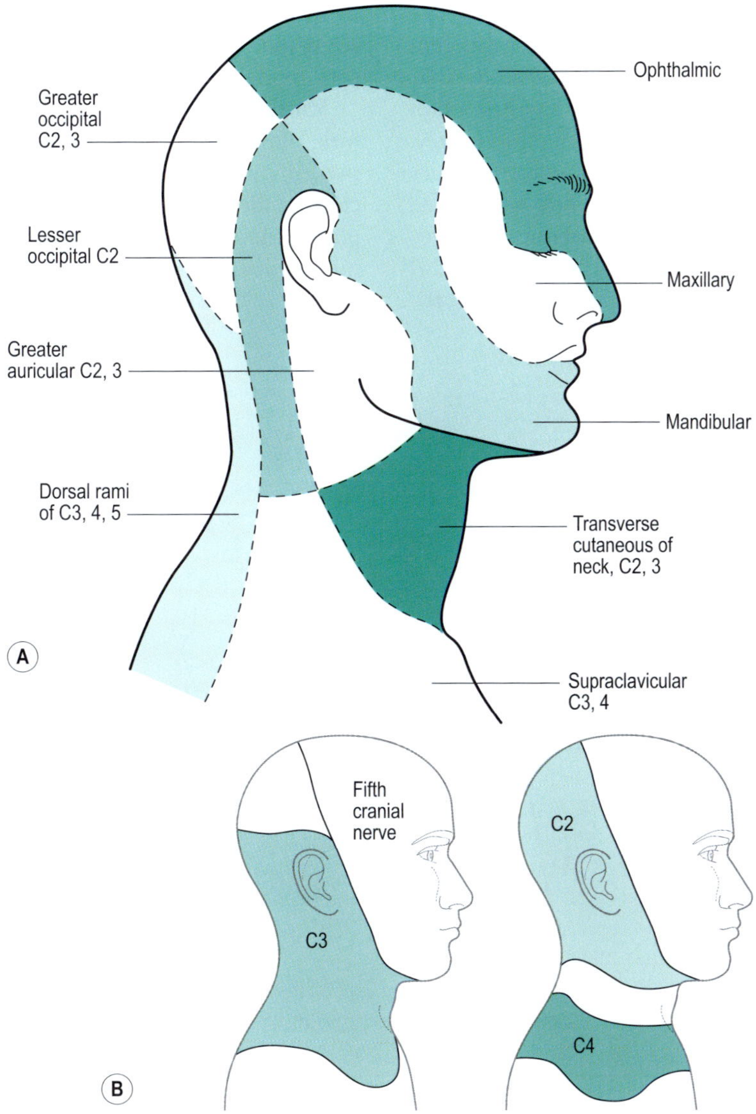

Fig. 4.12 (A) Cutaneous nerve supply to the face, head and neck. (B) Dermatomes of the head and neck. (A, From Williams et al. 1995, with permission. B, Grieve 1981, with permission.)

clinician needs to explain each test and apply it to an unaffected area of the skin first so that the patient knows what to expect and to establish what is normal. There are five aspects of sensation that can be examined (Fuller, 2004; Gardner, 2021; Cook et al., 2022):

1. Light touch: tests patency of Aβ fibres and dorsal column.
2. Vibration: tests patency of Aβ fibres and dorsal column.
3. Joint position sense: tests patency of Aβ fibres and dorsal column.
4. Pinprick: tests patency of Aδ fibres and spinothalamic tract.
5. Temperature: tests patency of Aδ and C fibres, as well as the spinothalamic tract.

Light touch is often tested with cotton wool for consistency. The clinician lightly strokes across the skin of the area being assessed. This is done in a circular motion around the limb, across the dermatomes. The patient is asked whether it feels the same as or different from an unaffected area, for instance, the opposite side. An alternative and graded method of assessment of touch is to use a set of monofilaments (von Frey, Semmes–Weinstein or West), which range from very thin to thick. Each monofilament delivers a specified amount of pressure, so testing is repeatable and provides quantitative information about the loss (or gain) of touch sensation (Hunter, 2002). The clinician needs to identify and map accurately the area of diminished sensation. The next step may be to explore other sensory modalities which may have been affected.

Vibration sense can be tested using a 128 Hz tuning fork. Lower frequencies reduce the chance that the patient can hear the vibration. With the patient's eyes closed, the clinician strikes the tuning fork before placing its flat end on a bony prominence such as the medial malleolus, testing from distal to proximal. The patient is asked to confirm when they feels vibration

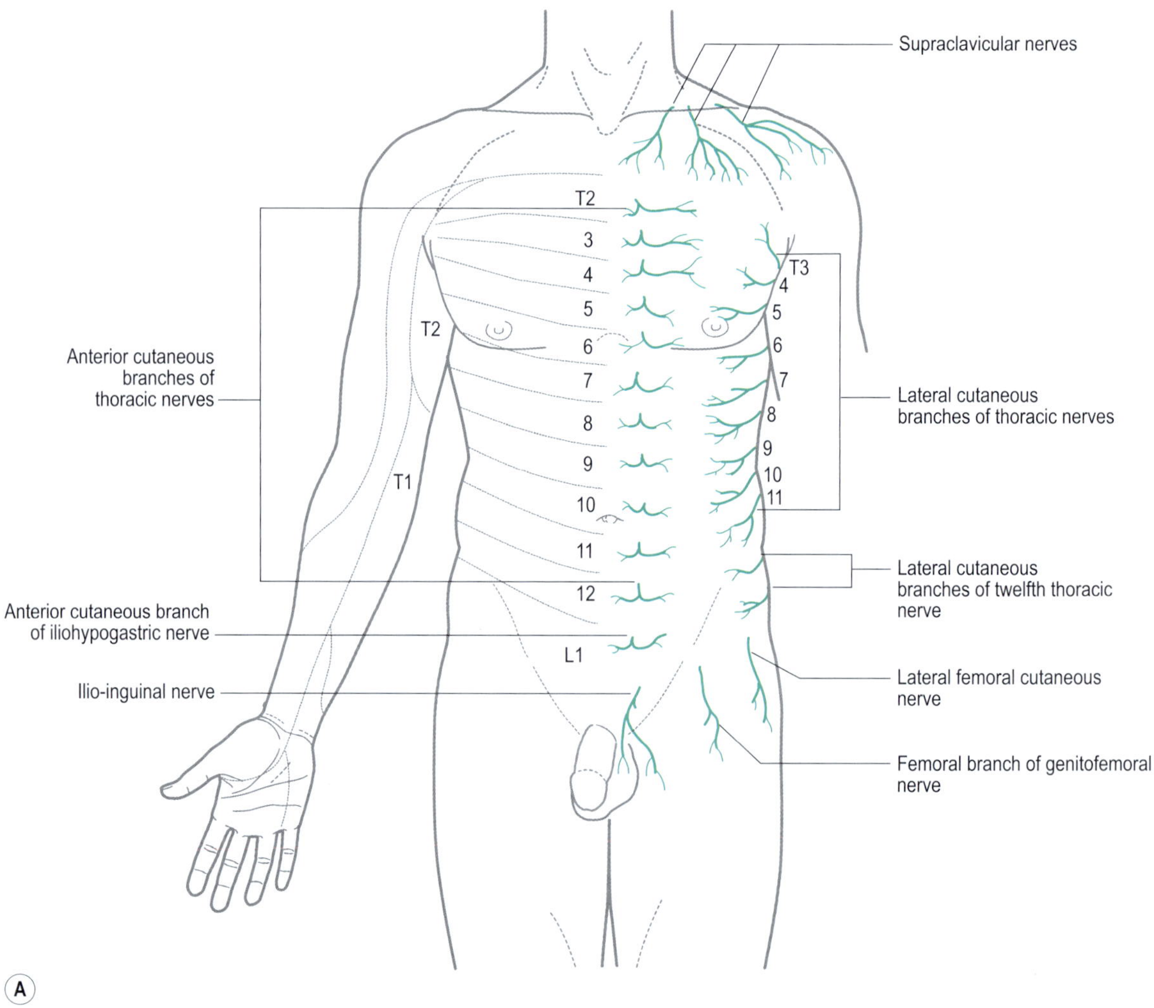

Fig. 4.13 (A) Cutaneous nerve supply to the trunk.

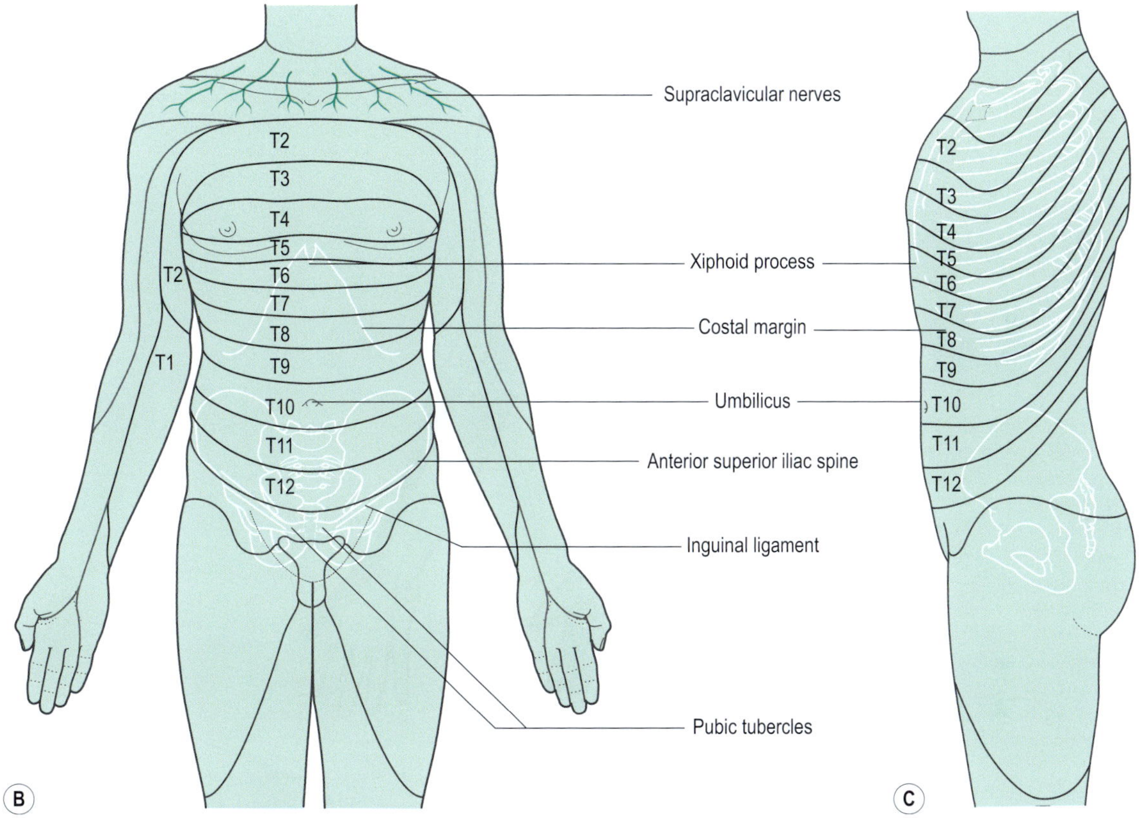

Fig. 4.13, cont'd (B) Anterior view of thoracic dermatomes associated with thoracic spinal nerves. (C) Lateral view of dermatomes associated with thoracic spinal nerves. (A, From Williams et al. 1995, with permission. C, Drake et al., 2005.)

(Leak, 1998; Fuller, 2004). The patient confirms when they can no longer feel the vibration, and the clinician records the time as the *vibration disappearance threshold* (VDT) (O'Connaire et al., 2011). This is compared with the other limb.

Joint proprioception can be tested by asking the patient to close their eyes, positioning their limb and asking them to identify whether it is being moved in a particular direction. Alternatively, the patient can be asked to mirror movement with the other limb. For example, with the patient lying prone the clinician flexes their right knee, and the patient has to copy the movement with their left knee.

Small fibre testing. Sensory integrity tests investigate a reduction in patency of large fibres (Aβ). These fibres mediate touch, vibration and proprioception. However, neuropathic pain and small fibre neuropathy may have their origin in thin nerve fibres (Aδ and C). If these conditions are suspected but the sensory tests above are negative, the clinician can apply the protocol as shown in Fig. 4.16 (Ridehalgh et al., 2018).

Pinprick sensation can be tested with a disposable *neurotip* using a gentle stabbing motion. The patient is told to close their eyes and the clinician touches many areas, moving from distal to proximal with the neurotip and not forgetting the trunk. The patient is asked to confirm when they can feel the sharp sensation.

The simplest way to test **temperature sensation** is with a cool metal object such as a teaspoon and compare it with an identical object at room temperature. The patient is asked to report what they feel. Warmth sensation can be tested with a coin from a trouser pocket.

Areas of sensory abnormality should be documented on the body chart. Mapping an area needs to be accurate, as a change, particularly an enlargement of the

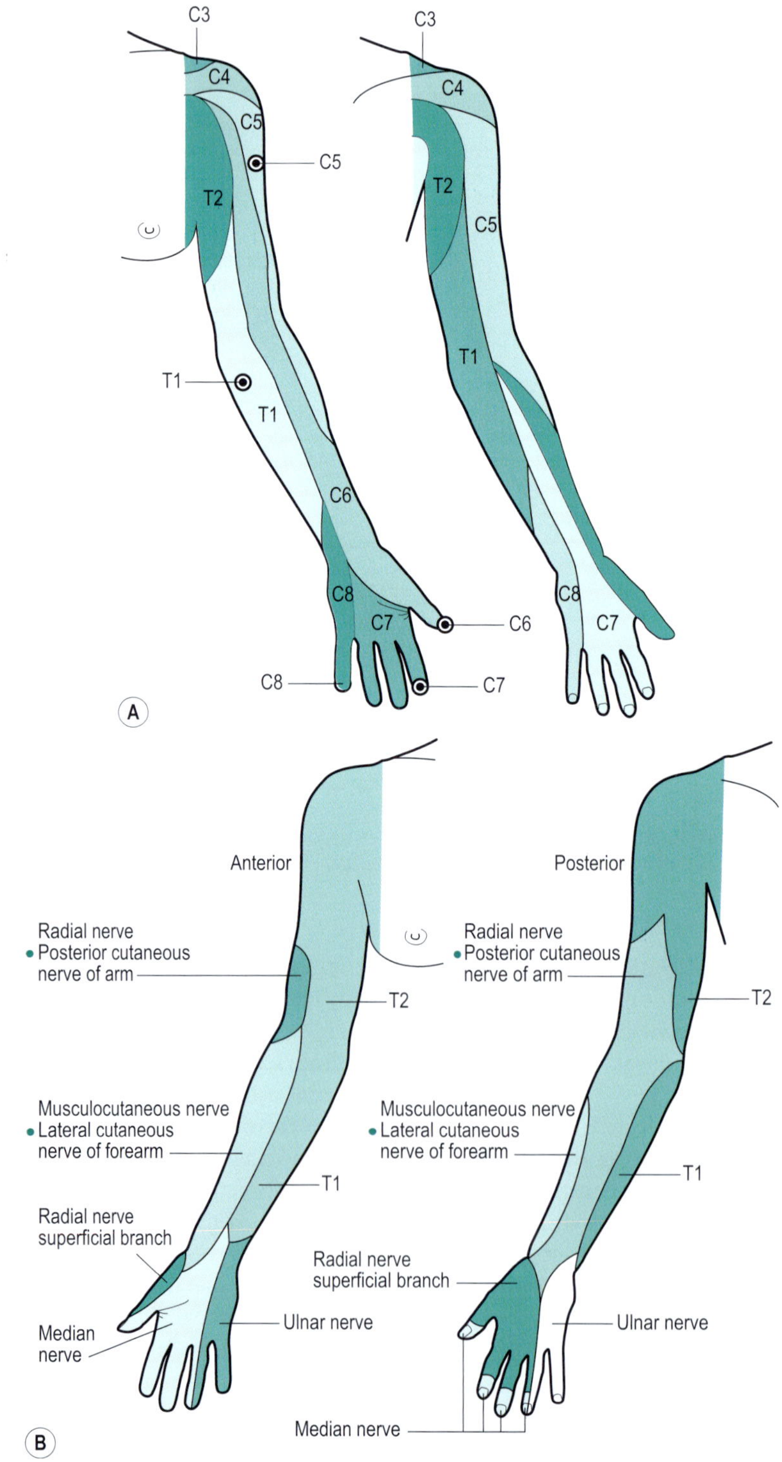

Fig. 4.14 Cutaneous innervation of the upper limbs (A) Nerve roots/Dermatomes Ai Anterior Aii Posterior (B) Peripheral nerves of the upper limb. Bi anterior Bii Posterior. Dots indicate areas of minimal overlap. (From Drake et al., 2005.)

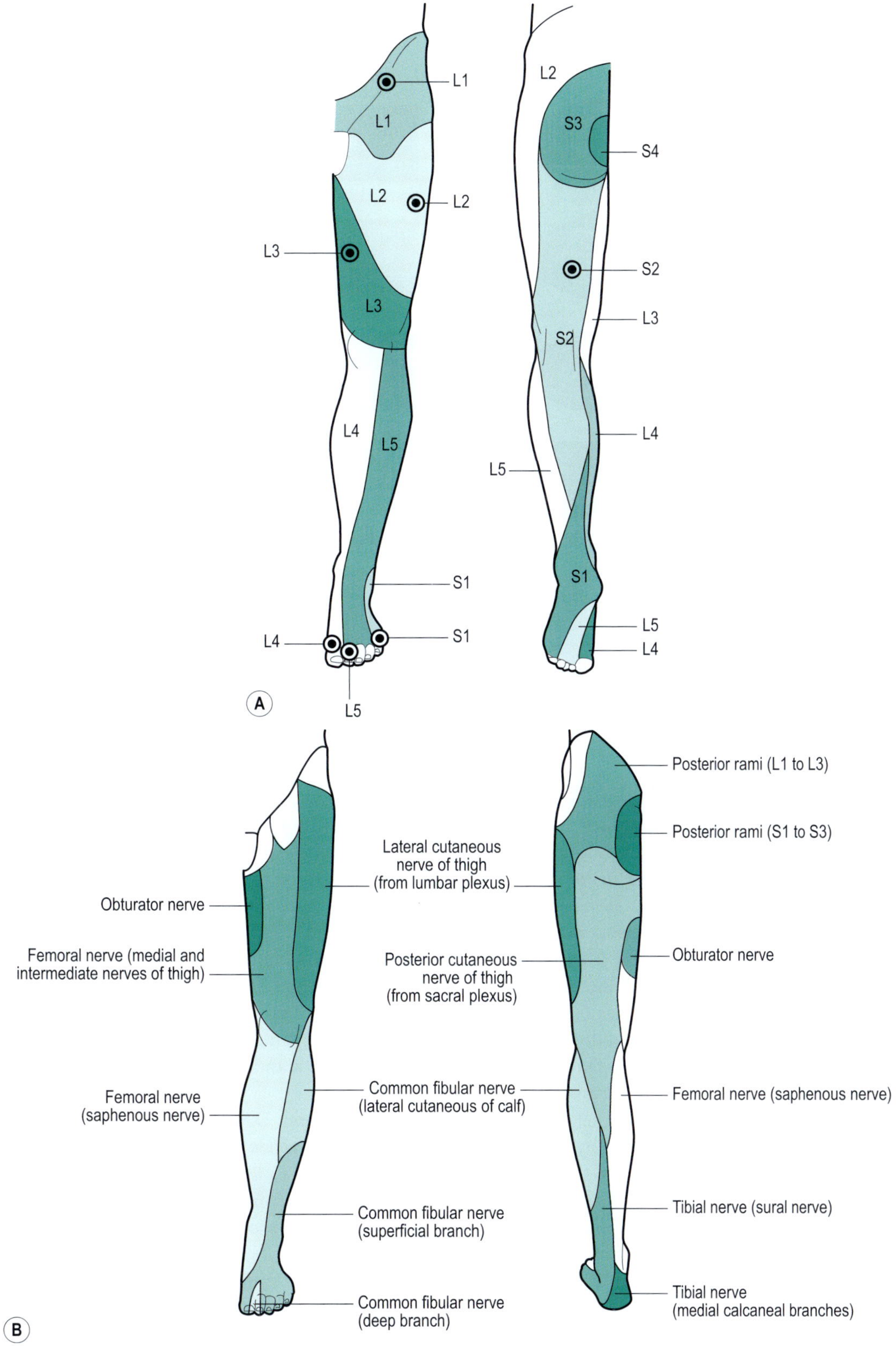

Fig. 4.15 Cutaneous innervation of the lower limbs (A) Nerve roots/Dermatomes Ai Anterior Aii Posterior (B) Peripheral nerves of the lower limb. Bi anterior Bii Posterior. Dots indicate areas of minimal overlap. (From Drake et al., 2005.)

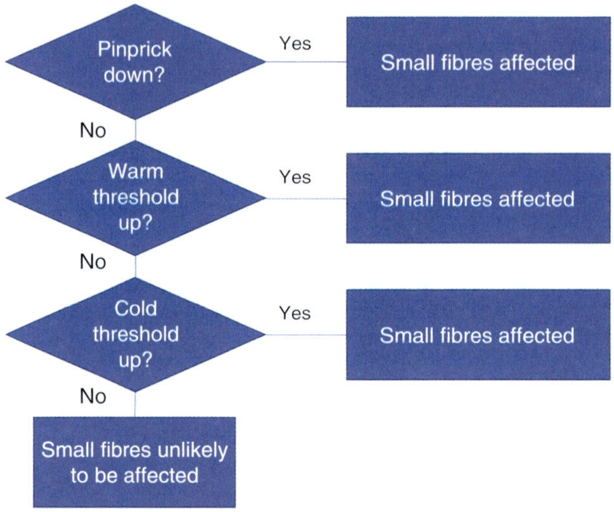

Fig. 4.16 Protocol for confirming small nerve fiber degeneration.

affected area, indicates a worsening neurological state and may require the patient to be referred to a medical practitioner. For this reason, sensation is often reassessed at each appointment, until it is established that the altered sensation is stable.

Motor changes. A loss of muscle strength is indicative of either a lesion of the motor neurones in the peripheral or central nervous system or a lesion of the muscle itself. If the lesion occurs at the nerve root, then any of the muscles supplied by the nerve root (the myotome) can be affected. If the lesion occurs in a peripheral nerve, then the muscles that it supplies can be affected. A working knowledge of the nerves and nerve roots supplying specific muscles enables the clinician to differentiate between motor loss due to a root lesion and a peripheral nerve lesion. The peripheral nerve distribution and myotomes are shown in Table 4.8 and Figs. 4.17–4.19. It should be noted that most muscles in the limbs are innervated by more than one nerve root (myotome) and that only the predominant segmental origin is given.

Motor nerve impairment will lead to muscle atrophy and weakness over time, e.g. in the thenar eminence due to median nerve entrapment in carpal tunnel syndrome.

Muscle strength testing consists of an isometric contraction of a muscle group for a few seconds. The patient must be in a supported position to minimize compensatory strategies. The muscle is placed in mid-position, and the patient is asked to hold the position against the resistance of the clinician. The resistance is applied slowly and smoothly to enable the patient to give the necessary resistance. The amount of force applied must be appropriate to the specific muscle group and the patient. Myotome testing is shown in Figs. 4.20 and 4.21. If a peripheral nerve lesion is suspected, the clinician may test the strength of individual muscles supplied by the nerve using the MRC scale mentioned earlier. Further details of peripheral nerve injuries are beyond the scope of this text, but they can be found in standard orthopaedic and neurological textbooks.

Reflex changes. Deep tendon reflexes test the integrity of the spinal reflex arc consisting of an afferent or sensory neurone, an efferent or motor neurone and spinal cord neurons that connect these. Reflexes test individual nerve roots and spinal cord levels, as shown in Table 4.8.

Deep tendon reflexes are elicited by tapping the tendon a few times. The commonly used deep tendon

TABLE 4.8 Myotomes

Root	Joint Action	Reflex
V cranial (trigeminal N)	Clench teeth, note temporalis and masseter muscles	Jaw
VII cranial (facial N)	Wrinkle forehead, close eyes, purse lips, show teeth	
XI cranial (accessory N)	Shoulder girdle elevation and sternocleidomastoid	
C1	Upper cervical flexion	
C2	Upper cervical extension	
C3	Cervical lateral flexion	
C4	Shoulder girdle elevation	
C5	Shoulder abduction	Biceps jerk
C6	Elbow flexion	Biceps jerk
C7	Elbow extension	Triceps jerk and brachioradialis
C8	Thumb extension; finger flexion	
T1	Finger abduction and adduction	
T2–T1	No muscle test or reflex	
L2	Hip flexion	
L3	Knee extension	Knee jerk
L4	Foot dorsiflexion	Knee jerk
L5	Extension of the big toe	
S1	Eversion of the foot Contract buttock Knee flexion	Ankle jerk
S2	Knee flexion	
Toe Standing		
S3–S4	Muscles of pelvic floor, bladder and genital function	

Grieve (1991).

reflexes are the biceps brachii, triceps, patellar and tendo calcaneus (Fig. 4.22).

The reflex response may be graded and recorded as follows:

— or 0: absent
— or 1: diminished
+ or 2: average
++ or 3: exaggerated
+++ or 4: clonus.

If a reflex is difficult to elicit then the clinician can test again using the *reinforcement Jendrassik manoeuvre*, which will facilitate motor neurone activity in the spinal cord. For example, for upper limb testing ask the patient to clench their jaw, or for lower limbs ask the patient to lock their hands together, and try to pull them apart just before the tendon is struck.

A diminished reflex response can occur if there is a lesion of the sensory and/or motor pathways. Reflexes are commonly decreased in the elderly.

Reflex changes alone, without sensory or motor changes, do not necessarily indicate nerve root involvement. For example, ankle reflexes can be abolished by injection of the zygapophyseal joints with hypertonic saline and restored by a steroid injection, illustrating that pain can alter reflexes (Mooney & Robertson, 1976). For this reason, reflex changes alone may not be a relevant clinical finding.

An exaggerated reflex response suggests an upper motor lesion such as multiple sclerosis. This should prompt further UMN testing, but it should also be realized that all tendon reflexes can be exaggerated by tension and anxiety.

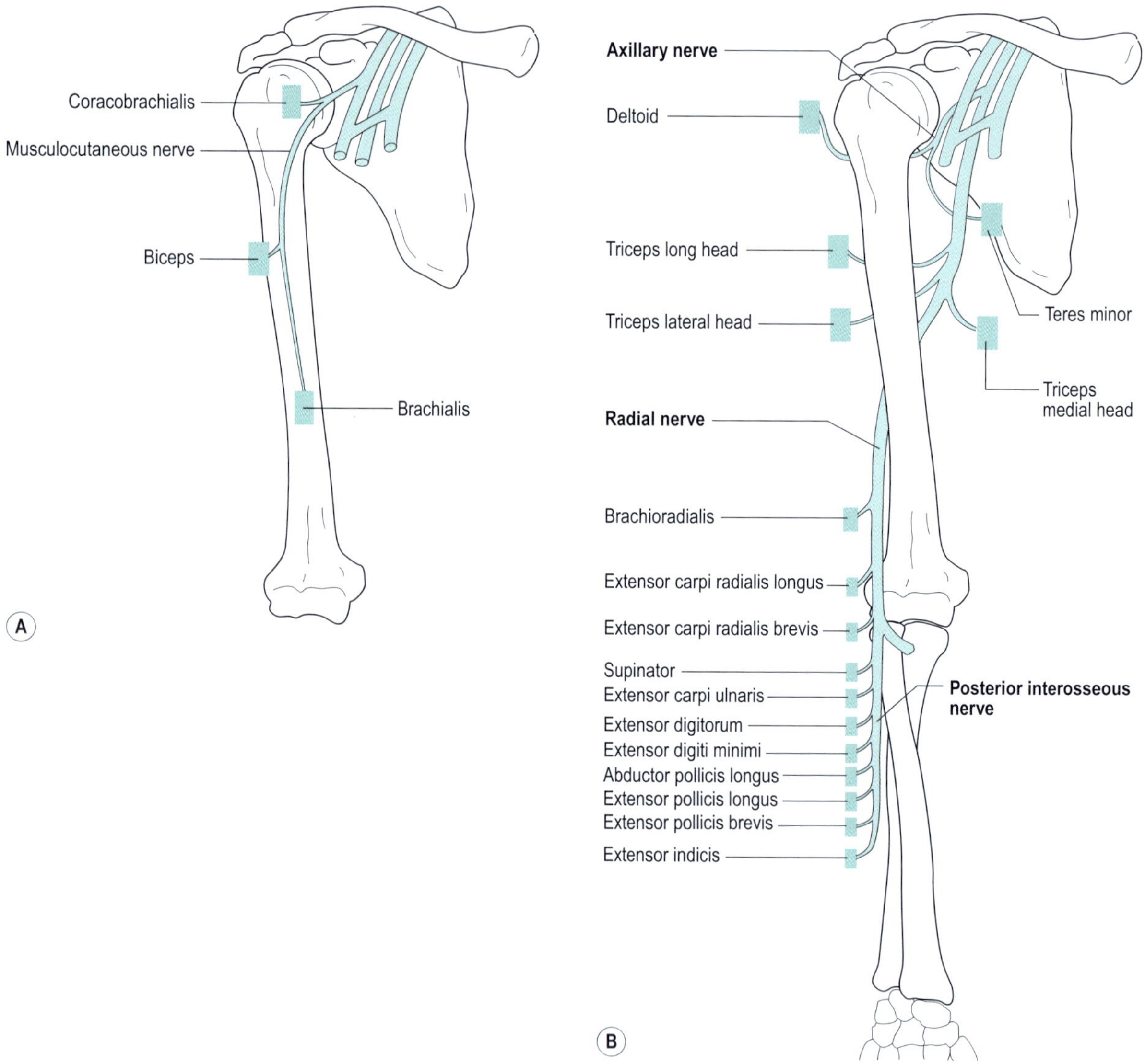

Fig. 4.17 The musculocutaneous (A), axillary and radial (B) nerves of the upper limb and the muscles that each supplies. (Medical Research Council 1976. Aids to the investigation of peripheral nerve injuries. HMSO, London. Reproduced with kind permission of the Medical Research Council.)

If an UMN lesion is suspected, the plantar response should also be tested. This is the most valid test for early detection of UMN lesions. This involves stroking the lateral plantar aspect of the foot and observing the movement of the toes. The normal response is for all the toes to flex, while an abnormal response consists of the extension of the great toe and abduction of the remaining toes, which is known as the extensor or Babinski response (Fig. 4.23).

Clonus is associated with exaggerated reflexes and is characterized by rapid, strong oscillating muscular contractions produced by sustained stretching of a muscle. It is most commonly tested in the lower limb, where the clinician sharply dorsiflexes the

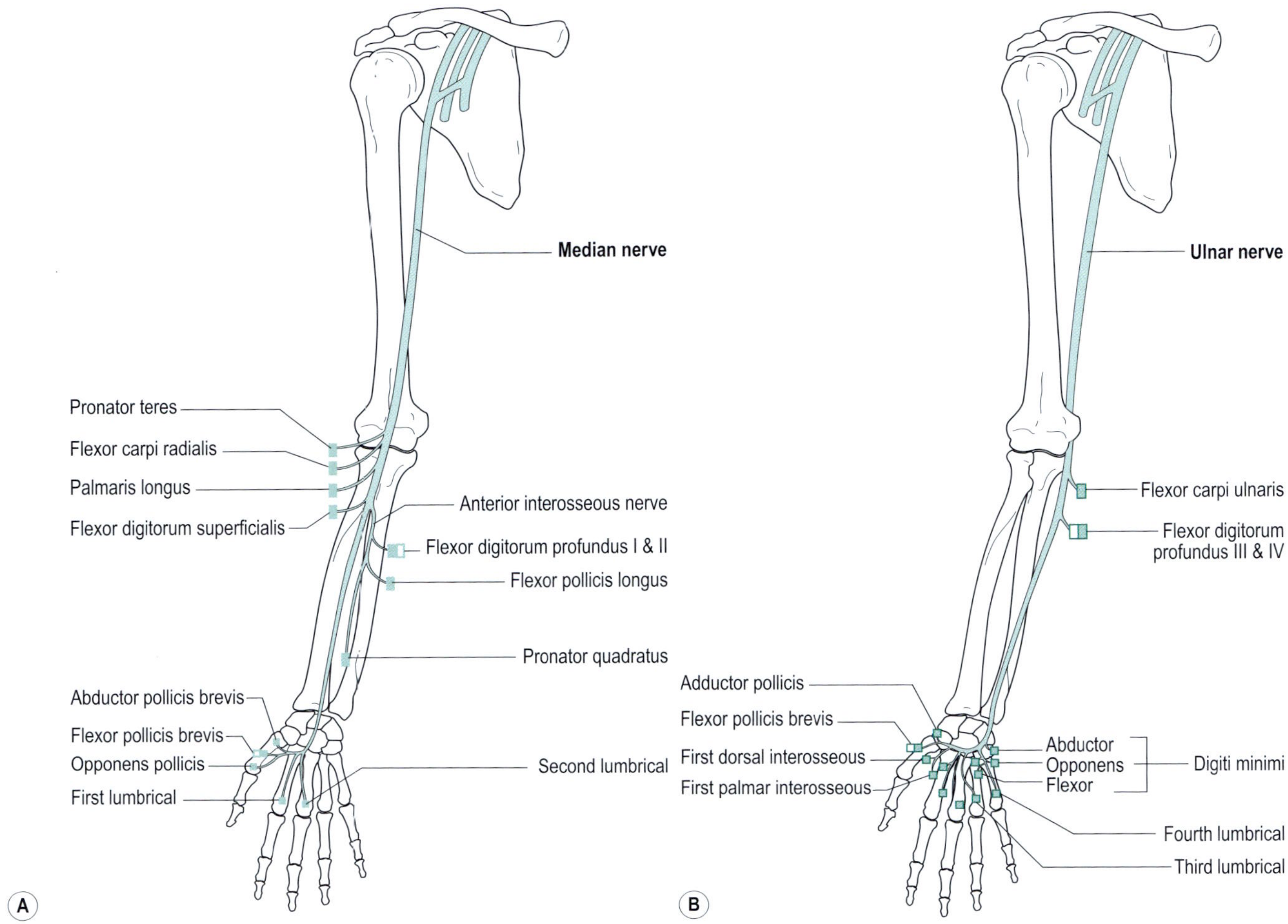

Fig. 4.18 Diagram of the (A) median and (B) ulnar nerves of the upper limb and the muscles that each supplies. (Medical Research Council 1976. Aids to the investigation of peripheral nerve injuries. HMSO, London. Reproduced with kind permission of the Medical Research Council.)

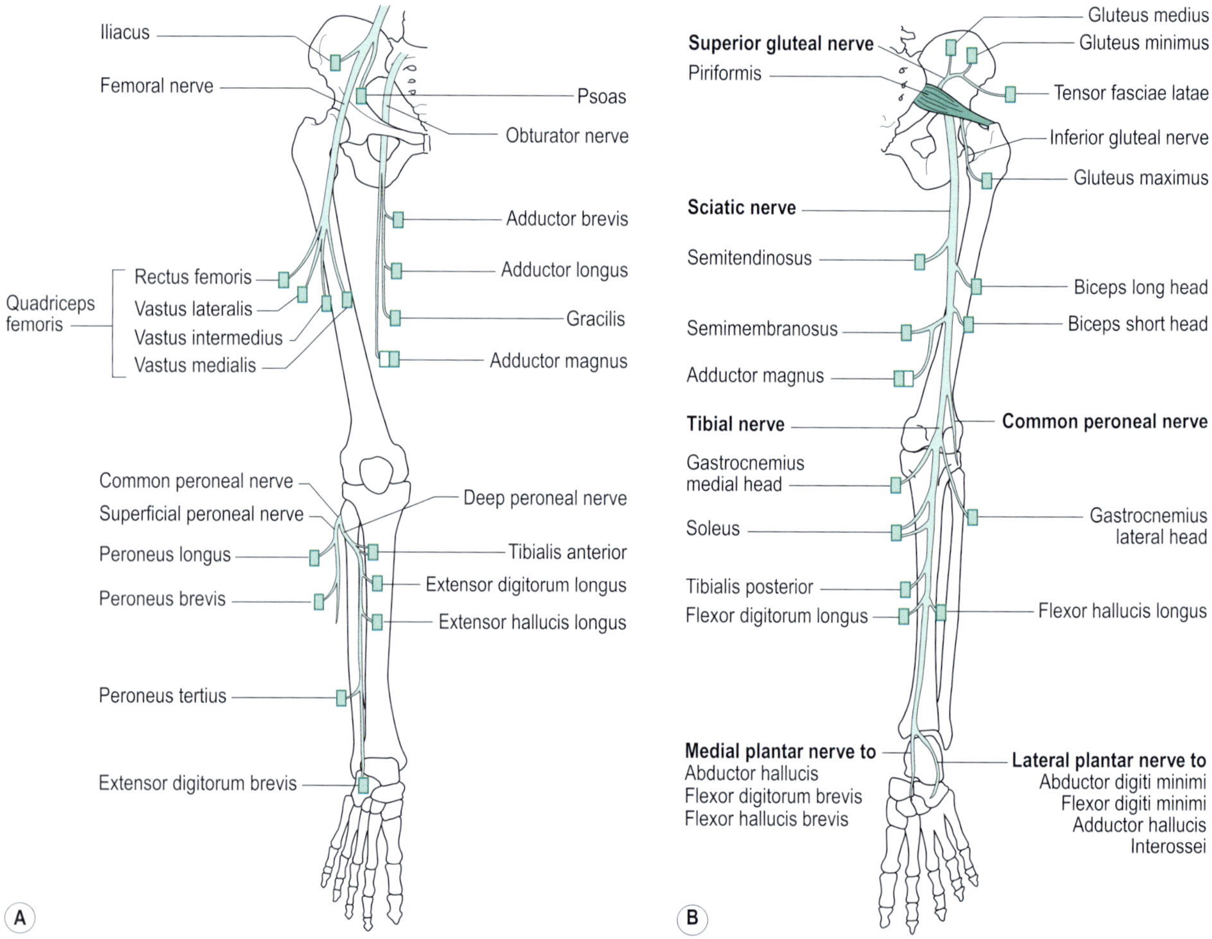

Fig. 4.19 Diagram of the nerves on the anterior (A) and posterior (B) aspects of the lower limb and the muscles that they supply. (Medical Research Council 1976. Aids to the investigation of peripheral nerve injuries. HMSO, London. Reproduced with kind permission of the Medical Research Council.)

patient's foot with the patient's knee semi-flexed and supported.

Additionally, tone defined as resistance to movement can be tested. Rigidity and spasticity indicating UMN involvement can be reliably screened using two quick upper limb tests:

- Wrist: Hold the patient's wrist with one hand and circumduct their hand (Donaghy, 1997).
- Pronator catch: From a pronated position abruptly supinate the patient's wrist (Donaghy, 1997).

Coordination. Quick screening tests include finger to nose for the upper limb and heel/shin test for the lower limb assessing for tremor, overshooting and 'trick' movements (Fig. 4.24).

KNOWLEDGE CHECK

1. What presenting symptoms in a patient's history might implicate a neural origin?
2. What is the difference between neural integrity and neural sensitivity? Can you offer examples?
3. How can you test for suspected upper motor neuron lesion (UMNL)?

Neural Sensitization Tests

Mechanosensitivity of the sensory nervous system is examined by carrying out neurodynamic tests (Butler, 2000). Some of these tests have been known for over 100 years (Dyck, 1984), but they have been an integral

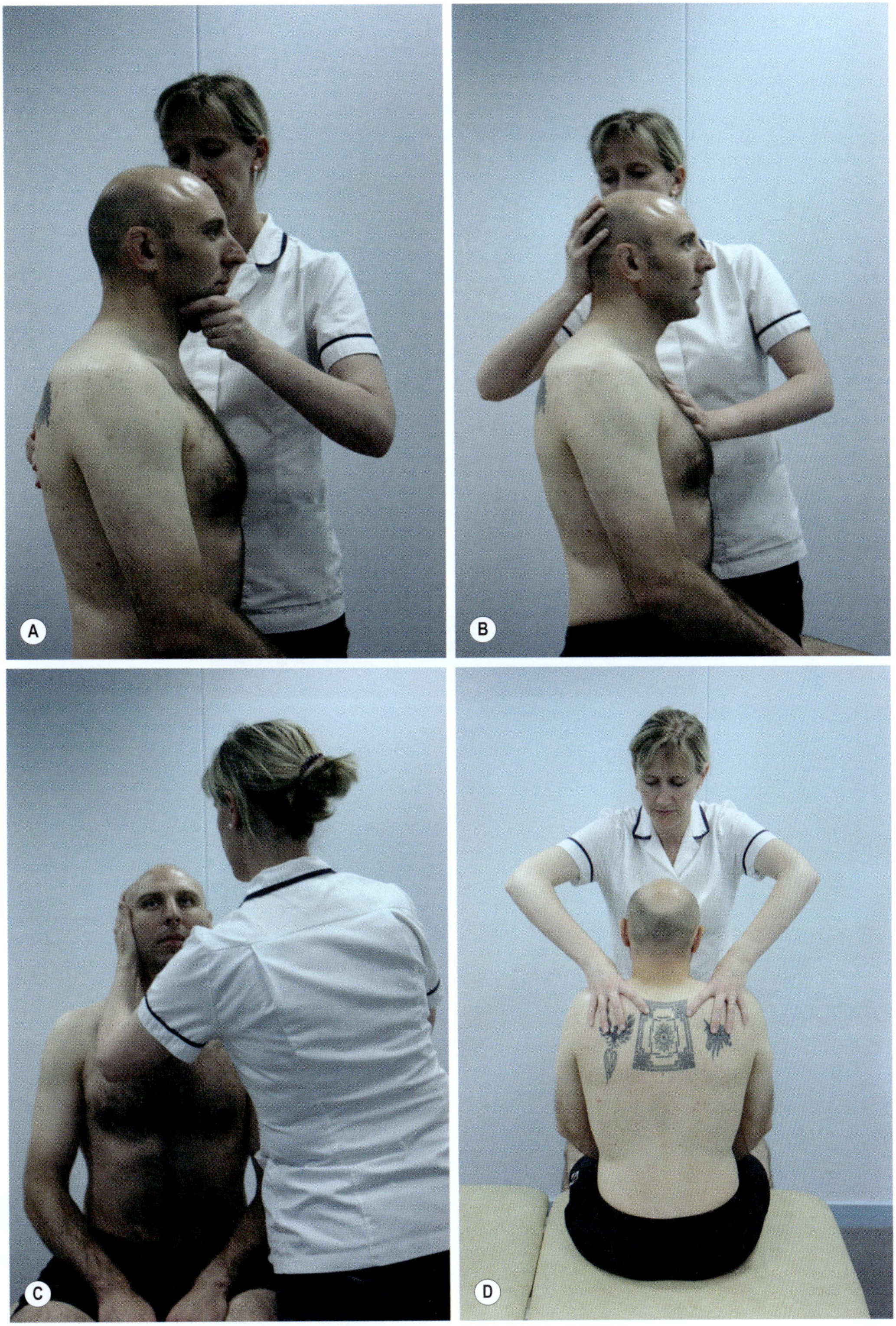

Fig. 4.20 Myotome testing for the cervical and upper thoracic nerve roots. The patient is asked to hold the position against the force applied by the clinician. (A) C1, Upper cervical flexion. (B) C2, Upper cervical extension. (C) C3, Cervical lateral flexion. (D) C4, Shoulder girdle elevation.

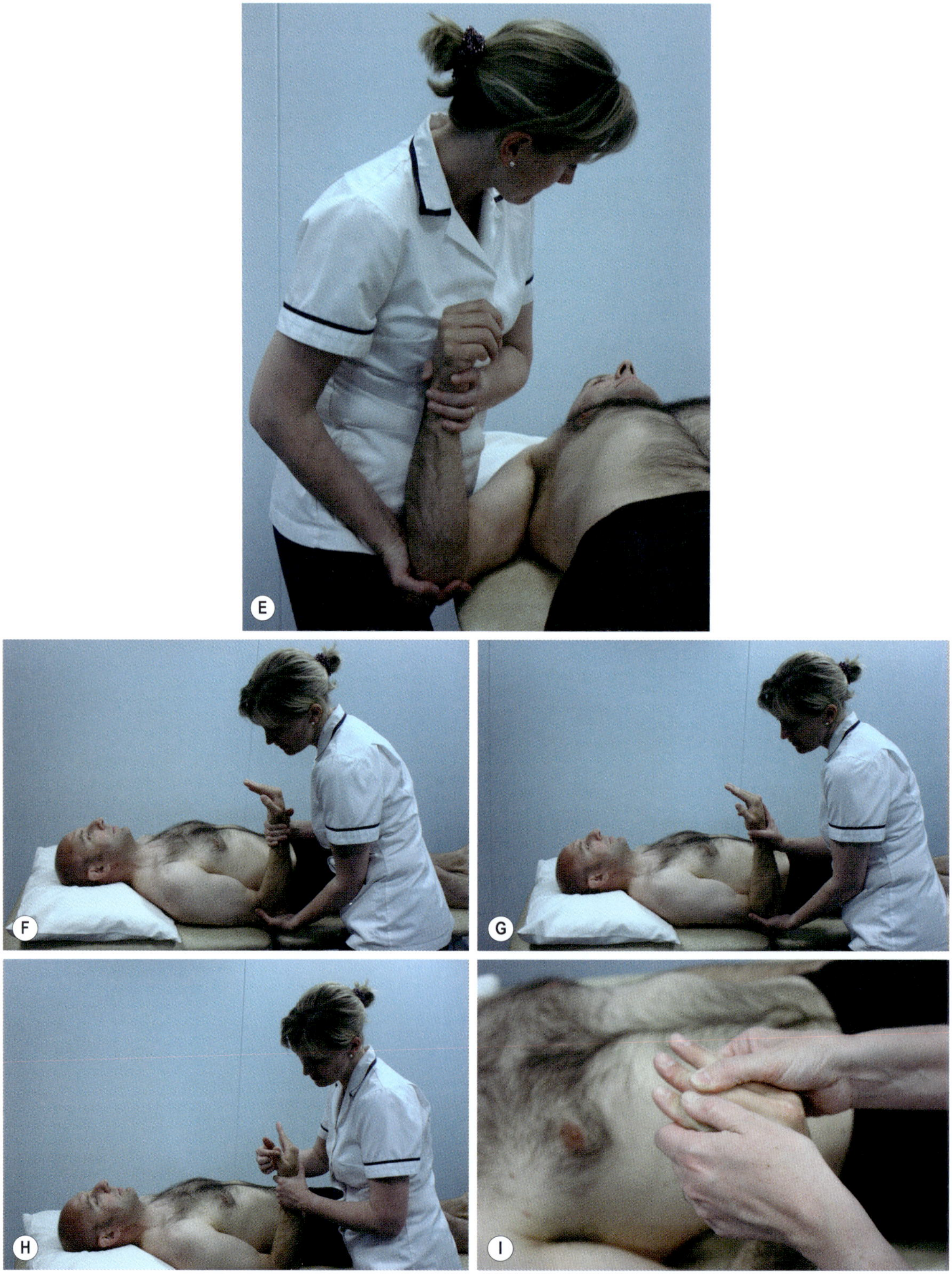

Fig. 4.20, cont'd (E) C5, Shoulder abduction. (F) C6, Elbow flexion. (G) C7, Elbow extension. (H) C8, Thumb extension. (I) T1, Finger adduction.

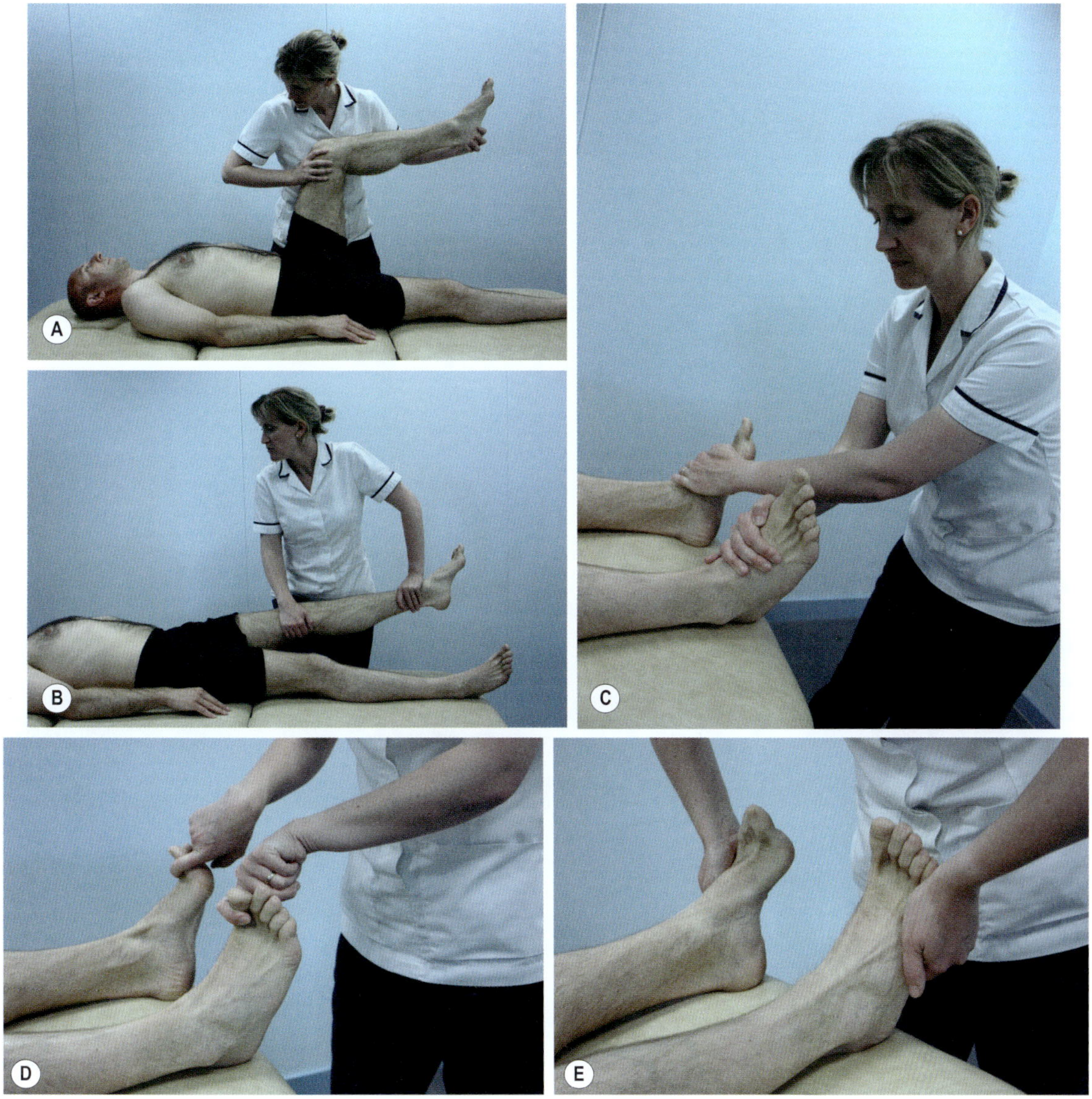

Fig. 4.21 Myotome testing for the lumbar and sacral nerve roots. (A) L2, Hip flexion. (B) L3, Knee extension. (C) L4, Foot dorsiflexion. (D) L5, Extension of the big toe. (E) S1, Foot eversion.

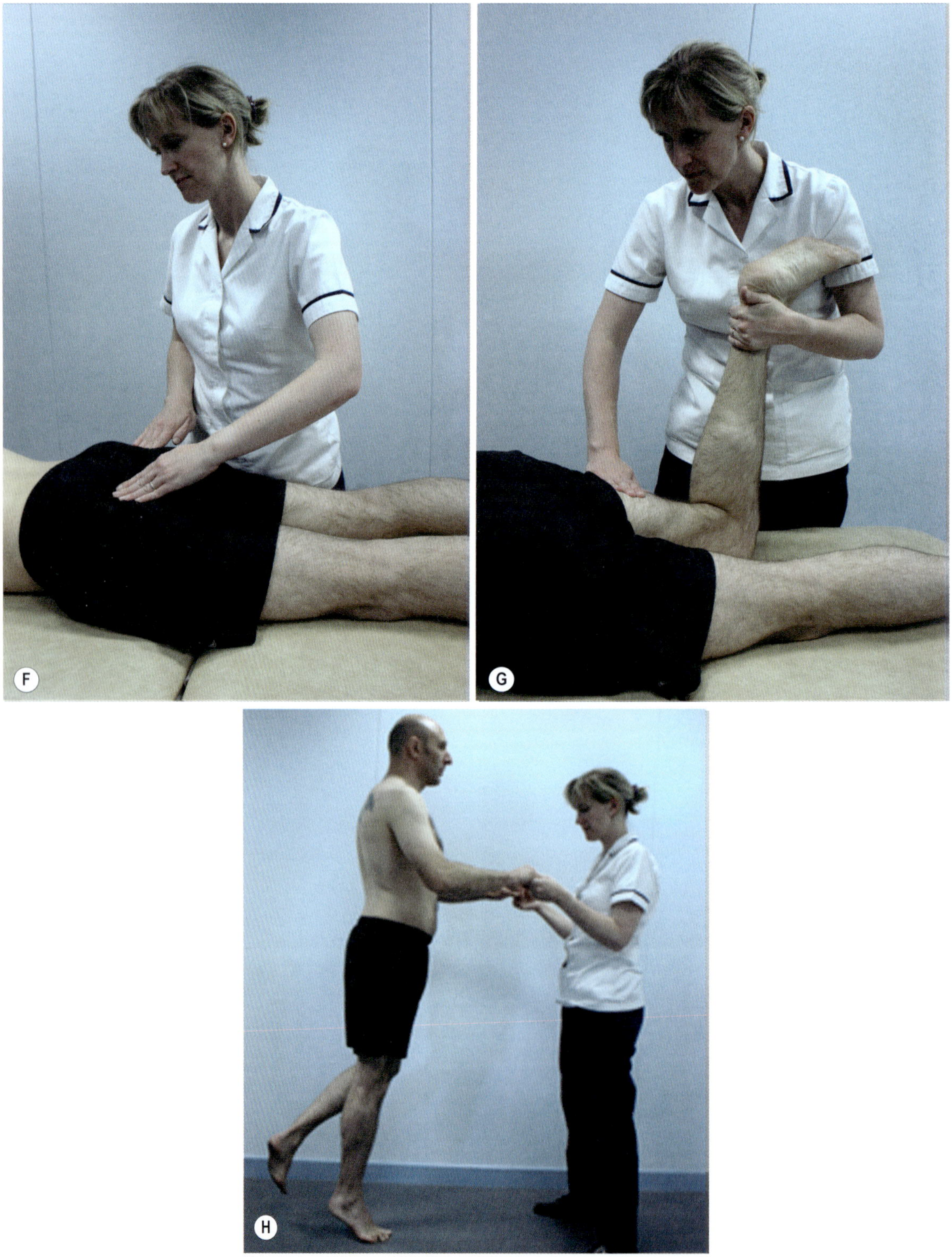

Fig. 4.21, cont'd (F) S1, Contract buttock. (G) S1 and S2, Knee flexion. (H) S2, Toe standing.

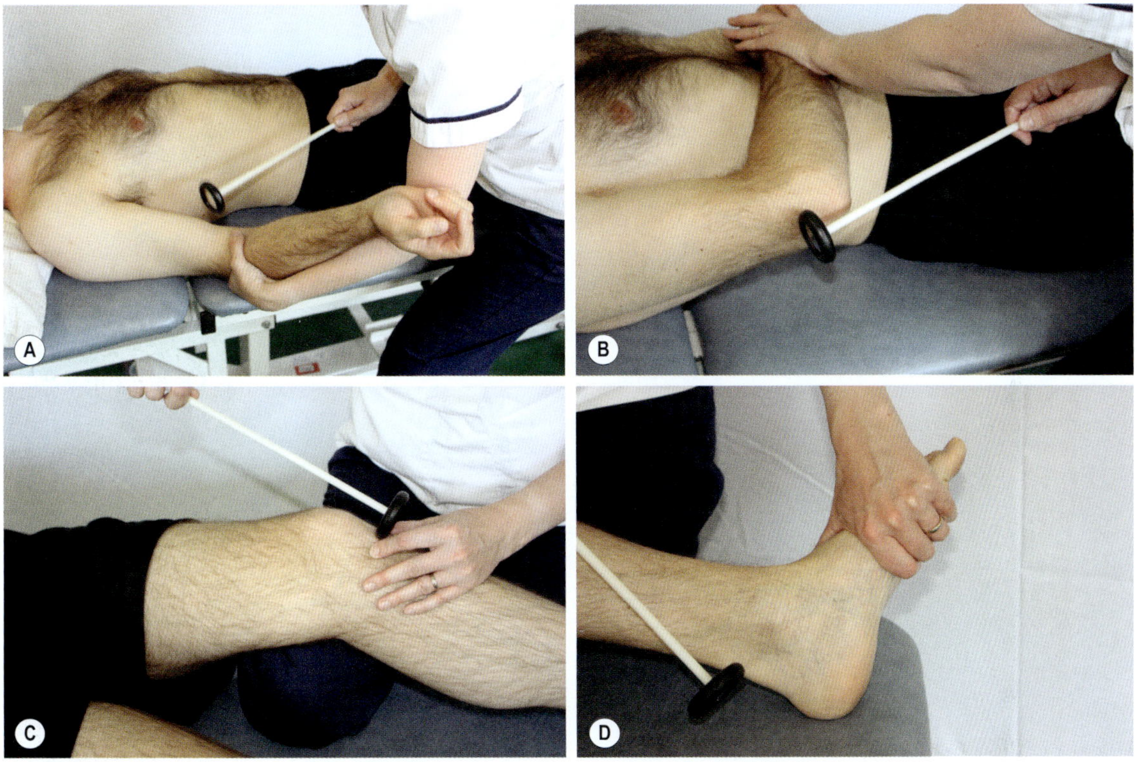

Fig. 4.22 Reflex testing. (A) Biceps jerk (C5 and C6). (B) Triceps jerk (C7). (C) Knee jerk (L3 and L4). (D) Ankle jerk (S1).

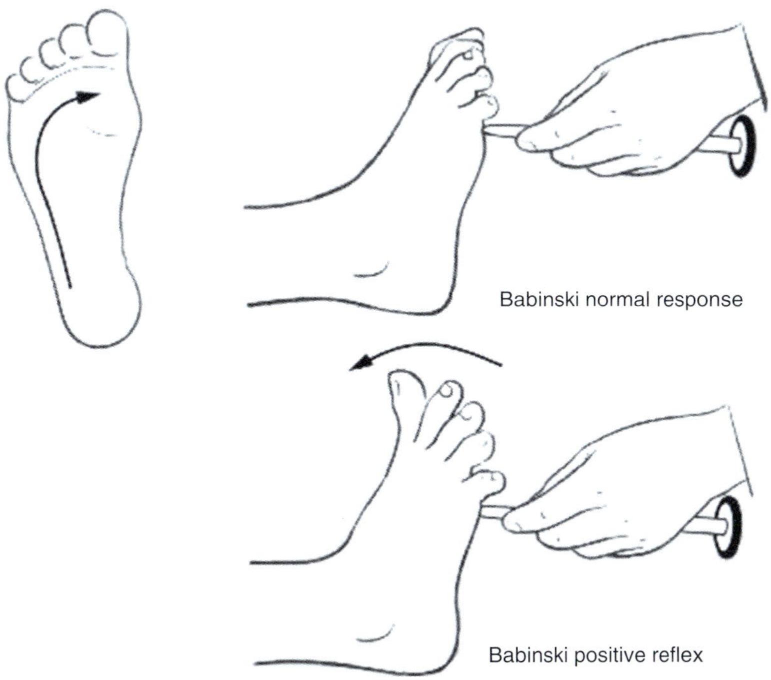

Fig. 4.23 Babinski's (plantar) reflex. (Moini, 2020).

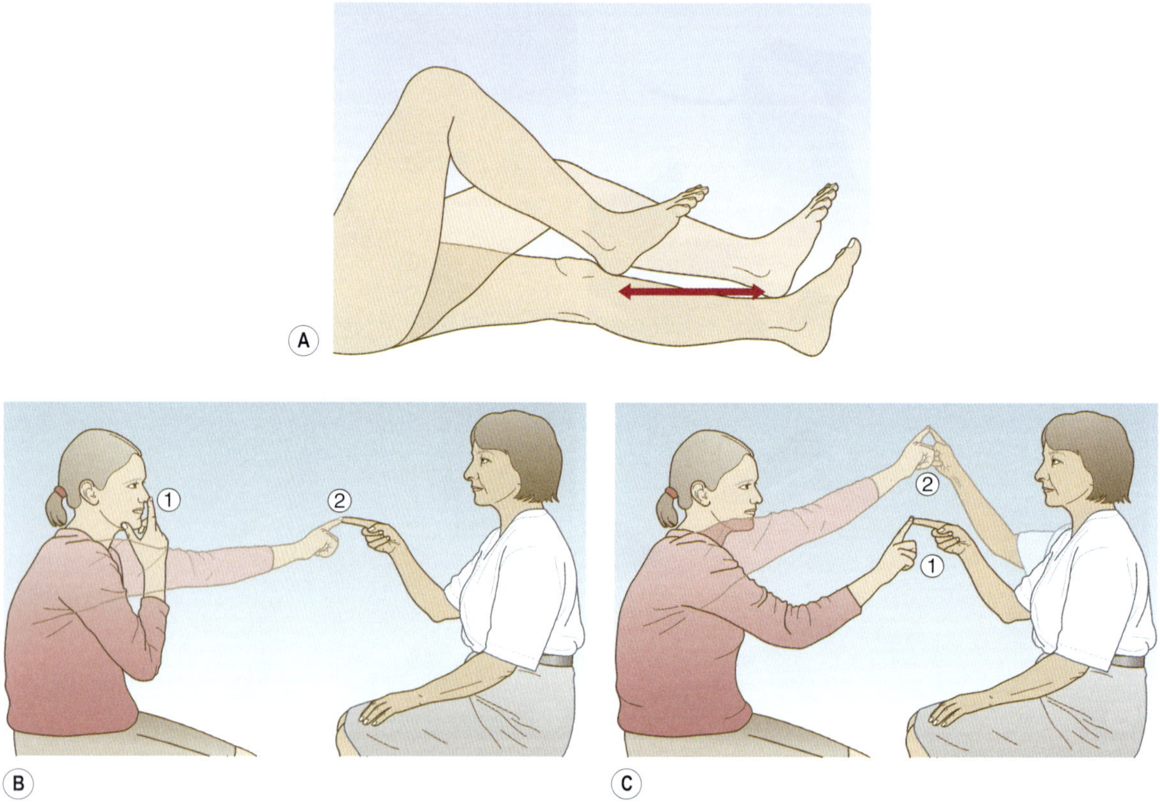

Fig. 4.24 Coordination Screening tests: (A) heel to shin; (B) finger-nose-finger test; (C) examiner moving the target finger. (1) Elbow flexed; (2) elbow extended. (Porter, 2021)

part of physiotherapy assessment for the last 30 years (Elvey, 1985; Butler, 2000). Research is ongoing in further understanding and refining the tests (Coppieters & Nee, 2015; Ridehalgh et al., 2015). A summary of the tests is given here, but details of their theoretical justification and how they are performed can be found in Butler (2000) and Shacklock (2005). In addition to the sensitization tests described here, the clinician can palpate peripheral nerves with and without the nerves being under tension; details are given under palpation in relevant chapters. Other common tests of mechanosensitivity of peripheral nerves include percussion (Tinel's sign) and compression such as Phalen's test, which will be covered in regional chapters where relevant.

Neurodynamic tests assess the presence of mechanosensitivity by applying tension to specific parts of the nervous system. By increasing and reducing tension at different points along peripheral nerves and the spinal cord and noting changes in symptoms, the clinician reasons whether mechanosensitivity may be present and in which neural structures.

Baseline neural integrity tests should be done prior to applying neurodynamic tests. Neurodynamic testing procedures follow the same format as those of joint movement, i.e. resting symptoms are established prior to any test and the following information is noted:

- Quality of movement.
- Range of movement.
- Resistance through the range and at the end of the range.
- Pain and pain location through the range.

Testing Principles

The following testing principles apply:

- As with all examination techniques, the tests selected should be justified and interpreted through sound clinical reasoning.

- Carefully note symptom response including the area and nature of the symptoms (Butler, 2000). The results are compared with the opposite side. The unaffected side is tested first.
- A positive test must reproduce at least part of the patient's symptoms.
- *Structural differentiation.* A test cannot be regarded as positive unless there is at least one joint between the symptomatic area and the joint that is moved to tension or offload the nerve(s). For example, upper arm symptoms may respond to changes in elbow position for a number of reasons. However, if they respond to extension in the wrist or side flexion of the cervical spine, they are suggestive of mechanosensitivity. Changing the testing position of the upper limb may suggest whether one, some or all of the peripheral nerves in the upper arm may be involved.
- Consistency. For a test to be positive, the response to structural differentiation to a specific part of the nervous system must be consistent. It is therefore important that the clinician is consistent in their application of the techniques (e.g. pillow under the neck).
- Tensioning sequence. A positive test should identify the same neural structure, independent of the order in which tension is applied (Nee et al., 2010). In the example above, tension could be built up from proximal to distal or vice versa.

The clinician should guard against false positive findings by bearing in mind that:

- It is important to not just hunt **for** symptoms, but rather to handle the limb with care, feeling for **tissue resistance** (Butler, 2000).
- Normal values for mechanosensitivity are not available (Nee et al., 2010).
- Most asymptomatic people get sensations at the end of the range of a neurodynamic test, such as stretch, aching, pain, burning and tingling (Walsh et al., 2007; Boyd, 2012; Martínez et al., 2014).
- Asymptomatic people vary considerably in their range of movement in neurodynamic tests (Herrington et al., 2008; Martínez et al., 2014).
- An asymmetry of 5%—10% in a neurodynamic range of movement may be normal (Boyd & Villa, 2012; Covill & Peterson, 2012).

In very sensitive and acute disorders it will not be necessary to perform the entire test. For example, if severe leg pain does not allow the patient to lie flat, the clinician can flex the opposite knee before testing the SLR, allowing a little more lateral migration of neural tissue in the spinal and IV canals (Butler, 2000).

The purpose of the test is explained to the patient and the patient is asked to tell the clinician what they feel during the test. Continuous monitoring of symptoms throughout the test is crucial to obtain useful subjective data. Single movements in one plane are slowly added, gradually taking the upper or lower limb through a sequence of movements. The order of the test movements will influence the tissue response (Coppieters et al., 2006). For example, in a chronic ankle sprain with a possible peroneal nerve component, plantar flexion and inversion may be applied first, before adding SLR with additional sensitizers at the hip. If the symptoms are very irritable, adding local components first may prove to be too provocative. Consistency in sequencing at each time of testing is essential. Each movement is added slowly and carefully. In order for a test to be valid, all other body parts are kept still. The clinician monitors the patient's symptoms continuously. If the patient's symptoms are reproduced then the clinician moves a part of the spine or limb that is at least one joint removed from the symptomatic area, in order to:

- Increase the tension on the affected part of the nervous system (sensitizing movement or tensioner technique),
- Decrease the tension (desensitizing movement).
- Examine the nerve's relationship with its interface and its ability to 'slide'.

The clinician may consider a test positive if a desensitizing movement eases the patient's symptoms. For example, shoulder abduction, lateral rotation and elbow extension may reproduce forearm pain in a patient. If shoulder girdle elevation reduces forearm symptoms this is a positive test suggesting a neurodynamic component.

The following may be included in neurodynamic testing:

- Passive neck flexion.
- Straight Leg Raise (SLR).
- Prone knee bend (PKB).
- Femoral nerve slump test.
- Saphenous nerve test.
- Slump.
- Obturator nerve test.
- Upper limb neurodynamic tests (ULNT) 1, 2a, 2b and 3.

Passive neck flexion. In the supine position, the neck is flexed passively by the clinician (Fig. 4.25). The

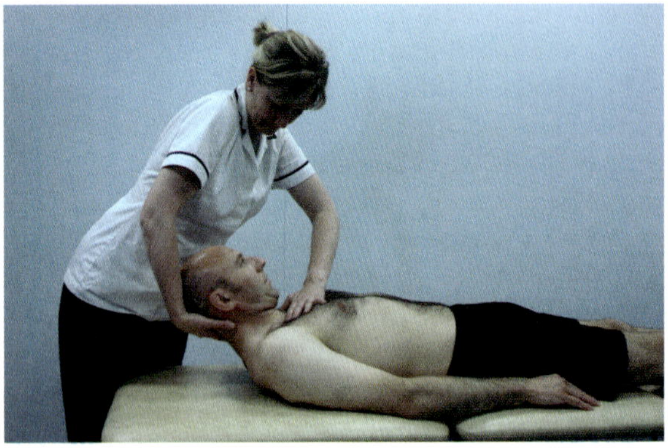

Fig. 4.25 Passive neck flexion.

normal response is a pain-free full-range movement. Sensitizing tests include the SLR or one of the ULNTs. Where symptoms are related to cervical extension, investigation of passive neck extension is necessary. Passive neck flexion is relevant because it produces movement and tension of the spinal cord and meninges of the lumbar spine and of the sciatic nerve (Breig, 1978; Tencer et al., 1985).

Straight leg raise. The SLR moves and tensions the nervous system (including the sympathetic trunk) from the foot to the brain (Breig, 1978).

The patient lies supine for this test. The way in which the SLR is carried out depends on where the patient's symptoms are. The component movements of the tests to bias the sciatic nerve are hip flexion, knee extension, hip adduction and hip medial rotation. The foot can be moved into any position, but ankle dorsiflexion/forefoot eversion sensitizes the tibial nerve, ankle plantarflexion/forefoot inversion the common peroneal nerve and dorsiflexion/inversion the sural nerve. Additional movements of the forefoot can bias the medial and lateral plantar nerves, which may be useful if symptoms are in the foot (Alshami et al., 2008). Neck flexion can be added to affect the spinal cord, meninges and sciatic nerve. Trunk lateral flexion may also be used, to lengthen the spinal cord on the contralateral side.

The normal response to hip flexion/adduction/medial rotation with knee extension and foot dorsiflexion is a strong feeling of tension or tingling in the posterior thigh, posterior knee, and posterior calf and foot (Miller, 1987; Slater, 1994). The clinician identifies what is normal for individual patients by comparing both limbs (Fig. 4.26).

Prone knee bend. This test has been shown to apply tension to the femoral nerve and mid-lumbar nerve roots (L2–4), and it is a good indicator of lateral disc pathology (L3–5) (Butler, 2000; Nadler et al., 2001; Kobayashi et al., 2003; Suri et al., 2011). The test is carried out in a prone position, with the clinician stabilizing the pelvis, as they passively maximally flex the patient's knee. It is considered a positive test if the patient's pain is reproduced in the lumbar spine, buttock, posterior or anterior thigh. If knee flexion is limited to below 90 degrees, a hip extension can be added to load the femoral nerve. Differentiation between neural tissue (femoral nerve) and rectus femoris stretch can be achieved through sensitizing movements of the ankle or head.

Femoral nerve slump test. The femoral nerve can be tested more selectively with the patient on side-lying with the symptomatic side uppermost and a pillow under the head (to avoid lateral flexion/rotation of the cervical spine). The neck and trunk are flexed, allowing cervical extension to be used as a desensitizing test (Fig. 4.27). The test movements are as follows:

- The clinician determines any resting symptoms and asks the patient to report immediately whether any of the symptoms are provoked during the test.

The patient is asked to hug both knees up on to the chest.

- The patient releases the uppermost knee to the clinician, who passively flexes the knee and then extends the hip, making sure the pelvis and trunk remain still. The clinician may add hip abduction/adduction to reproduce the patient's symptoms.
- At the point at which symptoms occur the patient is asked to slightly extend their neck while the clinician maintains the trunk, pelvis and leg position. A positive finding would be for the cervical extension to change, either increase or decrease the patient's symptoms.

Normal responses include tension over the anterior thigh which reduces with cervical extension, both in a

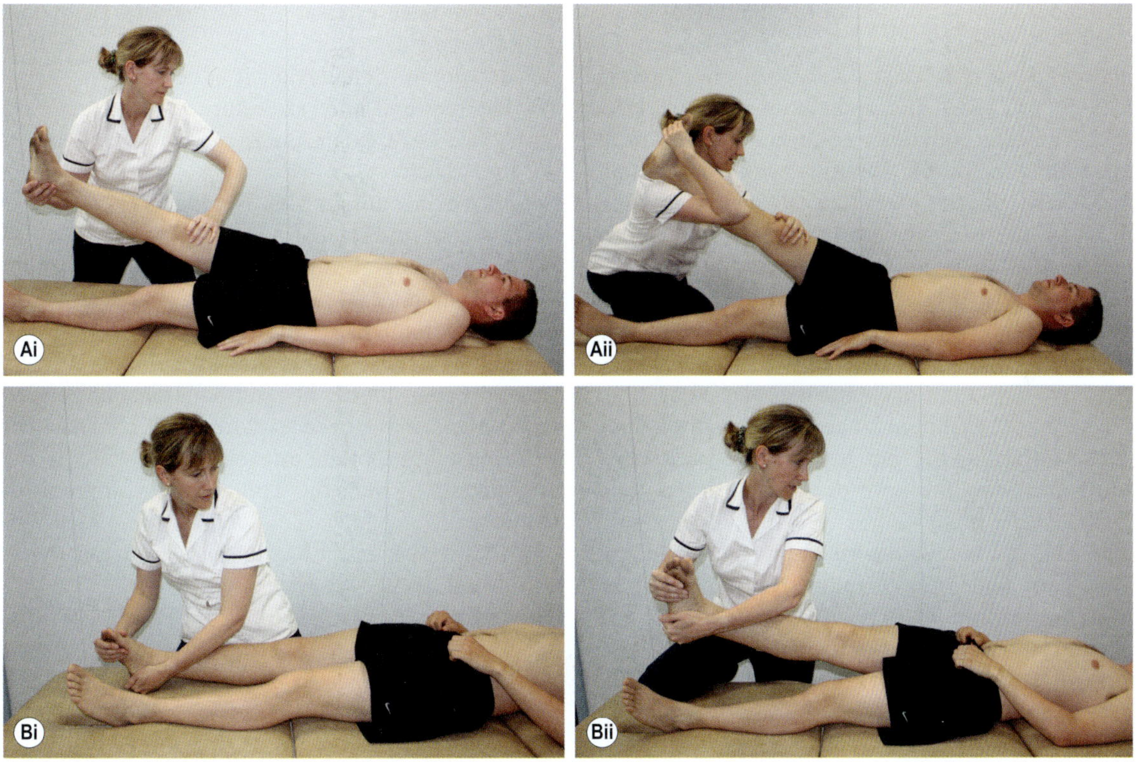

Fig. 4.26 (A) Straight-leg raise if, for example, symptoms are in the posterior thigh. (i) Hip adduction, medial rotation and then flexion to the onset of patient's posterior thigh symptoms. (ii) The clinician then adds ankle dorsiflexion and forefoot eversion. If the posterior thigh symptoms are increased (or decreased) with the dorsiflexion/eversion, this would be a positive test. (B) Straight-leg raise if, for example, symptoms are over lateral calf brought on with ankle plantarflexion and forefoot inversion. (i) Passive ankle plantarflexion and forefoot inversion to the onset of the patient's lateral calf symptoms. (ii) The clinician then adds hip adduction, medial rotation and flexion. If the lateral calf symptoms are increased (or decreased) with the addition of hip movements, this would be a positive test.

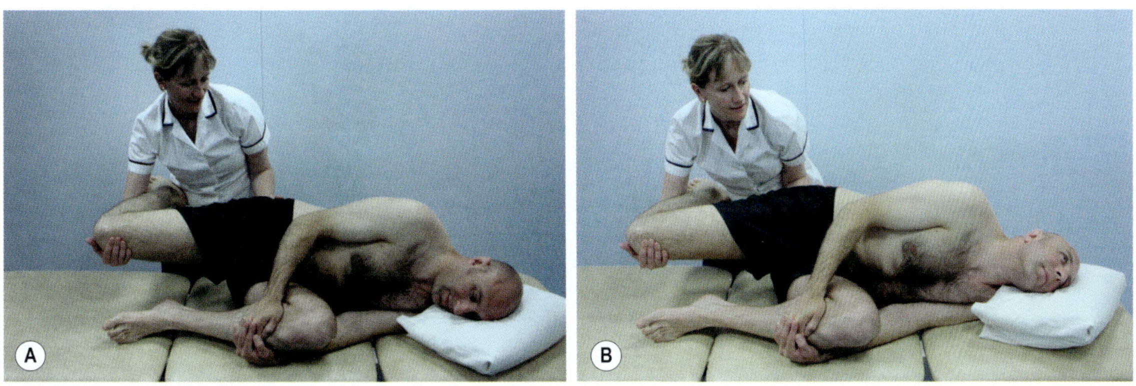

Fig. 4.27 Femoral nerve slump test (in side-lying). (A) With knee flexion, the clinician passively extends the hip to the point of onset of the patient's anterior thigh symptoms. (B) Patient extends the cervical spine. If the anterior thigh symptoms are reduced (or increased) with the neck movement, this would be a positive test.

slumped and a neutral position of the trunk (Lai et al., 2012).

Saphenous nerve test. The patient lies prone. The hip is placed in extension and abduction with the knee extended. The clinician adds passive lateral rotation of the hip, and dorsiflexion and inversion of the foot (Fig. 4.28A). Shacklock (2005) suggests medial rotation of the hip because of the position of the sartorius muscle but also advocates trying different positions. Butler (2000) suggests lateral rotation of the hip based on a study of saphenous nerve entrapments in adolescents (Nir-Paz et al., 1999). The clinician can sensitize the test by, for example, moving the foot into plantarflexion if symptoms are above the knee (Fig. 4.28B), moving the hip into medial rotation if symptoms are below the knee or adding contralateral side flexion of the spine.

Slump. This test is fully described by Hengeveld and Banks 2014 and Butler (2000) and is shown in Fig. 4.29.

The slump test can be carried out as follows:

- The clinician establishes the patient's resting symptoms and asks the patient to report any symptom provocation immediately.
- The patient sits with thighs fully supported at the edge of the plinth with hands behind their back. The lumbar spine is in a neutral position and the sacrum is horizontal.
- The patient is asked to flex the trunk by 'slumping the shoulders towards the groin'.
- The clinician monitors trunk flexion.
- Active cervical flexion is added and monitored by the clinician.
- Active knee extension is carried out on the asymptomatic side.
- Active foot dorsiflexion is added.
- The foot and knee are returned to neutral.
- Active knee extension is carried out on the symptomatic side.
- Active foot dorsiflexion is added.
- The foot and knee are returned to neutral.
- Active bilateral foot dorsiflexion is carried out.
- Active bilateral knee extension is added.
- The foot and knee are returned to neutral.

The clinician ensures that no compensatory movements occur. Once all combinations of lower limb movements have been explored, the clinician chooses the most appropriate movement to which to add a sensitizing movement. This would commonly be as follows:

- Active knee extension is carried out on the symptomatic side.
- Active foot dorsiflexion on the symptomatic side is added.
- The patient is asked to extend the neck to look up and report any change in symptoms. It is vital that there is no change in the position of the trunk and lower limbs when the cervical spine is extended. A change in the patient's symptoms on cervical extension would suggest a neurodynamic component.

The normal response might be:

- Pain or discomfort in the mid-thoracic area on trunk and neck flexion.
- Pain or discomfort behind the knees or in the hamstrings during flexion in the trunk and neck with

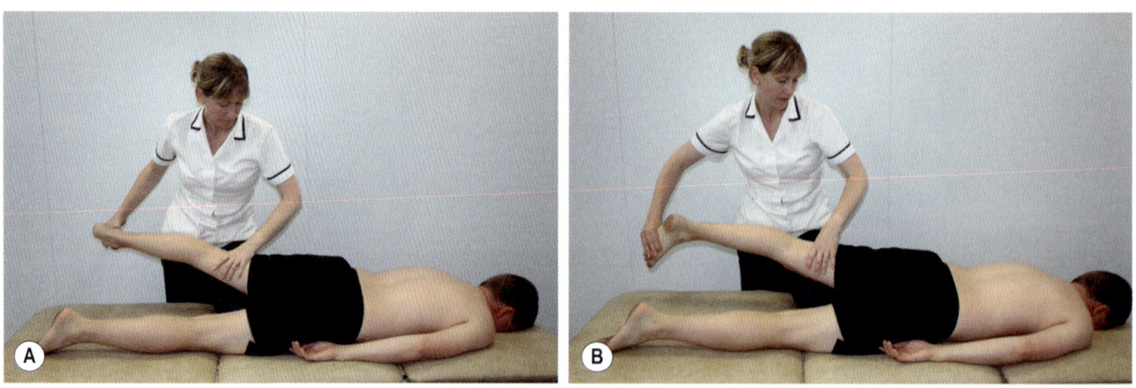

Fig. 4.28 Saphenous nerve test. (A) With the hip in extension abduction and lateral rotation and the knee extended, the clinician moves the foot into dorsiflexion and eversion. (B) If symptoms are above the knee the clinician can then move the foot into plantarflexion and inversion. If the symptoms are reduced (or increased) with foot movement, this would be a positive test.

knee extension. Symptoms are increased with ankle dorsiflexion.

- Some restriction of knee extension in the trunk and neck flexion position.
- Some restriction of ankle dorsiflexion during flexion in trunk and neck with knee extension. This restriction should be symmetrical.
- A decrease in pain in one or more areas with the release of the neck flexion.
- An increase in the range of knee extension and/or ankle dorsiflexion with the release of the neck flexion.

The sensitizing test is cervical extension. Sensitizing tests can include cervical rotation, cervical lateral flexion, hip flexion, hip adduction, hip medial rotation, thoracic lateral flexion and altering foot and ankle movements.

Most people have a sensory response to elements or all of the slump test. (Walsh et al., 2007). These include sensations of tightness, tension, paraesthesia and discomfort.

Obturator nerve test. The slump test can be utilized to differentiate muscle or nerve dysfunction as a cause of groin strain. After positioning the patient in sitting and abducting the hip to the onset of symptoms, slump and neck flexion are added. An increase in symptoms may suggest obturator nerve involvement, while no change in symptoms suggests a local groin strain.

Upper limb neurodynamic tests. There are four tests, each of which is biased towards a particular nerve:

1. ULNT 1—median nerve
2. ULNT 2a—median nerve
3. ULNT 2b—radial nerve
4. ULNT 3—ulnar nerve.

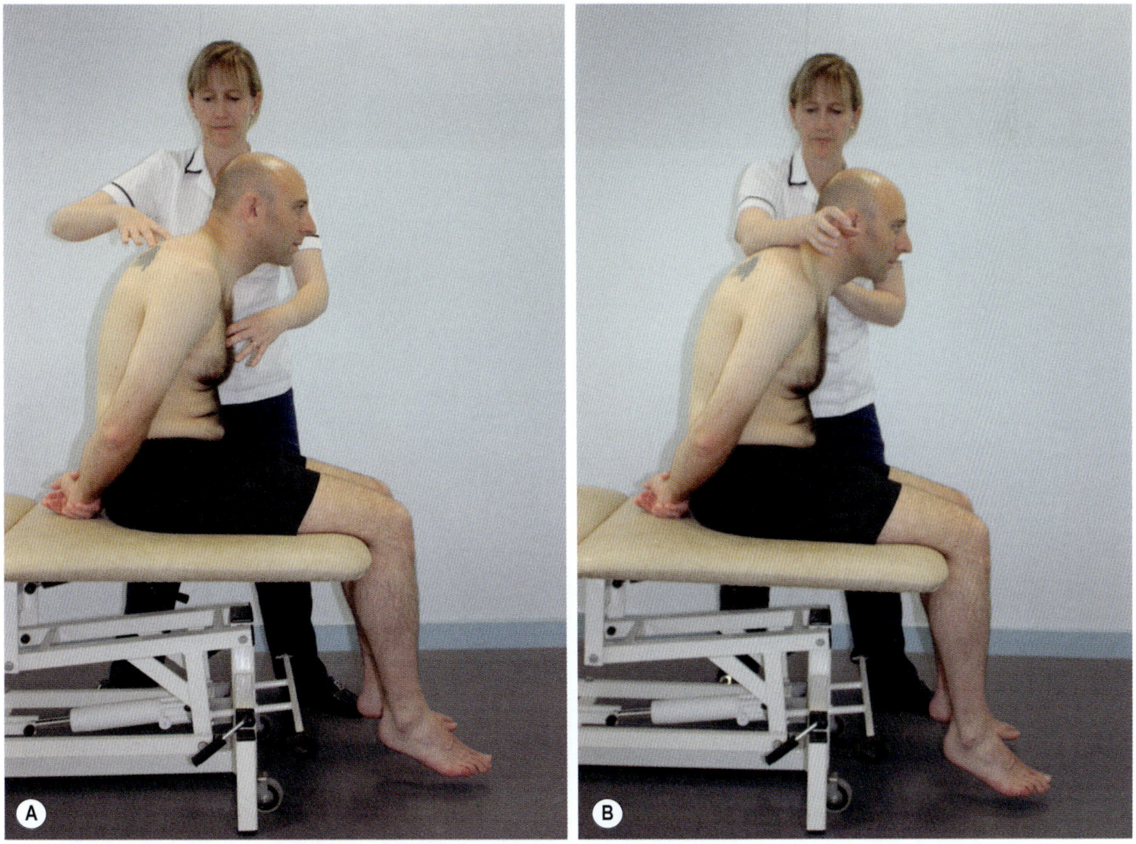

Fig. 4.29 Slump test. Demonstrated for a patient with left posterior thigh pain. (A) Active trunk flexion with arms behind back. (B) Monitoring trunk flexion.

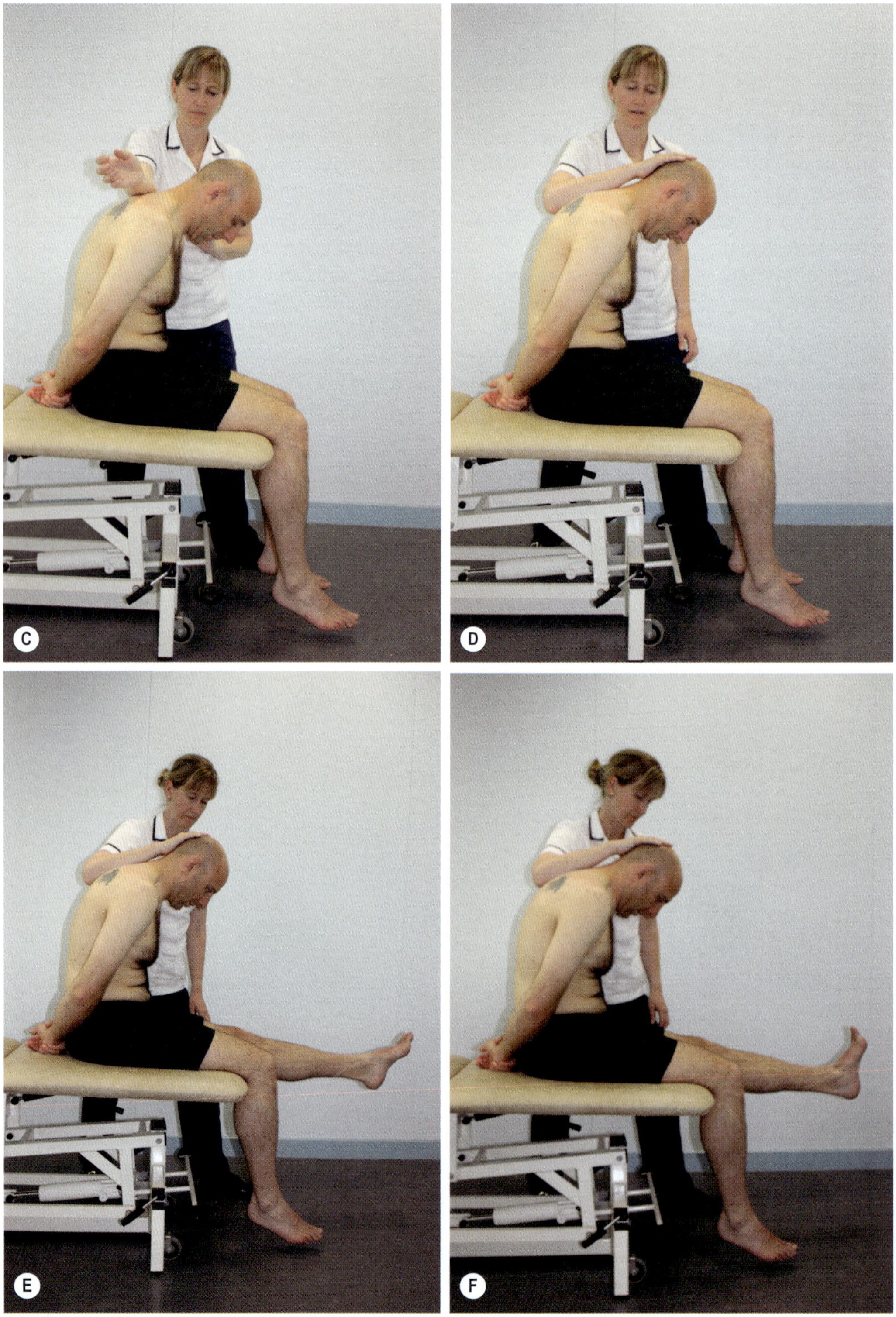

Fig. 4.29, cont'd (C) Active cervical flexion. (D) Monitoring of cervical flexion. (E) Left leg: knee extension. (F) Left leg: dorsiflexion.

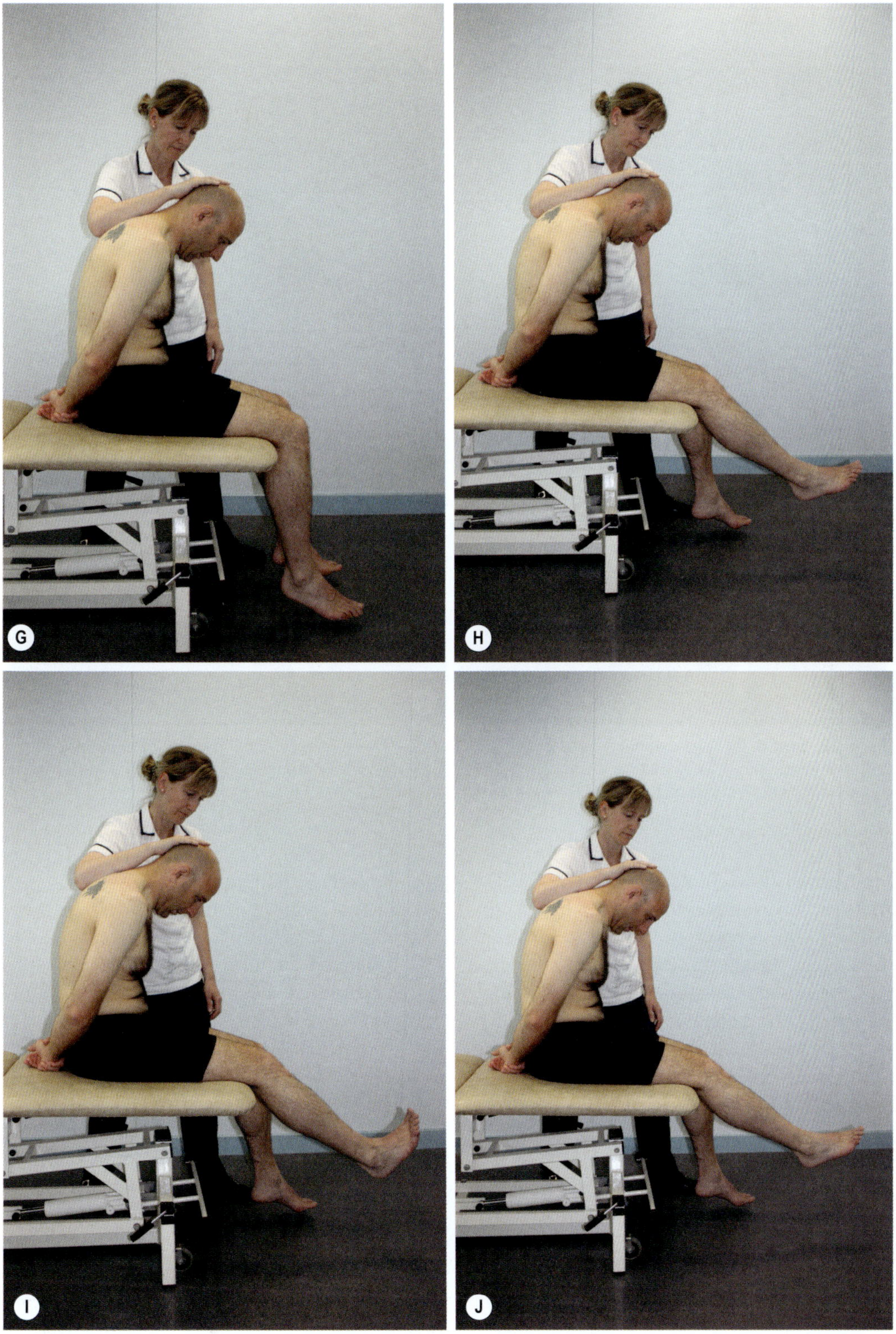

Fig. 4.29, cont'd (G) Return to start position. (H) Right leg: knee extension (reduced range due to onset of right thigh pain). (I) Right leg: knee extension (reduced range due to onset of left thigh pain); addition of dorsiflexion increases right thigh pain. (J) Right leg: release of dorsiflexion reduces right thigh pain.

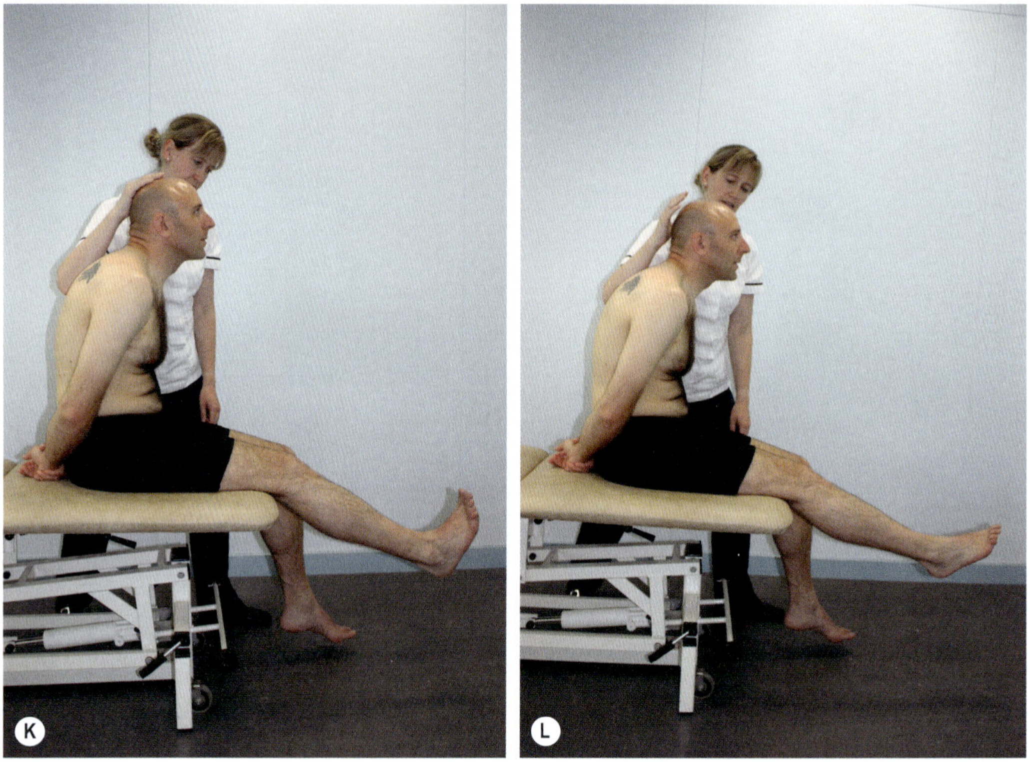

Fig. 4.29, cont'd (K) Active cervical extension. If cervical extension reduces (or increases) the patient's right posterior thigh pain, this would be a positive test. (L) Active cervical extension may produce an increase in range which would increase further on release of dorsiflexion.

The test movements are outlined below. The ULNTs are appropriate, if, for example, the patient has symptoms in the upper arm, forearm or hand. The order of the movements has been chosen so that the last movement is the easiest for the clinician to gauge visually. The area of the patient's symptoms will help the clinician to decide which is the most appropriate ULNT. For example, where symptoms are mainly in the distribution of the radial nerve, ULNT 2b would be carried out.

ULNT 1: median nerve bias (Fig. 4.30).

1. Neutral supine position of the body on the couch.
2. Contralateral lateral flexion of the cervical spine.
3. Shoulder girdle depression.
4. Shoulder abduction.
5. Wrist and finger extension.
6. Forearm supination.
7. Lateral rotation of the shoulder.
8. Elbow extension.
9. Ipsilateral lateral flexion of the cervical spine.

If symptoms are over the upper fibres of the trapezius then:

10. Wrist flexion would be used, instead of ipsilateral lateral flexion of the cervical spine.

The movement of ipsilateral lateral flexion of the cervical spine is used to test whether there is a neurodynamic component to the patient's symptoms. If there is a neurodynamic component, the patient's symptoms will be produced at some stage during the arm movements from 2 to 8. These symptoms will be reduced (or increased) by ipsilateral lateral flexion of the cervical spine. This principle also applies to each of the ULNT below.

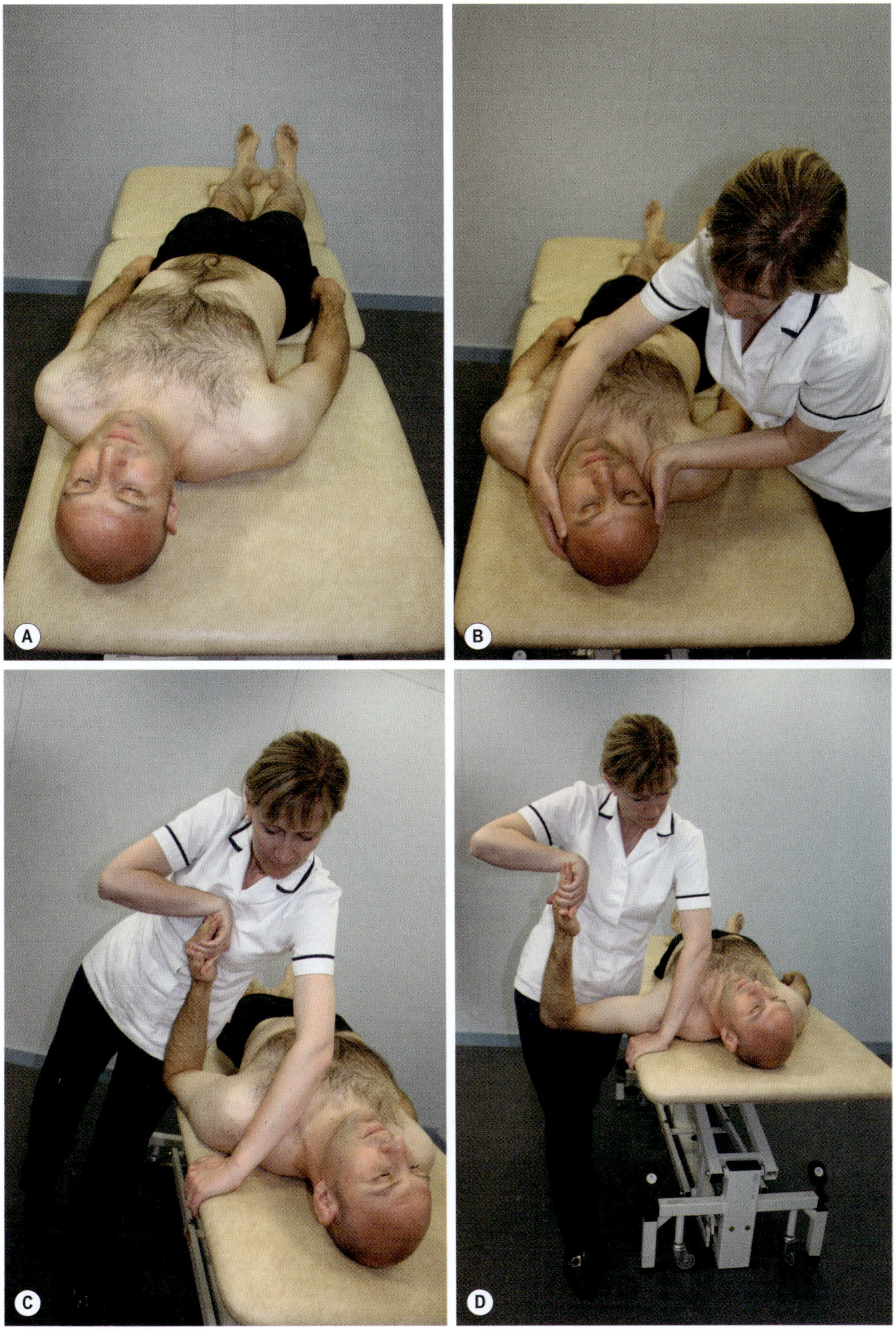

Fig. 4.30 Upper-limb neurodynamic test (ULNT 1). (A) Neutral start position. (B) Contralateral lateral flexion of the cervical spine. (C) Shoulder girdle depression. (D) Shoulder abduction.

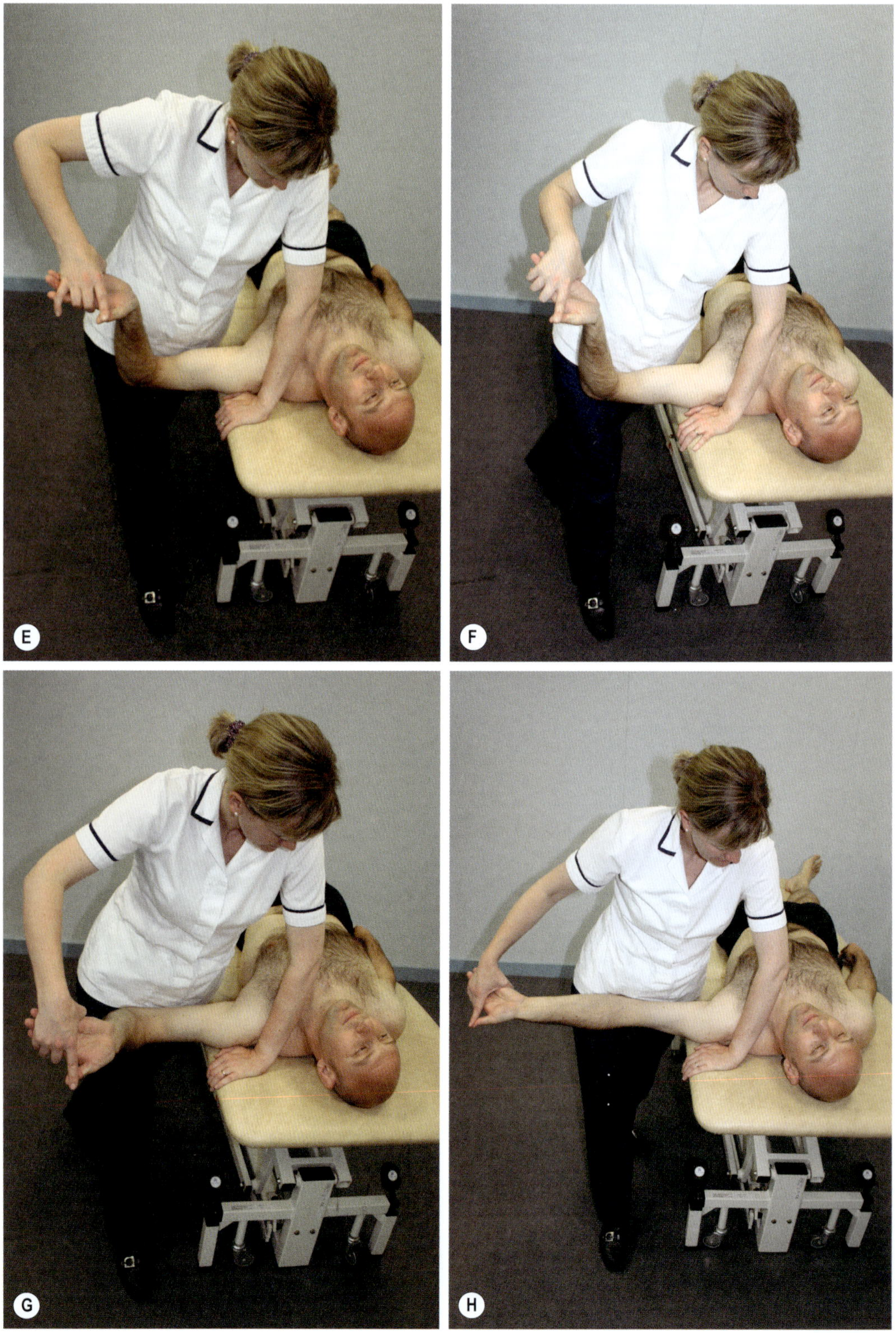

Fig. 4.30, cont'd (E) Wrist and finger extension. (F) Forearm supination. (G) Shoulder lateral rotation. (H) Elbow extension.

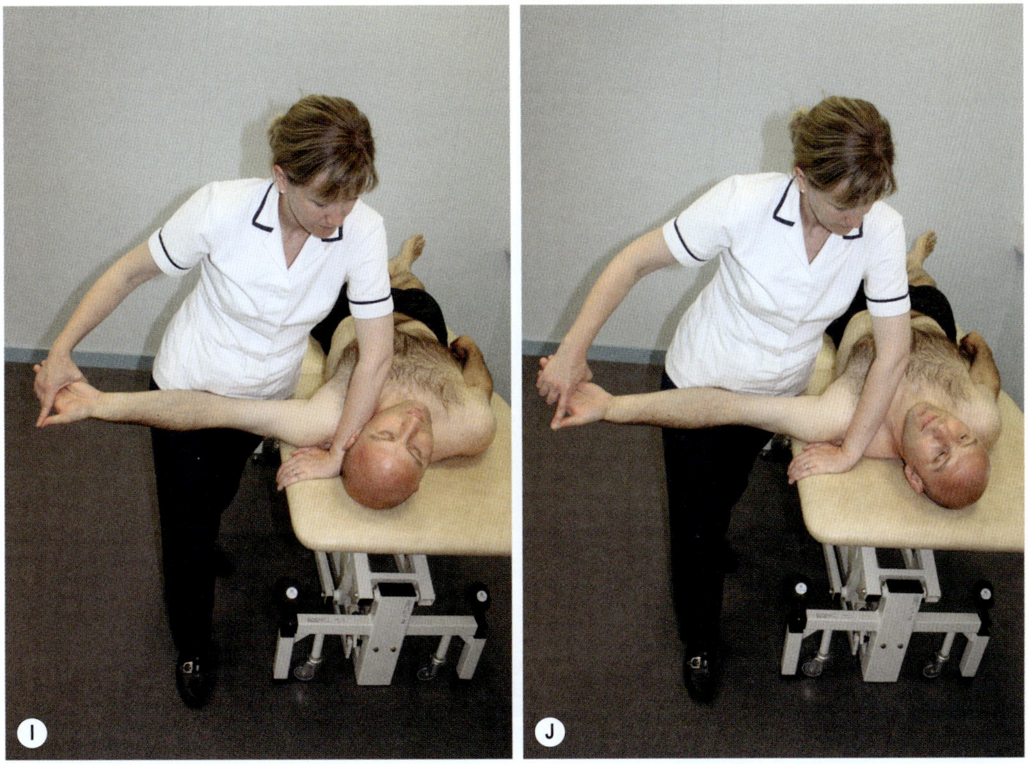

Fig. 4.30, cont'd (I) Ipsilateral lateral flexion of the cervical spine if symptoms are in the arm. If ipsilateral lateral flexion reduces (or increases) the patient's symptoms, this would be a positive test. (J) Wrist flexion may be used to desensitize the movement, if the patient's symptoms are close to the cervical spine such as over the upper fibres of trapezius. If wrist flexion reduces (or increases) the patient's neck symptoms this would be a positive test.

ULNT 2a: median nerve bias (Fig. 4.31). This test is useful as an alternative to ULNT1, if the patient has restricted glenohumeral range.

1. Neutral position of the body on the couch, with shoulder girdle over the edge.
2. Contralateral lateral flexion of the cervical spine.
3. Shoulder girdle depression.
4. Wrist, finger and thumb extension.
5. Forearm supination.
6. Elbow extension.
7. Shoulder lateral rotation.
8. Shoulder abduction.
9. Desensitizing movement of ipsilateral lateral flexion of the cervical spine.

If symptoms are near the cervical spine, e.g. upper fibres of the trapezius, the movement of wrist flexion could be used as the desensitizing movement, for example.

ULNT 2b: radial nerve bias (Fig. 4.32).

1. Neutral position of the body on the couch, with shoulder girdle over the edge.
2. Contralateral lateral flexion of the cervical spine.
3. Shoulder girdle depression.

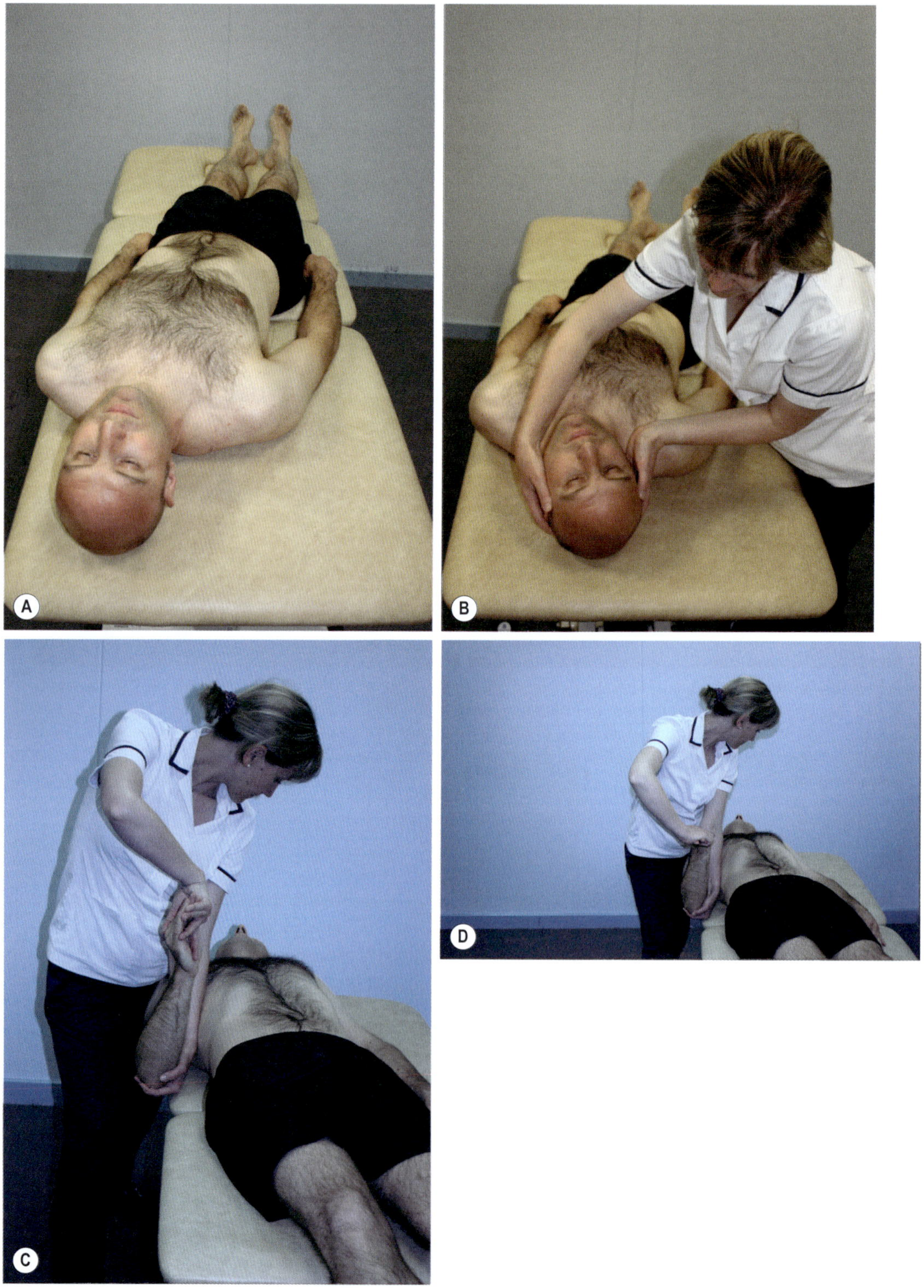

Fig. 4.31 Upper-limb neurodynamic test (ULNT) 2a. (A) Neutral position of body on couch, but with shoulder girdle overhanging the edge. (B) Contralateral lateral flexion of the cervical spine. (C) Shoulder girdle depression. (D) Wrist, finger and thumb extension.

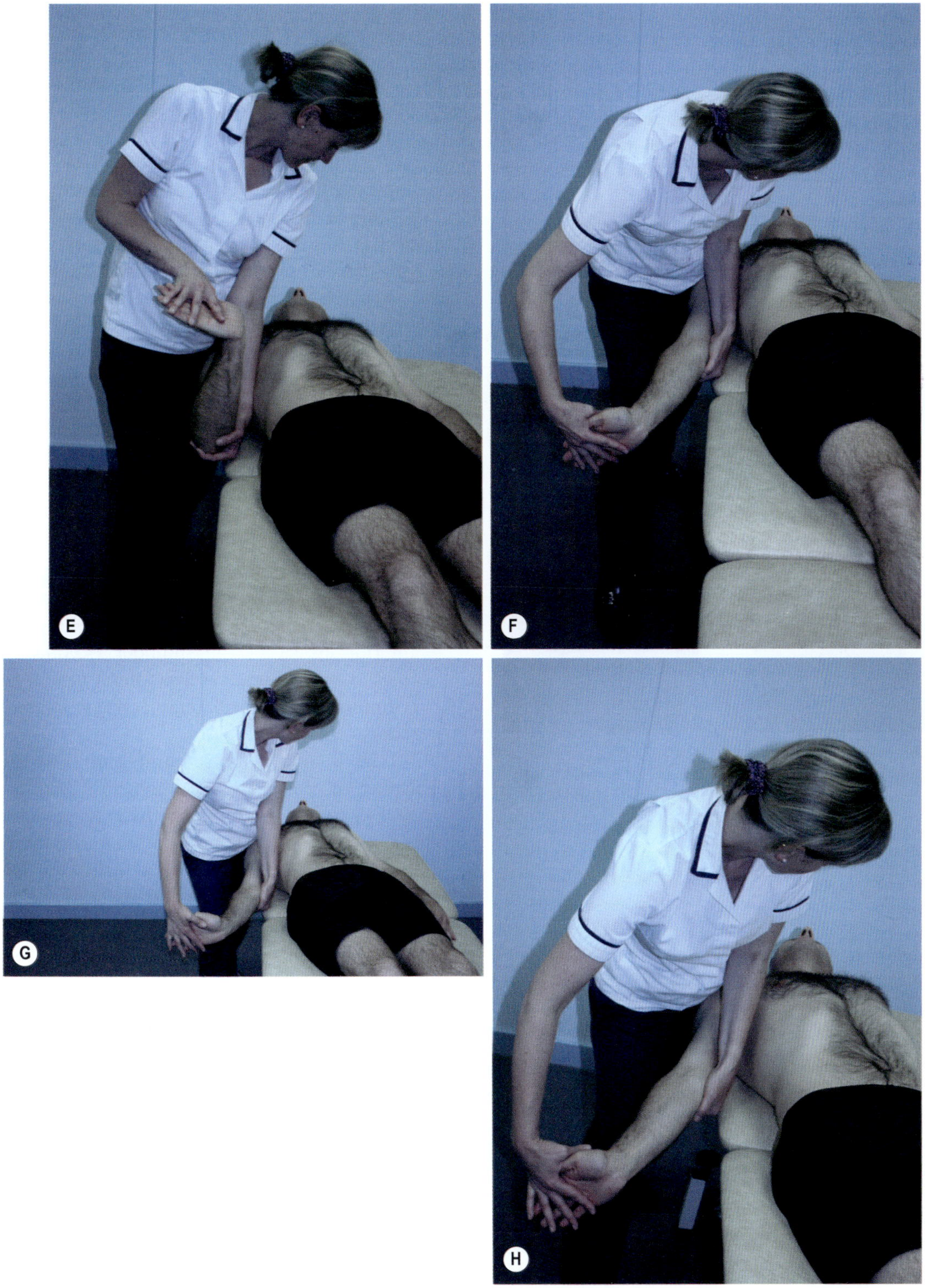

Fig. 4.31, cont'd (E) Forearm supination. (F) Elbow extension. (G) Shoulder lateral rotation. (H) Shoulder abduction.

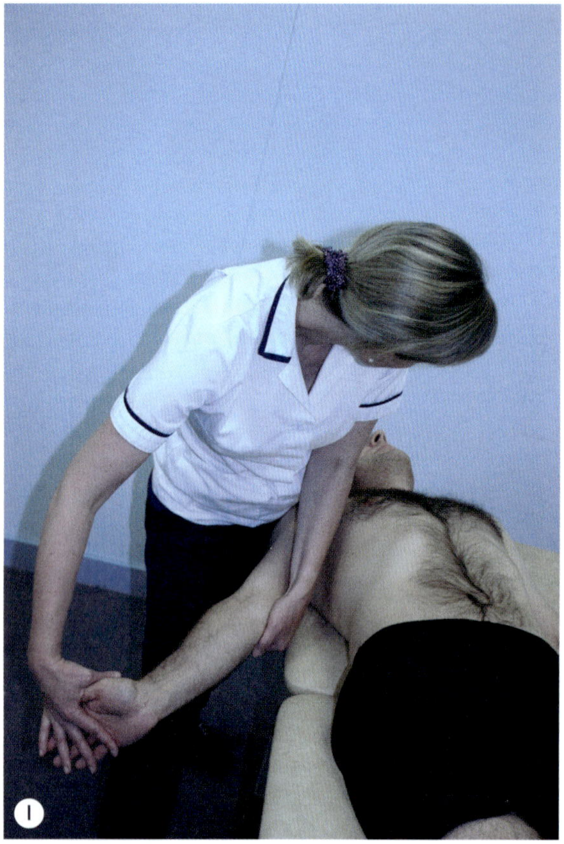

Fig. 4.31, cont'd (l) Desensitizing movement of ipsilateral lateral flexion of the cervical spine.

4. Wrist, finger and thumb flexion.
5. Shoulder medial rotation.
6. Elbow extension.
7. Desensitizing movement of ipsilateral lateral flexion of the cervical spine.
   or
8. Wrist extension if symptoms are near the cervical spine, e.g. upper fibres of the trapezius.

ULNT 3: ulnar nerve bias (Fig. 4.33).

1. Neutral position of the body on the couch.
2. Contralateral lateral flexion of the cervical spine.
3. Shoulder girdle stabilized.
4. Wrist and finger extension.
5. Forearm pronation.
6. Elbow flexion.
7. Shoulder abduction.
8. Shoulder lateral rotation.
9. Further shoulder abduction.
10. Desensitizing movement of ipsilateral lateral flexion of the cervical spine.
    or
11. Wrist flexion if symptoms are near the cervical spine, e.g. upper fibres of the trapezius.

Additional tests for the ULNT include placing the other arm in a ULNT position or adding in either the SLR or the slump test. The tests can also be carried out with the patient in other starting positions. For example, the ULNT can be performed with the patient prone, which allows accessory movements to be carried out at the same time. Other upper-limb movements can be carried out in addition to those suggested. For example, pronation/supination or radial/ulnar deviation can be added to ULNT 1.

Normal responses to ULNT tests on asymptomatic subjects are as follows:

ULNT 1: a deep ache or stretch in the cubital fossa extending to the anterior and radial aspects of the forearm and hand, tingling in the thumb and first three fingers, and a stretching feeling over the anterior aspect of the shoulder (Kenneally et al., 1988). Contralateral cervical lateral flexion increases symptoms while ipsilateral cervical lateral flexion reduces them.

ULNT 2b: a feeling of stretching pain over the radial aspect of the proximal forearm (Yaxley & Jull, 1993); these symptoms are usually increased with the addition of contralateral cervical lateral flexion.

ULNT 3: a stretching pain and paraesthesia over the hypothenar eminence, ring and little finger (Martínez et al., 2014).

Nerve Tissue Palpation

Clinicians can further confirm neural tissue involvement through direct palpation of the nerves where they are superficial and indirectly in and out of tension positions (Walsh & Hall, 2009). Palpation of nerves can elicit a variety of sensations. Where a nerve contains more fascicles and connective tissue it will be more difficult to elicit a neural response, e.g. the common peroneal nerve CPN as it winds around the head of the fibula. Normally nerves feel hard and round and are likened to guitar strings. When a nerve is under tension

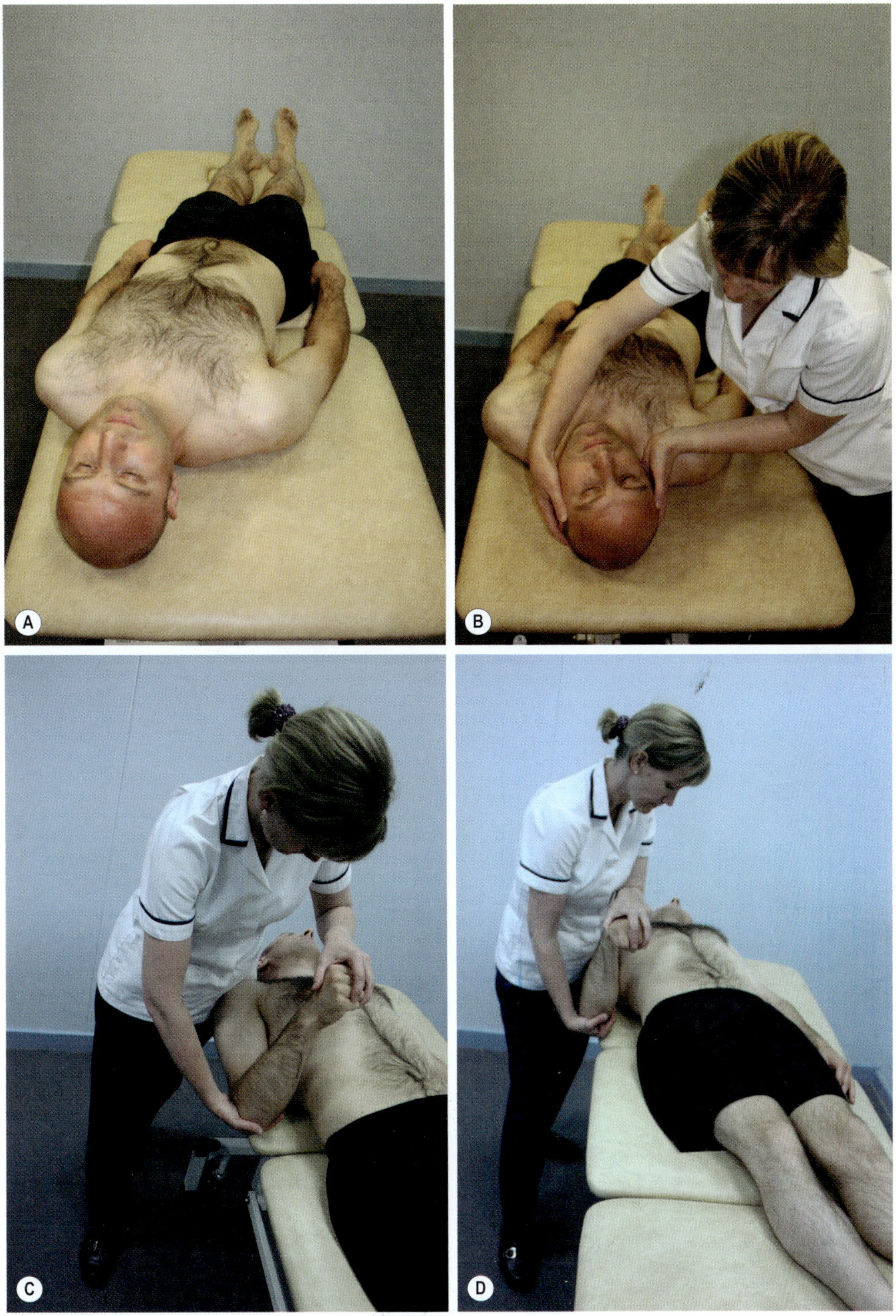

Fig. 4.32 Upper-limb neurodynamic test (ULNT) 2b. (A) Neutral position of body on couch, but with shoulder girdle overhanging the edge. (B) Contralateral lateral flexion of the cervical spine. (C) Shoulder girdle depression. (D) Wrist, finger and thumb flexion.

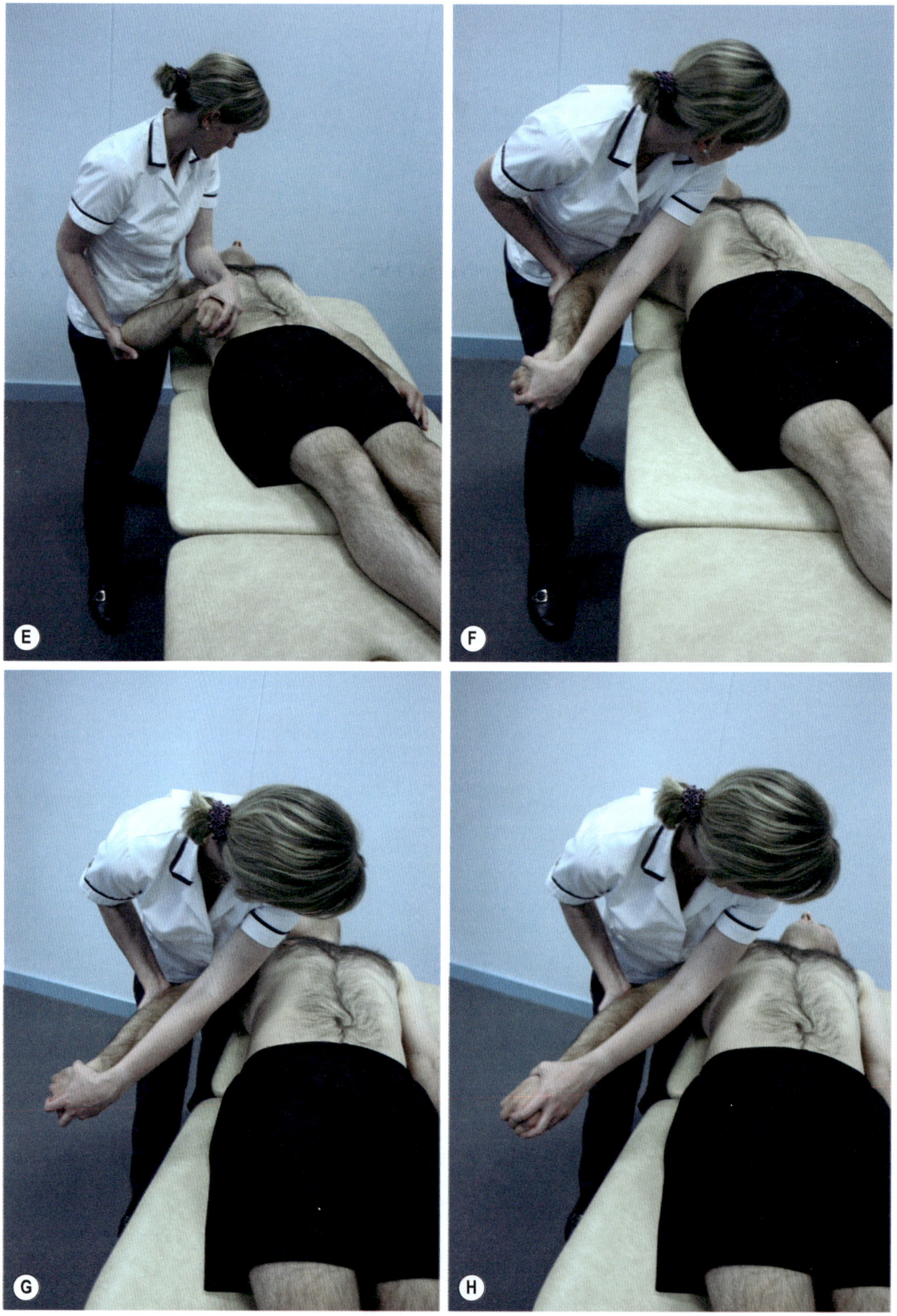

Fig. 4.32, cont'd (E) Shoulder medial rotation. (F) Elbow extension. (G) Desensitizing movement of ipsilateral lateral flexion of the cervical spine, or (H) wrist extension would be used as a desensitizing movement if symptoms are near the cervical spine, for example over the upper fibres of trapezius.

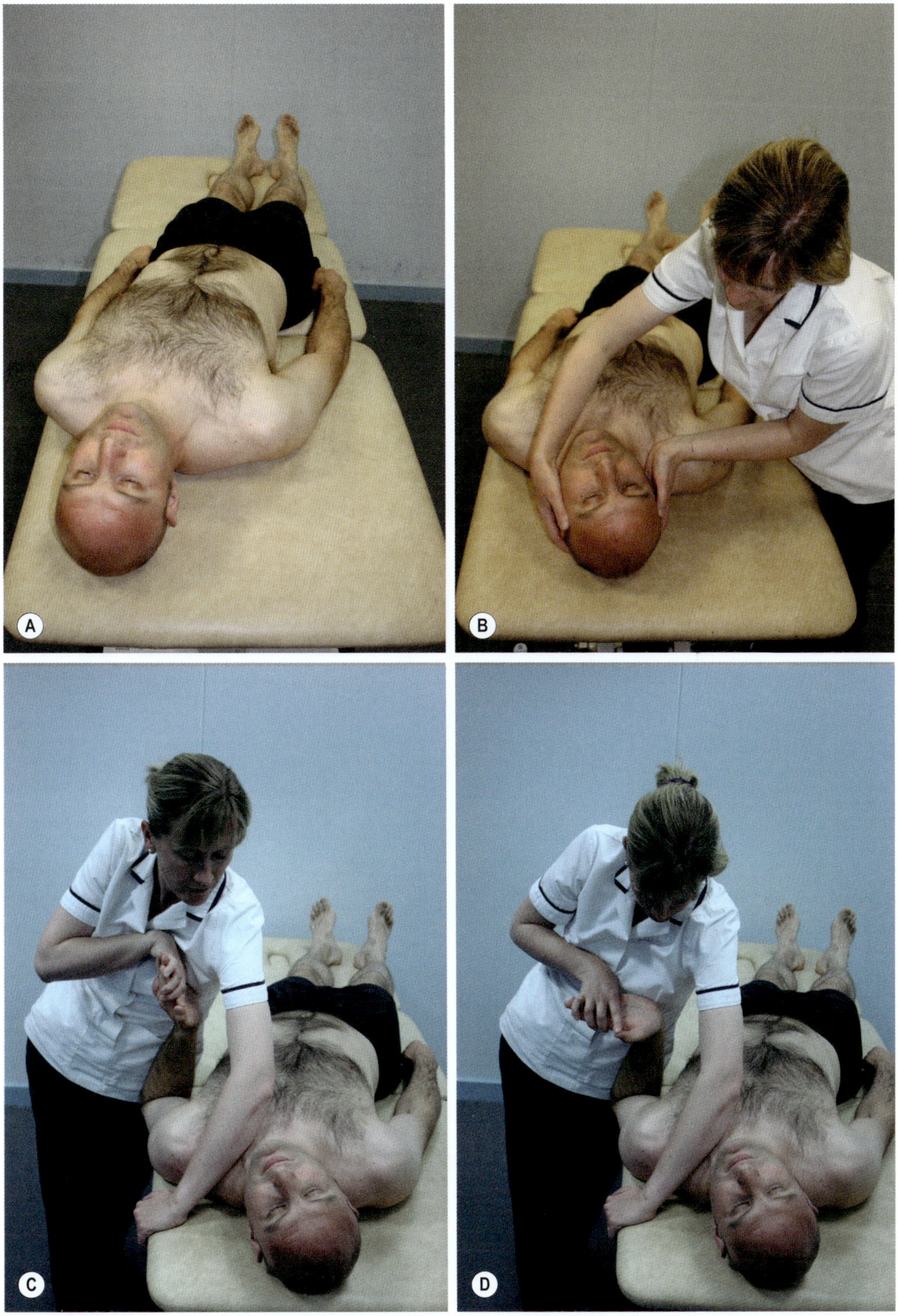

Fig. 4.33 Upper-limb neurodynamic test (ULNT) 3 (ulnar nerve bias). (A) Neutral position of body on couch. (B) Contralateral lateral flexion of the cervical spine. (C) Shoulder girdle stabilized. (D) Wrist and finger extension.

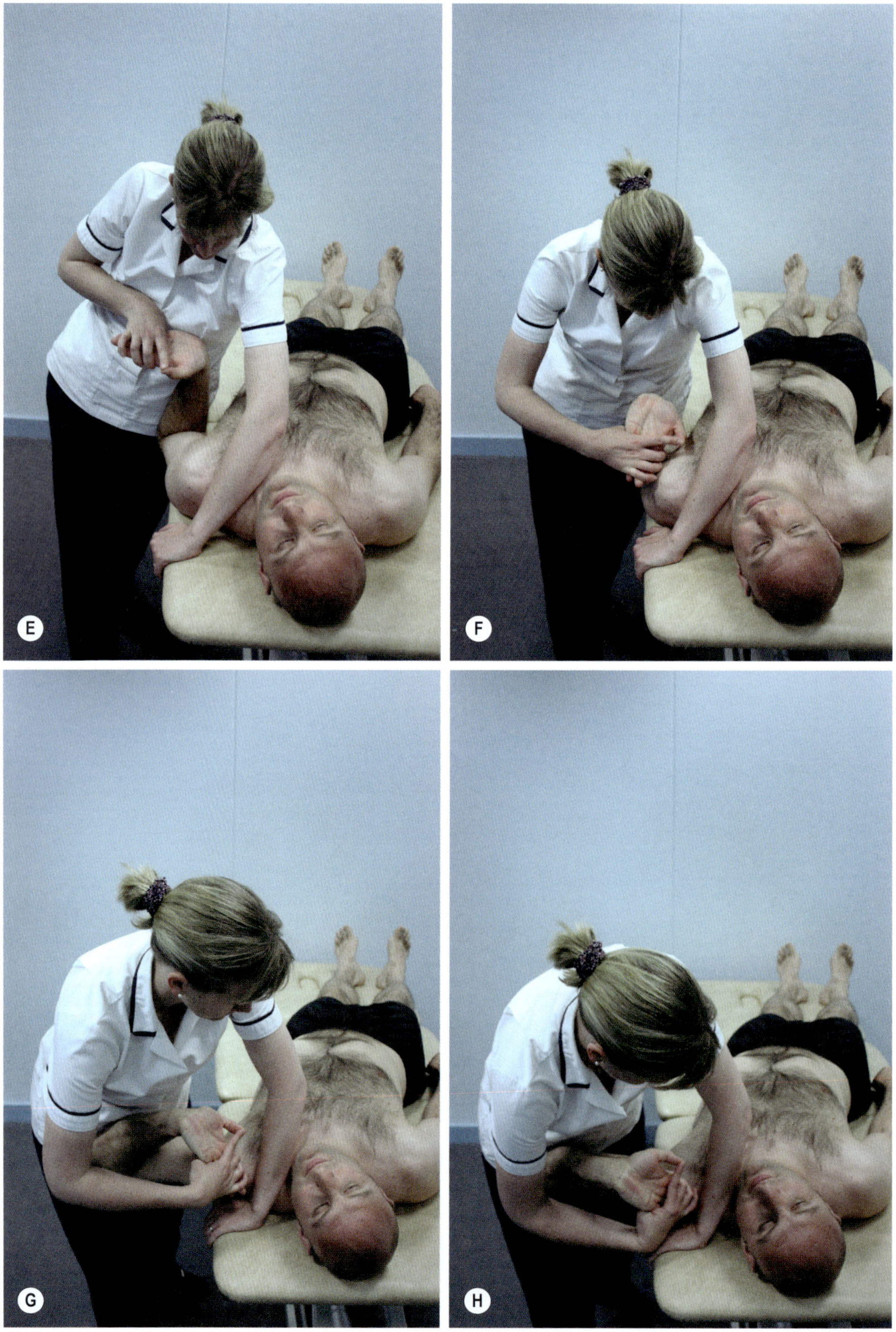

Fig. 4.33, cont'd (E) Pronation of forearm. (F) Elbow flexion. (G) Shoulder abduction. (H) Lateral rotation of shoulder.

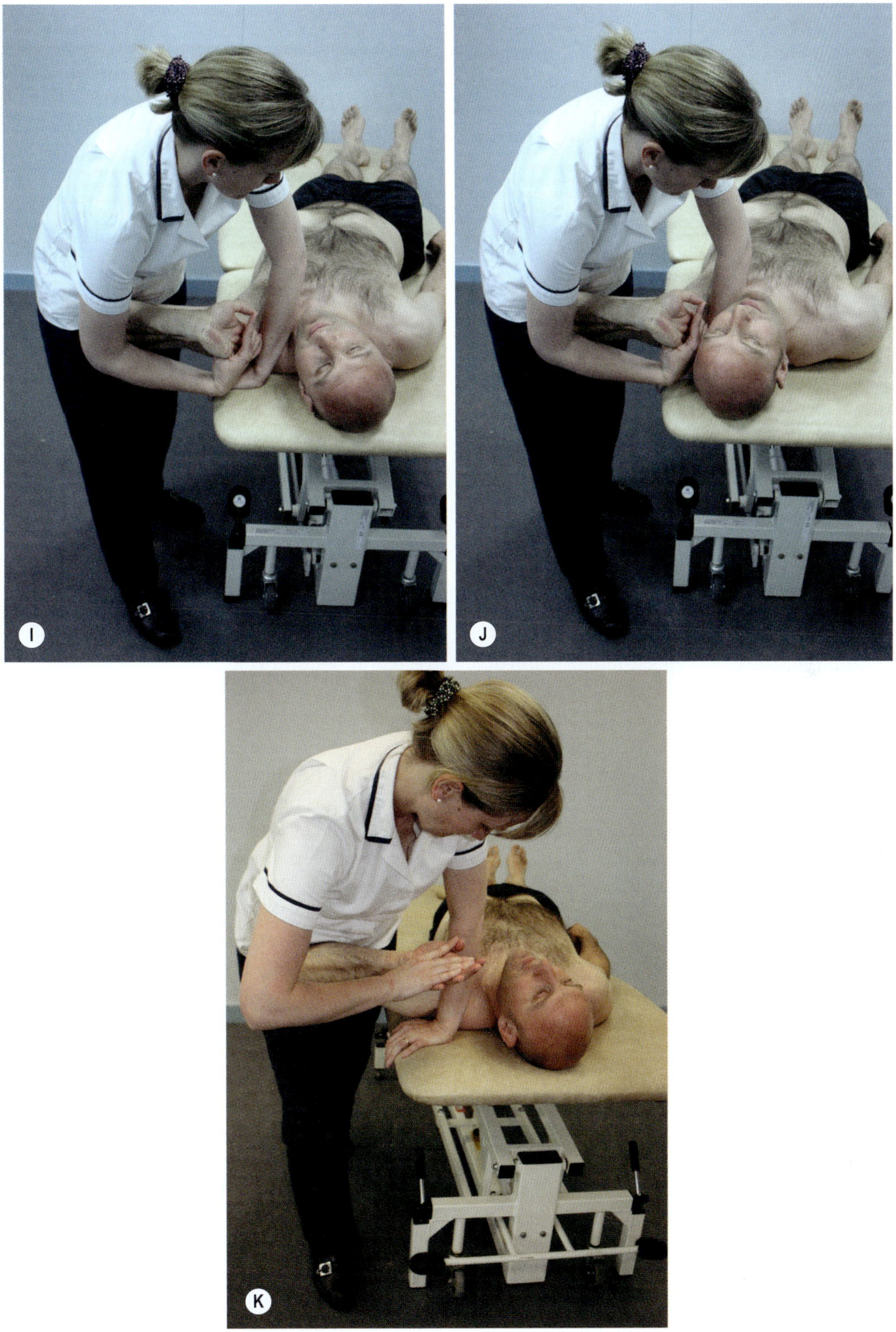

Fig. 4.33, cont'd (I) Further shoulder abduction. (J) Desensitizing movement of ipsilateral lateral flexion of the cervical spine (if symptoms are in the forearm or hand), or (K) wrist flexion if symptoms are near the cervical spine or shoulder.

or if the nerve is adhered to the surrounding interface structures, transverse movement will be reduced.

For further information on nerve palpation, the reader is referred to Butler (2000) and region-specific chapters in this text.

Other Neurological Tests

These tests include various tests for spinal cord and peripheral nerve damage and are discussed in the relevant chapters.

KNOWLEDGE CHECK

1. How can components of the SLR test be modified to test the sensitivity of different peripheral nerves of the lower limb?
2. Which lumbar nerve roots are tensioned by the Prone Knee Bend test?
3. Which nerve is loaded by ULNT3?

Palpation

The clinician must be aware of the psychological impact of touch on a patient. Palpation also has a neurophysiological effect which may produce a change in the patient's symptoms (Bjorbækmo & Mengshoel, 2016). Clear communication is required to ensure the patient is comfortable.

During the palpation of soft tissues and skeletal tissues, the following should be noted:

- The temperature of the area (increase is indicative of local inflammation).
- Localized increased or decreased skin moisture (indicative of autonomic disturbance).
- The presence of oedema and/or effusion.
- Mobility and feel of superficial tissues, e.g. ganglions or nodules.
- The presence or elicitation of muscle spasm.
- Tenderness of bone, ligament, muscle, tendon, tendon sheath and nerve.
  The presence of trigger points.
- Increased or decreased prominence of bones.
- Joint effusion or swelling of a limb. This can be measured using a tape measure, comparing the left and right sides.
- Pain provoked or reduced on palpation.

Hints on the method of palpation are given in Box 4.2. Further guidance on palpation of the soft tissues can be found in Hunter (1998). Palpation can be used to inform clinicians about tissue states. The diagnostic use of palpation has been questioned. There are issues of reliability and validity due to its subjectivity, but within a clinically reasoned examination palpation can yield useful information, especially when skillfully applied. Palpation findings can be recorded on a body chart (see Fig. 3.2) and/or palpation chart for the vertebral column (Fig. 4.34).

BOX 4.2 Hints on Palpation

- Have the patient comfortably positioned and ensure they understand the purpose of the test
- Adjust the plinth to a comfortable height
- Palpate the unaffected side first and compare this with the affected side
- Palpate from superficial to deep
- Use just enough force to feel—excessive force can reduce feel
- Never assume that a relevant area does not need palpating

Trigger Points

Trigger points are described in Chapter 3. Trigger points may be either latent or active. Both can produce allodynia and referred pain. In a latent trigger point this is only when evoked, for instance by palpation, while an active trigger point produces symptoms spontaneously (Dommerholt, 2011). In order to examine for a trigger point, the muscle is put on a slight stretch, and the clinician searches for trigger points by mild to moderate pressure with the fingers over the muscle. A trigger point can be considered to be present if two out of the following three signs are found: a small spot with marked hypersensitivity, a taut band in the muscle, and referred pain (Fernández-de-las-Peñas & Dommerholt, 2018). It should only be classed as active if palpation reproduces the patient's symptoms.

Accessory Movements

Accessory movements are movements which a person cannot perform actively but which can be performed on that person by an external force (Hengeveld and Banks 2014). They take the form of gliding (sometimes referred to as translation or sliding) of the joint surfaces (medially, laterally, anteriorly or posteriorly),

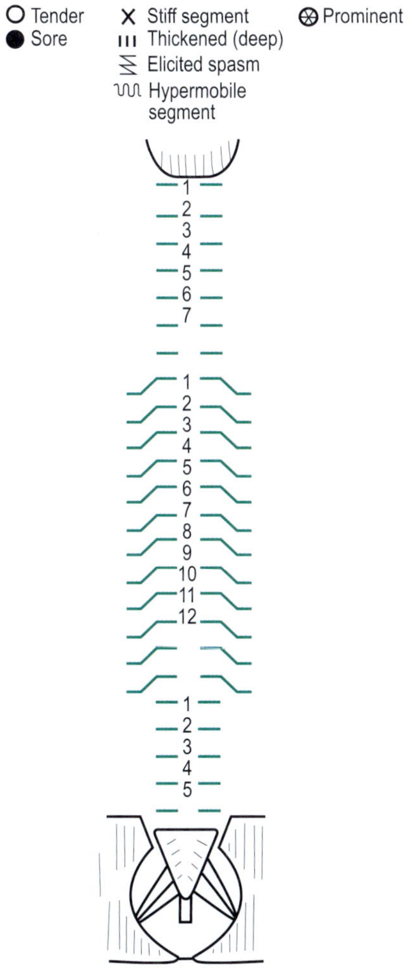

Fig. 4.34 Palpation chart. (From Grieve 1991, with permission.)

distraction and compression of the joint surfaces and in some joints, rotation movements where this movement cannot be performed actively, e.g. rotation at the metacarpal and interphalangeal joints of the fingers. These movements are possible because all joints have a certain amount of play or slack in the capsule and surrounding ligaments (Kaltenborn, 2002).

Limitation in the physiological range of movement may be associated with a limitation of the accessory range of movement at the joint. Application of biomechanical models proposing the *concave-convex rule* for the assessment of peripheral joints (Fig. 4.35) and theories of spinal coupling have been adapted in recent years, because evidence suggests that joint surfaces move differently in the presence of pathology (Schohmacher, 2009).

Indeed, evidence supporting a purely biomechanical basis for testing is limited. An increased understanding of the neurophysiological effects of accessory movement testing has broadened reasoning and thinking to appreciate the complex interactions that occur within the central nervous system (Bialosky et al., 2009). These effects are also psychological as the patient's response to hands-on testing will be influenced by their mood, expectation and conditioning (Bialosky et al., 2011). This means clinicians must be aware of the context within which testing takes place, reasoning all aspects of the complex interaction between body and mind.

Accessory assessment can:

- Identify a symptomatic joint.

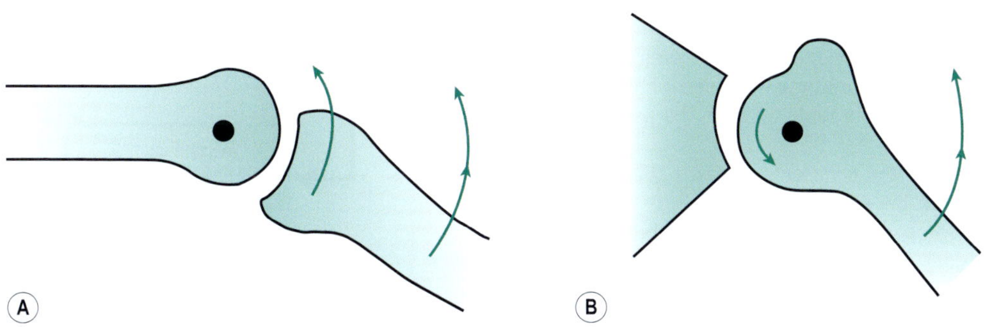

Fig. 4.35 The concave-convex rule. Movement of articular surfaces during physiological movements. The single arrow depicts the direction of movement of the articular surface and the double arrow depicts the physiological movement. **A** A concave surface moving on a convex surface. **B** A convex surface moving on a concave surface (From Kaltenborn 2002, with permission.)

- Explore the nature of a joint motion abnormality.
- Provide a basis for the selection of treatment techniques.

Hints on performing an accessory movement are given in Box 4.3.

During accessory movement testing, pressure is applied to a bone close to the joint line. The clinician increases movement progressively through the range and notes:

- Quality of movement.
- Range of movement.
- Pain (local and referred) through the range, which may be provoked or reduced.
- Resistance through the range and at the end of the range.
- Muscle spasm.

Accessory movements are carried out on each joint that may be a source of the symptoms. After this has been done for each joint, all relevant asterisks are reassessed to determine the effect on the signs and symptoms. For example, in a patient with cervical spine, shoulder and elbow pain, it may be found that there is an increase in range and reduction in pain in both the cervical spine and the shoulder joint following accessory movements to the cervical spine, but that there is no change in elbow movement. Accessory movements to the elbow joint, however, may improve the elbow's range of movements. Such a scenario suggests that the cervical spine is giving rise to the pain in the cervical spine and the shoulder, but the local tissues around the elbow are responsible for producing the pain at the elbow. This process had been termed the *analytical assessment* by Maitland et al. (2001) and is shown in Fig. 4.36.

BOX 4.3 Hints on Performing an Accessory Movement

- Have the patient comfortably positioned and ensure they understand the purpose of the test
- Adjust the plinth to a comfortable height
- Examine the joint movement on the unaffected side first and compare this with the affected side
- Obtain feedback through continuous communication with the patient throughout
- Have as large an area of skin contact as possible for maximum patient comfort
- The force is applied utilising the body weight of the clinician and not the intrinsic muscles of the hand, which can be uncomfortable for both the patient and the clinician
- Where possible, the clinician's forearm should lie in the direction of the applied force
- Apply the force smoothly and slowly through the range with or without oscillations
- At the end of the available movement, apply small oscillations to feel the resistance at the end of the range
- Use just enough force to feel the movement—the harder you press, the less you feel

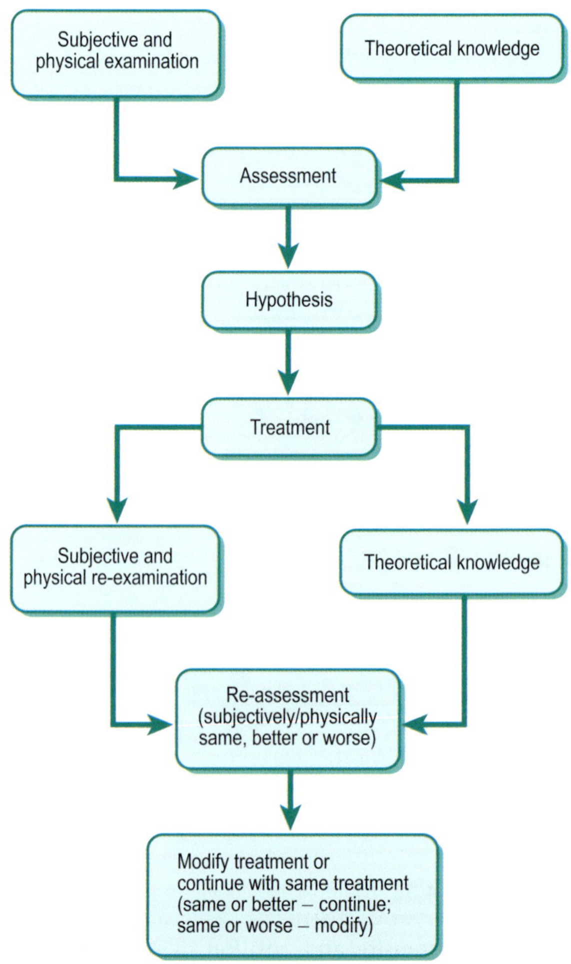

Fig. 4.36 Analytical assessment.

Modifications to Accessory Movement Examination

Accessory movements can be modified by altering the:

- Speed of applied force. Pressure can be applied slowly or quickly, and may or may not be oscillated through the range.
- Direction of the applied force.
- Point of application of the applied force.
- Resting position of the joint.

The joint can be placed in different start positions. The clinician should use clinical reasoning to select an appropriate start position, based on known aggravating and easing factors, as well as irritability and severity. For example, accessory movements can be applied to the patella with the knee anywhere between full flexion and full extension. Accessory movements to any part of the spine can be performed in flexion, extension, lateral flexion, rotation or any combination of these positions. This positioning alters the effect of the accessory movement. For example, central posteroanterior pressure on C5 causes the superior articular facets of C5 to slide upwards on the inferior articular facets of C4, a movement similar to cervical extension; this upward movement can be enhanced with the cervical spine positioned in extension. This would be appropriate for a patient who has low irritability and severity of symptoms on cervical spine extension.

KNOWLEDGE CHECK

1. How would you define an accessory movement?
2. How can accessory movement testing inform clinical reasoning?

Movement Diagrams

A movement diagram can be used to record the relationship of pain, resistance or muscle spasm within the available range of movement. A movement diagram is a useful tool when learning how to examine joint movement. It is also a quick and easy way of recording information about joint movement. It was initially described by Geoffrey Maitland. For full details of compiling a movement diagram with clinical examples, refer to Hengeveld and Banks (2014).

A movement diagram is a graph that describes the behaviour of pain, resistance and muscle spasm, showing the intensity and position in range at which each is felt during a passive accessory or passive physiological movement of a joint (Fig. 4.37).

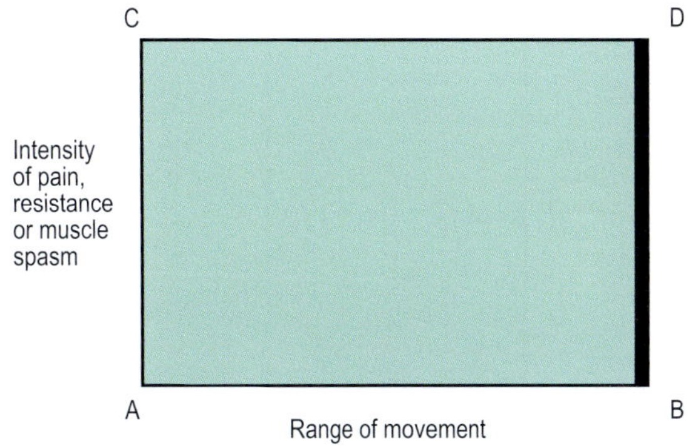

Fig. 4.37 A movement diagram. The baseline AB is the range of movement of any joint and the vertical axis AC depicts the intensity of pain, resistance or muscle spasm.

The baseline AB represents the range of movement of the joint. Point A represents the starting point of movement and can be anywhere in range. Point B is the end of the passive range of movement.

The vertical axis AC represents the severity, irritability and nature of the factors being plotted. Point A is the absence of any pain, resistance or spasm, while Point C is the maximum intensity that the clinician is prepared to provoke. The clinician needs to judge irritability and the underlying cause of the patient's symptoms to reason the acceptable levels of provocation. The horizontal line CD is where the limit of movement is marked.

Procedure for Drawing a Movement Diagram

To draw resistance (Fig. 4.38). The first point at which firm resistance is felt is called R_1 and is marked on baseline AB. A normal joint, when moved passively, has the feel of being well-oiled and friction-free until near the end of the range, when some resistance begins to be felt. As mentioned, the resistance to further movement at the end of the range may be due to bony apposition, increased tension in the surrounding ligaments and apposition of muscles and other soft tissues.

The joint is then taken to the limit of the range, and the point of limitation is marked by L on the line AB. If resistance limits the range, the point of limitation is marked by R_2 vertically above L on the CD line to indicate that resistance is limiting the range. R_2 is the point beyond which the clinician is not prepared to go. A line is drawn between R_1 and R_2, to depict the behaviour of the resistance.

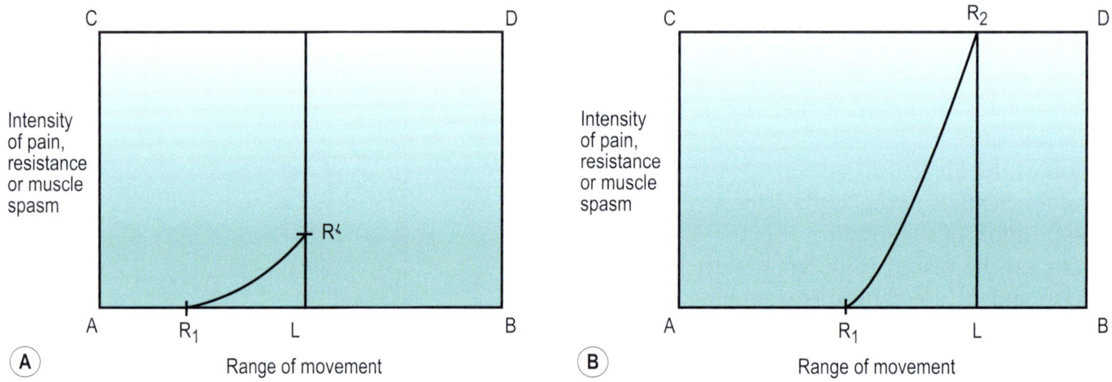

Fig. 4.38 Resistance depicted on a movement diagram for physiological movements. (A) The diagram describes a joint movement that is limited (L) to half range. Resistance is first felt at around one-quarter of full range (R_1) and increases a little at the end of the available range (R′). (B) The diagram describes a joint movement that is limited (L) to three-quarters range. Resistance is first felt at around half of full range (R_1) and gradually increases to the limit range of movement (R_2).

If the range of movement is limited by pain, an estimate of the intensity of resistance is made at the end of the available range and is plotted vertically above L as R'. The behaviour of the resistance between R_1 and R' is visualized by drawing a line between the two points.

The resistance curve of the movement diagram, representing physiological movements, is essentially part of the load-displacement curve of soft tissue and is shown in Fig. 4.39 (Panjabi, 1992; Lee & Evans, 1994). In a normal joint, the initial range of movement has minimal resistance, and this part is known as the toe region (Lee & Evans, 1994). As the joint is moved further into the range, resistance increases; this is known as the linear region (Lee & Evans, 1994). R_1 is the point at which the therapist perceives an increase in the resistance, generally somewhere between the toe region and the linear region.

The ease with which this change in resistance can be felt may depend on the range of joint movement and the type of movement being examined. It is likely that it is easier to feel R_1 when the range of movement is large and the toe region is relatively long, e.g. in elbow flexion. By contrast, accessory movements may only have a few millimetres of movement and no clear toe region (Petty et al., 2002). In this case, R_1 may be perceived at the beginning of the range, as shown in Fig. 4.40. A complication in finding R_1 also occurs with

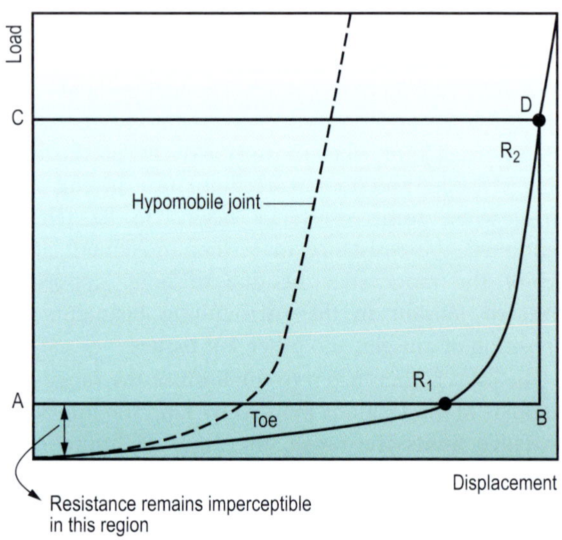

Fig. 4.39 Relationship of movement diagram (ABCD) to a load–displacement curve. (From Lee & Evans 1994, with permission.)

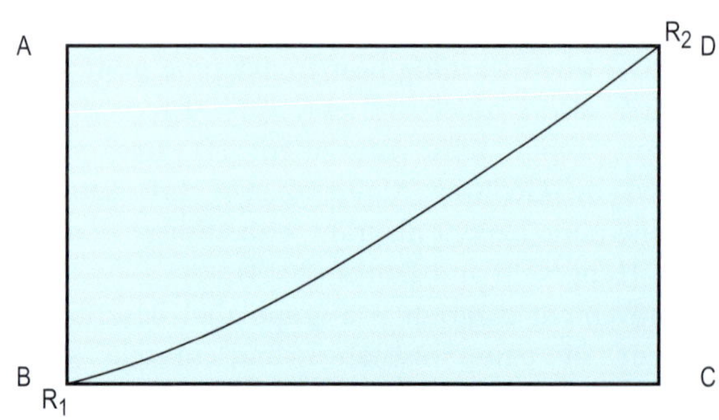

Fig. 4.40 A movement diagram of an accessory movement, where R_1 starts at the beginning of range (at A).

spinal accessory movements, because the movement cannot be localized to any one joint but produces a general movement of the spine (Lee & Svensson, 1990).

To draw pain (Fig. 4.41). In this case, the clinician must establish whether the patient has resting pain before moving the joint. The patient is asked to report any discomfort immediately.

The joint is then moved passively through the range. Several small oscillatory movements are carried out, gradually moving further into the range up to the point where the pain is first felt. The exact position in the range at which pain first occurs is marked as P1 on the baseline AB.

Next, the joint is moved passively beyond P_1, to determine the behaviour of the pain through the available range of movement. If pain limits range, the point of limitation is marked as L on baseline AB. Vertically above L, P_2 is marked on the CD line to indicate pain limits the range. The behaviour of the pain between P_1 and P_2 has now been drawn.

If, however, it is resistance that limits the range of movement, an estimate of the intensity of pain is made at the end of the range and plotted vertically above L as P'. The behaviour of the pain between P_1 and P' is then represented by drawing a line between the two points.

To draw muscle spasm (Fig. 4.42). The joint is taken through the range and the point at which resistance due to muscle spasm is first felt is marked on baseline AB as S_1.

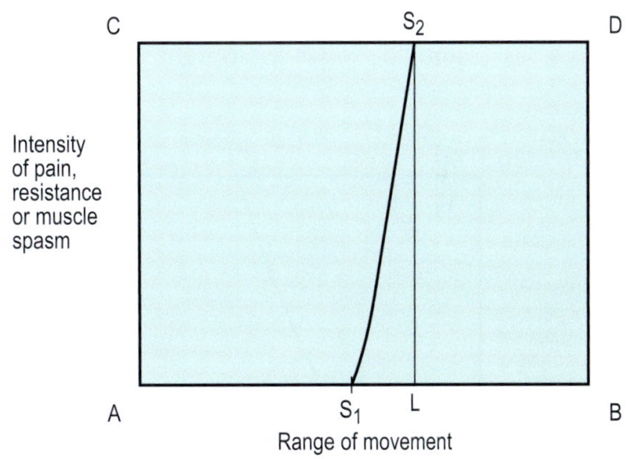

Fig. 4.42 Muscle spasm depicted on a movement diagram. The diagram describes a joint movement that is limited to three-quarters range (L). Muscle spasm is first felt just before three-quarters of full range (S_1) and quickly increases to limit the range of movement (S_2).

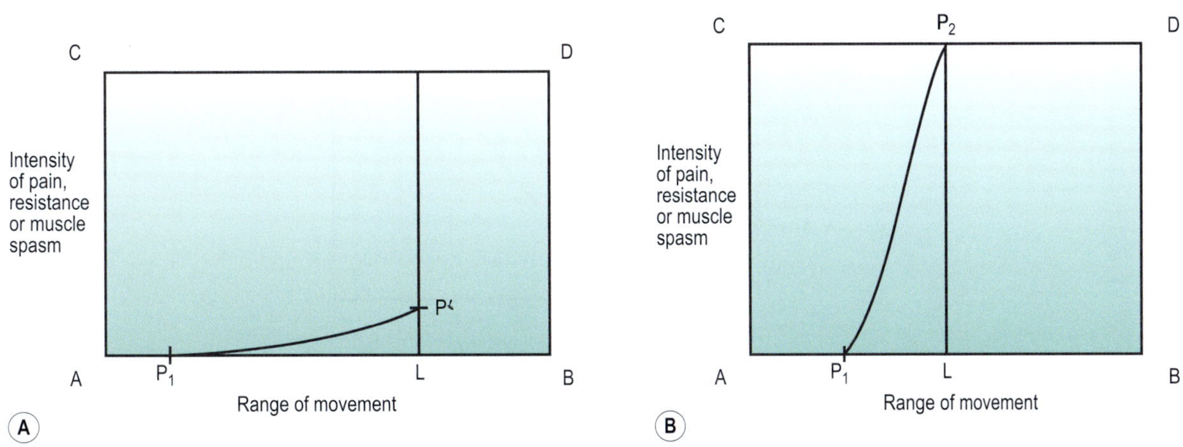

Fig. 4.41 Pain depicted on a movement diagram. (A) The diagram describes a joint movement that is limited to three-quarters range (L). Pain is first felt at around one-quarter of full range (P_1) and increases a little at the end of available range (P′). (B) The diagram describes a joint movement that is limited to half range (L). Pain is first felt at around one-quarter of full range (P_1) and gradually increases to limit range of movement (P_2).

The joint is then taken to the limit of the range. If muscle spasm limits range, the point of limitation is marked as L on baseline AB. Vertically above L, S_2 is marked on the CD line to indicate that muscle spasm is limiting the range. The behaviour of spasm is then plotted between S_1 and S_2. Spasm limiting range reaches its maximum quickly and is represented on the line as more or less a straight line almost vertically upwards. The resistance from muscle spasm varies depending on the speed at which the joint is moved—as the speed increases, so the resistance increases.

Examples of movement diagrams are given in Fig. 4.43.

A few examples of movement diagrams are shown in Fig. 4.44.

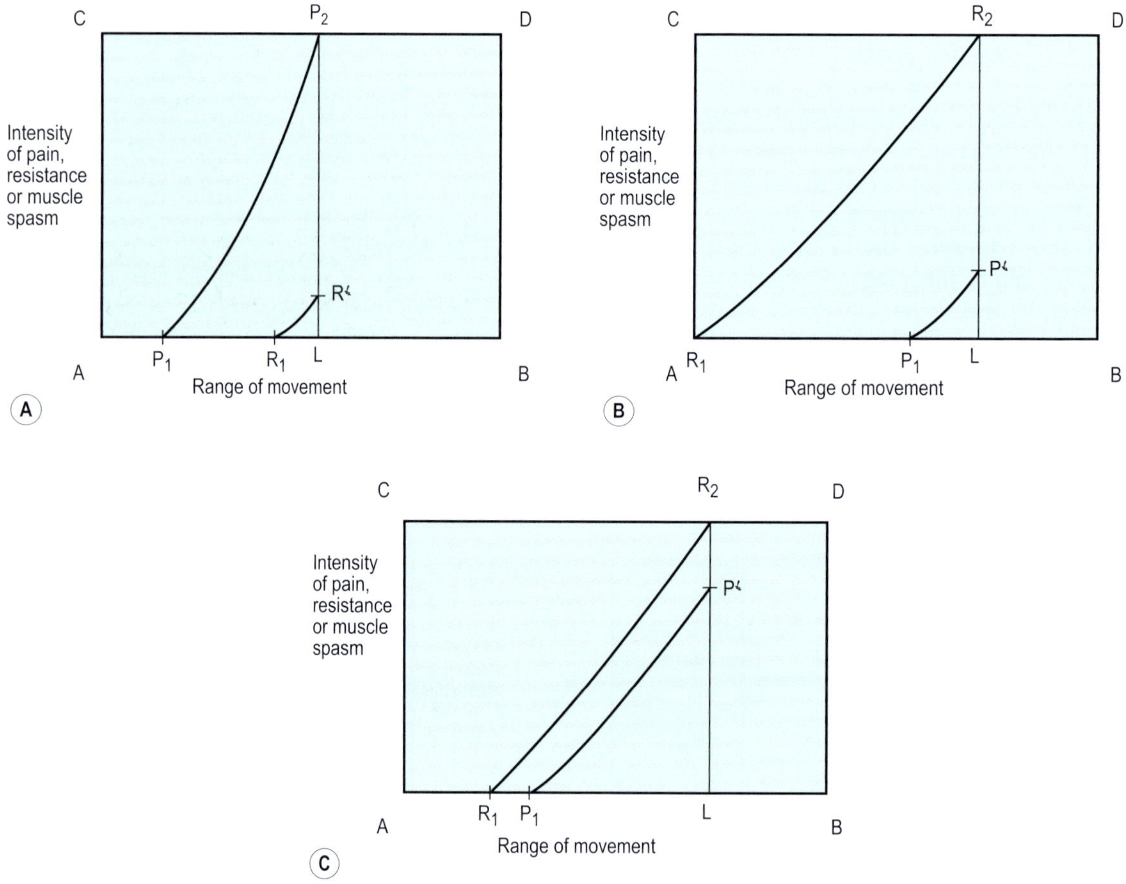

Fig. 4.43 Examples of completed movement diagrams. (A) Shoulder joint flexion. Interpretation: shoulder joint flexion is limited to just over half range (L). Pain first comes on at about one-quarter of full range (P_1) and increases to limit the range of movement (P_2). Resistance is first felt just before the end of the available range (R_1) and increases a little (R′). The movement is therefore predominantly limited by pain. (B) Central posteroanterior (PA) pressure on L3. Interpretation: the PA movement is limited to three-quarters range (L). Resistance is felt immediately, at the beginning of range (R_1), and increases to limit the range of movement (R_2). Pain is first felt just before the limit of the available range (P_1) and increases slightly (P′). The movement is therefore predominantly limited by resistance. (C) Left cervical rotation. Interpretation: left cervical rotation is limited to three-quarters range (L). Resistance is first felt at one-quarter of full range (R_1) and increases to limit range of movement (R_2). Pain is felt very soon after resistance (P_1) and increases (P′) to an intensity of about 8/10 (where 0 represents no pain and 10 represents the maximum pain ever felt by the patient). Cervical rotation is therefore limited by resistance, but pain is a significant factor.

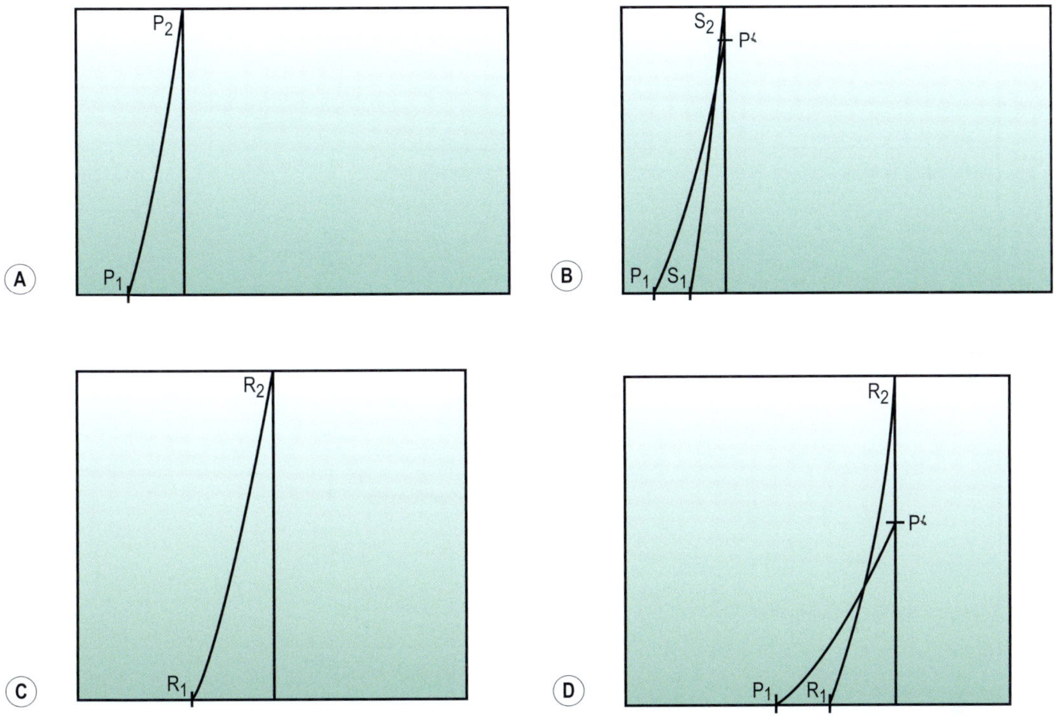

Fig. 4.44 Comparison of movement diagrams and joint pictures. (A) Pain limits movement early in the range. (B) Spasm and pain limit movement early in range. (C) Resistance limits movement halfway through range. (D) Limitation of movement to three-quarters range because of resistance, with some pain provoked from halfway through range.

COMPLETION OF THE PHYSICAL EXAMINATION

Once all steps have been carried out, the physical examination is complete. It is important to record the examination accurately and to highlight with an asterisk (*) the important findings from the examination (Hengeveld, 2014). These findings must be reassessed at and during subsequent treatment sessions, to evaluate the effects of treatment on the patient's condition. An outline examination chart that summarizes the physical examination is shown in Fig. 4.45.

The physical testing procedures which specifically indicate joint, nerve or muscle tissues as a source of the patient's symptoms are summarized in Table 5.2.

Findings at one end of the scale represent strong evidence and at the other end weak evidence. A variety of presentations between these two extremes may be found. For further information, the reader is directed to Chapter 5.

Clinicians may find the treatment and management planning form shown in Fig. 4.46 helpful as a guide to what is often a complex clinical reasoning process.

On completion of the physical examination the clinician:

- Gives the patient the opportunity to ask questions. Any misconceptions should be cleared up at this stage.
- Explains to the patient the findings of the physical examination and how these relate to their symptoms, using appropriate language.
- Warns the patient of possible exacerbation up to 24–48 hours following the examination. With severe and/or irritable conditions, the patient may have increased symptoms following examination.
- Requests that the patient reports at the next attendance details of their symptoms following examination.
- Evaluates the findings, using clinical reasoning forms to refine the primary hypothesis. This includes

Observation	Isometric muscle testing
Joint integrity tests	Other muscle tests
Active and passive physiological movements	Neurological integrity tests
	Neurodynamic tests
	Other nerve tests
	Miscellaneous tests
Muscle strength	
	Palpation
Muscle control	
	Accessory movements and reassessment of each relevant region
Muscle length	

Fig. 4.45 Physical Examination Chart

List the patient's subjective reassessment asterisks (*) you will use	
Subjective	Physical

What outcome measures will you use to evaluate management interventions?

Indicate your primary hypothesis (H1) regarding the cause of the patient's complaint and identify evidence to support this decision				
Primary hypothesis (H1)	Alternative	Alternative	Alternative	Alternative
Evidence				

List the positive and negative factors (from both subjective and physical examination findings) in considering the patient's prognosis	
Positive	Negative

Management options
1.1. Based on your primary hypothesis briefly outline a clinically reasoned treatment programme
1.2. What would your management be on day 1? Why was this chosen over other options?
1.3. What is your expectation of the patient's response over the next 24 hours?
If the patient returned better, how would you modify your treatment?
If the patient returned the same, how would you modify your treatment?
If the patient returned worse, how would you modify your treatment?
Comment on this patient's prognosis. (Include your estimation of the % improvement for this patient, the number of treatments required to achieve this and the time period over which it will occur)

Fig. 4.46 Management planning form (to be completed after the physical examination). (After Maitland 1985.)

1. Activity and participation capabilities/restrictions

Activity capability	Restriction
Participation capability	Restriction

2. Patient's perspectives on their experience

Examples:
- Their understanding
- Their feelings
- Their coping strategies
- Attitude to self-management and physical activity
- Their beliefs/what does this experience mean to them?
- Their expectations
- Their goals

3. Pathobiological mechanisms

3.1 Tissue sources/tissue healing, e.g., at what stage of the inflammatory/healing process would you judge the principal disorder to be?

3.2 Pain mechanisms. List the subjective evidence which supports each specific mechanism of symptoms

Input mechanism		Processing mechanism	Output mechanism
Nociceptive symptoms	Neuropathic symptoms	Nociplastic changes	Behaviour, motor function, thoughts, beliefs, cognition, autonomic nervous system

Reflect on this pie chart the proportional involvement of the pain mechanisms

Nociceptive
Peripheral neuropathic
Nociplastic changes
Autonomic nervous system

4. The sources of the symptoms

List in order of likelihood the possible structures at fault for each area/component of symptoms

Tissue sources	Symptom 1:	Symptom 2:	Symptom 3:	Symptom 4:
Local				
Referred				
Neurogenic				
Vascular				
Visceral				

Fig. 4.47 Clinical reasoning form revisited.

5. **Contributing factors**

Examples:
- Physical
- Environmental
- Psychosocial
- Health related

6. **History of symptoms**

Onset/physical impairment/stage/implications for physical examination

7. **List for each area of symptoms**

	Aggravating activity	Time to aggravate	Stops the activity	Easing the activity	Time to ease	Irritability Yes/No	Severity Yes/No
Symptoms 1 (P_a)							
Symptoms 2 (P_a)							

8. **Give an indication of the proportion of inflammatory to mechanical components in this patient's pain presentation, together with the clinical features that support or negate your hypothesis**

Mechanical	Inflammatory
Justification	Justification

9. **Health considerations, precautions and contraindications to physical examination and management**

9.1 **Does the patient have any health, red flag or precaution to limit your physical examination?**

Consider the following in relation to red flags

9.2 **Is reproduction of symptoms easy or difficult to reproduce? How vigorously would you examine this patient for each area of symptoms?**

Symptom	Short of P_1	To P_1 only	25% reproduction of pain	Full reproduction of pain
P_1				
P_2				
P_3				

9.3 **Will a neurological integrity examination be necessary**

Yes No

Justify your decision

Fig. 4.47, cont'd

10. Indicate your primary (working) hypothesis (H1) regarding the cause of the patient's complaint and identify evidence to support this decision

Primary hypothesis (H1)	Alternative H	Alternative H	Alternative H	Alternative H
Evidence:				

To test Neurointegrity Yes No		Expected findings
Must	→	
Should	→	
Could	→	

Fig. 4.47, cont'd

writing a problem list, i.e. a concise numbered list of the patient's problems at the time of the examination. Signs and symptoms of patellofemoral dysfunction, for example, could include pain over the knee and difficulty ascending and descending stairs, secondary to reduced lateral gluteal control and eccentric quadriceps function. Problem lists should also reflect contributing factors such as general fitness, poor ergonomics and lack of sleep, as these will all impact on the patient's symptoms.

- Identify the agreed long- and short-term goals in collaboration with the patient. Short-term goals for the above example might be relief of knee pain on stairs. A long-term goal may be to return to sport.
- Devise an initial treatment plan in order to achieve the short- and long-term objectives through discussion with the patient. This includes a discussion of the options for management including the option to do nothing, to be active participant in their management discussing approaches and frequency of treatment. In the patellofemoral example, this might include using symptom modification on step up/down to justify prescription of exercises targeting proximal muscle strength and endurance of lateral glutei; passive accessory movements to the patella; taping to facilitate patellar malalignment; and specific exercises with biofeedback to facilitate vastus medialis oblique contraction in squat standing, progressing to steps and specific functional exercises and activities.

By the end of the physical examination, the clinician will be able to revisit and further develop the hypotheses categories generated from the subjective examination (see Fig. 4.47) (Jones & Rivett, 2004).

For further information on the treatment and management of patients with musculoskeletal dysfunction, please see the companion to this text: *Principles of Musculoskeletal Treatment and Management* (Barnard & Ryder, 2024).

REVIEW AND REVISE QUESTIONS

1. How can postural observations inform clinical reasoning?
2. How would you test joint stability? Can you offer examples of commonly used tests?
3. What are you looking for when examining active physiological movements?
4. What does the abbreviation PPIVM represent?
5. How can the examination of light touch sensation be assessed in the clinic, and which fibres and tracts are being tested?
6. When you test for motor changes, how can you differentiate a lesion of a spinal nerve root and from a peripheral nerve lesion?
7. How would you document a diminished reflex?
8. How can you test for nerve tissue sensitization?
9. What can be recorded on a movement diagram?
10. What do examination findings marked with an * (asterisk) indicate?

REFERENCES

Alshami, A.M., Souvlis, T., Coppieters, M.W., 2008. A review of plantar heel pain of neural origin: differential diagnosis and management. Man. Ther. 13, 103–111.

Beighton, P.H., Solomon, L., Soskolne, C.L., 1973. Articular mobility in an African population. Ann. Rheum. Dis. 32, 413–418.

Bergmark, A., 1989. Stability of the lumbar spine. A study in mechanical engineering. Acta Orthop. Scand. 230 (Suppl. l.), 20–24.

Bialosky, J.E., Bishop, M.D., George, S.Z., Robinson, M.E., 2011. Placebo response to manual therapy: something out of nothing? J. Man. Manip. Ther. 19 (1), 11–19.

Bialosky, J.E., Bishop, M.D., Price, D.D., Robinson, M.E., George, S.Z., 2009. The mechanisms of manual therapy in the treatment of musculoskeletal pain: a comprehensive model. Man. Ther. 14, 531–538.

Binkley, J.M., Stratford, P.W., Lott, S.A., Riddle, D.L., 1999. The lower extremity functional scale (LEFS): scale development, measurement properties, and clinical application. North American orthopaedic rehabilitation research network. Phys. Ther. 79, 371–383.

Bjorbækmo, W.S., Mengshoel, A.M., 2016. 'A touch of physiotherapy'—the significance and meaning of touch in the practice of physiotherapy. Physiother. Theory Pract. 32 (1), 10–19. https://doi.org/10.3109/09593985.2015.1071449.

Boyd, B.S., Villa, P.S., 2012. Normal inter-limb differences during the straight leg raise neurodynamic test: a cross sectional study. BMC Musculoskelet. Disord. 13, 245.

Boyd, B.S., 2012. Common interlimb asymmetries and neurogenic responses during upper limb neurodynamic testing: implications for test interpretation. J. Hand Ther. 25, 56–64.

Breig, A., 1978. Adverse Mechanical Tension in the Central Nervous System. Almqvist and Wiksell, Stockholm.

Butler, D.S., 2000. The Sensitive Nervous System. Neuro Orthopaedic Institute, Adelaide.

Cole, J.H., Furness, A.L., Twomey, L.T., 1988. Muscles in Action: An Approach to Manual Muscle Testing. Churchill Livingstone, Edinburgh.

Comerford, M.J., Mottram, S.L., 2013. Kinetic Control the Management of Uncontrolled Movement. Churchill Livingstone Elsevier, Edinburgh, pp. 23–42.

Comerford, M.J., Mottram, S.L., 2001. Movement and stability dysfunction—contemporary developments. Man. Ther. 6, 15–26.

Cook, N., van Griensven, H., Jesson, T., in press. Neuropathic pain and complex regional pain syndrome. In: van Griensven, H., Strong, J. (Eds.), Pain. A Textbook for Health Professionals. Churchill Livingston, Edinburgh.

Coppieters, M., Nee, R., 2015. Neurodynamic management of the peripheral nervous system. In: Jull, G., Moore, A., Falla, D., Lewis, J., McCarthy, C., Sterling, M., Khan, K. (Eds.), Grieves Modern Musculoskeletal Physiotherapy, fourth ed. Elsevier, Edinburgh, pp. 287–297.

Coppieters, M.W., Alshami, A.M., Babri, A.S., Souvlis, T., Kippers, V., Hodges, P.W., 2006. Strain and excursion of the sciatic, tibial, and plantar nerves during a modified straight leg raising test. J. Orthop. Res. 24, 1883–1889.

Covill, L.G., Peterson, S.M., 2012. Upper extremity neurodynamic tests: range of motion asymmetry may not indicate impairment. Physiother. Theory Into Pract. 28, 535–541.

Cyriax, J., 1982. Textbook of Orthopaedic Medicine—Diagnosis of Soft Tissue Lesions, eighth ed. Baillière Tindall, London.

Dankaerts, W., O'Sullivan, P.B., Strakera, L.M., Burnett, A.F., Skouen, J.S., 2006. The inter-examiner reliability of a classification method for nonspecific chronic low back pain patients with motor control impairment. Man. Ther. 11 (1), 28–39.

Dommerholt, J., 2011. Dry needling—peripheral and central considerations. J. Man. Manip. Ther. 19 (4), 223–237.

Donaghy, M., 1997. Neurology. Oxford University Press, Oxford.

Downs, M.B., Laporte, C., 2011. Conflicting dermatome maps: educational and clinical implications. J. Orthop. Sports Phys. Ther. 41, 427–434.

Drake, R.L., Vogl, W., Mitchell, A.W.M., 2005. Gray's Anatomy for Students. Churchill Livingstone, Philadelphia.

Duncan, P.W., Weiner, D.K., Chandler, J., Studenski, S., 1990. Functional reach: a new clinical measure of balance. J. Gerontol. 45 (6), 192–197.

Dyck, P., 1984. Lumbar nerve root: the enigmatic eponyms. Spine 9, 3–6.

Edwards, B.C., 1999. Manual of Combined Movements: Their Use in the Examination and Treatment of Mechanical Vertebral Column Disorders, second ed. Butterworth-Heinemann, Oxford.

Elvey, R.L., 1985. Brachial plexus tension tests and the pathoanatomical origin of arm pain. In: Glasgow, E.F., Twomey, L.T., Scull, E.R. (Eds.), Aspects of Manipulative Therapy, second ed. Churchill Livingstone, Melbourne, p. 116.

Fernández-De-Las-Peñas, C., Dommerholt, J., 2018. International consensus on diagnostic criteria and clinical considerations of myofascial trigger points: a Delphi study. Pain Med. 19, 142–150.

Fuller, G., 2004. Neurological Examination Made Easy. Churchill Livingstone, Edinburgh.

Galindo, H., 2005. Assessment of function. In: van Griensven, H. (Ed.), Pain in Practice: Theory and Treatment Strategies for Manual Therapists. Butterworth Heinemann, Edinburgh, pp. 153–180.

Gardner, E., 2021. Receptors of the somatosensory system. In: Kandel, E., Koester, J., Mack, S., Siegelbaum, S. (Eds.), Principles of Neural Science. McGraw Hill, New York.

Gerhardt, J.J., 1992. Documentation of Joint Motion, third ed. Isomed, Oregon.

Grieve, G.P., 1981. Common Vertebral Joint Problems. Churchill Livingstone, Edinburgh.

Grieve, G.P., 1991. Mobilisation of the Spine, fifth ed. Churchill Livingstone, Edinburgh.

Harding, V.R., de C. Williams, A.C., Richardson, P.H., Nicholas, M.K., Jackson, J.L., Richardson, I.H., Pither, C.E., 1994. The development of a battery of measures for assessing physical functioning of chronic pain patients. Pain 58, 367–375.

Hengeveld, E., 2014. Recording. In: Hengeveld, E., Banks, K. (Eds.), Maitlands's Vertebral Manipulation. Churchill Livingston, Edinburgh, pp. 433–443.

Hengeveld, E., Banks, K., 2014. Maitlands's Vertebral Manipulation. Churchill Livingston, Edinburgh.

Herrington, L., Bendix, K., Cornwell, C., Fielden, N., Hankey, K., 2008. What is the normal response to structural differentiation within the slump and straight leg raise tests? Man. Ther. 13, 289–294.

Hunter, J.M., 2002. Rehabilitation of the Hand and Upper Extremity, fifth ed. Mosby, St. Louis.

Hunter, G., 1998. Specific soft tissue mobilization in the management of soft tissue dysfunction. Man. Ther. 3, 2–11.

Inman, V.T., Saunders, J.B.D.M., 1944. Referred pain from skeletal structures. J. Nerv. Mental Dis. 99, 660–667.

Institute for Work and Health, 2006. The QuickDASH Outcome Measure. A Faster Way to Measure Upper-Extremity Disability and Symptoms. Information for Users. Institute for Work and Health, Toronto.

Ivanusic, J.J., 2007. The evidence for the spinal segmental innervation of bone. Clin. Anat. 20, 956–960.

Janda, V., 1993. Muscle strength in relation to muscle length, pain and muscle imbalance. In: Harms-Ringdahl, K. (Ed.), Muscle Strength. Churchill Livingstone, Edinburgh, p. 83.

Janda, V., 1994. Muscles and motor control in cervicogenic disorders: assessment and management. In: Grant, R. (Ed.), Physical Therapy of the Cervical and Thoracic Spine, second ed. Churchill Livingstone, Edinburgh, p. 195.

Janda, V., 2002. Muscles and motor control in cervicogenic disorders. In: Grant, R. (Ed.), Physical Therapy of the Cervical and Thoracic Spine, third ed. Churchill Livingstone, New York, p. 182.

Jones, M.A., Rivett, D.A., 2004. Clinical Reasoning for Manual Therapists. Butterworth-Heinemann, Edinburgh.

Jull, G.A., Janda, V., 1987. Muscles and motor control in low back pain: assessment and management. In: Twomey, L.T., Taylor, J.R. (Eds.), Physical Therapy of the Low Back. Churchill Livingstone, Edinburgh, p. 253 (Chapter 10).

Jull, G.A., Richardson, C.A., 1994. Rehabilitation of active stabilization of the lumbar spine. In: Twomey, L.T., Taylor, J.R. (Eds.), Physical Therapy of the Low Back, second ed. Churchill Livingstone, Edinburgh, p. 251.

Kaltenborn, F.M., 2002. Manual Mobilization of the Joints In: The Extremities, sixth ed., vol. I. Olaf Norli, Oslo.

Kendall, F.P., McCreary, E.K., Provance, P.G., 1993. Muscles: Testing and Function, fourth ed. Lippincott, Williams & Wilkins, Baltimore.

Kendall, F.P., McCreary, E.K., Provance, P.G., Rodgers, M., Roamni, W., 2010. Muscles: Testing and Function with Posture and Pain, fifth ed. Lippincott, Williams & Wilkins, Baltimore.

Kenneally, M., Rubenach, H., Elvey, R., 1988. The upper limb tension test: the SLR test of the arm. In: Grant, R. (Ed.), Physical Therapy of the Cervical and Thoracic Spine. Churchill Livingstone, Edinburgh, p. 167.

Kobayashi, S., Suzuki, Y., Asai, T., Yoshizawa, H., 2003. Changes in nerve root motion and intraradicular blood flow during intraoperative femoral nerve stretch test. Report of four cases. J. Neurosurg. 99 (3), 298–305.

Lai, W.-H., Shih, Y.-F., Lin, P.-L., Chen, W.-Y., Ma, H.-L., 2012. Normal neurodynamic responses of the femoral slump test. Man. Ther. 17, 126–132.

Leak, S.V., 1998. Measurement of physiotherapists' ability to reliably generate vibration amplitudes and pressures using a tuning fork. Man. Ther. 3, 90–94.

Lee, M., Svensson, N.L., 1990. Measurement of stiffness during simulated spinal physiotherapy. Clin. Phys. Physiol. Meas. 11, 201–207.

Lee, R., Evans, J., 1994. Towards a better understanding of spinal posteroanterior mobilisation. Physiotherapy 80, 68–73.

Lewis, J.S., 2009. Rotator cuff tendinopathy/subacromial impingement syndrome: is it time for a new method of assessment? Br. J. Sports Med. 43, 259–264.

Magee, D., Manske, R., 2021. Orthopedic Physical Assessment, seventh ed. Saunders Elsevier, St. Lois.

Martínez, M.D., Cubas, C.L., Girbés, E.L., 2014. Ulnar nerve neurodynamic test: study of the normal sensory response in asymptomatic individuals. J. Orthop. Sports Phys. Ther. 44, 450–456.

May, S., Clare, H., 2015. The McKenzie method of mechanical diagnosis and therapy—an overview. In: Jull, G., Moore, A., Falla, D., Lewis, J., McCarthy, C., Sterling, M., Khan, K. (Eds.), Grieves Modern Musculoskeletal Physiotherapy, fourth ed. Elsevier, Edinburgh, pp. 460–462.

Medical Research Council, 1976. Aids to the Investigation of Peripheral Nerve Injuries. HMSO, London.

Miller, A.M., 1987. Neuro-meningeal limitation of straight leg raising. In: Dalziel, B.A., Snowsill, J.C. (Eds.), Manipulative Therapists Association of Australia. 5th Biennial Conference Proceedings, Melbourne, pp. 70–78.

Moini, J., Piran, P., 2020. Functional and Clinical Neuroanatomy: A Guide for Health Care Professionals, first ed. Elsevier, Edinburgh.

Mooney, V., Robertson, J., 1976. The facet syndrome. Clin. Orthop. Relat. Res. 115, 149–156.

Muscolino, J., 2016. The Muscle Bone Palpation Manual, second ed. Elsevier Mosby, Missouri.

Nadler, S.F., Malanga, G.A., Stitik, T.P., Keswani, R., Foye, P.M., 2001. The crossed femoral nerve stretch test to improve diagnostic sensitivity for the high lumbar radiculopathy: 2 case reports. Arch. Phys. Med. Rehab. 82, 522–523.

Nee, R.J., Yang, C.H., Liang, C.C., Tseng, G.F., Coppieters, M.W., 2010. Impact of order of movement on nerve strain and longitudinal excursion: a biomechanical study with implications for neurodynamic test sequencing. Man. Ther. 15, 376–381.

Nir-Paz, R., Luder, A.S., Cozacov, J.C., Shahin, R., 1999. Saphenous nerve entrapment in adolescence. Paediatrics 103, 161–163.

Norkin, C., White, D.J., 2016. Measurement of Joint Motion A Guide to Goniometry. F.A. Davis, Philadelphia.

O'Connaire, E., Rushton, A., Wright, C., 2011. The assessment of vibration sense in the musculoskeletal examination: moving towards a valid and reliable quantitative approach to vibration testing in clinical practice. Man. Ther. 16, 296–300.

Panjabi, M.M., 1992. The stabilizing system of the spine. Part II. Neutral zone and instability hypothesis. J. Spinal Disord. 5, 390–396.

Petty, N.J., Maher, C., Latimer, J., Lee, M., 2002. Manual examination of accessory movements—seeking R1. Man. Ther. 7, 39–43.

Porter, S., Wilson, J., 2020. A Comprehensive Guide to Sports Physiology and Injury Management: An Interdisciplinary Approach, first ed. Elsevier, St. Louis.

Ridehalgh, C., Moore, A., Hough, A., 2015. Sciatic nerve excursion during a modified passive straight leg raise test in asymptomatic participants and participants with spinally referred leg pain. Man. Ther. 20, 564–569.

Ridehalgh, C., Sandy-Hindmarch, O.P., Schmid, A., 2018. Validity of clinical small-fiber sensory testing to detect small-nerve fiber degeneration. J. Orthop. Sports Phys. Ther. 48, 767–774.

Roland, M., Fairbank, J., 2000. The Roland–Morris disability questionnaire and the oswestry disability questionnaire. Spine 25 (24), 3115–3124.

Russek, L.N., Stott, P., Simmonds, J., 2019. Recognizing and effectively managing hypermobility-related conditions. Phys. Ther. 99, 1189–1200.

Sahrmann, S.A., 2002. Diagnosis and Treatment of Movement Impairment Syndromes. Mosby, St Louis.

Schmid, A.B., 2015. The peripheral nervous system and its compromise in entrapment neuropathies. In: Jull, G., Moore, A., Falla, D., Lewis, J., McCarthy, C., Sterling, M., Khan, K. (Eds.), Grieves Modern Musculoskeletal Physiotherapy, fourth ed. Elsevier, Edinburgh, pp. 78–89.

Schmid, A.B., Fundaun, J., Tampin, B., 2020. Entrapment neuropathies: a contemporary approach to pathophysiology, clinical assessment, and management. Pain Rep 5 (4), e829.

Schmid, A.B., Nee, R.J., Coppieters, M.W., 2013. Reappraising entrapment neuropathies—mechanisms, diagnosis and management. Man. Ther. 18, 449–457.

Schohmacher, J., 2009. The convex-concave rule and the lever law. Man. Ther. 14, 579–582.

Shacklock, M., 2005. Clinical Neurodynamics. Churchill Livingstone, Edinburgh.

Singh, S.J., Morgan, M.D., Scott, S., Walters, D., Hardman, A.E., 1992. Development of a shuttle walking test of disability in patients with chronic airways obstruction. Thorax 47 (12), 1019–1024.

Slater, H., 1994. The Sensitive Nervous System. Neuro Orthopaedic Institute, Adelaide.

Slater, D., Korakakis, V., O'Sullivan, P., Nolan, D., O'Sullivan, K., 2019. 'Sit up straight': time to re-evaluate. Orthop. Sports Phys. Ther. 49 (8), 562–564.

Sterling, M., Rebbeck, T., 2005. The neck disability index (NDI). Aust. J. Physiother. 51 (4), 271.

Sueki, D.G., Cleland, J.A., Wainner, R.S., 2013. A regional interdependence model of musculoskeletal dysfunctions: research, mechanisms, and clinical implications. J. Man. Manip. Ther. 21 (2), 90–102.

Suri, P., Rainville, J., Ktaz, J., Jouve, C., Hartigan, C., Limke, J., Pena, E., Li, L., Swaim, B., Hunter, D.J., 2011. The accuracy of the physical examination for the diagnosis of mid-lumbar and low lumbar nerve root impingement. Spine (Phila Pa 1976 36 (1), 63–73.

Tencer, A.F., Allen Jr., B.L., Ferguson, R.L., 1985. A biomechanical study of thoracolumbar spine fractures with bone in the canal. Part III. Mechanical properties of the dura and its tethering ligaments. Spine 10, 741–747.

Threlkeld, A.J., 1992. The effects of manual therapy on connective tissue. Phys. Ther. 72 (12), 893–902.

Valdes, K., LaStayo, P., 2013. The value of provocative tests for the wrist and elbow: a literature review. J. Hand Ther. 26, 32–43.

Van Dillen, L.R., Maluf, K.S., Sahrmann, S.A., 2009. Reliability of physical examination items used for classification of patients with low back pain. Man. Ther. 14, 52–60.

Walsh, J., Hall, T., 2009. Reliability, validity and diagnostic accuracy of palpation of the sciatic, tibial and common peroneal nerves in the examination of low back related leg pain. Man. Ther. 14, 623–629.

Walsh, J., Flatley, M., Johnston, N., Bennett, K., 2007. Slump test: sensory responses in asymptomatic subjects. J. Man. Manip. Ther. 15, 231–238.

Walton, J.H., 1989. Essentials of Neurology, sixth ed. Churchill Livingstone, Edinburgh.

Wernli, K., O'Sullivan, P., Smith, A., Campbell, A., Kent, P., 2020. Movement, posture and low back pain. How do they relate? A replicated single-case design in 12 people with persistent, disabling low back pain. Eur. J. Pain 24, 1831–1849.

Williams, P.L., 1995. In: Williams, P.L., Bannister, L.H., Berry, M.M. (Eds.), Gray's Anatomy, thirty-eighth. Churchill Livingstone, Edinburgh.

Yaxley, G.A., Jull, G.A., 1993. Adverse tension in the neural system. A preliminary study of tennis elbow. Aust. J. Physiother. 39, 15–22.

5

Clinical Reasoning and Assessment: Making Sense of Examination Findings

Dionne Ryder, Matthew Low, and Neil Langridge

LEARNING OUTCOMES

After studying this chapter, you should be able to:

- Explain what is understood by the term clinical reasoning and describe different models of reasoning.
- Discuss how clinical reasoning informs decision making and possible errors in the process.
- Explore how evidence, guidelines classification and prediction rules inform reasoning.
- Identify the importance of keeping the patient central to the reasoning process.
- Explain how information from the subjective and physical examinations contributes to the clinical reasoning process.
- Identify the skills and attributes the clinician needs to continually develop their reasoning skills.
- Identify how clinicians can use reasoning to identify those at risk of developing persistent symptoms.
- Utilise clinical reasoning to ensure appropriate management options are identified and offered to the patient.

CHAPTER CONTENTS

Introduction, 143
Clinical Reasoning, 144
Developments in Decision-Making, 146
Entering Into a Person's Story, 150
Activity and Participation Capabilities and Restrictions, 151
Patient's Perspectives on Their Experience, 152
Pathobiological Mechanisms, 152
Tissue Responses and Healing, 152
Pain Mechanisms, 153
Physical Impairments and Associated Structure/Tissue Sources, 154
Contributing Factors to the Development and Maintenance of the Problem, 156
Precautions/Contraindications to Physical Examination, Treatment and Management, 157
Severity and Irritability, 158
Management Strategy and Treatment Planning, 160
Prognosis, 166
Conclusion, 166
References, 167

INTRODUCTION

The previous chapters describe a step-by-step approach to the subjective and physical examination. This chapter aims to revisit some of the information included within the preceding chapters to explore how data is interpreted by the clinician. It is hoped that taken together, these chapters will provide an overview of the broad clinical reasoning processes that underpin effective, robust treatment and management decisions.

CLINICAL REASONING

Clinical reasoning could be described as the process by which the clinician interprets information from the patient and their history along with physical examination findings, in order to identify the most appropriate management plan for individual patients. However, this description belies a far more complex process that involves interpreting multiple perspectives, and understanding oneself with respect to managing one's bias whilst all the while aiming to create a therapeutic relationship with the patient. Throughout the clinical encounter, the clinician needs to come to terms with evidence from both verbal and nonverbal cues to gain an understanding of the clinical presentation, its impact, the rehabilitation goals and also ensure safety. The collaboration of decision-making across the patient interview and into the physical examination is now recognized as a co-constructed shared management plan with agreed goals (Politi & Street, 2011). Musculoskeletal physiotherapy has moved from an empirico-analytical model which results in distancing the patient from the clinician; for example, the clinician asks the question and interprets the answers as opposed to one that embraces the social context of the examination and offers a focus on health-related behaviour change, psychological and contextual factors rather than purely focusing on physical symptoms (Houtman et al., 1994; Petty et al., 2012a, 2012b; Vargas-Prada & Coggon, 2015).

Successful reasoning requires the ability to interpret and process multiple pieces of information concurrently, whilst prioritizing patients' needs within a healthcare framework and ensuring diagnosis, prognosis and planning are reached in a collaborative way that enhances outcomes, or informs the next step in the patient journey. There are numerous influences on the reasoning process, and it is important for clinicians to be aware of these and adapt appropriately when faced with complexity. Clinical reasoning is a core competency of musculoskeletal practice and requires the clinician to systematically address a range of challenges in the assessment of patients, clients and service users (Higgs, 1992; Cruz et al., 2012; Wijbenga et al., 2019).

Effective communication skills are essential to gather information, negotiate and collaborate with the patient in exploring possible solutions. Advanced cognitive skills are necessary to incorporate a range of knowledge and, where available, relevant research evidence to support thinking. Interactions with patients do not take place within a vacuum so an ability to identify the patient's human context and reflect on how clinical practice is shaped and influenced by the clinician's own life experiences is also central to effective reasoning (Higgs & Jones, 2008).

Clinical reasoning is the foundation of effective patient care. It is through this process of critical thinking, incorporating the best available evidence and reflecting on the process, that collaborative decisions are made with the patient about the most appropriate care for each individual patient (Higgs & Jones, 2008).

The complex process of clinical reasoning has been studied and presented in the form of a number of theoretical models (Jones, 1995; Gifford, 1998; Edwards et al., 2004; Jones & Rivett, 2004; Danneels et al., 2011) which have developed over time in response to new knowledge, so allowing the clinical practice to evolve.

Early models in musculoskeletal practice have been heavily influenced by the hypothetico-deductive model. Such models have a history within medicine and ask that practitioners draw upon prior knowledge of possible causes of symptoms and generate a range of potential hypotheses. The use of the hypothetico-deductive model of reasoning in healthcare was identified in 1978 by Elstein et al., who suggested that diagnostic problems are solved by generating a number of hypotheses or problem formulations, which then guide clinical data collection. The model focuses on the processes of cue acquisition, hypothesis generation, cue interpretation, and hypothesis evaluation (Loftus & Smith, 2008). This technique of collecting data and then generating hypotheses is a method that structures a problem into possible solutions. A systematic approach is then applied via tests or questions that either support or refute the possible solutions. These hypotheses are then tested either through questions, physical tests, or combinations to draw out a potential diagnosis that is often based upon a pathoanatomical model and therefore tissue source such as disc, facet, arthritis or nerve, as a cause of the symptoms. Whilst these models seek to represent how clinicians function in practice, research has shown that clinicians, whether expert or novice, often use a number of different reasoning strategies in parallel (Doody & McAteer, 2002). Experienced clinicians have been found to use pattern recognition reasoning early on in a patient encounter. Pattern recognition requires the clinical examiner to make assumptions that are fast and effective and are related to the structure of a person's memory (Patel et al., 1997). This has been developed from cognitive psychology and involves the clinicians using 'illness scripts' which are presentations of conditions that are supported by the clinician's previous experience (Arocha et al., 1993). Schmidt and Rikers (2007) suggest that pattern recognition is the matching of memory to previously seen presentations. It is thought that expert clinicians use their well-organized and extensive knowledge base to search quickly for familiar patterns to forward or inductively reason. It is thought that using illness scripts to create patterns offers the opportunity to identify presenting features of frequently encountered conditions quickly (Feltowich & Barrows, 1984) (Fig. 5.1).

Although pattern recognition allows for fast and efficient inductive reasoning, it is vulnerable to errors including the tendency for the clinician to make the features fit (Maitland et al., 2005). This can result in the bias sifting of information, whereby data supporting a favoured or familiar pattern are accepted, whilst contradictory data are rejected. This was the first of three types of reasoning errors identified by Grant (2008), the others being errors in interpreting the meaning and misjudging the relevance of information.

Due to the high risk of error, experienced clinicians do not rely entirely on pattern recognition but seek to explore/test further initial hypotheses that have been generated through pattern recognition. Using this deductive reasoning process, working hypotheses are confirmed or refuted through gathering data by further questioning and selected physical examination testing. Although more time-consuming than pattern recognition, the hypothetico-deductive reasoning process is considered more robust. However, this is dependent on the ability of clinicians to interpret subjective and physical findings.

How clinicians interpret information will depend on their propositional and nonpropositional knowledge base. Propositional knowledge is identified as scientific/theoretical knowledge derived from the literature. Nonpropositional knowledge can be further subdivided into professional craft knowledge, accumulated through experience or from formal teaching and personal knowledge. These forms of knowledge anchor a frame of reference for all individual clinicians, including their beliefs and values which have been shaped by their experiences (Higgs & Titchen, 1995) (Fig. 5.2).

Pattern recognition and hypothetico-deductive reasoning are considered forms of diagnostic reasoning and do not encompass the cognitive, psychological, social and intellectual context in which care is being given (Kerry, 2010). Through an interpretive approach, the clinician seeks to decipher and understand the patient's problem through the use of narrative reasoning by listening to the patient's story (Edwards et al., 2006). Intuitive practice may occur when the clinician empathizes, seeks to understand and

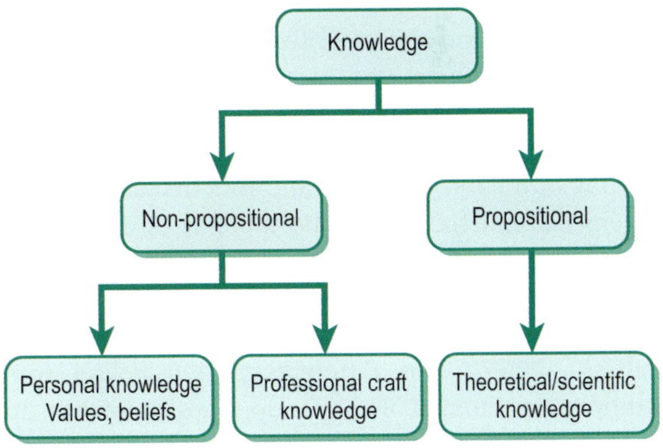

Fig. 5.2 Knowledge flow diagram. (From Higgs & Titchen, 1995, with permission.)

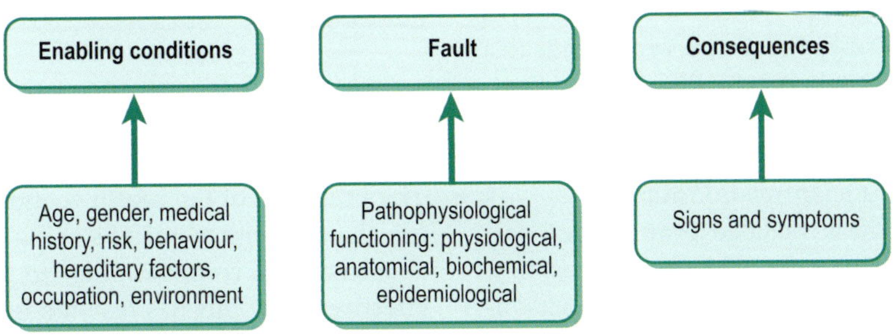

Fig. 5.1 Illness scripts. Experts will have an illness script for each condition/disease they know. How complete they are will depend on how often they have encountered patients with the condition. (From Feltowich & Barrows, 1984, with permission.)

communicates with the patient, and so attention to the social context is needed (Orme & Maggs, 1993). Gut-feeling is well documented in the literature in medicine and is normally associated with decision-making around a sense of alarm or concern (Langridge et al., 2016). Intuitive thought and gut-feeling both seem to sit well with the definition of subconscious decisions that are difficult to explain (Hammond, 1996). It remains largely invisible as it is not articulated (Standing, 2008). The Lens model (Cooksey, 1996) offers a structure that may explain how intuition and gut-feeling differ from pattern recognition. The model takes an uncertain situation (intangible state) and uses the cues from that situation to build into patterns of prioritized information. If enough of these pieces of information can be grouped, they may form a heuristic (rule of thumb), this will generate a behaviour or outcome. The model shows that the accuracy of a decision is affected by many indicators and how those indicators are integrated and judged. These cues may mean very little without context, yet as a group or pattern they mean a course of action is needed. It is therefore not just the recognition of the patterns but the prioritization of these that differentiates the three modes of thinking. The 'Lens model' takes the intangible state (such as intuition) and validates it to a judgement via knowledge and understanding of the relevance of indicators that support that judgement. Gut-feeling can be thought of as intuitive thought that has created concern; the patterns are such that it creates a neuro-physiological response in the clinician as it raises alarm in some way (Bechara & Damasio, 2005). This differentiates gut-feeling from intuition, i.e. thought without awareness, and has not raised that awareness in a physiological way, as the cues have not grouped to arouse the tacit skills of the clinician to a physical response (Stolper et al., 2010). The gut-feeling response has potentially produced a neurophysiological prioritized response which leads to a raised awareness (McCutcheon & Pincombe, 2001). The overarching theory referred to what was described as a 'synergy' which linked the described factors involving the patient/clinician relationship.

In contrast, the patient is included as an integral part of the decision-making process. This model has now been further reconstructed and described as person-centred (Fig. 5.3). This person-centred collaborative model really links the two perspectives (clinician and patient) towards a purposeful design of the factors that might be contributing to the symptoms or the reason for the clinical encounter. The clinician then looks to link these causal factors in collaboration with the patient into a bespoke model that represents the patient's perspectives, requirements and finally leads to a co-constructed management plan which is ultimately built on the patient's story (Low, 2017).

This revised model acknowledges that the patient's thoughts and beliefs are integral to the process of reasoning and so should be incorporated through interpretive reasoning in order to encompass patient/person-centred care (Cooper et al., 2008).

Clinical expertise should not be measured in terms of years qualified but on how effective reflection is on the development of dialectical reasoning skills which encompass both diagnostic and interpretive paradigms (Terry & Higgs, 1993; Jones & Rivett, 2004; Wainwright et al., 2011). Recognizing that clinical reasoning and expert practice is an ongoing journey that supports the importance of continuing professional development through self-reflection (Higgs & Jones, 2008). A powerful tool for developing reflective skills is through engagement with case studies, peer coaching, completion of clinical reasoning templates or the development of mind maps. The reader is directed to section six of Higgs and Jones (2008) book, *Clinical reasoning in the health professions*, for an in-depth exploration of strategies to develop clinical reasoning skills.

KNOWLEDGE CHECK

1. List the different models of clinical reasoning that are commonly referred to in musculoskeletal physiotherapy practice.
2. Describe the different forms of knowledge that can be drawn from when participating in the clinical reasoning process.
3. What tools may be helpful for developing reflective skills relevant to the development of clinical reasoning?

DEVELOPMENTS IN DECISION-MAKING

The pressures of the health economy have been a driver for change, with clinicians being increasingly accountable to service commissioners to provide the most cost-effective care. This has resulted in the development of a whole series of adjuncts to clinical reasoning, such as clinical guidelines, clinical prediction rules (CPRs), treatment protocols and diagnostic/treatment classification systems.

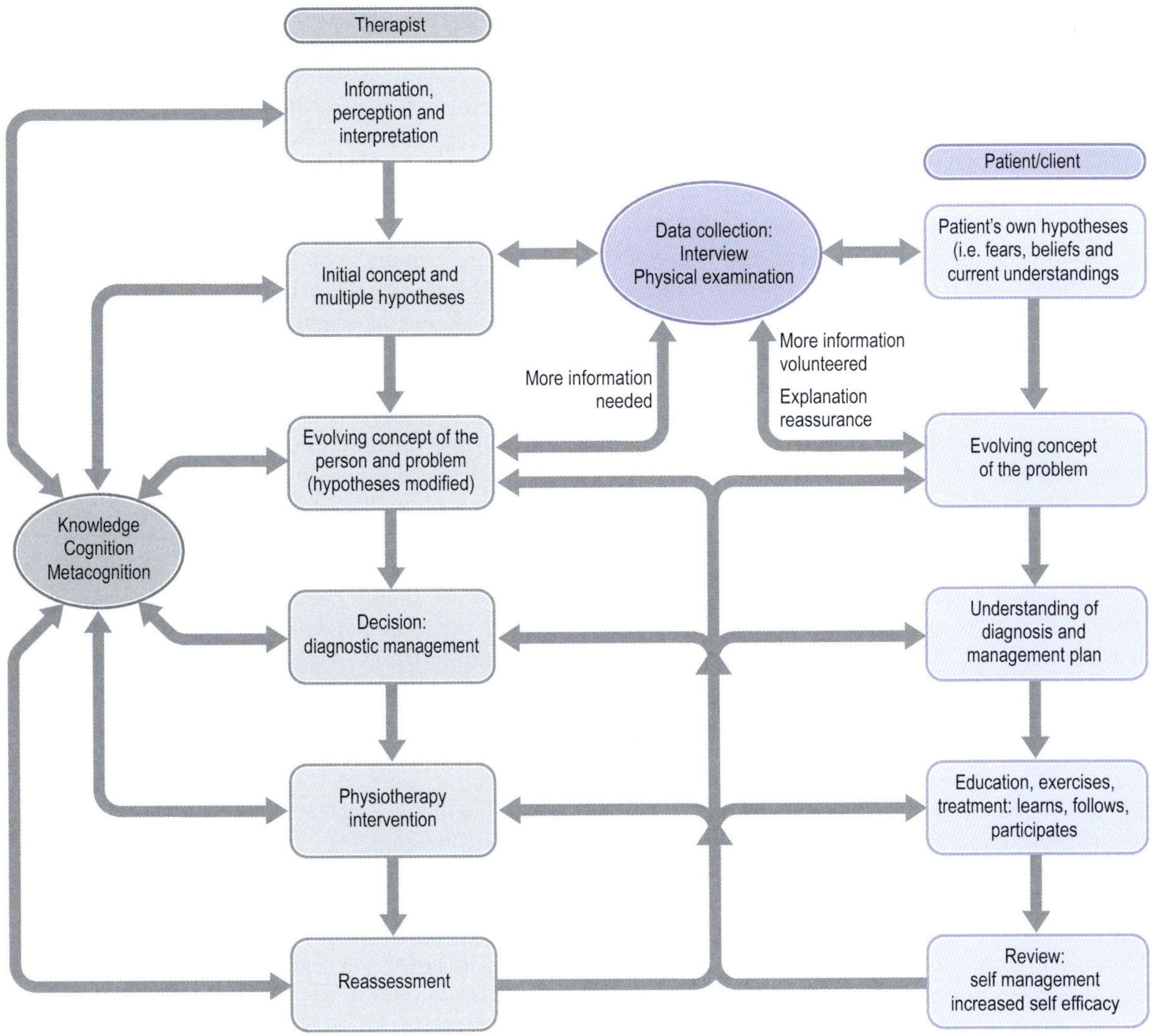

Fig. 5.3 Clinical reasoning process. (From Jones, 1995, with permission.)

Clinical guidelines seek to synthesize what is a potentially overwhelming evidence base to identify best practice. In 1994 the Clinical Standards Advisory Group developed guidelines on the management of low-back pain aimed at reducing the burden of persistent low-back pain on health services and the economy. The 2016 National Institute for Health and Care Excellence (NICE) guidelines on the management of low-back pain are used by commissioners in the UK to purchase musculoskeletal services.

In a similar way, CPRs have been developed to inform clinical decision-making. CPRs are tools that use a combination of patient history and physical examination findings to identify the likelihood of a particular condition being present (diagnostic) or to predict a particular outcome (prognostic) or to select the most effective management option (prescriptive). CPRs have been developed from practice through patient profiling or subgrouping of patients. An example of a diagnostic CPR is the Ottawa ankle rules (Stiell et al., 1993). These rules help clinicians to exclude the likelihood of a fracture in patients presenting with an ankle sprain. The decision to refer for an x-ray is based on specific areas of bony tenderness and the patient's ability to weight-bear. The rules have been found to be accurate in excluding fractures of the ankle and mid-foot, in patients over 18 years of age, with a sensitivity of 100% and also offer economic and patient benefits by reducing unnecessary radiographs by 30%–40% (Bachmann et al., 2003).

A prognostic CPR for the management of acute nonspecific low-back pain was developed by Flynn et al. (2002). This is an example of a rule whereby it has been found that patients fitting a profile matching four out of five criteria were identified as being most likely to respond favourably to spinal manipulation (Table 5.1).

The prediction rule included within these criteria a psychological measure, the fear avoidance belief questionnaire (FABQ). Fear-avoidance has been recognized as a poor prognostic indicator: patients demonstrating fear-avoidance behaviours were less likely to respond to a specific manual therapy intervention (Leeuw et al., 2007). Of course, CPRs should be evaluated critically; for example, it can be argued that a single intervention such as manipulation does not reflect practice, whereby manual therapy is integrated within a package of care, usually including functionally relevant exercises, education and advice (Moore & Jull, 2010). An example of this are treatment-based algorithms. Stanton et al. (2011) developed a treatment-based protocol that used CPRs to subgroup patients and therefore predict which treatment would be best placed for that particular presentation. However, the four categories of manipulation, stabilizations, specific exercise and traction had underpinning gaps. The manipulation group had to have pain for 16 days or less to be applicable, the stabilization group required patients to have what was described as 'aberrant movement', the specific exercise group applied a range of modalities and traction was based on a study that showed benefits for 2 weeks only. Therefore, although purported to be a selective treatment protocol, it presented with gaps within the underpinning evidence. This protocol also was further followed up and highlighted that 25% of LBP patients did not fall into any of the categories, whilst 25% met the criteria across two of them (Stanton et al., 2013). Therefore, although potentially helpful in defining how money may be spent for specific groups, generally these systems do not represent all patient groups, and while CPRs have been identified as useful adjuncts in clinical reasoning, there is concern that their indiscriminate use could harm patients if clinicians no longer rely on their own clinical reasoning skills (Learman et al., 2012).

TABLE 5.1 Criteria for Clinical Prediction Rules of Spinal Manipulation

Less than a 16-day symptom duration
A score of 19 or less on the fear-avoidance beliefs questionnaire
Lumbar hypomobility
Hip internal rotation range of >35 degrees motion
No symptoms distal to the knee

Flynn et al. (2002).

There are examples of more complex classification systems, such as the McKenzie method of mechanical diagnosis and therapy, based on repeated movements (May & Clare, 2015). As implied in the title, this classification is biomechanically based and so may be suitable for some patients, though not all. In contrast, classification-based cognitive functional therapy for people with persistent nonspecific low-back pain, first proposed by O'Sullivan (2005), classifies patients into groups based on the primary driver of their symptoms. Patients are assessed across a range of different domains, including physical impairment, pain, functional loss, activity limitation and psychological adaptation. This classification system continues to be developed into a clinical reasoning framework for the targeted assessment and management of low-back pain (O'Sullivan et al., 2015) and acknowledges that, for those with persistent symptoms and psychological factors, such as fear and anxiety, these factors will result in behaviours that will be the primary driver of their symptoms. These psychological drivers will require acknowledgement and management if successful outcomes are to be achieved (McCarthy et al., 2004).

The recognition that patients with the same complaint, such as persistent nonspecific low-back pain, will present differently and therefore need different management approaches is now widely accepted. Stratifying patients into more specific subgroups is evident in the development of the STarT Back tool (Hill & Fritz, 2011). This algorithm categorizes patients with low-back pain into one of three groups. Those identified by an initial questionnaire as being at 'low risk' of developing persistent pain receive advice; those at 'medium risk' are referred for standard musculoskeletal care and those identified as 'high risk' receive psychologically informed care.

Whilst all of these approaches inform practice, the challenge for individual clinicians is the decision-making that is required to incorporate them into their reasoning so that they are able to offer safe, evidence-informed, person-centred care.

It is evident from developments in clinical reasoning theories that practice continues to evolve. There has been a shift from a biomedical approach, seeking a diagnosis based on underlying pathobiological processes, to incorporate the psychosocial paradigms with the recognition that body and mind cannot be separated (Chapman et al., 2008) (Fig. 5.4).

So how do clinicians make sense of all the data collected in the subjective and physical examination to identify 'wise action' for their patients? The World Health Organization (2001) *International Classification of Functioning, Disability and Health* (ICF), introduced in Chapter 3 (see Fig. 3.1), provides a useful starting point, as this framework incorporates all factors capable of impacting an individual's health and well-being (Atkinson & Nixon-Cave, 2011).

Building on this framework are the reasoning categories developed by Jones et al. (2002), also introduced in Chapter 3 (see Box 3.1) and revisited at the end of Chapter 4.

These reasoning categories are included in the clinical reasoning documentation at the end of Chapter 4. The planetary model of reasoning (Danneels et al., 2011) is a vertical representation of the World Health Organization (2001) ICF framework showing the continuum of the influence of pain and psychosocial factors as orbiting planets around other components of the ICF framework (Fig. 5.5).

KNOWLEDGE CHECK

1. What are the differences between clinical prediction rules, classification strategies and stratification models?
2. What is the fear-avoidance belief questionnaire?
3. What are the limitations of clinical prediction rules?

This chapter will use these reasoning categories as a framework to review some of the data gathered within the previous two chapters in order to explore how the information guides clinical reasoning.

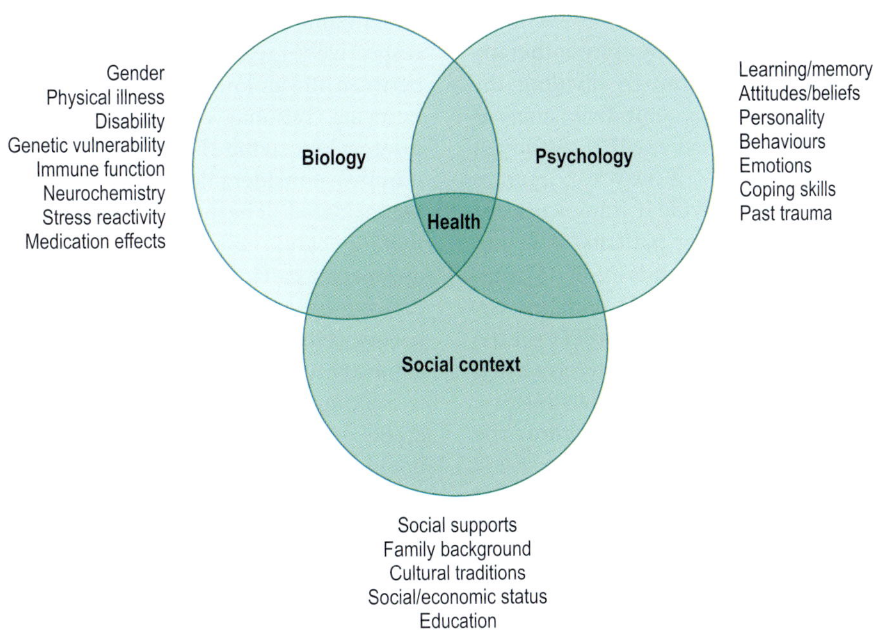

Fig. 5.4 Biopsychosocial model of health.

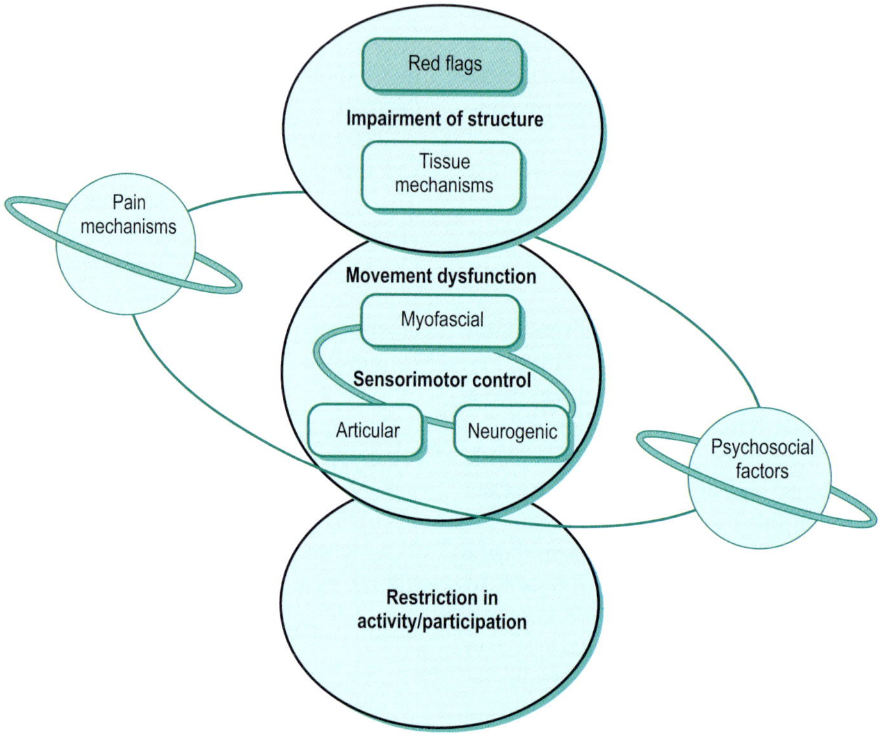

Fig. 5.5 Planetary model. (From Danneels et al., 2011, with permission.)

ENTERING INTO A PERSON'S STORY

A conventional method of recording physiotherapy records in a systematic way is through dividing the clinical encounter into subjective, objective, analysis and plan (or SOAP) (Jaroudi & Payne, 2019). Although this method of approach allows a way to organize complicated information and provide a framework for clinicians to follow when assessing patients, it is not without problems. This approach lends itself to fragment the clinical encounter into separate domains being the clinician on the one side and the patient on the other. The subjective aspects of the encounter are often attributed to the patient domain (such as their history, thoughts, feelings and behaviours), in other words the experiences of the patient. The clinician's perspective is often seen as objective, such as the measurements that have been taken, the thought processes, physical examination findings and analysis and plan. The concerning issue about conceiving the therapeutic encounter in this way is that subjectivity is seen as purely existing within the patient's domain which is problematic. Looking at the relationship between a patient and a clinician as being subjective and objective respectively creates and maintains a power difference between the unknowing, irrational patient and the all-knowing rational clinician and is entirely inappropriate. Conceiving the clinical encounter in such a way requires considerable reflection and may need to be reconsidered. The process of clinical reasoning, sense-making and the formulation of a therapeutic approach calls toward stepping away from this convention because the encounter is intersubjective in nature (Øberg et al., 2015; Low, 2017). Human intersubjectivity refers to the fact that more than one person is making sense of a particular situation and is inseparable from the other when communicating between people. Healthcare demands that the interpretation and negotiated understanding of the patient's predicament is almost entirely intersubjective. Seeing the clinical encounter in this way values patient stories or narratives as these rich perspectives direct, guide and facilitate the clinical reasoning process, physical examination and collaborative decision-making.

The primary aim of receiving a history from a patient is to enter into a therapeutic relationship by building a rapport with the patient (Roberts et al., 2013). The clinician will ask the patient why they have come for assessment and what their goals and expectations are for the initial session (Chester et al., 2014). Open questions, such as, 'What would be a successful outcome for you?' can be helpful in identifying what the patient may be seeking. Usually, the patient will indicate having some functional or physical difficulty often, though not always, as a result of pain. This early discussion provides the clinician with very useful insights into the patient's lifestyle, level of physical activity and the impact of the condition on their life (Opsommer & Schoeb, 2014). It offers the patient an opportunity to tell their story and for the clinician to engage in a narrative reasoning approach with the patient (Fleming & Mattingly, 2008). This type of reasoning will require the clinician to demonstrate active listening using cues such as head nodding, eye contact, making use of pauses and asking reflective questions (Maguire & Pitceathly, 2002). The role of communication is explored more fully in Chapter 2.

The clinician will have the opportunity to indicate what can be offered in terms of the diagnosis and treatment as well as wider healthcare management, with the focus on restoring function and promoting healthy living (Chartered Society of Physiotherapy, 2008; Middleton, 2008; Banks & Hengeveld, 2014). An appreciation of the patient's expectations at the outset will help foster a collaborative partnership between the patient and clinician. Offering treatment choices and setting agreed goals are thought to enhance a patient's motivation and compliance. Patients who share in decision-making take greater responsibility for their own management and are more likely to achieve better outcomes (Jones et al., 2008; Main et al., 2010).

ACTIVITY AND PARTICIPATION CAPABILITIES AND RESTRICTIONS

Using the World Health Organization (2001) framework the clinician explores the impact of the patient's condition on their life by considering her level of activity, what the patient is able and unable to do, e.g. walking, lifting, sitting, and their ability/inability to participate in life situations, i.e. work, family and leisure activities.

From the outset the clinician should be reasoning from a biopsychosocial perspective, initially using forward or inductive reasoning of the possible causes of the patient's symptoms (Rivett & Jones, 2004). This will assist in developing hypotheses on possible tissues/structures, to examine in the physical examination that may be restricting the patient's activities or participation in life. Alternatively, psychological factors may be limiting the patient, as a result of fear and hypervigilant behaviours. Identification of these at this point would provide a cue for the clinician to modify their language, seeking not to dismiss fears but to interpret and understand the patient's beliefs about their symptoms (Barker et al., 2009; Darlow et al., 2013). At this stage, the clinician may begin to formulate management strategies in terms of initial advice and education aimed at promoting normal activity and participation. Sharing information with patients may enhance the therapeutic relationship as they become active participants in their own care. Answering patients' specific questions and tailoring information to suit their situation will encourage empowerment, a vital component of person-centred care (Moseley et al., 2004; Caladine & Morris, 2015).

Similarly, information about the patient's ability to participate in everyday activities will be very relevant, for example, the financial pressures of being self-employed and unable to work, or the social isolation that may result from being unable to participate in leisure activities (Froud et al., 2014). The implications of loss on the individual and family can be significant and should be acknowledged (Nielsen, 2014).

Seeking information on what patients are still capable of doing is equally important. Gifford (2005) labelled these 'pink flags'. He argued that there can be a preoccupation, on the part of the clinician, to focus on what patients cannot do in the desire to problem solve. He promoted identifying positively all the things they are able to do, for example, encouraging patients to continue to work, using normal activity to promote recovery. The assessment of activity and participation capabilities offers an opportunity for the clinician to encourage activity and deliver a positive message of hope, reducing the potential for medicalizing patients (MacKereth et al., 2014).

PATIENT'S PERSPECTIVES ON THEIR EXPERIENCE

Patients often seek treatment because of pain, and so seeking to understand what pain may mean from the patient's perspective will increase the likelihood of achieving a therapeutic rapport.

Pain is 'an unpleasant sensory and emotional experience associated with, or resembling that associated with, actual or potential tissue damage' (www.iasp-pain.org).

A patient's response to pain is unique and is influenced by beliefs, cultural and social constructs, and memories of past experience (Main et al., 2010). Patients' beliefs are learned and are considered modifiable, with evidence demonstrating that pain education can be effective in reframing the patient's pain experience (Moseley et al., 2004; Louw et al., 2011). It is also recognized that persistent pain may influence mood, with more widespread symptoms increasing the likelihood of depression. The patient's response to simple screening questions such as:

- In the past month, has your pain been bad enough to stop you from doing many of your day-to-day activities?
- In the past month, has your pain been bad enough to make you feel worried or low in mood (Aroll et al., 2003; Barker et al., 2014)?

will assist the clinician in reasoning whether the patient should be referred to an appropriately trained mental health professional to offer additional support alongside musculoskeletal management (Main & Spanswick, 2000; Kent et al., 2014).

It is acknowledged that pain and beliefs will influence a patient's behaviour. In the acute stages avoidance strategies, referred to as adaptive, can assist in protecting tissues from further harm, allowing tissue healing to take place. However, in patients with persistent pain, avoidance behaviours are unhelpful and defined as maladaptive. Maladaptive movement patterns and altered loading may result in proprioceptive deficits and altered body schema (Luomajoki & Moseley, 2011). Changes in muscle activity associated with guarding or deconditioning are thought to be responsible for pain production beyond the original symptomatic tissue. Using their knowledge of tissue healing, clinicians can reason whether behaviours are adaptive or maladaptive and use this to inform assessment and management decisions (Diegelmann & Evans, 2004). Increasingly, physiotherapy clinicians are being trained to integrate psychological therapy techniques such as cognitive behavioural therapy and acceptance commitment therapy within their practice to manage maladaptive behaviours (Henschke et al., 2010).

Adopting psychological therapy approaches will require the clinician to appreciate the emotional dimension of clinical reasoning. The clinician's reasoning of pain will also be influenced by their own constructs, which may be quite different to those expressed by the patient (Langridge et al., 2016). Much has been written on how faulty beliefs, such as pain equals harm, can be a barrier to patient recovery, but beliefs held by clinicians can also negatively influence clinical reasoning. Evidence indicates that clinicians holding negative beliefs are less likely to adopt best-practice clinical guidelines (Darlow et al., 2012; Nijs et al., 2013). Recognition of the existence of these beliefs will require clinicians to be self-reflective enough to recognize how their own attitudes and beliefs will impact on the decisions they make (Bishop et al., 2008; Nijs et al., 2013). Within the patient-centred model of reasoning (see Fig. 3.2), such reflection is termed metacognition and is essential if clinicians are to remain open-minded to allow their practice to evolve.

KNOWLEDGE CHECK

1. What are the strengths and limitations of SOAP notes?
2. What type of open question might you start a clinical encounter with and why?
3. What are adaptive and maladaptive movement behaviours?

PATHOBIOLOGICAL MECHANISMS

Although there has been a shift in emphasis from a purely biomedical focus, as indicated above, clinicians are still rightly concerned with what is happening at the tissue level. Pathobiological mechanisms can be considered in two parts: (1) tissue responses and healing; and (2) pain mechanisms.

Tissue Responses and Healing

Clinicians can use their knowledge of tissue healing to stage conditions as acute, subacute or chronic/

persistent. For example, in an acute ankle sprain, the clinician would initially seek to unload injured tissue, perhaps prescribing crutches, advising a regime of **PEACE**: protection, elevation, avoidance of anti-inflammatory modalities, compression and elevation, whilst encouraging movement within pain tolerance, before moving towards **LOVE** a progressive loading programme, optimism in recovery, vascularization and exercise (Dubois & Esculier, 2020). However, a patient who presents following an ankle sprain with persistent pain beyond normal tissue-healing timeframes and a continued reluctance to weight bear would, after having been screened to exclude other causes, be encouraged to 'trust' the ankle with a graded loading intervention aimed at restoring normal function (Woods & Asmundson, 2008).

Reasoning will also be influenced by the underlying health of the patient's tissues with comorbidities such as diabetes mellitus and lifestyle choices such as smoking potentially negatively impacting on the tissue-healing process. Comorbidities may slow recovery, so reasoning about tissue health is specific to the individual patient. This reasoning will guide the advice given and assist in the selection of interventions and staging of rehabilitation strategies.

Pain Mechanisms

Identifying pain mechanisms may inform what may be happening at the tissue level, peripheral neuropathic and central nervous system levels. They serve as 'rules of thumb' to support the clinical reasoning process. Using Gifford's mature organism model of reasoning (Fig. 5.6) may allow the clinician to consider pain in terms of inputs from peripheral tissues, including nociception, which can be identified as mechanical, inflammatory or ischaemic, depending on characteristics (see Box 3.2) or as peripheral neuropathic, generated by somatosensory tissues such as nerve roots. There are other pain mechanisms that can be broadly described as forms of sensitization such as nociplastic that arises from altered nociception despite no clear evidence of actual or threatened tissue damage causing activation of peripheral nociceptors or evidence for disease or lesion of the somatosensory system (IASP, 2022), and central sensitization. Central sensitization is a 'neurophysiological phenomenon that is adaptive, activity-dependent, and dynamic consisting of neurobiological changes in dorsal horn neurons such as increased excitability, strengthened synaptic transmission and reduced inhibition' (Van Griensven et al., 2020.)

Understanding how pain mechanisms present are helpful for the clinician to direct toward a treatment and management plan.

Smart et al. (2012) identified clusters of symptoms that may help clinicians identify certain pain mechanisms. Although their work focused on patients with low back with or without leg pain their findings may generalize into other areas of the body. Van Griensven

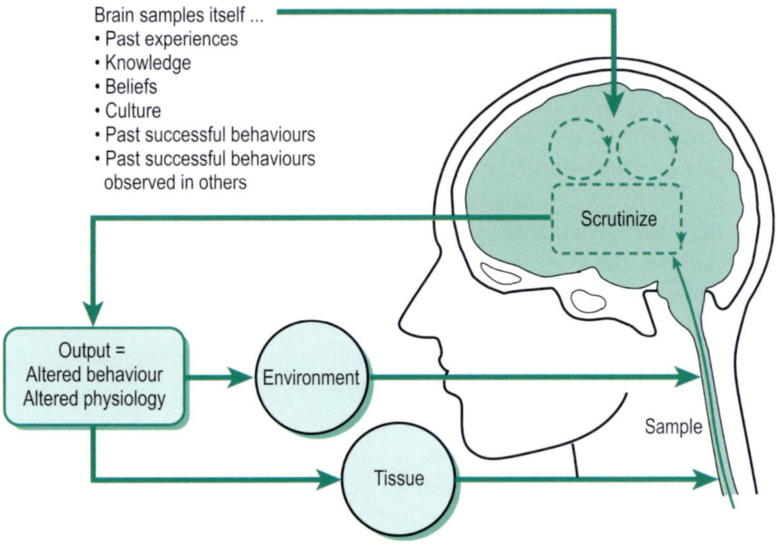

Fig. 5.6 Mature organism model. (From Gifford, 1998, with permission.)

BOX 5.1 Using Symptoms and Signs to Reason Pain Mechanisms

Pain Mechanism	Cluster of Symptoms and Signs
Nociceptive pain (Smart et al., 2012c)	Pain localized to the area of injury, clear proportionate mechanical/anatomical nature to aggravating and easing factors, usually intermittent and sharp with movement/mechanical provocation: may be a constant dull ache or throb at rest. Pain in association with other symptoms of inflammation The absence of pain in association with other dysesthesias, the absence of night pain/sleep disturbance
Peripheral neuropathic pain (Smart et al., 2012b)	Pain referred in a dermatomal or cutaneous distribution, pain/symptom provocation with mechanical/movement tests (e.g. active/passive, neural provocation e.g. SLR) that move/load/compress neural tissue
Nociplastic pain—one neurophysiological mechanism is central sensitization (Smart et al., 2012; Van Griensven et al., 2020).	Disproportionate, nonmechanical, unpredictable pattern of pain provocation in response to multiple/nonspecific aggravating/easing factors Ongoing, spontaneous and widespread pain. Severe, and prolonged pain despite a seemingly innocuous stimulus The presence of secondary hyperalgesia (increased pain sensitivity in undamaged tissue away from the site of a painful lesion) Tertiary hyperalgesia (increased pain sensitivity on the contralateral side of a painful lesion)

et al. (2020) clearly articulated the challenges of diagnosis, identification, treatment and management of patients presenting with features of central sensitization, particularly how it may be becoming lost in translation in clinical practice (see Box 5.1).

It is evident that patients with persistent pain can become trapped in a vicious cycle (Main et al., 2010). In an effort to seek a tissue diagnosis, for example, lumbar disc, patients may consult numerous practitioners navigating the 'sea of endless professionals' (Butler & Moseley, 2003). This can further complicate the patient's pain journey, as the patient is left juggling numerous different diagnoses and opinions. Directing treatment to localized tissue is likely to be unsuccessful even though the problem may have originated peripherally. So it can be reasoned for these patients their management focus will include a psychological approach to reduce abnormal central processing and impact on centrally mediated pain alongside other physical interventions.

Pain also results in output mechanisms resulting in altered motor responses, linked to maladaptive movement or suboptimal movement patterns, for example, due to increased muscle tone.

Autonomic system activation is linked with upregulation and protective mechanisms in the presence of pain, resulting in neuroendocrine changes such as raised cortisol levels. Raised cortisol over an extended period has been linked to depression, poor tissue healing and loss of sleep (Hannibal & Bishop, 2014). So when patients report they are not sleeping then this information needs to be linked to their stress biology (Sapolsky, 2004).

To reason the aspects of a patient's presentation successfully, clinicians will require sound physiological knowledge of body systems and how they interact and impact on one another.

PHYSICAL IMPAIRMENTS AND ASSOCIATED STRUCTURE/TISSUE SOURCES

Patients' descriptions and location of their symptoms will assist in reasoning symptomatic underlying tissue. Whilst completing the body chart the clinician will be using anatomical and pain mechanism knowledge to consider all the structures lying beneath and capable of referring into symptomatic areas (Woolf, 2004; Bogduk, 2009). This information, matched with reported limitations in activity, will be explored in an analysis of the aggravating and easing factors reported by the patient. These cues in the subjective will provide justification for the 'must, should and could' lists in planning the physical examination. Based on this, the clinician will prioritize testing, seeking to confirm or refute primary working hypotheses. In order to deliver effective treatment, the clinician will hypothesize on the possible target tissues capable of producing the patient's symptoms.

From the outset, the clinician will be developing hypotheses of the likely cause of the patient's symptoms. These hypotheses are then tested using hypothetico-deductive reasoning and refined through further subjective and physical examination data collection. The clinician will be making judgements about the existence of tissue pathology based on information from the history of the present condition. If the patient can identify a specific mechanism of injury, such as an ankle inversion injury, this allows for hypothesis generation of tissue trauma. This would include all structures likely to be stressed and capable of producing the lateral ankle symptoms reported by the patient and mapped on to the body chart. This hypothesis would also include consideration of the extent of injury, for example, the likelihood of a fracture. This would prompt follow-up questions about the velocity of the fall, the ability of the patient to weight bear afterwards (Stiell et al., 1993) and the extent of swelling. This is an example of how clinicians might use pattern recognition or forward reasoning of a familiar condition such as an ankle sprain.

As already discussed in Chapter 4, physical tests are often not tissue-specific and will require the clinician to use diagnostic reasoning to synthesize responses from a number of physical tests in order to identify the possible source of symptoms. If meaningful conclusions are to be drawn the clinician will need to weigh up the sensitivity and specificity of tests selected, as well as critically reflect on the accuracy of their own handling skills (Christensen et al., 2008).

Further medical investigations may or may not be the solution to identifying specific tissue sources of symptoms. Blood tests can confirm the existence of an inflammatory condition such as rheumatoid arthritis or can be used to exclude sinister pathologies. Imaging is helpful where clinically reasoned, for example, an x-ray if a fracture is suspected or to confirm a diagnosis or for example, an ultrasound to identify a Morton neuroma, for which a further intervention may be appropriate (Bignotti et al., 2015). Patients with persistent pain may believe that scans will indicate tissue faults and so diagnose the cause of their pain; however, there is often a poor correlation between what is reported on scans and how patients may present in the clinic (Brinjikji et al., 2015). This can be difficult for patients to accept. Indeed, evidence has shown that magnetic resonance imaging results, given without the epidemiological data of what is found in a normal asymptomatic population, increase dependence on narcotic medication in patients with persistent nonspecific low-back pain (McCullough et al., 2012). Requests for investigations should be based on very sound clinical reasoning, with the clinician providing clear justification.

In some patients it is possible to identify specific tissue sources; for example, reactive Achilles tendinopathy presents with a recognized pattern of localized pain and swelling and is usually linked to specific provocative activities (Kountouris & Cook, 2007). The underlying pathological processes of tissue healing can be hypothesized using the available evidence to stage the condition (Cook et al., 2016). The clinician reasons why the tissue has become symptomatic.

- Is it related to a change in activity? This should be detected in the patient's history of the present complaint such as a change in load or training.
- Is there a problem elsewhere in the kinetic chain increasing load on the tendon? Perhaps a previous injury has restricted range or strength, resulting in altered loading patterns (Cook & Purdam, 2012)?
- Are the patient's gender, age and lifestyle choices factors? Achilles tendinopathy is more common in males and is associated with a change in levels of activity (Cook et al., 2007; Gaida et al., 2010).

Using a knowledge of tissue healing to clinically reason all possible factors contributing to the development of tissue symptoms will assist the clinician in the selection of appropriate management strategies.

KNOWLEDGE CHECK

1. What does the acronym LOVE mean?
2. What are the pain mechanisms described in this chapter, and how might they present in clinical practice?
3. Offer examples of factors that are thought to delay tissue healing.

CONTRIBUTING FACTORS TO THE DEVELOPMENT AND MAINTENANCE OF THE PROBLEM

Throughout the subjective examination, the clinician is seeking to identify factors contributing to the development and/or persistence of the patient's symptoms, e.g. environmental, behavioural and physical.

Consideration of the patient's environment has been highlighted as an important aspect in disability (World Health Organization, 2011), so it is often useful to explore this early in the subjective examination.

- How does the patient function at home?
- Does the patient have family support? Is this helpful or unhelpful?
- What does the patient's job involve?
- Could work be a cause of tissue stress?
- How adaptable is the patient's work situation?

This information will assist the clinician in selecting management options that are realistic and patient-specific. See also black flags in Table 3.2 (Waddell, 2004; Linton & Shaw, 2011). Related to this will be patients' perception of their work. Patients may believe work has been the cause of their symptoms or that their colleagues or managers are unsympathetic or unsupportive. These thoughts could impact on their motivation to return to work if signed off sick. In order to offer patient-centred advice the clinician may need to ask additional questions, such as:

- Are you concerned that the physical demands of your job might delay your return to work?
- Do you expect your work could be modified temporarily so you could return to work sooner? (Nicholas et al., 2011)

Psychosocial factors may also contribute to symptom development or persistence, and these are identified as yellow flags (see Table 3.2). These are summarized under seven headings, ABCDEFW with examples for each:

- Attitudes: guarding or fear of movement, catastrophizing, external locus of control
- Behaviours: rest, reduced activity, poor pacing—boom-bust cycle
- Compensation issues: history of claims, no incentive to return to work, long-term sick leave
- Diagnosis and treatment: conflicting diagnosis, seeking a cure, passive recipient of care
- Emotion: fear, anxiety, feeling of hopelessness, low mood
- Family: overprotective or lacking in support
- Work: low-skilled manual work, belief work is harmful, shift work, job dissatisfaction.

It is important that the clinician is aware that different psychological flags may be significant at different points in the patient's journey. This should prompt a regular reassessment of these factors through narrative reasoning. Clinicians can use their intuition, supported through information from the subjective examination, to assess for yellow flags (Beales et al., 2016). In addition, the use of brief validated questionnaires such as STarT Back tools (Hill & Fritz, 2011) or Orebro musculoskeletal pain questionnaire (Linton & Boersma, 2003) can help confirm the clinician's judgements. Screening tools can produce false positives and false negatives whereby patients without psychological risk factors may be identified as high-risk or vice versa (Nicholas et al., 2011). Screening is not diagnostic but rather a predictor of chronicity. Results from screening tools should be viewed and reasoned in the context of the full examination (Beales et al., 2016) and used to inform rather than direct clinical reasoning.

Psychological factors have the potential to drive behaviours that can impact on physical function. These behaviours can lead to possible avoidance of activity resulting in deconditioning at one end of the spectrum or, in the case of those endurance copers, suppressing thoughts, resulting in overconditioning at the other end (Hasenbring et al., 2012).

Resulting physical factors may contribute to symptoms. The clinician will use their knowledge of normal movement in order to clinically reason the impact of altered muscle activation patterns on movement dysfunction. Observations along with reported aggravating and easing factors will inform the examination of selected active movements. Muscle lengths, strength and control tests will further inform the clinician's thinking. Testing of passive movements will examine the involvement of associated articular components as the clinician feels for available range and tissue response. However, it should not be assumed that areas judged to be hyper- or hypomobile are a cause of the patient's symptoms as these may be incidental findings. Cause and effect should be supported with modification or mini treatments producing a change in the patient's symptoms. One such approach is the shoulder symptom modification procedure. This involves a systematic assessment of the influence of thoracic posture, scapular position and humeral head position on shoulder symptoms (Lewis, 2016). An alternative example is an assessment of repeated movements using the concept advocated by McKenzie whereby clinicians use their clinical reasoning to select repeated movements. The patient's response to repeated movements allows the clinician to classify low-back pain patients into subgroups: derangement, dysfunction, postural syndrome or other (May & Clare, 2015). In this example, the clinician will be seeking to confirm or refute a hypothesis of physical impairment.

It is worth noting that a patient's response to hands-on testing may be influenced by a placebo which will depend on the patient's mood, expectation and conditioning (Bialosky et al., 2011). This means clinicians must be aware of the context within which testing takes place in order to reason about all aspects of the complex interaction between body and mind. For further details the reader is directed to Chapter 9 Understanding and Managing Persistent Pain by Hubert Van Griensven in the companion text (Barnard & Ryder, 2024).

PRECAUTIONS/CONTRAINDICATIONS TO PHYSICAL EXAMINATION, TREATMENT AND MANAGEMENT

In order to ensure wise action for patients, clinicians must be able to reason clinically when assessment and treatment are contraindicated and when precautions require modification in the extent and vigour of the physical examination.

As autonomous practitioners, clinicians must be able to screen their patients for red flags, identified as indicators of serious pathology, such as neoplasms. This is more than asking a standard list of questions but requires associated reasoning to identify the relative weight and suspected index of suspicion (Goodman et al., 2018). The context in which these screening questions are asked is also significant; clinicians need to be mindful not to alarm patients. Clear explanations are required so that patients understand the relevance of questions as they will be reasoning alongside the clinician and may subconsciously or consciously withhold information that they may feel is not relevant (Greenhalgh & Selfe, 2004).

The red-flag system continues to evolve over time (see Table 3.4 for an updated list; Greenhalgh & Selfe, 2010) and clinicians must continue to update their knowledge base on how serious pathologies present. Clinicians also need to be aware of 'red herrings' due to misattribution of symptoms, biomedical masqueraders and overt illness behaviour that may lead to reasoning errors.

To inform reasoning and screen for precautions and contraindications clinicians will also seek information about family history asking about cancer, for example. Heredity factors play a part in the development of some musculoskeletal conditions, such as ankylosing spondylitis and rheumatoid arthritis. A diagnosis of inflammatory joint disease such as rheumatoid arthritis would contraindicate accessory and physiological movements to the upper cervical spine, and care is needed in applying forces to other joints. For further reasoning of serious pathologies see Chapter 11 (Barnard & Ryder, 2024).

Identifying specific pathologies can assist in identifying the need for caution. Fractures are probably the most straightforward example. How vigorously techniques are applied will depend on the stage of fracture healing. The patient's general health and the presence of comorbidities such as osteoporosis will impact on the quality and healing time frames (Gandhi et al., 2005; Marsell & Einhorn, 2011). Osteoporosis can be caused by a number of factors, including long-term use of steroids, early menopause or hysterectomy, so careful questioning is required (NICE, 2012).

Diabetes can also cause delayed healing; especially if poorly controlled, diabetes is also associated with peripheral neuropathies (Brem & Tomic-Canic, 2007). Patients may complain of bilateral pins and needles or numbness in both hands and/or both feet, leading to reduced mobility. There are many reasons why a patient may report sensory changes or have difficulty walking. Of concern would be the possibility of red flag pathologies such as spinal cord, cauda equina compression or an upper motor neurone lesion such as a stroke.

Early features of cervical artery dysfunction can mimic a musculoskeletal pain presentation, as patients often present with neck/occipital pain and unusual or severe headaches. In order to make a differential diagnosis, follow-up questions should seek details of risk factors and information about any features indicating ischaemia or bleeding, such as visual disturbance, balance or gait disturbance, speech/swallowing difficulties or limb weakness or paraesthesia (Rushton et al., 2014). (See Upper Cervical spine Chapter 7 in this text and Chapter 8 Considering vascular flow limitations in Barnard and Ryder, 2024, for more in-depth discussion of this topic area.)

The presence of spinal spondylolysis or spondylolisthesis would contraindicate strong direct pressure to the affected vertebral level as this might compromise neural tissue.

If a patient is pregnant or postpartum, hormonal changes may cause a reduction in joint stiffness and an increase in the range of joint movement, particularly around the pelvis, so contraindicating excessive forces being applied (Calguneri et al., 1982; Stuber et al., 2012). Excessive forces would be contraindicated too in hypermobile patients with hypermobility spectrum disorder (HSD) and Erhlers-Danlos syndrome (hEDS) (Russek et al., 2019)

Anticoagulant therapy causes an increase in the time for blood to clot, so the clinician would need to be aware that this may cause soft tissues to bruise when force is applied. Conversely, oral contraceptives and smoking are associated with an increased risk of thrombosis.

Heart or respiratory disease may preclude some treatment positions; for example, the patient may not tolerate lying flat.

In order to reason safely, clinicians require knowledge of a wide range of pathological conditions, their clinical presentation as well as a working knowledge of the side-effects of commonly prescribed medications. The reader is referred to a pathology textbook such as (Goodman et al., 2018) for further information.

KNOWLEDGE CHECK

1. What is the acronym ABCDEFW?
2. What are 'red flags'?
3. What is the difference between a precaution and a contraindication?

SEVERITY AND IRRITABILITY

The clinician's judgement of the severity and irritability for each symptom, as defined in Chapter 3, will also guide the extent and vigour of the physical examination.

Whether the symptoms are constant or intermittent, they are deemed to be severe if the patient reports that a single movement, which increases pain, is so severe that the movement has to be stopped. Severe symptoms may limit the extent of the physical examination. The clinician would, in this situation, aim to examine the patient as fully as possible, but within the constraints of the patient's symptoms and so will have decided how much of the symptoms to provoke, e.g. to stop short of the point of pain (P_1) (see Fig. 4.41).

The effect of severe pain on active and passive movement testing is given below as an example of how a physical test is adapted.

Active movements would involve the patient moving to a point just before the onset of (or increase in) the symptom, or just to the point of onset (or increase), and would then immediately return to the starting position. No overpressures would be applied. This requires the clinician to give clear instructions to the patient.

For passive movements, patients may be asked to say as soon as they think they are about to feel their symptom (intermittent), or, if their symptom is constant, are about to feel an increase in their symptom. In both cases, the significant increase in pain is avoided. Alternatively, the patient may be able to tolerate movement just to the onset (or increase) of the symptom. The clinician would carry out the passive movement and, under the instruction of the patient, take the movement to only the first point of pain—and then immediately move away from the point of symptom reproduction. In both situations, the clinician should give clear instructions to the patient. The clinician must be able to control the movement and carry it out very slowly. This is necessary in order to avoid causing unnecessary symptoms and to obtain an accurate measure of the range of movement for reassessment purposes (Box 5.2).

The irritability of symptoms is the time taken for symptoms to increase with provocation and subside once the provocation is stopped. When a movement is performed, and pain is provoked, for example, and this provoked pain continues to be present for a length of time, even though the movement is stopped, then the pain is said to be irritable. In the context of a physical examination, any period of time that is required for symptoms to return to their resting level is classified as irritable. If symptoms are provoked and require a pause before the examination can recommence in order to settle sufficiently, this will increase the appointment time, which may be a problem in a busy department. As

BOX 5.2 Communication Suggestions When Assessing a Patient With Severe Conditions

Active Movements	Passive Movements
For example, if active shoulder flexion is being examined the clinician may instruct the patient in the following way (emphasis is in italics):	For example, for passive shoulder flexion, the clinician may instruct the patient in the following way (emphasis is in italics):
Intermittent severe symptom: 'Lift your arm up in front of you, *and as soon as you think you are about to get your arm pain, bring your arm down again'* or 'Lift your arm up in front of you, *and as soon as you get your arm pain, bring your arm down again'.*	Intermittent severe symptoms: 'I want to move your arm, but I want you to tell me *as soon as you think you are about to get your arm pain*, and I'll bring your arm down'. 'I want to move your arm, but I want you to tell me *as soon as you get your arm pain*, and I will bring your arm down'.
Constant severe symptom: 'Lift your arm up in front of you, *and as soon as you think your arm pain is going to increase, bring your arm down again'* or 'Lift your arm up in front of you, *and as soon as your arm pain increases, bring your arm down again'*	Constant severe symptoms: 'I want to move your arm, but I want you to tell me *as soon as you think you are about to get more of your arm pain*, and I'll bring your arm down'. 'I want to move your arm up, but I want you to tell me *as soon as you get more of your arm pain*, and I will bring your arm down'

well as this, repeatedly provoking symptoms and then waiting for them to settle will add little to the clinician's understanding of the patient's condition and result in a bad experience for the patient. For this reason, an alternative strategy is used whereby movements are carried out within the symptom-free range; irritable symptoms are not provoked at all.

For the examination of active movements for a patient with intermittent symptoms, the patient would move to a point just before the onset of the symptoms and then immediately return to the start position. In this way, symptoms are not provoked, and therefore there will be no lingering symptoms. For passive movements, patients may be asked to say as soon as they think they are about to feel the symptom (intermittent), or feel that it is about to increase (constant). In both cases, further pain provocation is avoided. The clinician must give clear instructions to the patient (Box 5.3).

For irritable symptoms, whether intermittent or constant, it is particularly important that the clinician clarifies after each movement the patient's resting symptoms to avoid exacerbating symptoms. In patients where symptoms are severe but not irritable the

BOX 5.3 Communication Suggestions When Assessing a Patient With Irritable Conditions

Active Movement	Passive Movement
Intermittent symptoms (emphasis is in italics): 'Lift your arm up in front of you, and *as soon as you think you are about to get your arm pain*, bring your arm down again'.	For example, for passive shoulder flexion, the clinician may instruct the patient in the following way (emphasis is in italics): Intermittent symptoms: 'I want to move your arm, but I want you to tell me *as soon as you think you are about to get your arm pain*, and I'll bring your arm down'
Constant symptoms: 'Lift your arm up in front of you, and *as soon as you think your arm pain is going to increase*, bring your arm down again'	Constant symptoms: 'I want to move your arm, but I want you to tell me *as soon as you think you are about to get more of your arm pain*, and I'll bring your arm down'

clinician will identify the tolerable level of symptom reproduction with the patient and so may seek to reproduce 25% of symptoms (see Fig. 4.41).

The clinician's reasoning of underlying pain mechanisms will also inform the assessment of severity and irritability. For patients reasoned to have a neuropathic presentation with high levels of pain, tissues are likely to be irritable (Butler, 2000). To confirm a hypothesis of a neuropathic pain driver the clinician would use subjective and physical examination findings (see Box 3.2 for typical characteristics) (Hansson & Kinnman, 1996; Cook & van Griensven, 2013). The clinician could confirm a hypothesis of neuropathic pain through the application of validated screening tools and the use of sensorimotor tests to assess the baseline conductivity of the system (Bennett et al., 2007). Neuropathic pain states would cue the clinician to handle with care, requiring careful assessment of severity and irritability. Strategies to reduce rather than reproduce symptoms would further confirm a neuropathic hypothesis. Unloading positions to ease neural tissue sensitivity would reassure the patient and inform the reasoning of management decisions (Butler, 2000).

KNOWLEDGE CHECK

1. Describe the difference between severity and irritability.
2. Why is it important to consider the severity and irritability of a presenting case?
3. What does P1 mean?

MANAGEMENT STRATEGY AND TREATMENT PLANNING

Management options will be formulated on the basis of reasoning all strands of the subjective and physical examinations and can be considered in two phases: the initial appointment on day 1 and follow-up appointments.

The first step in this process occurs between the subjective and physical examinations. In the subjective examination, in seeking to make sense of the patient's symptoms, a primary hypothesis and other possible alternative hypotheses are formulated. Using hypothetico-deductive reasoning these hypotheses will be confirmed, refined or refuted during the physical examination (Jones et al., 2008). The process then involves putting the possible structures at fault in priority order to develop a 'must, should and could' plan for the physical examination whilst also taking into account any precautions or contraindications.

The aims of the physical examination are to:

- Confirm, if necessary, any precautions or contraindications
- Identify the most likely source of the patient's symptoms
- Explore further, if relevant, any factors contributing to the patient's condition.

In order to identify the source of the symptoms the clinician uses the information from the subjective examination to forward reason the findings of the physical examination. This includes:

- The structures thought to be at fault
- Which tests are likely to reproduce/alter the patient's symptoms
- How the tests need to be performed to reproduce/alter the patient's symptoms, for example, which combined movements may be required
- What other structures need to be examined in order to disprove them as a source of the symptoms.

The physical testing procedures which indicate joint, nerve or muscle tissues as a source of the patient's symptoms are summarized in Table 5.2.

At one end of the scale, the findings may provide strong evidence, and at the other end, they may provide weak evidence. Of course, there may be a variety of presentations between these two extremes.

The strongest evidence that a joint is the primary source of the patient's symptoms is that active and passive physiological movements, passive accessory movements and joint palpation all reproduce the patient's symptoms, and that, following a joint-based treatment, reassessment identifies an improvement in the patient's signs and symptoms. For example, let us assume a patient has lateral elbow pain caused by a radiohumeral joint dysfunction. In the physical examination, there are limited elbow flexion and extension movements with some resistance due to the reproduction of the patient's elbow pain. Active movement is very similar to passive movement in terms of range, resistance and pain reproduction. Accessory movement examination of the radiohumeral joint reveals limited posteroanterior and anteroposterior glide of the radius due to the reproduction of the patient's elbow pain with some resistance. Following the application of accessory

TABLE 5.2 **Physical Tests Which, if Positive, Indicate Joint, Nerve and Muscle as a Source of the Patient's Symptoms**

Test	Strong Evidence	Weak Evidence
Joint		
Active physiological movements	Reproduces patient's symptoms	Dysfunctional movement: reduced range, excessive range, altered quality of movement, increased resistance, decreased resistance
Passive physiological movements	Reproduces patient's symptoms; this test same as for active physiological movements	Dysfunctional movement: reduced range, excessive range, increased resistance, decreased resistance, altered quality of movement
Accessory movements	Reproduces patient's symptoms	Dysfunctional movement: reduced range, excessive range, increased resistance, decreased resistance, altered quality of movement
Palpation of joint	Reproduces patient's symptoms	Tenderness
Reassessment following therapeutic dose of accessory movement	Improvement in tests which reproduce patient's symptoms	No change in physical tests which reproduce patient's symptoms
Muscle		
Active movement	Reproduces patient's symptoms	Reduced strength
Passive physiological movements	Patient's symptoms not reproduced	
Isometric contraction	Reproduces patient's symptoms	Reduced strength
Passive lengthening of muscle	Reproduces patient's symptoms	Reduced range Increased resistance Decreased resistance
Palpation of muscle	Reproduces patient's symptoms	Tenderness
Reassessment following therapeutic dose of muscle treatment	Improvement in tests which reproduce patient's symptoms	No change in physical tests which reproduce patient's symptoms
Nerve		
Passive lengthening and sensitizing movement, i.e. altering length of nerve by a movement at a distance from patient's symptoms	Reproduces patient's symptoms and sensitizing movement alters patient's symptoms	Reduced range Increased resistance
Palpation of nerve	Reproduces patient's symptoms	Tenderness

movements, reassessment of the elbow's physiological movements is improved, in terms of range and pain. This scenario would indicate that there is a dysfunction at the radiohumeral joint—first, because elbow movements, both active and passive physiological, and accessory movements, reproduce the patient's symptoms, and, second, because, following accessory movements, the active elbow movements are improved. Even if the active movements are made worse, this would still suggest a joint dysfunction because it is likely that the accessory movements would predominantly affect the joint, with much less effect on nerve and muscle tissues around the area. Collectively, this evidence would suggest that there is primarily a joint dysfunction.

The strongest evidence that a muscle is the primary source of a patient's symptoms is if active movements, an isometric contraction, passive lengthening and palpation of a muscle all reproduce the patient's symptoms, and that, following a treatment, reassessment identifies an improvement in the patient's signs and symptoms. For example, let us assume that a patient has lateral elbow pain caused by lateral epicondylalgia. In this case, reproduction of the patient's lateral elbow pain is found on active wrist and finger extension, isometric/isotonic/eccentric contraction of the wrist extensors and/or finger extensors and passive lengthening of the extensor muscles to the wrist and hand. These signs and symptoms are found to improve following soft-tissue mobilization examination, sufficient to be considered a treatment dose. Collectively, this evidence would suggest that there is a muscle dysfunction, as long as this is accompanied by negative joint and nerve tests.

The strongest evidence that a nerve is the source of the patient's symptoms is when active and/or passive physiological movements reproduce the patient's symptoms, which are then increased or decreased with an additional neurally sensitizing movement, at a distance from the patient's symptoms. In addition, there is a reproduction of the patient's symptoms on palpation of the nerve, and following treatment directed at neural tissue an improvement in the above signs and symptoms occurs. For example, let us assume this time that the lateral elbow pain is caused by a neurodynamic dysfunction of the radial nerve supplying this region. The patient's lateral elbow pain is reproduced during the component movements of the upper-limb neurodynamic test (ULNT) 2b and is eased with ipsilateral cervical lateral flexion desensitizing movement. There is tenderness over the radial groove in the upper arm and, following testing of the ULNT 2b, sufficient to be considered a treatment dose, an improvement in the patient's signs and symptoms. Collectively, this evidence would suggest that there is a neurodynamic dysfunction, as long as this is accompanied by negative joint and muscle tests.

It can be seen that the common factor for identifying joint, nerve and muscle dysfunction as a source of the patient's symptoms is the reproduction of the patient's symptoms, an alteration in the patient's signs and symptoms following targeted treatment and a lack of evidence from other potential sources of symptoms. It is assumed that if a test reproduces a patient's symptoms then it is somehow stressing the structure at fault. As mentioned earlier, each test is not purely a test of one structure—every test, to a greater or lesser degree, involves other structures. For this reason, it is imperative that, whatever treatment is given, it is proved to be of value by altering the patient's signs and symptoms. The other factor common in identifying joint, nerve or muscle dysfunction is the lack of positive findings in the other possible tissues; for example, a joint dysfunction is considered when joint tests are positive and muscle and nerve tests are negative. Thus the clinician collects evidence to implicate tissues and evidence to negate tissues—both are equally important.

An ongoing analysis of the evidence as indicated above facilitates the clinician in reasoning the main driver underlying the patient's symptoms so that treatment can be correctly targeted. For example, the source of symptoms may be a hypermobile motion segment of the lumbar spine which may be symptomatic as a result of a neighbouring hypomobile segment. In this instance, it could be hypothesized that treatment directed at the hypomobile segment should improve symptoms. This analysis would also need to be accompanied by consideration of other components of the movement system such as muscle activity, normal movement patterns and associated behaviours.

The clinician's primary hypothesis can be summarized in a statement of a clinical diagnosis or clinical impression. Rather than identifying a particular structure, this statement will include detail on presenting symptoms, associated movement dysfunction, underlying pain mechanism, psychosocial considerations and key physical examination findings. For example:

A 15-year-old hockey player presents with nonsevere/nonirritable mechanical nociceptive anterior knee pain, secondary to a tight lateral retinaculum tracking the patella laterally during eccentric control of knee flexion. Pain is eased with a medial glide of the patella.

A 45-year-old female dentist presents with right C4–C5 zygapophyseal joint dysfunction, inflammatory and mechanical, nociceptive pain, right side of the neck and lateral upper arm, not severe and not irritable.

There are regular compression pattern cervical movements plus a positive ULNT 2a, biasing the median nerve.

Alternatively, read the clinical impression statements below. Although both cases have sustained the same injury, treatment priorities, treatment and goals will differ markedly. This shows that one size does not fit all.

Case 1: Clinical Impression

A 28-year-old female track and field athlete has a 3-week history of mechanical and inflammatory nociceptive pain of left lateral ankle origin, anterior talofibular ligament, following a grade 2 inversion injury. Reduced talocrural dorsiflexion/inversion, active and passive range with proprioceptive and strength deficits. Keen to resume training as soon as possible.

Case 2: Clinical Impression

A 45-year-old policeman, deconditioned, body mass index of 27, has a left ankle inversion injury. Six-month history, persistent discomfort over the lateral aspect, reduced talocrural dorsiflexion/inversion, active and passive range proprioceptive, strength deficits, reluctant to move, deconditioned and anxiety about upcoming fitness test.

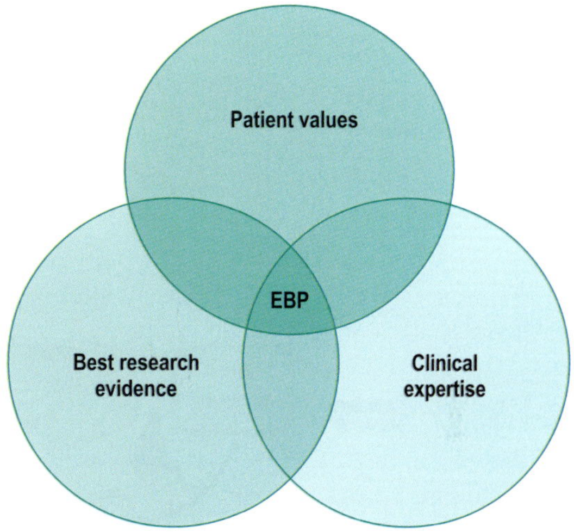

Fig. 5.7 Evidence-based practice (EBP). (From Sackett et al., 2000, with permission.)

S	Specific
M	Measurable
A	Attainable
R	Relevant
T	Time-bound

Fig. 5.8 SMART goals.

Through procedural reasoning, the clinician will use the identification of functional problems to offer the patient choice on possible management strategies (Fleming, 1991). Interventions offered should be evidence-based and justified (Sackett, 2000) (Fig. 5.7). Knowledge of how tissues respond to injury and disease underpins the explanation of the mechanism by which treatment will have an effect.

The clinician will need to be competent in the skilful application of the agreed intervention (Banks & Hengeveld, 2014) and all options should be presented to the patient so that an agreed plan can be negotiated in order to achieve agreed SMART goals—specific, measurable, attainable, relevant and time-bound (Fig. 5.8).

Achievement of treatment goals will also be dependent on the patient's ability to engage in the process fully. Treatment may be unsuccessful if the patient is not ready or able to change behaviours that may be barriers to recovery. The stages-of-change model described by Prochaska and DiClemente (1982) can be used to help people make changes that will have a positive impact on their well-being, for example, being more physically active, taking on board advice (Fig. 5.9 and Table 5.3).

Is the patient contemplating change but not yet ready to move on to the action stage? The patient's level of confidence or self-efficacy in achieving behaviour change to reach agreed goals is also a factor in engagement (Nicholas, 2007; Menezes Costa et al., 2011). Management should ideally be tailored to promoting self-efficacy, accommodating the patient's degree of motivation, interest and stage of readiness if the benefits of interventions are to be maximized (Rollnick et al., 1993). For further details see Chapter 2.

Clinical reasoning continues to refine hypotheses about the cause of the patient's symptoms throughout

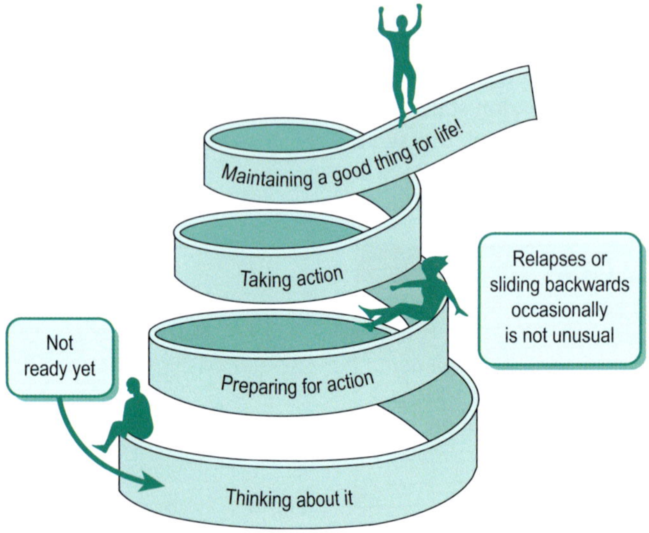

Fig. 5.9 Stages-of-change model. (Data from Prochaska, J.O., DiClemente, C.C., 1982. Transtheoretical therapy: toward a more integrative model of change. Psychotherapy 19 (3), 276–288.)

TABLE 5.3 Stages of Change

Precontemplation	The person is not considering change—this is the 'ignorance is bliss' stage
Contemplation	The person appears ambivalent about change—the individual is 'sitting on the fence'
Preparation	The person has had some experience with change and is trying to change. The individual is 'testing the waters'
Action	The person has taken steps towards changing behaviour and has made changes to his or her lifestyle to work towards the desired outcome
Maintenance	The person is working to stay on track and avoid relapse. Positive experience is reaffirming that the person can succeed
Relapse	Although not part of the original model, this refers to a person falling back into old harmful behaviours after going through the other stages

Prochaska et al. (1992).

the management of the patient in what Maitland termed 'analytical assessment' (Banks & Hengeveld, 2014; p. 33). Following treatment, both within and between treatment sessions, the clinician will critically evaluate responses to treatment through the reassessment of subjective and physical markers or asterisks (Maitland used the term comparable signs), seeking to identify change. These individual markers/* used for reassessment come from the subjective examination and can relate to symptoms on the body chart, functional deficits, evaluation of severity and irritability and the volume of medication required to manage symptoms. Physical examination markers (*) indicate retesting of functional activities, active and passive movement, muscle reassessment and neural responses to tests.

An improvement in subjective asterisks seems to be fairly strong evidence that there has been a change. For example, a patient who is able to increase the time ironing or walking, or is able to sleep better although the response will depend, in part, on the patient's attitude to the problem, to the clinician and towards treatment, which may positively or negatively affect the patient's response. Further questioning of any change is always needed to clarify that it is the condition that has improved and not something else. For example, if sleeping has improved, the clinician checks the details of the nature of that improvement, and whether there is any other explanation, such as a change in analgesia that may explain the improvement.

Changes in physical findings also need careful and unbiased reasoning by the clinician. A test must be carried out in a reliable way for the clinician to consider that a change in the test is a real change. Clearly, some of the tests carried out are easier to replicate than others. For example, a change in an active movement is rather easier to quantify than the clinician's 'feel' of a passive physiological movement. Clinicians will do well to evaluate critically their reassessment asterisks and consider carefully how much weight they can place upon them when they interpret a change.

Reassessment of both subjective and physical aspects includes a combination of the patient's and the clinician's views to increase validity (Cook et al., 2015). These markers provide individual patient-specific outcome measures that can be linked to validated outcome tools to measure the impact of interventions on the patient, and on the patient's health and well-being (Banks & Hengeveld, 2014). Outcomes that measure across a range of domains, such as function, generic health status, work disability, patient satisfaction, as well as pain, are best placed to capture the multidimensional nature of patients attending for musculoskeletal treatment (Bombadier, 2000).

At each attendance, the clinician obtains a detailed account of the effect of the last treatment on the patient's signs and symptoms. This will involve the immediate effects after the last treatment, the relevant activities of the patient since the last treatment and enquiring how the patient is presenting on the day of treatment. Patients who say they are worse since the last treatment should be questioned carefully, as this may be due to some activity they have been involved with, or an increase in stress in their life rather than any treatment that has been given. Patients who say they feel better also need to be questioned carefully, as the improvement may not be related to treatment. If the patient remains the same, following the subjective and physical reassessment, the clinician may consider altering the treatment approach. The process of assessment, treatment and reassessment is depicted in Fig. 5.10.

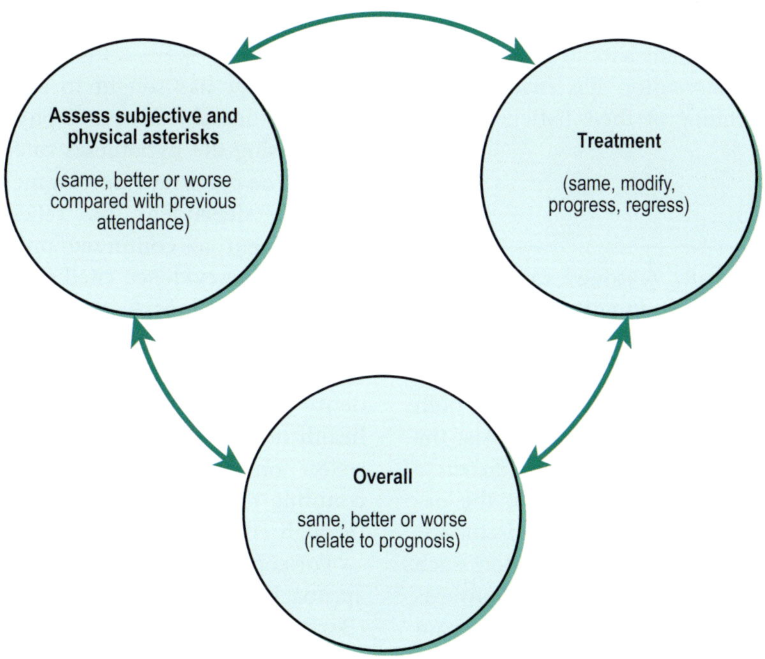

Fig. 5.10 Modification, progression and regression of treatment.

Retrospective assessment at regular intervals allows the clinician the opportunity to reflect and clinically reason with the patient on overall progress, comparing the subjective and physical markers, at a follow-up appointment with the findings of the initial assessment. Reflective reasoning taking into account the patient's view of what has worked and the progress made towards agreed goals will allow the clinician to consider whether additional interventions are required. This continuous analytical assessment would identify when improvement has plateaued, prompting a collaborative review on why this might be. Is there a fault with the selection of reassessment parameters? What is the patient's view? Has treatment been directed towards the right source? Is there an issue with self-management strategies? Is there an indication for additional medical interventions? For further information, the reader is referred to Banks and Hengeveld (2014).

Finally, analysis at the end of a course of treatment will consider overall what has been learned by the clinician but also by the patient. What is the possibility of recurrent problems in the future? Is it likely that the patient will be able to self-manage any remaining functional deficits? This will depend on the patient's level of participation and empowerment to take ownership. Increasingly clinicians should also consider the contribution their intervention has made to the future healthy life expectancy of their patients (Middleton, 2008).

PROGNOSIS

Having agreed on a clinically reasoned management plan, patients will often ask how long it will take them to recover and how often they will need to attend for treatment.

A number of positive and negative factors from both the subjective and physical examination will assist the clinician in reasoning a predictive response to these questions. Factors to consider might include the patient's age; general health; lifestyle; levels of self-efficacy; personality; expectations and psychosocial factors such as their attitude towards their condition, towards themselves and towards the clinician, as well as pain drivers; severity and irritability of the symptoms; extent of tissue damage; the natural history and progression of the condition. Physical factors predicting prognosis may include predominant pain mechanisms, the extent of physical limitation, the number of systems involved, response to movement and manual assessment and proprioceptive awareness.

By considering all of these individual factors, the clinician is then able to predict to what extent, in percentage terms, symptoms will respond to treatment and the anticipated number of treatment sessions required to achieve this improvement. At discharge, it is useful for the clinician to compare the final outcome with the predicted outcome, as this reflection will help clinicians to learn and enhance their ability to hypothesize about prognoses in the future.

KNOWLEDGE CHECK

1. What are the aims of the physical examination?
2. What does SMART refer to, and why might it be useful in the therapeutic process?
3. What shapes the prognosis?

CONCLUSION

This chapter has sought to explore clinical reasoning through the subjective and physical examination processes using the hypotheses categories (Jones & Rivett, 2004). The continued development of clinical reasoning skills is dependent on reflective practice and a commitment to continued professional development. Much of the evidence cited in this chapter is extrapolated from the nonspecific low-back pain literature. The challenge for the future is for clinicians to adapt to the currently incomplete and constantly developing evidence base in order to contribute to the improved health of their patients. This will require the ability to reflect on each and every interaction in order to continue to reason, question and learn from patients through effective communication.

For consideration of the treatment and management approaches the reader is directed to the companion text (Barnard & Ryder, 2024).

REVIEW AND REVISE QUESTIONS

1. What skills and attributes does the clinician need to successfully clinically reason?
2. What is known about how experts clinically reason?
3. Nonpropositional knowledge includes personal and professional knowledge.
   True or False?
4. How would you explain the relevance and differences between gut feeling and intuition in clinical reasoning?
5. Offer examples of active listening cues that can reassure a patient they are being heard.
6. What factors can make a patient's response to pain so unique?
7. What are pink flags, and why are they useful to identify?
8. Pattern recognition is also known as backward or deductive reasoning.
   True or False?
9. What physical examination findings would support muscle dysfunction being the primary driver of a patient's symptoms?
10. What is understood by the term continuous analytical assessment, and what is its significance?

REFERENCES

Aroll, B., Khin, N., Kerse, N., 2003. Screening for depression in primary care with two verbally asked questions: cross sectional study. Br. Med. J. 327, 1144–1146.

Arocha, J.F., Patel, V.L., Patel, Y.C., 1993. Hypothesis Generation and the Coordination of Theory and Evidence in Novice Diagnostic Reasoning. Med Decis Making 13 (3), 198–211. https://doi.org/10.1177/0272989X9301300305.

Atkinson, H.L., Nixon-Cave, K., 2011. A tool for clinical reasoning and reflection using the international classification of functioning, disability and health (ICF) framework and patient management model. Phys. Ther. 91, 416–430.

Bachmann, L.M., Kolb, E., Koller, M.T., Steurer, J., ter Riet, G., 2003. Accuracy of Ottawa ankle rules to exclude fractures of the ankle and mid-foot: systematic review. Br. Med. J. 326, 417.

Banks, K., Hengeveld, E., 2014. The Maitland concept as a clinical practice framework for neuromusculoskeletal disorders. In: Hengeveld, E., Banks, K. (Eds.), Maitland's Peripheral Manipulation. Churchill Livingstone, Edinburgh (Chapter 1).

Barker, C., Taylor, A., Johnson, M., 2014. Problematic pain—redefining how we view pain? Br. J. Pain 8, 9–15.

Barker, K.L., Reid, M., Minns Lowe, C.J., 2009. Divided by a lack of common language? A qualitative study exploring the use of language by health professionals treating back pain. BMC Musculoskelet. Disord. 10, 123.

Barnard, K., Ryder, D., 2024. Principles of Musculoskeletal Treatment and Management: A Handbook for Therapists, fourth ed. Elsevier, Edinburgh.

Beales, D., Kendell, M., Chang, R.P., Håmsø, M., Gregory, L., Richardson, K., et al., 2016. Association between the 10 item Orebro musculoskeletal pain screening questionnaire and physiotherapists' perception of the contribution of biopsychosocial factors in patients with musculoskeletal pain. Man. Ther. 23, 48–55.

Bechara, A., Damasio, A.R., 2005. The somatic marker hypothesis: a neural theory of economic decision. Games Econ. Behav. 52 (2), 336–372.

Bennett, M.I., Attal, N., Backonja, M.M., Baron, R., Bouhassira, D., Freynhagen, R., et al., 2007. Using screening tools to identify neuropathic pain. Pain 127, 199–203.

Bialosky, J.E., Bishop, M.D., George, S.Z., Robinson, M.E., 2011. Placebo response to manual therapy: something out of nothing? J. Man. Manip. Ther. 19, 11–19.

Bignotti, B., Signori, A., Sormani, M.P., Molfetta, L., Martinoli, C., Tagliafico, A., 2015. Ultrasound versus magnetic resonance imaging for Morton neuroma: systematic review and meta-analysis. Eur. Radiol. 25, 2254–2262.

Bishop, A., Foster, N.E., Thomas, E., Hay, E.M., 2008. How does the self-reported clinical management of patients with low back pain relate to the attitudes and beliefs of health care practitioners? A survey of UK general practitioners and physiotherapists. Pain 135, 187–195.

Bogduk, N., 2009. On the definitions and physiology of back pain, referred pain, and radicular pain. Pain 147, 17–19.

Bombadier, C., 2000. Outcome assessments in the evaluation of treatment of spinal disorders. Introduction. Spine 25, 3097–3099.

Brem, H., Tomic-Canic, M., 2007. Cellular and molecular basis of wound healing in diabetes. J. Clin. Invest. 117, 1219–1222.

Brinjikji, W., Luetmer, P.H., Comstock, B., Bresnahan, B.W., Chen, L.E., Deyo, R.A., et al., 2015. Systematic literature review of imaging features of spinal degeneration in asymptomatic populations. AJNR Am. J. Neuroradiol. 36, 811–816.

Butler, D., 2000. The Sensitive Nervous System. NOI Group Publications, Adelaide.

Butler, D., Moseley, L., 2003. Explain Pain. NOI Group Publications, Adelaide.

Caladine, L., Morris, J., 2015. Patient education: a collaborative approach. In: Jull, G., Moore, A., Falla, D., Lewis, J., McCarthy, C., Sterling, M. (Eds.), Grieve's Modern Musculoskeletal Physiotherapy, fourth ed. Elsevier, Edinburgh, pp. 250—253.

Calguneri, M., Bird, H.A., Wright, V., 1982. Changes in joint laxity occurring during pregnancy. Ann. Rheum. Dis. 41, 126—128.

Chapman, R., Tuckett, R.P., Song, C.W., 2008. Pain and stress in a systems perspective: reciprocal neural, endocrine, and immune interactions. J. Pain 9, 122—145.

Chartered Society of Physiotherapy, 2008. Scope of physiotherapy practice. Available online at: http://www.clinicaledge.com.au/app/webroot/uploads/pd001_scope_of_practice_2008.pdf. (accessed 30 January 2017).

Chester, E.C., Robinson, N.C., Roberts, L.C., 2014. Opening clinical encounters in an adult musculoskeletal setting. Man. Ther. 19, 306—310.

Christensen, N., Jones, M., Higgs, J., Edwards, I., 2008. Dimensions of clinical reasoning capability. In: Higgs, J., Jones, M.A., Loftus, S., Christensen, N. (Eds.), Clinical Reasoning in the Health Professions. Elsevier Butterworth-Heinemann, Oxford, pp. 101—110.

Clinical Standards Advisory Group (CSAG), 1994. Report on Low Back Pain. HMSO, London.

Cook, C., Learman, K., Showalter, C., O'Halloran, B., 2015. The relationship between chief complaint and comparable sign in patients with spinal pain: an exploratory study. Man. Ther. 20, 451—455.

Cook, J., Purdam, C., 2012. Is compressive load a factor in the development of tendinopathy? Br. J. Sports Med. 46, 163—168.

Cook, J.L., Bass, S.L., Black, J.E., 2007. Hormone therapy is associated with smaller Achilles tendon diameter in active post-menopausal women. Scand. J. Med. Sci. Sports 17, 128—132.

Cook, J.L., Rio, E., Purdam, C.R., Docking, S.I., 2016. Revisiting the continuum model of tendon pathology: what is its merit in clinical practice and research? Br. J. Sports Med. 50 (19), 1187—1191. https://doi.org/10.1136/bjsports-2015-095422.

Cook, N., van Griensven, H., 2013. Neuropathic pain and complex regional pain syndrome. In: van Griensven, H., Strong, J., Unruh, A. (Eds.), Pain: A Textbook for Health Professionals, second ed. Churchill Livingstone, Edinburgh, pp. 137—158.

Cooksey, R., 1996. The Methodology of Social Judgement Theory Thinking & Reasoning, 2 (2—3), 141—173.

Cooper, K., Smith, B.H., Hancock, E., 2008. Patient-centredness in physiotherapy from the perspective of the chronic low back pain patient. Physiotherapy 94, 244—252.

Cruz, E.B., Moore, A.P., Cross, V., 2012. A qualitative study of physiotherapy final year undergraduate students' perceptions of clinical reasoning. Man. Ther. 17 (6), 549—553.

Danneels, L., Beernaert, A., De Corte, K., Descheemaeker, F., Vanthillo, B., Van Tiggelen, D., et al., 2011. A didactical approach for musculoskeletal physiotherapy: the planetary model. J. Musculoskelet. Pain 19, 218—222.

Darlow, B., Dowell, A., Baxter, G.D., Mathieson, F., Perry, M., Dean, S., 2013. The enduring impact of what clinicians say to people with low back pain. Ann. Fam. Med. 11, 527—534.

Darlow, B., Fullen, B.M., Dean, S., Hurley, D.A., Baxter, G.D., Dowell, A., 2012. The association between health care professional attitudes and beliefs and the attitudes and beliefs, clinical management, and outcomes of patients with low back pain: a systematic review. Eur. J. Pain 16, 3—17.

Diegelmann, R.F., Evans, M.C., 2004. Wound healing: an overview of acute, fibrotic and delayed healing. Front. Biosci. 9, 283—289. https://doi.org/10.1097/ACM.0000000000002483.

Doody, C., McAteer, M., 2002. Clinical reasoning of expert and novice physiotherapists in an outpatient orthopaedic setting. Physiotherapy 88, 258—268.

Dubois, B., Esculier, J., 2020. Soft-tissue injuries simply need PEACE and LOVE. Br. J. Sports Med. 54, 72—73.

Edwards, I., Jones, M., Carr, J., Braunack-Mayer, A., Jensen, G.M., 2004. Clinical reasoning strategies in physical therapy. Phys. Ther. 84, 312—330.

Edwards, I., Jones, M., Hillier, S., 2006. The interpretation of experience and its relationship to body movement: a clinical reasoning perspective. Man. Ther. 11, 2—10.

Feltowich, P.J., Barrows, H.S., 1984. Issues of generality in medical problems solving. In: Schmidt, H.G., Volder, M.I. (Eds.), Tutorials in Problem Based Learning: A New Direction in Teaching the Health Professional. van Gorcum, Assen, the Netherlands, pp. 128—141.

Fleming, M., Mattingly, C., 2008. Action and narrative: two dynamics of clinical reasoning. In: Higgs, J., Jones, M.A., Loftus, S., Christensen, N. (Eds.), Clinical Reasoning in the Health Professions, third ed. Butterworth Heinemann, Elsevier, Amsterdam (Chapter 5).

Fleming, M.H., 1991. The therapist with the three track mind. Am. J. Occup. Ther. 45, 1007—1014.

Flynn, T., Fritz, J., Whitman, J., Wainner, R., Magel, J., Rendeiro, D., et al., 2002. A clinical prediction rule for classifying patients with low back pain who demonstrate short-term improvement with spinal manipulation. Spine 27, 2835—2843.

Froud, R., Patterson, S., Eldridge, S., Seale, C., Pincus, T., Rajendran, D., et al., 2014. A systematic review and meta-synthesis of the impact of low back pain on people's lives. BMC Musculoskelet. Disord. 15, 50.

Gaida, J., Alfredson, H., Kiss, Z.S., Bass, S.L., Cook, J.L., 2010. Asymptomatic Achilles tendon pathology is associated with a central fat distribution in men and a peripheral fat distribution in women: a cross sectional study of 298 individuals. BMC Musculoskelet. Disord. 11, 41.

Gandhi, A., Beam, H.A., O'Connor, J.P., Parsons, J.R., Lin, S.S., 2005. The effects of local insulin delivery on diabetic fracture healing. Bone 37, 482–490.

Gifford, L., 1998. Pain, the tissues and the nervous system: a conceptual model. Physiotherapy 84, 27–36.

Gifford, L.S., 2005. Editorial. Now for pink flags. PPA News 22, 3–4.

Goodman, C.C., Heick, J., Lazaro, R., 2018. Differential Diagnosis for Physical Therapists: Screening for Referral, sixth ed. Elsevier, St Louis.

Grant, J., 2008. Using open and distance learning to develop clinical reasoning skills. In: Higgs, J., Jones, M.A., Loftus, S., Christensen, N. (Eds.), Clinical Reasoning in the Health Professions. Elsevier Butterworth-Heinemann, Oxford, pp. 441–450.

Greenhalgh, S., Selfe, J., 2004. Margaret: a tragic case of spinal red flags and red herrings. Physiotherapy 90, 73–76.

Greenhalgh, S., Selfe, J., 2010. Red Flags II: A Guide to Solving Serious Pathology of the Spine. Elsevier, Edinburgh.

Hannibal, K.E., Bishop, M.D., 2014. Chronic stress, cortisol dysfunction, and pain: a psychoneuroendocrine rationale for stress management in pain rehabilitation. Phys. Ther. 94, 1816–1825.

Hansson, P., Kinnman, E., 1996. Unmasking mechanisms of chronic peripheral neuropathic pain in a clinical perspective. Pain Rev. 3, 272–292.

Hammond, K.R., 1996. Human Judgment and Social Policy: Irreducible Uncertainty, Inevitable Error, Unavoidable Justice. Oxford University Press, London.

Hasenbring, M.I., Hallner, D., Klasen, B., Streitlein-Böhme, I., Willburger, R., Rusche, H., 2012. Pain-related avoidance versus endurance in primary care patients with subacute back pain: psychological characteristics and outcome at a 6-month follow-up. Pain 153, 211–217.

Henschke, N., Ostelo, R.W., van Tulder, M.W., Vlaeyen, J.W., Morley, S., Assendelft, W.J., et al., 2010. Behavioural treatment for chronic low-back pain. Cochrane Database Syst. Rev. 7, CD002014.

Higgs, J., 1992. Developing clinical reasoning competencies. Physiotherapy 78 (8), 575–581.

Higgs, J., Jones, M.A., 2008. Clinical decision making and multiple problem spaces. In: Higgs, J., Jones, M.A., Loftus, S., Christensen, N. (Eds.), Clinical Reasoning in the Health Professions. Elsevier Butterworth-Heinemann, Oxford, pp. 3–18.

Higgs, J., Titchen, A., 1995. The nature, generation and verification of knowledge. Physiotherapy 81, 521–530.

Hill, J., Fritz, J.M., 2011. Psychosocial influences on low back pain, disability, and response to treatment. Phys. Ther. 91, 712–721.

Houtman, I.L., Bongers, P.M., Smulders, P.G., Kompier, M. A., 1994. Psychosocial stressors at work and musculoskeletal problems. Scand. J. Work. Environ. Health 20, 139–145.

Jaroudi, S., Payne, J.D., 2019. Remembering Lawrence Weed: a pioneer of the SOAP note. Acad. Med. 94 (1), 11.

Jones, M., Edwards, I., Gifford, L., 2002. Conceptual models for implementing biopsychosocial theory in clinical practice. Man. Ther. 7, 2–9.

Jones, M., Jensen, G., Edwards, I., 2008. Clinical reasoning in physiotherapy. In: Higgs, J., Jones, M.A., Loftus, S., Christensen, N. (Eds.), Clinical Reasoning in the Health Professions, third ed. Butterworth Heinemann/Elsevier, Amsterdam, pp. 245–256.

Jones, M.A., 1995. Clinical reasoning and pain. Man. Ther. 1, 17–24.

Jones, M.A., Rivett, D.A., 2004. Clinical Reasoning for Manual Therapists. Butterworth-Heinemann, Edinburgh.

Kent, P., Mirkhil, S., Keating, J., Buchbinder, R., Manniche, C., Albert, H.B., 2014. The concurrent validity of brief screening questions for anxiety, depression, social isolation, catastrophization, and fear of movement in people with low back pain. Clin. J. Pain 4, 479–489.

Kerry, R., 2010. The theory of clinical reasoning in combined movement therapy. In: McCarthy, C. (Ed.), Combined Movement Theory: Rational Mobilization and Manipulation of the Vertebral Column. Churchill Livingstone, Edinburgh, pp. 19–47.

Kountouris, A., Cook, J., 2007. Rehabilitation of Achilles and patellar tendinopathies. Clin. Rheumatol. 21, 295–316.

Langridge, N., Roberts, L., Pope, C., 2016. The role of clinician emotion in clinical reasoning: balancing the analytical process. Man. Ther. 14, 277–281.

Learman, K., Showalter, C., Cook, C., 2012. Does the use of a prescriptive clinical prediction rule increase the likelihood of applying inappropriate treatments? A survey using clinical vignettes. Man. Ther. 17, 538–543.

Leeuw, M., Goossens, M.E., Linton, S.J., Crombez, G., Boersma, K., Vlaeyen, J.W., 2007. The fear-avoidance model of musculoskeletal pain: current state of scientific evidence. J. Behav. Med. 30, 77–94.

Lewis, J., 2016. Rotator cuff related shoulder pain: assessment, management and uncertainties. Man. Ther. 23, 57–68.

Linton, S.J., Boersma, K., 2003. Early identification of patients at risk of developing a persistent back problem: the predictive validity of the Örebro musculoskeletal pain questionnaire. Clin. J. Pain 19, 80–86.

Linton, S.J., Shaw, W.S., 2011. Impact of psychological factors in the experience of pain. Phys. Ther. 91, 700–711.

Loftus, S., Smith, M., 2008. A history of clinical reasoning. In: Clinical Reasoning in the Health Professions, third ed. Elsevier, London, pp. 205–212.

Louw, A., Diener, I., Butler, D.S., Puentedura, E.J., 2011. The effect of neuroscience education on pain, disability, anxiety, and stress in chronic musculoskeletal pain. Arch. Phys. Med. Rehabil. (12), 2041–2056. https://doi.org/10.1016/j.apmr.2011.07.198.

Low, M., 2017. A novel clinical framework: the use of dispositions in clinical practice. A person centred approach. J. Eval. Clin. Pract. 23 (5), 1062–1070. https://doi.org/10.1111/jep.12713.

Luomajoki, H., Moseley, G.L., 2011. Tactile acuity and lumbopelvic motor control in patients with back pain and healthy controls. Br. J. Sports Med. 45, 437–440.

MacKereth, P., Carter, A., Stringer, J., 2014. Complementary therapy approaches to pain. In: van Griensven, H., Strong, J., Unruh, A. (Eds.), Pain: A Textbook for Health Professionals, second ed. Churchill Livingstone, Edinburgh, pp. 237–253.

Maguire, P., Pitceathly, C., 2002. Key communication skills and how to acquire them. Br. Med. J. 325, 697–700.

Main, C.J., Buchbinder, R., Porcheret, M., Foster, N., 2010. Addressing patient beliefs and expectations in the consultation. Best Pract. Res. Clin. Rheumatol. 24, 219–225.

Main, C.J., Spanswick, C.C., 2000. Pain Management: An Interdisciplinary Approach. Churchill Livingstone, Edinburgh.

Maitland, G.D., Hengeveld, E., Banks, K., English, K., 2005. Maitland's Vertebral Manipulation, seventh ed. Butterworth-Heinemann, London, p. 57.

Marsell, R., Einhorn, T., 2011. The biology of fracture healing. Injury 42, 551–555.

May, S., Clare, H., 2015. The McKenzie method of mechanical diagnosis and therapy—an overview. In: Jull, G., Moore, A., Falla, D., Lewis, J., McCarthy, C., Sterling, M. (Eds.), Grieve's Modern Musculoskeletal Physiotherapy, fourth ed. Elsevier, Edinburgh, pp. 460–462.

McCarthy, C.J., Arnall, F.A., Strimpakos, N., Freemont, A., Oldham, J.A., 2004. The biopsychosocial classification of nonspecific low back pain: a systematic review. Phys. Ther. Rev. 9, 17–30.

McCullough, B.J., Johnson, G.R., Martin, B.I., Jarvik, J.G., 2012. Lumbar MR imaging and reporting epidemiology: do epidemiologic data in reports affect clinical management? Radiology 262, 941–946.

McCutcheon, H.H., Pincombe, J., 2001. Intuition: an important tool in the practice of nursing. J. Adv. Nurs. 35 (3), 342–348.

Menezes Costa, L., Maher, C.G., McAuley, J.H., Hancock, M.J., Smeets, R.J., 2011. Self-efficacy is more important than fear of movement in mediating the relationship between pain and disability in chronic low back pain. Eur. J. Pain 15, 213–219.

Middleton, K., 2008. Framing the Contribution of Allied Health Professionals Delivering High Quality Health Care. UK Department of Health, London, pp. 1–38.

Moore, A., Jull, G., 2010. The primacy of clinical reasoning and clinical practical skills. Man. Ther. 15, 513.

Moseley, G.L., Nicholas, M.K., Hodges, P.W., 2004. A randomized controlled trial of intensive neurophysiology education in chronic low back pain. Clin. J. Pain 20, 324–330.

National Institute for Health and Care Excellence (NICE), 2012. Osteoporosis: assessing the risk of fragility fracture. Available online at: https://www.nice.org.uk/.

National Institute for Health and Clinical Excellence (NICE), 2006. Guidelines on the management of low back pain. Available online at: https://www.nice.org.uk/.

Nicholas, M.K., 2007. The pain self-efficacy questionnaire: taking pain into account. Eur. J. Pain 11, 153–163.

Nicholas, M.K., Linton, S.J., Watson, P.J., Main, C.J., 'Decade of the Flags' Working Group, 2011. Early identification and management of psychological risk factors ("yellow flags") in patients with low back pain: a reappraisal. Phys. Ther. 91, 737–753.

Nielsen, M., 2014. The patient's voice. In: van Griensven, H., Strong, J., Unruh, A.M. (Eds.), Pain: A Textbook for Health Professionals, second ed. Churchill Livingstone, Edinburgh, pp. 9–20.

Nijs, J., Roussel, N., Paul van Wilgen, C., Köke, A., Smeets, R., 2013. Thinking beyond muscles and joints: therapists' and patients' attitudes and beliefs regarding chronic musculoskeletal pain are key to applying effective treatment. Man. Ther. 18, 96–102.

Øberg, G., Normann, B., Gallagher, S., 2015. Embodied-enactive clinical reasoning in physical therapy. Physiother. Theory Pract. 21 (4), 244–252. https://doi.org/10.3109/099593985.2014.1002873.

Opsommer, E., Schoeb, V., 2014. 'Tell me about your troubles': description of patient–physiotherapist interaction during initial encounters. Physiother. Res. Int. 19, 205–221.

Orme, L., Maggs, C., 1993. Decision-making in clinical practice: how do expert nurses, midwives and health visitors make decisions? Nurse Educ. Today 13 (4), 270–276.

O'Sullivan, P., 2005. Diagnosis and classification of chronic low back pain disorders: maladaptive movement and motor control impairments as underlying mechanism. Man. Ther. 10, 242–255.

O'Sullivan, P., Dankaerts, W., O'Sullivan, K., Fersum, K., 2015. Multidimensional approach for targeted management of low back pain. In: Jull, G., Moore, A., Falla, D., Lewis, J., McCarthy, C. (Eds.), Grieve's Modern Musculoskeletal Physiotherapy, fourth ed. Edinburgh, Edinburgh, pp. 465–470.

Patel, V.L., Groen, G.J., Patel, Y.C., 1997. Cognitive aspects of clinical performance during patient workup: the role of medical expertise. Adv. Health Sci. Educ. 2, 95–114.

Petty, N.J., Thomson, O.P., Stew, G., 2012a. Ready for a paradigm shift? Part 2: introducing qualitative research methodologies and methods. Man. Ther. 17 (5), 378–384.

Petty, N.J., Thomson, O.P., Stew, G., 2012b. Ready for a paradigm shift? Part 1: introducing the philosophy of qualitative research. Man. Ther. 17 (4), 267–274.

Politi, M., Street, R., 2011. The Importance of Communication in Collaborative Decision Making: Facilitating Shared Mind and the Management of Uncertainty. J. Eval. Clin. Pract. 17 (4), 579–584. https://doi.org/10.1111/j.1365-2753.2010.01549.x.

Prochaska, J.O., DiClemente, C.C., 1982. Transtheoretical therapy: toward a more integrative model of change. Psychother. Theory Res. Pract. 19, 276–287.

Prochaska, J.O., DiClemente, C.C., Norcross, J.C., 1992. In search of how people change. Applications to addictive behaviors. Am. Psychol. 47, 1102–1114.

Rivett, D., Jones, M., 2004. Improving clinical reasoning in manual therapy. In: Higgs, J., et al. (Eds.), Clinical Reasoning in the Health Professions, third ed. Butterworth Heinemann/Elsevier, Amsterdam, pp. 403–419.

Roberts, L., Whittle, C.T., Cleland, J., Wald, M., 2013. Measuring verbal communication in initial physical therapy encounters. Phys. Ther. 93, 479–491.

Rollnick, S., Kinnersley, P., Stott, N., 1993. Methods of helping patients with behaviour change. Br. Med. J. 307, 188–190.

Rushton, A., Rivett, D., Carlesso, L., Flynn, T., Hing, W., Kerry, R., 2014. International framework for examination of the cervical region for potential of cervical arterial dysfunction prior to orthopaedic manual therapy intervention. Man. Ther. 19, 222–228.

Russek, L.N., Stott, P., Simmonds, J., 2019. Recognizing and effectively managing hypermobility-related conditions. Phys. Ther. 99, 1189–1200.

Sackett, D.L., 2000. Evidence-Based Medicine: How to Practice and Teach EBM, second ed. Churchill Livingstone, Edinburgh.

Sapolsky, R., 2004. Why Zebras Don't Get Ulcers. St Martin's Press, New York.

Schmidt, H.G., Rikers, R.M., 2007. How expertise develops in medicine: knowledge encapsulation and illness script formation. Med. Educ. 41 (12), 1133–1139.

Smart, K.M., Blake, C., Staines, A., Thacker, M., Doody, C., 2012a. Mechanisms-based classifications of musculoskeletal pain: part 1 of 3: symptoms and signs of central sensitisation in patients with low back (± leg) pain. Man. Ther. 17 (4), 336–344. https://doi.org/10.1016/j.math.2012.03.013.

Smart, K.M., Blake, C., Staines, A., Thacker, M., Doody, C., 2012b. Mechanisms-based classifications of musculoskeletal pain: part 2 of 3: symptoms and signs of peripheral neuropathic pain in patients with low back (± leg) pain. Man. Ther. 17 (4), 345–351. https://doi.org/10.1016/j.math.2012.03.003.

Smart, K.M., Blake, C., Staines, A., Thacker, M., Doody, C., 2012c. Mechanisms-based classifications of musculoskeletal pain: part 3 of 3: symptoms and signs of nociceptive pain in patients with low back (± leg) pain. Man. Ther. 17 (4), 352–357. https://doi.org/10.1016/j.math.2012.03.002.

Standing, M., 2008. Clinical judgement and decision-making in nursing - nine modes of practice in a revised cognitive continuum. J. Adv. Nurs. 62 (1), 124–134.

Stanton, T.R., Fritz, J.M., Hancock, M.J., Latimer, J., Maher, C.G., Wand, B.M., et al., 2011. Evaluation of a treatment-based classification algorithm for low back pain: a cross-sectional study. Phys. Ther. 91 (4), 496–509.

Stanton, T.R., Hancock, M.J., Apeldoorn, A.T., Wand, B.M., Fritz, J.M., 2013. What characterizes people who have an unclear classification using a treatment-based classification algorithm for low back pain? A cross-sectional study. Phys. Ther. 93 (3), 345–355.

Stiell, I.G., Greenberg, G.H., McKnight, R.D., Nair, R.C., McDowell, I., Reardon, M., et al., 1993. Decision rules for the use of radiography in acute ankle injuries. Refinement and prospective validation. J. Am. Med. Assoc. 269, 1127–1132.

Stolper, E., van Royen, P., Dinant, G., 2010. The 'sense of alarm' ('gut feeling') in Clinical Practice. A Survey Among European General Practitioners on Recognition and Expression. Eur. J. Gen. Pract. 16 (2), 72–74. https://doi.org/10.3109/13814781003653424.

Stolper, E., van Royen, P., Dinant, G.J., 1996. The 'sense of alarm' ('gut feeling') in clinical practice. A survey among European general practitioners on recognition and expression. Acute renal infections. Radiol. Clin. North Am. 34 (5), 965–995.

Stuber, K.J., Wynd, S., Weis, C.A., 2012. Adverse events from spinal manipulation in the pregnant and postpartum periods: a critical review of the literature. Chiropr. Man. Therap. 20, 8.

Terry, W., Higgs, J., 1993. Educational programmes to develop clinical reasoning skills. Aust. J. Physiother. 39, 47–51.

Van Griensven, H., Schmid, A., Trendafilova, T., Low, M., 2020. Central sensitization in musculoskeletal pain: lost in translation? J. Orthop. Sports Phys. Ther. 50 (11), 592–596.

Vargas-Prada, S., Coggon, D., 2015. Psychological and psychosocial determinants of musculoskeletal pain and associated disability. Best Pract. Res. Clin. Rheumatol. 29 (3), 374–390.

Waddell, G., 2004. The Back Pain Revolution, second ed. Churchill Livingstone, Edinburgh.

Wainwright, S.F., Shepard, K.F., Harman, L.B., Stephens, J., 2011. Factors that influence the clinical decision making of novice and experienced physical therapists. Phys. Ther. 91, 87–101.

Wijbenga, M.H., Bovend'Eerdt, T.J.H., Driessen, E.W., 2019. Physiotherapy students' experiences with clinical reasoning during clinical placements: a qualitative study. Health Professions Educ. 5 (2), 126–135.

Woods, M.O., Asmundson, G.J.G., 2008. Evaluating the efficacy of graded in vivo exposure for the treatment of fear in patients with chronic back pain: a randomized controlled clinical trial. Pain 136, 271–280.

Woolf, C.J., 2004. Pain: moving from symptom control toward mechanism-specific pharmacologic management. Ann. Intern. Med. 140, 441–451.

World Health Organization, 2001. International Classification of Functioning, Disability and Health. World Health Organization, Geneva.

World Health Organization, 2011. World Report on Disability. World Health Organization, Geneva.

6

Examination of the Temporomandibular Region

Helen Cowgill

LEARNING OUTCOMES

After studying this chapter, you should be able to:

- Describe the key anatomical structures and biomechanics of the temporomandibular joint (TMJ) and understand the relationship between the TMJ and other anatomical structures.
- Understand the signs and symptoms of temporomandibular dysfunction (TMD) and the classification of TMD using the Diagnostic Criteria.
- Describe the common signs and symptoms of TMD and be able to discuss the relevance of other structures and conditions which may mimic TMD.
- Understand the role of parafunctional habits in relation to TMD and understand the relationship between dental issues and chewing in relation to TMD.
- Understand the multifactorial nature of TMD.
- List the key constituents of a thorough examination of the TMJ.
- Be able to inspect the intraoral environment in relation to TMD and understand the precautions when examining the face and intraoral environment.
- Explain how the physical examination findings contribute to the reasoning of common TMD presentations and appreciate the importance of the Multidisciplinary Team (MDT) in the examination of the TMD.

CHAPTER CONTENTS

Introduction, 174
Anatomy Review, 174
Temporomandibular Joint Dysfunction, 174
Subjective Examination/Taking the Patient's History, 176
Patient's Perspective on Their Experience, 176
Body Chart, 176
Behaviour of Symptoms, 177
Special/Screening Questions, 178
History of the Present Condition, 180
Past Medical History, 180
Plan of the Physical Examination, 180
Physical Examination, 181
Observation, 181
Active Physiological Movements, 182
Passive Physiological Movements, 185
Muscle Testing, 186
Neurological Testing, 186
Miscellaneous Tests, 188
Palpation, 188
Accessory Movements, 188
Other Tests for the Temporomandibular Joint, 189
Completion of the Examination, 189
Validity of Clinical Tests, 189
Multidisciplinary Team Approach to Temporomandibular Dysfunction, 189
Case Study, 192
References, 194

INTRODUCTION

The masticatory system is primarily responsible for chewing, speaking and swallowing. The temporomandibular joint (TMJ) plays an integral role within the masticatory system and is one of the most complex and used joints of the body (Okeson, 2020; Magee & Manske, 2021).

Anatomy Review

The TMJ is composed of the condylar head of the mandible and the glenoid or mandibular fossa of the temporal bone of the skull (Okeson, 2020). The right and left TMJ, along with their associated ligaments and muscles, create a bilateral articulation between the U-shaped mandible and the temporal bone of the cranium (Pertes & Gross, 1995). There is no bony attachment of the mandible to the cranium, and the articulation of these two bones is separated by the intraarticular disc and supported by a joint capsule and various ligaments. The disc divides the TMJ into upper and lower articular compartments, which gives the TMJ the capability to perform a variety of complex movements involving a combination of hinging and gliding movements (Pertes & Gross, 1995; Okeson, 2020) and is considered a ginglymoarthrodial joint (Okeson, 2020).

The TMJ is classified as a synovial joint with the presence of synovial lining and fluid which helps the joint withstand both frictional and compressive forces whilst keeping the joint lubricated (Okeson, 2020). The articular disc is attached to the mandible via the capsular ligaments, the posterior aspect of the disc is attached to the retrodiscal tissue and the lateral pterygoid muscle attaches to the anterior part of the articular disc. The retrodiscal tissue is a loose elastic connective tissue which is highly vascularized and innervated and attaches posteriorly to the tympanic plate (Okeson, 2020).

Movement of the mandible bone occurs as a series of rotational and translatory movements and is reliant on the combined simultaneous movement of both TMJs (Pertes & Gross, 1995). Therefore, the movement of one joint cannot occur in isolation or without influence from the other. The main muscles involved in the movement and function of the TMJ are the muscles of mastication which include the masseter, temporalis and medial and lateral pterygoid. Problems with the muscles of mastication and the mobility of the intraarticular disc can be major sources of pain, limitation of movement and dysfunction. It is important, during an examination, that both TMJs are evaluated to determine the dysfunctional side as pain is not always associated with the side of dysfunction (Cowgill, 2014). The TMJ is the only joint in the body where limitation of movement is restricted by the teeth (Magee & Manske, 2021) and it is, therefore, important to consider the dental occlusion or bite when assessing the TMJ.

Temporomandibular Joint Dysfunction

Like all other joints, the TMJ has the capacity to adapt to functional demand and depends on many factors, such as loading of the joint, systemic disease and age. Any damage to the TMJ structures may interfere with normal function and thus cause dysfunction. Temporomandibular joint dysfunction (TMD) is a collective term that encompasses pain arising from the muscles of mastication along with disorders of the TMJ, including capsulitis, degenerative joint disease and internal derangement (Schiffman et al., 1990, 2014; Dimitroulis, 1998). Limitation of function, persistent pain and disability are the three main consequences of TMD (Sharma & Ohrbach, 2019).

The aetiology of TMD is not clearly understood; however, it appears to be multifactorial and reflects an interaction between physical, functional and psychosocial factors and is more likely the result of multiple risk factors rather than a single isolated disorder (Slade et al., 2016). Risk factors for developing TMD include trauma, malocclusion, gender, bruxism, headache and migraine, clenching or grinding, catastrophizing and depression, genetic factors, smoking and obesity (Kumar et al., 2019). TMD may be caused by macrotrauma due to an acute single event, or chronic microtrauma involving frequent low-grade events to the TMJ over time. Parafunctional habits, including clenching and bruxism (nocturnal grinding), are examples of microtrauma (Okeson, 2020). Any force that overloads the joint complex may cause damage to joint structures or disturb the normal functional relationship between the condyle, disc and articular eminence of the temporal bone, resulting in pain, dysfunction or both.

To appreciate the causes of potential dysfunction and clinical presentation of arthrogenic TMD, it is important to understand the disc–condylar relationship. Displacement of the articular disc is characterized by an abnormal relationship between the articular disc, mandibular condyle and articular eminence of the temporal bone. The two main types of disc displacement are with or without reduction (Pertes & Gross, 1995; Okeson, 2020).

- Disc displacement with reduction occurs when the disc is displaced in an anterior or anteromedial position when the mouth is closed and returns to a more normal position relative to the condyle on mouth opening.
- Disc displacement without reduction is characterized by displacement of the disc permanently and the condyle does not recapture or recentre under the disc during mandibular movement.

Signs and Symptoms of Temporomandibular Joint Dysfunction

Dysfunction of the TMJ can present in a variety of ways and the main signs and symptoms include facial pain, joint sounds, jaw activity aggravating factors, mandibular deviation during movement and restricted movement (Pertes & Gross, 1995; Okeson, 2020; Magee & Manske, 2021). TMD is often associated with aural fullness, otalgia, tinnitus, disequilibrium and perceived hearing loss (Porto De Toledo, 2016), and therefore it is important for the patient to have a full hearing test to exclude any non-TMD pathology.

TMD is often associated with headaches, and headaches are closely associated with TMD; The International Classification of Headache Disorder ICHD-3 (2018) classify TMD as a secondary headache (headache attributed to TMD ICHD-3, 11.7) and a specific subclassification of temporal headache is included in the Diagnostic Criteria (DC) (Schiffman et al., 2014). TMD and headaches are described further later in this chapter.

Classification of Temporomandibular Joint Dysfunction

There are lots of various classifications for TMD (International Classification of Orofacial Pain, 2020; Schiffman et al., 2014; Michelotti & Svensson, 2019). A reliable and valid system that broadly classifies TMD is the DC published by Schiffman et al. (2014). The DC was initially used for research and is a comprehensive package to help with diagnosis and screening for patients with TMD. The most common disorders within the DC are outlined in Table 6.1.

TABLE 6.1 Most Common Pain and Intraarticular Temporomandibular Dysfunction (TMD)

Most Common Pain-Related TMD	Most Common Intraarticular TMD
Myalgia • Local myalgia • Myofascial pain • Myofascial pain with referral • Arthralgia • Headache attributed to TMD	• Disc displacement with reduction • Disc displacement with reduction with intermittent locking • Disc displacement without reduction with limited opening • Disc displacement without reduction without limited opening • Degenerative joint disease • Subluxation

Schiffman et al. (2014).

The DC highlights the importance of an accurate diagnosis when treating TMD due to its complex and multifactorial nature. This is because, frequently, a patient does not fit into one classification and can present with more than one disorder. This may make the treatment and management of TMD complicated, as frequently patients with TMD are treated simultaneously and referred to more than one speciality (Ahmed et al., 2014). It is important to identify the primary and secondary diagnoses and any contributing factors which may be driving the patient's pain or disorder.

Relationship Between the Cervical Spine, Thoracic and Temporomandibular Joint Dysfunction

There is a functional relationship between TMJ, cervical and thoracic spine due to their close anatomical proximities and associated biomechanical correlation, for example; during mouth opening approximately 50% of the movement will come from lifting the mouth via the maxilla involving cervical extension (Eriksson et al., 1998). There is a neurophysiological relationship between the head, TMJ and cervical spine via the trigeminal nerve and nucleus. Symptoms in the frontal, retroorbital, temporal and occipital areas of the head can be mediated by both the upper cervical spine and the TMJ due to neural convergence in the trigeminocervical nucleus in the brainstem (Bogduk & Bartsch, 2008; Bogduk & Govind, 2009; Cairns, 2019). Therefore, it is important to accompany examination of the TMJ with an examination of the cervical and thoracic spine.

Other Nontemporomandibular Joint Causes

It is vital always to have a differential diagnosis as part of a comprehensive clinical reasoning process. Diseases which may be of vascular origin, e.g. arteritis, or neural origin, e.g. trigeminal neuralgia, as well as craniocervical disorders and ear, nose and throat pathology may mimic TMD and can coexist with TMD; therefore full examination and reproduction of a patient's symptoms are paramount. Where a diagnosis is unclear and non-musculoskeletal, an onward referral to an appropriate specialist is indicated.

Further details of the questions asked during the subjective examination and the tests carried out during the physical examination can be found in Chapters 3 and 4, respectively. This chapter focuses on the TMJ; therefore the subjective and objective assessment will be tailored towards this.

The order of the subjective questioning and the physical tests described below can be altered as appropriate for the patient being examined.

KNOWLEDGE CHECK

1. Which three main attachments does the intraarticular disc have?
2. Name the four main muscles of mastication.
3. What are the three main consequences of temporomandibular dysfunction?
4. Name three risk factors of temporomandibular dysfunction.

SUBJECTIVE EXAMINATION/TAKING THE PATIENT'S HISTORY

Patient's Perspective on Their Experience

For general questions to explore patient's perspectives on their condition, the reader is directed to Chapter 3. Factors from this information may indicate direct and/or indirect mechanical influences on the TMJ.

The patient's occupation should be determined, and its relevance to the patient's presentation, including psychosocial aspects, needs to be considered. It is well established that patient's individual cognitive, behavioural and emotional responses in relation to their pain are independent of the actual source of their pain (Schiffman et al., 2014). TMD does have significant psychosocial associations and contributing factors, and the clinician may ask the types of questions to elucidate psychosocial factors that are outlined in Chapter 3. It is useful to use appropriate outcome measures to review any potential psychological factors which are prevalent in patients with TMD (Kraus, 2014; Ohrbach & Knibbe, 2016), and readers are referred to the DC axis II for further information (Schiffman et al., 2014). The information gained from this screening can be used appropriately within the session, and onward referral can be made where indicated.

Occupations that are commonly associated with TMD are singers or actors, telephonists and musicians. Students of all ages need to be considered due to the stress associated with examinations and assessments.

Body Chart

It is recommended that a separate facial chart is used to be precise when recording head and facial symptoms (Fig. 6.1).

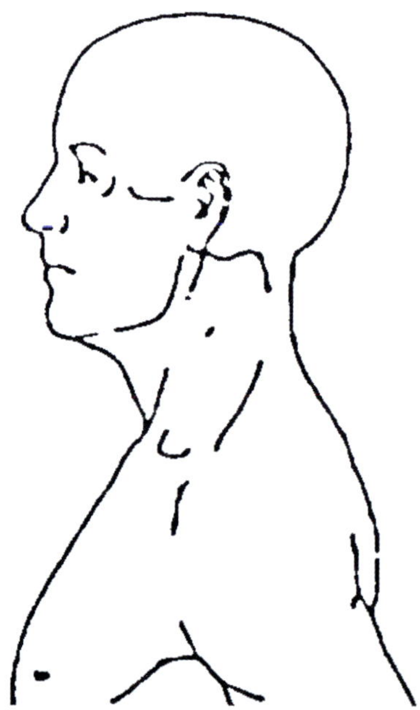

Fig. 6.1 Facial chart for recording head and facial symptoms.

Area of Current Symptoms

Be exact when recording the area of the symptoms. Symptoms associated with TMD are discussed earlier in this chapter and include pain located in the ears, eyes and teeth and radiate into the mandibular and temporal regions (Feinstein et al., 1954; Rocabado, 1983), neck pain and headaches (Kraus, 2014). The clinician always needs to check for red flags and precautions to an assessment of the affected area (see Table 3.3 and Table 7.3).

Ask whether the patient has ever experienced disequilibrium, dizziness or other symptoms associated with cervical arterial dysfunction (CAD) or vertebrobasilar insufficiency (Kerry, 2013). Please refer to Chapter 7 in this book and to Chapter 8 in the companion textbook (Barnard & Ryder, 2024) for further reading on this subject. The reader is also directed to the Taylor and Kerry (2010) masterclass. Suspicious presentations need to be referred for medical investigation (Bogduk, 1994; Kerry & Taylor, 2006).

Areas Relevant to the Region Being Examined

All other relevant areas need to be checked for symptoms including the cervical and thoracic spine as discussed earlier. It is important to ask about pain or even stiffness, as this may be relevant to the patient's main symptom. Mark unaffected areas with ticks (✓) on the body chart.

Quality of Pain

Establish the quality of the pain. Orofacial pain may arise from musculoskeletal, neurologic or neurovascular changes, each of these having distinctive characteristics of pain. This is important information when attempting to determine the primary source of pain during differentiation between different structures.

Intensity of Pain

The intensity of pain can be measured using, for example, a visual analogue scale, as shown in Fig. 3.4. A pain diary (see Chapter 3) may be useful for patients to determine pain patterns and triggering factors over a period of time.

Abnormal Sensation

Check for any altered sensation locally over the temporomandibular region and face and, if appropriate, over the cervical spine, upper thoracic spine or upper limbs (see Chapter 4).

Constant or Intermittent Symptoms

Ascertain the frequency of the symptoms, and whether they are constant or intermittent. If symptoms are constant, check whether there is variation in the intensity of the symptoms, as constant unremitting pain is indicative of neoplastic disease (Greenhalgh & Selfe, 2010).

Relationship of Symptoms

Determine the relationship between the symptomatic areas—do they come together or separately? For example, the patient may have pain over the jaw without neck pain, or the pains may always be present together. This can assist with clinical reasoning and can assist with planning the physical examination.

Behaviour of Symptoms

Aggravating Factors

Common aggravating factors for the temporomandibular region are mouth opening, prolonged talking, yawning, singing, shouting and chewing challenging food groups. For aggravating factors for other regions, which may be relevant, the reader is directed to the appropriate chapter in this book.

Consider the function of chewing and whether the patient is able to chew through pain, able to get food into their mouth, how long has their diet been altered and whether they are chewing bilaterally. This information is important when considering joint loading, muscle activation and function.

For further information regarding severity, irritability and nature with regard to assessment planning, the reader is directed to Chapter 3.

The clinician ascertains how the symptoms affect function and how function affects symptoms; for example, a forward head posture will change the resting position of the mandible and possibly alter muscle activity and tone (Olivo et al., 2006) which may be relevant in office workers.

For detailed information on how to note aggravating and easing factors please refer to Chapter 3.

Easing Factors

The clinician asks the patient about theoretically known easing factors for structures that could be a source of the symptoms. For example, symptoms from the TMJ may be eased by placing the joint in a particular position, whereas symptoms from the upper cervical spine may be eased by supporting the head or neck. The clinician can then analyse the position or movement that eases the symptoms, to help determine the structure at fault.

Parafunctional Habits

Activities of the muscles of mastication can be broadly divided into two main types: functional activities such as chewing and talking and parafunctional activities such as grinding or clenching the teeth, which are nonfunctional activities (Okeson, 2020). Parafunctional habits can occur in the daytime and also during sleep and can be either in single activities (clenching) or rhythmic contractions (bruxing). They can occur in isolation or together and can be hard to separate, and therefore termed as bruxing events. Clinical signs which indicate bruxism and/or excessive functional or parafunctional activity are tongue scalloping, frictional keratosis or linea alba of the buccal mucosa and tooth wear on the posterior molars or canines observed on intraoral examination (Okeson, 2020). Examples of common parafunctional habits are detailed in Table 6.2.

Twenty-Four-Hour Behaviour

The reader is referred to Chapter 3 regarding questions to ask to determine the 24-hour behaviour of symptoms. The following additional questions may be useful in patients with TMD.

Night symptoms.

- Do you grind or clench your teeth at night? Usually, the patient will be unaware of bruxism, and their partner may be able to provide this information.
- Do you suffer from sleep apnoea?

TABLE 6.2 Common Functional and Parafunctional Habits

Functional Habits	Parafunctional Habits
Mastication or chewing food	Grinding
Swallowing	Clenching
Speech	Chewing gum excessively
	Tongue thrusting
	Sucking cheeks
	Biting nails
	Biting the lip or cheek
	Excessive positional clicking of the joint (party tricks)

- Do you currently wear or have you ever worn a splint at night? If so, then the following questions need to be considered:
  - What effect did it have on your symptoms?
  - Current state of the splint (where possible, view the splint for signs of wear).
  - When was the last time it was replaced? This can indicate the strength of the patient's bruxism.
- In patients undergoing orthodontic treatment: Do you use elastic bands overnight or a plastic retainer?

Morning and evening symptoms. Patients who grind their teeth at night may wake up with a headache and/or facial, jaw or tooth symptoms (Kraus, 1994). However, if patients have strong parafunctional habits, they may have pain during the day which can worsen as the day progresses. If stress or the work/study environment is thought to be a contributing factor, it is worthwhile exploring the pattern of symptoms on a working/study versus nonworking/nonstudy day.

Special/Screening Questions

Special questions must always be asked, as they may identify certain precautions or contraindications to the physical examination and/or treatment (see Table 3.3). Readers are referred to Greenhalgh and Selfe (2010) and Chapter 3 for further information. The following additional special questions need to be considered for TMJ patients.

Clicking

Clicking is usually associated with abnormal disc–condylar mechanics (Okeson, 2020; Magee & Manske, 2021), and establishing the nature of a click can assist in diagnosis and prognosis. A click may be heard on auscultation with a disc displacement with reduction, and a disc displacement without reduction may or may not be associated with a click (Pertes & Gross, 1995; Magee & Manske, 2021).

It is important to remember that anatomical evidence of disc displacement is not always associated with patient symptoms. More often than not, disc displacement is accompanied by a clicking sound and restriction in mandibular movement; however, a painless click is not always indicative of a joint dysfunction (Okeson, 2020; Schiffman et al., 2014; Magee & Manske, 2021).

Bruxism

The extent and nature of teeth grinding need to be established, and its relationship to the present condition considered. The mechanical forces produced during grinding can contribute to TMD. Bruxism is often a manifestation of stress and as such it is important to consider associated psychological factors which may be causing, contributing to and/or mediating the present condition.

Clenching

Clenching can occur at night and also during the day. The normal resting position for the mandible is with the posterior teeth slightly apart and the tip of the tongue in the roof of the mouth. Clenching causes overactivity in the muscles of mastication responsible for this action and can lead to myogenic pain.

Dental Disorders

The association between upper and lower tooth contact (occlusion) and forces through the TMJ should be considered. A thorough history of all dental disorders, including surgery, tooth extraction, orthodontic history, tooth fractures (may indicate bruxism) and prolonged opening during dental examination/treatment, should be noted. Note should be taken if the patient has any loose dentition or wears dentures as this will be relevant when planning the objective examination. Asymmetrical occlusion or the absence of teeth can have an effect on TMJ loading and the muscles of mastication (Magee & Manske, 2021), which may lead to pathomechanical changes within and around the TMJ.

Trismus

Trismus, or a limitation of mouth opening, is common with TMD. It should be noted that it can also be a primary presenting sign of malignancy (Beddis et al., 2014). Beddis et al. (2014) suggest that a 30 mm mouth opening is the upper limit for trismus.

Cranial Nerve Disorders

Signs and symptoms associated with TMJ dysfunction can be similar to those arising from frank cranial nerve disorders. It is therefore essential to establish whether or not there are cranial nerve disorders present which would require further medical investigation (Okeson, 2020). Alternatively, known cranial nerve disorders may result in, or contribute to, TMJ dysfunction, and vice versa. The relevance of any disorder needs to be established, for example:

- pain and/or altered sensation in the forehead and face needs to be differentiated from trigeminal (cranial nerve [CN] V) neuralgia
- for difficulties in opening and closing, consideration should be given to the trigeminal nerve innervation of masticating muscles
- facial asymmetries need to be differentiated from facial nerve (CN VII) palsies
- aural symptoms should be differentiated from vestibulocochlear nerve (CN VIII) palsies, which may be related to serious neoplastic pathology
- swallowing problems should be differentiated from glossopharyngeal (CN IX) and vagus (CN X) nerve palsies
- tongue asymmetries should be differentiated from hypoglossal nerve (CN XII) disorder (Kerry, 2013). Table 7.6 details cranial nerve assessment.

Cervical Arterial Dysfunction

The clinician identifies symptoms suggestive of vasculopathy related to either the vertebral arteries (e.g. vertebrobasilar insufficiency) or the internal carotid arteries. Pathology of these vessels can mimic craniofacial signs and symptoms associated with TMJ dysfunction (see Chapter 7). Symptoms include disequilibrium, dizziness, altered vision (including diplopia), nausea, ataxia, drop attacks, altered facial sensation, difficulty speaking, difficulty swallowing, sympathoplegia, hemianaesthesia and hemiplegia (Bogduk, 1994; Kerry & Taylor, 2006). Ptosis (drooping eyelid) is associated with internal carotid artery pathology and may be mistaken for facial asymmetry. Specifically, jaw claudication related to carotid pathologies can mimic mechanical TMJ dysfunction. If present, the clinician determines in the usual way the aggravating and easing factors. Similar symptoms can also be related to upper cervical instability and diseases of the inner ear. It is important to remember that, in their pre-ischaemic stage, cervical vasculopathies can present with just upper cervical and head pain (Kerry & Taylor, 2006; Bogduk & Govind, 2009), as shown in Fig. 7.8. Awareness of predisposing factors to vascular injury and information regarding the patient's blood pressure can assist in the diagnosis (Kerry & Taylor, 2006, 2008, 2009). See Table 7.5 for screening associated with CAD and Chapter 7 for guidance on testing for CAD. The reader is also directed to Chapter 8 in the companion text (Barnard & Ryder, 2024). For presentations of temporofrontal headache, the clinician needs also to consider temporal arteritis as a differential diagnosis.

Ear Symptoms

Aural symptoms, otalgia and tinnitus are common complaints alongside TMJ symptoms and any concerns that the TMJ is not the source of ear symptoms should prompt an onward referral to the appropriate specialist. See earlier chapter for further information.

Headaches

Headaches are highly prevalent in patients with TMD (Franco et al., 2010), can worsen TMD symptoms (Costa et al., 2017) and can increase the likelihood of TMD (Tchivileva et al., 2017). TMD-related headaches are usually located in the temple region and are aggravated by jaw movement, function and/or parafunction, and provocation of the masticatory system can reproduce the headache (Schiffman et al., 2014). The International Headache society has further classified TMD and TMD with headaches in the International Classification of Orofacial Pain (2020) Code 3.

History of the Present Condition

A detailed section on general questions to be asked for a history of the present condition can be found in Chapter 3. For each symptomatic area, the clinician needs to discover how long the symptom has been present, whether there was a sudden or slow onset and whether there was a known cause that provoked the onset of the symptom, such as trauma, stress, surgery or occupation. If the onset was slow, the clinician needs to find out if there has been any change in the patient's lifestyle, e.g. a new diet, recent dental treatment or other factors. The onset of symptoms may be insidious, due to a specific event or trauma, including whiplash, direct trauma to the jaw, prolonged dental treatment or surgery (Kraus, 2014). It is important to find out about previous consultations with other healthcare professionals as it has been reported that patients with TMD on average will have consulted with 3.2 healthcare professionals prior to their initial physiotherapy consultation (Kraus, 2014).

Past Medical History

The following additional PMH information is obtained from the patient and/or dental/medical notes:

- The details of any relevant dental/medical history, particularly involving the teeth, jaw, cranium or cervical spine.
- The history of any previous episodes: how many episodes? When were they? What was the cause? What is the frequency? What was the duration of each episode? Did the patient fully recover between episodes?
- Ascertain the results of any past treatment for the same or a similar problem.
- Is the patient taking any medication or trialled medication for the problem, and what is its effect on symptoms?
- Has the patient had any recent aesthetic cosmetic work completed which may be relevant, such as facial fillers? Fillers can move during the physical assessment, so the clinician needs to clarify where the facial filler has been injected and avoid this area.

> **KNOWLEDGE CHECK**
> 1. What may clicking of the temporomandibular joint indicate?
> 2. Describe three parafunctional habits.
> 3. What is bruxism and what would you expect on a 24-h pattern?

Plan of the Physical Examination

When all this information has been collected, the subjective examination is complete. The reader is referred to Chapter 3 for general considerations of planning the physical examination.

Points to consider when planning the physical examination specific to the temporomandibular region:

- TMJ examination should always be accompanied by an examination of the cervical and thoracic spine.
- Are there any precautions and/or contraindications to elements of the physical examination that need to be explored further, such as vertebrobasilar insufficiency, neurological involvement, recent fracture, trauma, steroid therapy or rheumatoid arthritis? There may also be contraindications to further examination and treatment, e.g. symptoms of cord compression. Consider

precautions such as loose dentition, dentures or fear of the dentist as the examination will include intraoral assessment. Consider medical history, including epilepsy, as it would not be recommended to assess accessory movements due to hand positioning which may be dangerous during an epileptic fit where the teeth may be heavily clenched.
- Be aware of any recent aesthetic cosmetic work such as facial fillers to avoid movement during the physical examination.

PHYSICAL EXAMINATION

The order and detail of the physical tests described below should be appropriate to the patient being examined. Ohrbach et al. (2013) provide a very detailed procedure of examination as part of the DC (Schiffman et al., 2014). Novice clinicians may initially want to copy what is shown, but then quickly adapt to what is best for them (Kerry, 2013). The clinician should always gain consent from the patient and explain the physical examination, including intraoral examination.

Observation

Informal Observation

Informal observation will have begun from the moment the clinician begins the subjective examination; for example, observing articulation during speech or parafunctional habits present, and observation will continue until the end of the physical examination. Chapter 4 provides further information regarding informal observation.

Formal Observation

The clinician needs to observe the patient in dynamic and static situations; the quality of cervical and jaw movement is noted, as are the postural characteristics and facial expressions.

Observation of Posture

The clinician observes the general posture and cervical posture. The myofascial relationships between the neck and the jaw mean that postural dysfunction in one may influence the other. For craniofacial observation, the clinician observes facial symmetry using the anatomical landmarks shown in Fig. 6.2.

Check whether the optic, bipupital, otic and occlusive lines of the face are parallel (Fig. 6.2). Additionally, the length (posterior-anterior) of the mandible can be measured from the TMJ line to the anterior notch of the chin, and any side-to-side differences noted. The clinician notes any paralysis such as drooping of the mouth, which may indicate Bell's palsy.

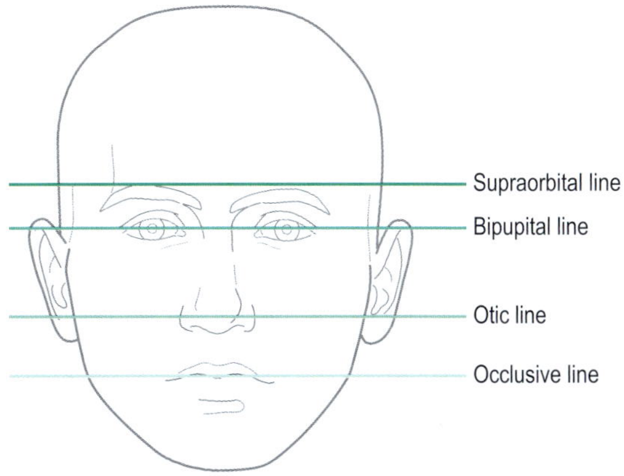

Fig. 6.2 Symmetry of the face can be tested by comparing the supraorbital, bipupital, otic and occlusive lines, which should be parallel. (From Magee 2014, with permission.)

The clinician checks the bony and soft-tissue contours of the face and TMJ. The clinician observes the resting position of the mandible, also known as the upper postural position of the mandible. In the resting position of the mandible, the back teeth are slightly apart, the mandible is in a relaxed position and the tip of the tongue lies against the palate just posterior to the inner surface of the upper central incisors. The clinician checks the intercuspal position, in which the back teeth are closed together, and observes the patient's teeth for malocclusion, such as:

- underbite (mandibular teeth anterior to maxillary teeth) or class III occlusion (Okeson, 2020)
- overbite (maxillary teeth anterior to mandibular teeth—2 mm of overbite is normal) or class II (Okeson, 2020). If an overbite is apparent, the degree of overjet (how far the maxillary incisors close down over the mandibular incisors) is measured with a ruler and noted (Ohrbach et al., 2013; Okeson, 2020)
- crossbite (deviation of the mandible to one side—use the interincisor gap between the two central incisors as reference points on both mandibular and maxillary sets).

Malocclusion and occlusal interference are noted and usually seen when teeth are missing, poorly formed, or when a dental brace, dentures or implants are being worn.

Observation of Muscle Form

The main muscles of mastication are the masseter, temporalis, medial pterygoid and lateral pterygoid and of these muscles, only the masseter and temporalis are visible and may be enlarged or atrophied. If there is a postural abnormality that is thought to be due to a muscle imbalance, then the muscles around the cervical spine and shoulder girdle may need to be inspected.

Observation of the Intraoral Environment

The clinician looks at the health of the patient's gums and also inspects the intraoral environment for any signs of clenching or bruxism. The three common clinical signs which indicate bruxism or bruxing events are:

1. linea alba or frictional keratosis of the buccal mucosa (ridging of the inner cheek) (Fig. 6.3)
2. deterioration of the wear facets on the posterior molars (Fig. 6.3)
3. tongue scalloping (indentations of the teeth on the tongue) (Fig. 6.4).

A torch and tongue depressor are helpful when observing the intraoral environment but are not essential. Clinical signs seen on intraoral examination may indicate excessive functional or parafunctional activity (Okeson, 2020). If patients have a diurnal variation in their symptoms, it is important to establish if their parafunctional habits are nocturnal or are continuing during the day by asking them to observe the clinical signs on waking, at midday and in the evening.

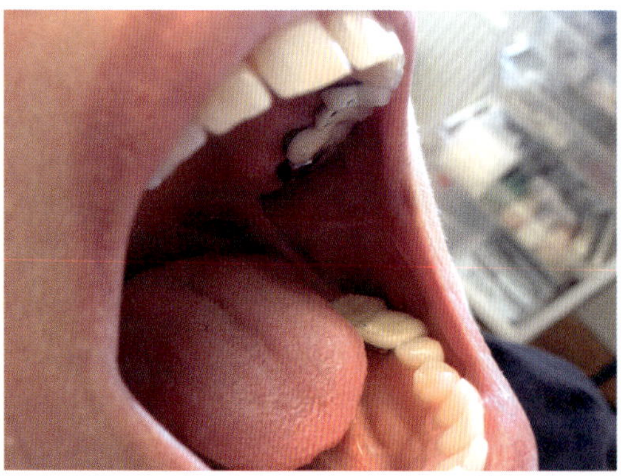

Fig. 6.3 Linea alba (frictional keratosis of the buccal mucosa) of the inner cheek and deterioration or flattening of the wear facets on the posterior molars can be noted on intraoral examination. These are indicative of bruxing events.

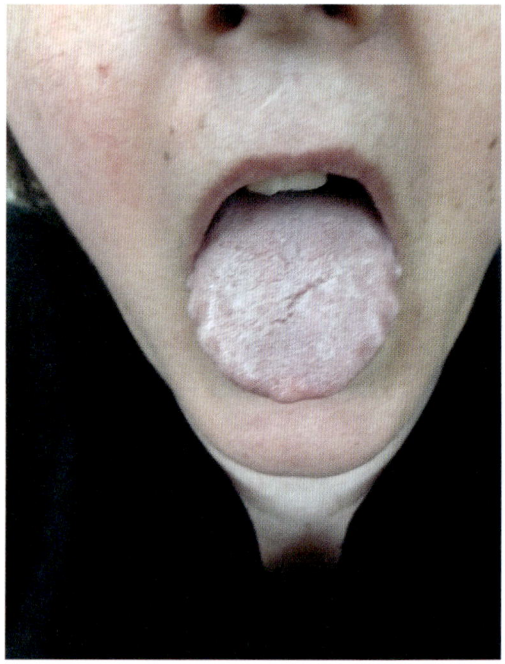

Fig. 6.4 Tongue scalloping can be noted on intraoral examination which is indicative of bruxing events or tongue thrusting.

Observation of Soft Tissues

The clinician observes the colour of the patient's skin and any swelling over the TMJ, face or gums, and takes cues for further examination. The clinician observes the lymph glands and nodes and when palpated, if an abnormality is felt or suspected, refers on appropriately.

Active Physiological Movements

For active passive physiological movements, the clinician should take note of the common procedures and considerations noted in Chapter 4. In addition, the clinician needs to consider the following in relation to TMD:

- Evaluate the quality of movement: minor subluxation, crepitus or a click on opening and/or closing the mouth.
- Assess the range of movement: excessive range, particularly opening, may indicate hypermobility of the TMJ.
- Observe any overactivity of the anterior cervical muscles, particularly with mouth opening.
- Observe for any alteration in the opening pathway:
  - Deviation is where the mandible deviates during mouth opening but returns to normal midline relationship at maximum mouth opening (Okeson, 2020).

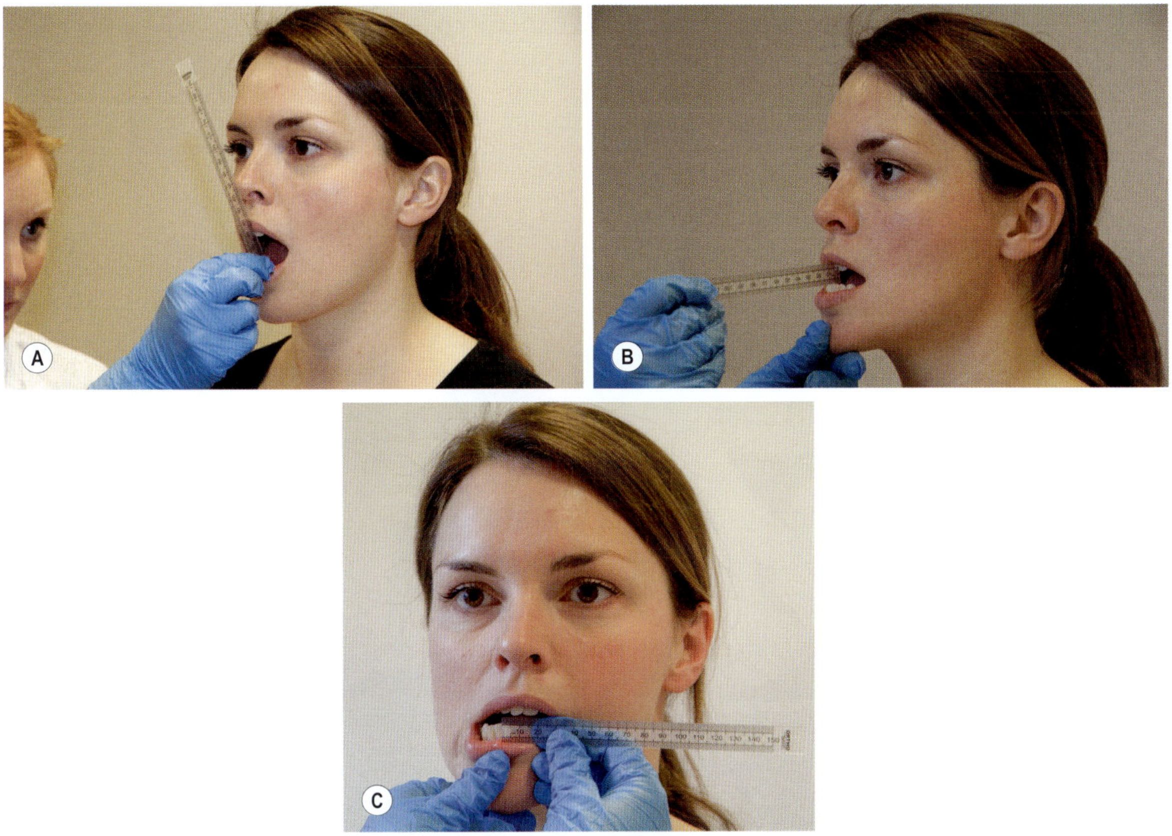

Fig. 6.5 Measuring mouth movement and temporomandibular joint active range of motion with a ruler. (A) Maximal comfortable and maximal mouth or incisal opening. The patient is asked to open the mouth just before pain is felt which is termed maximal comfortable opening. This measurement is the distance between the incisal edges of the anterior teeth. This is repeated with the patient opening as wide as she can even in the presence of pain, which is termed maximal mouth opening. (B) Protrusion. (C) Lateral deviation.

- Deflection is where the mandible is shifted to one side on opening and does not return to the normal midline relationship (Okeson, 2020).

TMJ movements can be measured with a ruler; the distance between the incisal edges of the anterior teeth is measured as shown in Fig. 6.5. Pain-free mouth opening as measured by the interincisal distance has proven reliability and validity (de Wijer et al., 1995; Beltran-Alacreu et al., 2014) and acceptable interrater reliability when measured in millimetres (Dworkin et al., 1990; Walker et al., 2000).

TMJ movements can be recorded as shown in Fig. 6.6 or in an active range of motion chart. The active movements of opening/closing, protraction/retraction and lateral deviation with overpressure listed in Table 6.4 are shown in Fig. 6.7 and can be tested with the patient sitting (Kerry, 2013) or lying

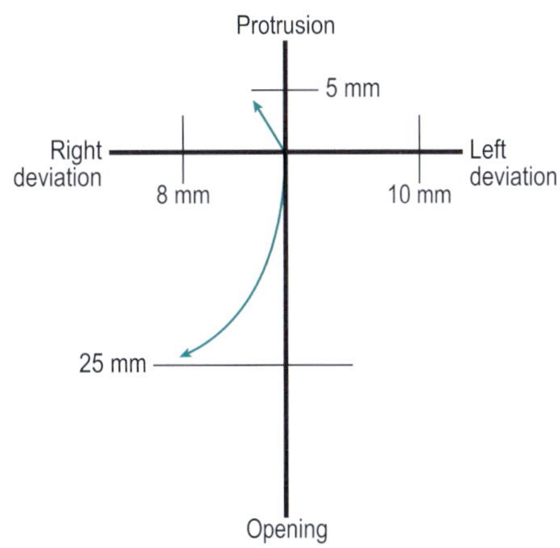

Fig. 6.6 Example of recording movement findings for the temporomandibular joint. Normally opening is around 35–45 mm. The joint mechanics normally function in a 4:1 ratio, i.e. 4 mm of opening to every 1 mm of lateral deviation/protrusion. (From Rocabado, 2004.)

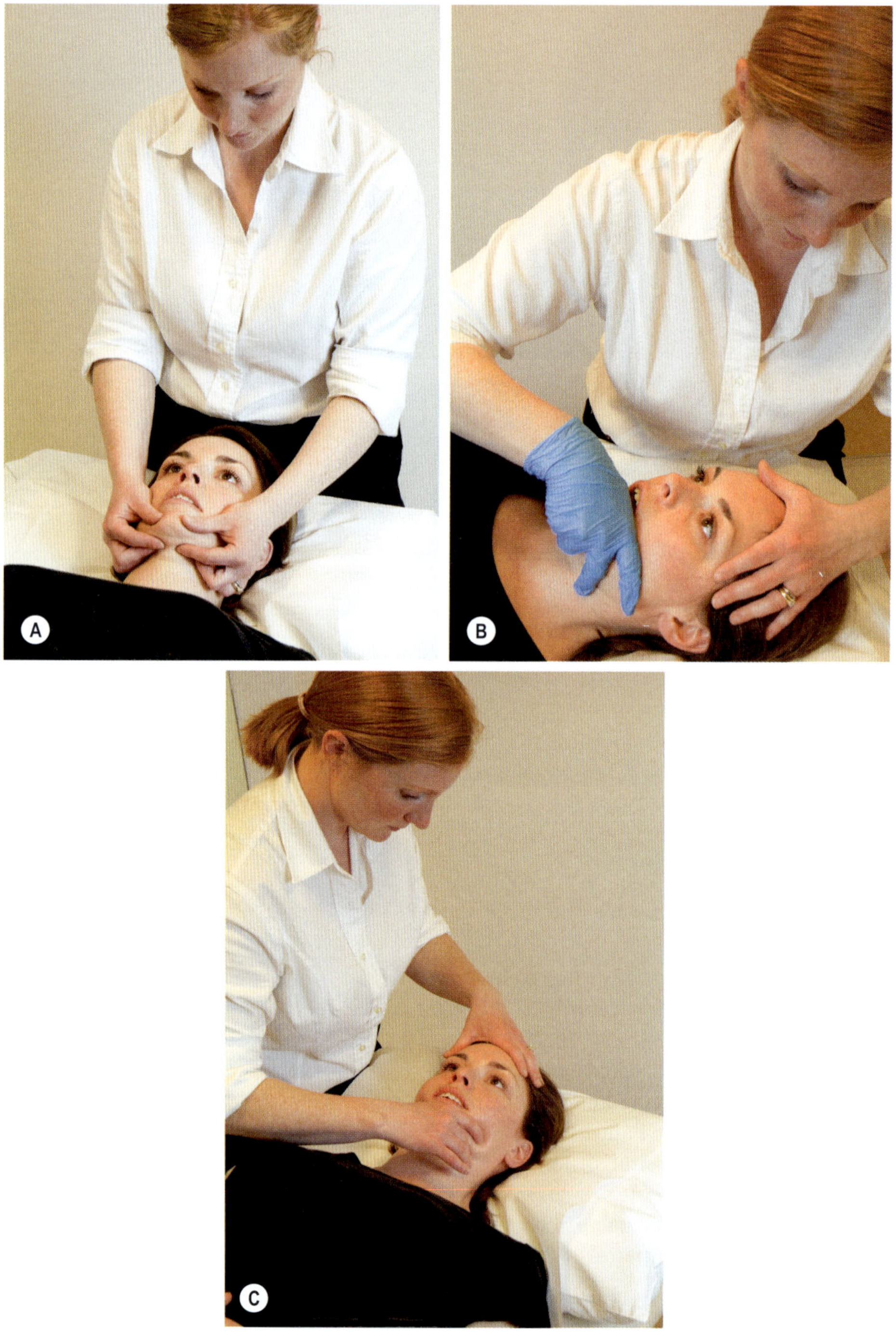

Fig. 6.7 Overpressures to the temporomandibular joint. (A) Depression (opening) and elevation (closing). The fingers and thumbs of both hands gently grasp the mandible to depress and elevate the mandible. (B) Protraction and retraction. A gloved thumb is placed just inside the mouth on the posterior aspect of the bottom front teeth. Thumb pressure can then protract and retract the mandible. (C) Lateral deviation. The left hand stabilizes the head while the right hand cups around the mandible and moves the mandible to the left and right.

supine. The clinician establishes the patient's symptoms at rest and prior to each movement and corrects any movement deviation to determine its relevance to the patient's symptoms. A normal opening has been cited as between 53 and 58 mm (Okeson, 2020), some suggest the lower limit for maximal opening is 35 and 40 mm for women and men respectively (Beddis et al., 2014); therefore above 35 mm could be considered normal taking into consideration the patient's age, gender and general size.

Palpation of the movement of the condyles during active movements can be useful to feel the quality of the movement (Ohrbach et al., 2013) and also to appreciate the biomechanics of the joint, with the first 20–25 mm mouth opening being a rotational movement, followed by a translatory movement. Excessive anterior movement of the lateral pole of the mandibular condyle may indicate TMJ hypermobility. Auscultation of the joint during jaw movements enables the clinician to listen to any joint sounds, including clicking or crepitus, as shown in Fig. 6.8.

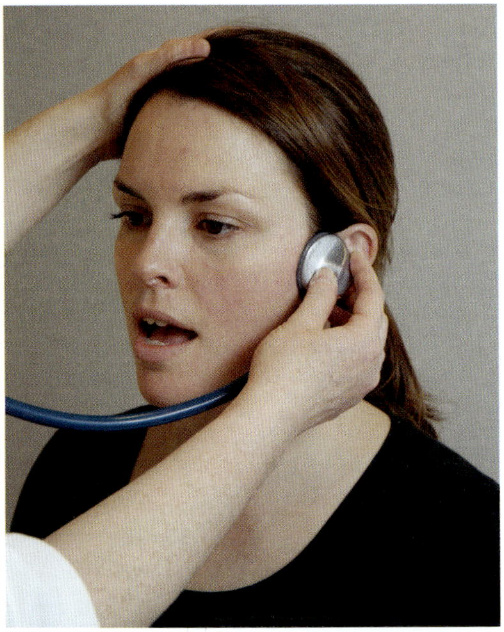

Fig. 6.8 Auscultation of temporomandibular joint (TMJ) noises. The clinician places the stethoscope over the TMJ and listens during TMJ active range of motion, mouth opening/closing, protrusion and lateral deviation, listening for clicking or crepitus.

TABLE 6.3 Summary of Active Movements and Their Possible Modification

Active Movements	Modifications to Active Movements
Temporomandibular joint	Repeated
Depression (opening)	Speed altered
Elevation (closing)	Combined, e.g.
Protraction	• Opening then lateral deviation
Retraction	• Lateral deviation then opening
Depression in retracted position	• Protraction then opening
Left lateral deviation	• Retraction then opening
Right lateral deviation	Sustained
?Upper cervical spine movements	Differentiation tests
Injuring movement	Functional ability
?Cervical spine movement	
?Thoracic spine movements	

Movements of the TMJ and the possible modifications are given in Table 6.3. Various differentiation tests (Rocabado, 2004; Hengeveld & Banks, 2014; Magee & Manske, 2021) can be performed; the choice depends on the patient's signs and symptoms.

Some functional ability has already been tested by the general observation of jaw movement as the patient has talked during the subjective examination. Any further testing can be carried out at this point in the examination. Clues for appropriate tests can be obtained from the subjective examination findings, particularly the aggravating factors.

KNOWLEDGE CHECK

1. What are the three clinical signs of bruxism?
2. How do you determine if the temporomandibular joint is clicking?
3. Which test could you use to help determine whether the pain is articular or myogenic in nature?

Passive Physiological Movements

The clinician can move the TMJ passively with the patient in the supine position. A comparison of the response of symptoms to the active and passive movements can help to determine the structure at fault.

Passive physiological movements can also determine the side of dysfunction, which may not always be the symptomatic side. Other regions may need to be examined to determine their relevance to the patient's symptoms.

Muscle Testing

Muscle tests include examining muscle strength, control, endurance and isometric contraction.

Muscle Strength

The clinician may test muscle groups that depress, elevate, protract, retract and laterally deviate the mandible, as shown in Fig. 6.9, and, if applicable, the cervical musculature. Kraus (1994), however, considers mandibular muscle weakness to be rare in TMJ disorders and difficult to determine manually. It is important to consider the lateral pterygoid muscle, which has attachments to the anterior disc and mandibular condyle, which may cause pain or spasm in patients with disc dysfunction.

Muscle Control

Excessive masticatory muscle activity is thought to be a factor in TMJ conditions. The muscles of the cervical spine, and in particular the deep neck flexors, should be tested due to their synergistic relationship with the muscles of mastication.

Isometric Muscle Testing

Test the muscle groups that depress, elevate, protract, retract and laterally deviate the mandible in the resting position, as shown in Fig. 6.9, and, if indicated, in various parts of the physiological ranges. Also, if applicable, test the cervical musculature. In addition, the clinician observes the quality of the muscle contraction necessary to hold this position (this can be done with the patient's eyes shut). The patient may, for example, be unable to prevent the joint from moving or may hold with excessive muscle activity; either of these circumstances would suggest a neuromuscular dysfunction (Kerry, 2013).

Endurance Testing

Here the clinician can test the muscle with repeated movement with or without resistance and observe the quality of movement and the distance. This is particularly important in patients who are constantly using their TMJ, such as singers and actors.

Neurological Testing

Neurological examination includes neurological integrity testing, neurodynamic tests and some other nerve tests.

Integrity of Nervous System

Generally, if symptoms are localized to the upper cervical spine and head, the neurological examination can be limited to cranial nerves and C1–C4 nerve roots (see Table 7.6).

Dermatomes/Peripheral Nerves

Light touch and pain sensation of the face, head and neck are tested using cotton wool and pinprick respectively, as described in Chapter 4. Knowledge of the cutaneous distribution of nerve roots (dermatomes) and peripheral nerves enables the clinician to distinguish the sensory loss due to a root lesion from that due to a peripheral nerve lesion.

Myotomes/Peripheral Nerves

The following myotomes are tested and are shown in Chapter 4 and Table 4.8:

- trigeminal (CN V)
- facial (CN VII)
- accessory (CN XI)
- C1–C2
- C2
- C3
- C4 and CN XI.

Reflex Testing

The jaw jerk (CN V) is elicited by applying a sharp downward tap on the chin with a reflex hammer with the mouth slightly open. A slight jerk is normal; an excessive jerk suggests a bilateral upper motor neuron lesion.

Neurodynamic Tests

The following neurodynamic tests may be carried out if indicated, in order to ascertain the degree to which neural tissue is responsible for the production of the patient's symptom(s):

- passive neck flexion
- upper-limb neurodynamic tests
- straight-leg raise
- slump.

These tests are described in detail in Chapter 4.

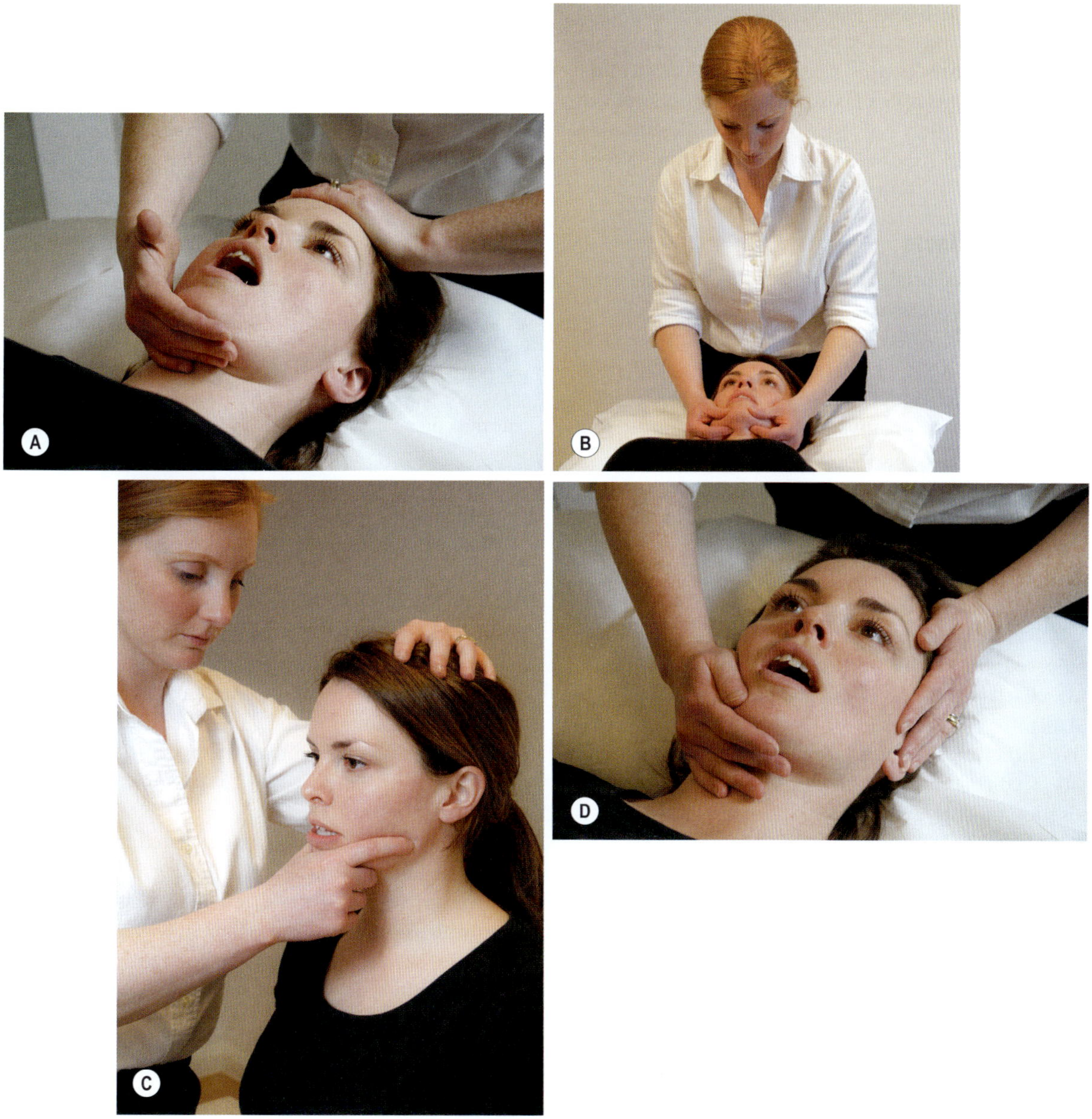

Fig. 6.9 Strength testing for temporomandibular joint movements. (A) Resisted mouth opening. The clinician places one hand under the chin to provide resistance and the other hand stabilizes the head. (B) Resisted mouth closing. The clinician places both hands over the chin and resists the patient closing her mouth. (C) Resisted protrusion. The clinician places the web space of her hand over the patient's chin and resists a forward movement of the chin into protrusion. (D) Resisted lateral deviation. The clinician places one hand over the mandible and the other hand stabilizes the head; the lateral movement of the mandible is resisted.

Lingual Mandibular Reflex (CN V)

The tongue is actively placed against the soft palate and a normal response is the relaxation of masticatory muscles. Loss of this reflex is not necessarily serious, but rather an indication of sensorimotor dysfunction related to the TMJ/upper cervical dysfunction (Kerry, 2013).

Miscellaneous Tests

To facilitate differential diagnosis, further testing may be undertaken as follows:

- Vertebral and carotid arterial examination (Kerry & Taylor, 2006, 2009) (see Chapter 7).
- Palpation of the temporal artery for suspected temporal arteritis. A positive finding is a painful and exaggerated pulse (Kerry, 2013).
- Further cranial nerve examination. Refer for medical investigation if frank nerve pathology is suspected (see Chapter 7).

Palpation

The TMJ and the upper cervical spine (see Chapter 7) are palpated. It is useful to record palpation findings on a body chart (see Fig. 6.1) and/or palpation chart (see Fig. 4.34).

The clinician is referred to Chapter 4 for general palpation considerations and guidelines (see Box 4.2). In addition to this general palpation, the following is specific to the TMJ region:

- position and prominence of the mandible and TMJ
- the presence or elicitation of any muscle spasm in the muscles of mastication
- tenderness of bony landmarks (zygomatic arch, mandibular ramus and condyle), ligament, muscle (masseter, temporalis, medial and lateral pterygoids, splenius capitis, suboccipital muscles, trapezius, sternocleidomastoid, digastric) and tendons. Check for tenderness of the hyoid bone and thyroid cartilage.
- the tendon of the temporalis as it inserts onto the coronoid process of the mandible, as shown in Fig. 6.10.
- the deep fibres of the masseter can also be palpated intraorally.
- the medial pterygoid can also be palpated intraorally; however, this is very uncomfortable in the normal population
- lymph glands for any enlargement

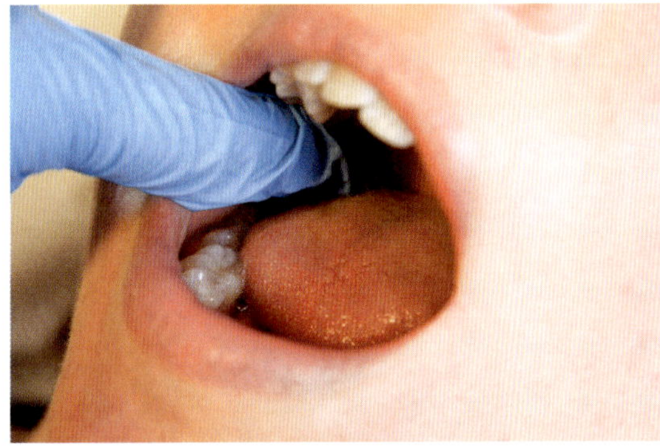

Fig. 6.10 Palpation of the coronoid process for the insertion of the tendon of temporalis muscle on intraoral examination. The clinician's finger is moved up the anterior border of the ramus until the coronoid process and tendon of the temporalis are felt.

- there is controversy as to whether the lateral pterygoid can be palpated. It is believed to be palpated indirectly intraorally (Rocabado & Iglarsh, 1991).

Accessory Movements

It is useful to use the palpation chart and movement diagrams (or joint pictures) to record findings. These are explained in detail in Chapter 4. The clinician is referred to Chapter 4 for general considerations when performing accessory movements. Consideration of the following is specific to the TMJ region in addition to general considerations.

TMJ accessory movements are listed in Table 6.4 and shown in Fig. 6.11, and are as follows:

- anteroposterior (not commonly assessed due to compression of the highly innervated retrodiscal area)—see Kerry (2013) for positioning for this test
- posteroanterior
- medial transverse
- lateral transverse
- longitudinal caudad
- longitudinal cephalad.

Accessory movements can be performed in supine, as shown in Fig. 6.11, or in a semi-sitting position, as demonstrated by Kerry (2013). Following accessory movements to the TMJ, the clinician reassesses all the physical asterisks (movements or tests that have been found to reproduce the patient's symptoms) in order to establish the effect of the accessory movements on the patient's signs and symptoms. Accessory movements can then be tested for other regions suspected to be a source of the symptoms.

TABLE 6.4 Accessory Movements, Choice of Application and Reassessment of the Patient's Asterisks

Accessory Movements	Choice of Application	Identify Any Effect of Accessory Movements on Patient's Signs and Symptoms
Temporomandibular joint ↕ Anteroposterior ↕ Posteroanterior ↔ Med Medial transverse ↔ Lat Lateral transverse ↔ Caud Longitudinal caudad ↔ Ceph Longitudinal cephalad	Start position, e.g. with the mandible depressed, elevated, protracted, retracted, laterally deviated or a combination of these positions Speed of force application Direction of the applied force Point of application of applied force	Reassess all asterisks
?Upper cervical spine	As above	Reassess all asterisks
?Cervical spine	As above	Reassess all asterisks
?Thoracic spine		Reassess all asterisks

Other Tests for the Temporomandibular Joint

Dynamic Loading and Distraction

The clinician places a cotton roll between the upper and lower third molars on one side only, and the patient is asked to bite onto the roll, noting any pain produced. Pain may be felt on the left or right TMJ as there will be distraction of the TMJ on the side of the cotton roll and compression of the TMJ on the contralateral side (Hylander, 1979).

Bite Test (Biting on a Tongue Depressor Test) for Loading

When the patient bites unilaterally on a tongue depressor, the interarticular pressure is reduced in the TMJ of the side of the tongue depressor and raised in the contralateral TMJ. This can help determine whether the TMJ pain is articular or myogenic (Rocabado & Iglarsh, 1991; Okeson, 2020) (Fig. 6.12).

Palpation via External Auditory Meatus

The TMJ can be palpated slightly anterior to the tragus and posteriorly via the external auditory meatus (De Wijer & Steenks, 2009), as shown in Fig. 6.13. The TMJ can be palpated during mandibular movement and the clinician feels whether there is equal rotation and translation of each condyle and whether there is equal movement on the return to a resting position (Magee & Manske, 2021). Correlation with the normal movement parameters and biomechanics needs to be made.

COMPLETION OF THE EXAMINATION

Having carried out the above tests, the examination of the temporomandibular region is now complete.

VALIDITY OF CLINICAL TESTS

Generally, individual tests for TMD have poor validity (Chaput et al., 2012; Julsvoll et al., 2016). However, a cluster of positive tests can assist with the diagnosis of an anterior disc displacement without reduction (Julsvoll et al., 2016). The new DC protocol (Schiffman et al., 2014) is ideal for identifying patients with simple to complex TMD and is seen as appropriate for use in both clinical and research settings. The reader is referred to the DC protocol (Schiffman et al., 2014) for physical (Axis I) and psychological (Axis II) screening instruments which have been validated.

MULTIDISCIPLINARY TEAM APPROACH TO TEMPOROMANDIBULAR DYSFUNCTION

It is essential when assessing and managing patients with TMD that a multidisciplinary team approach is considered due to the multifactorial nature of TMD and its associations. No single cause accounts for all the signs and symptoms of TMD described by a patient; therefore there is no one single treatment strategy that can be recommended for patients with TMD. A multimodal and multidisciplinary approach is proposed, which has

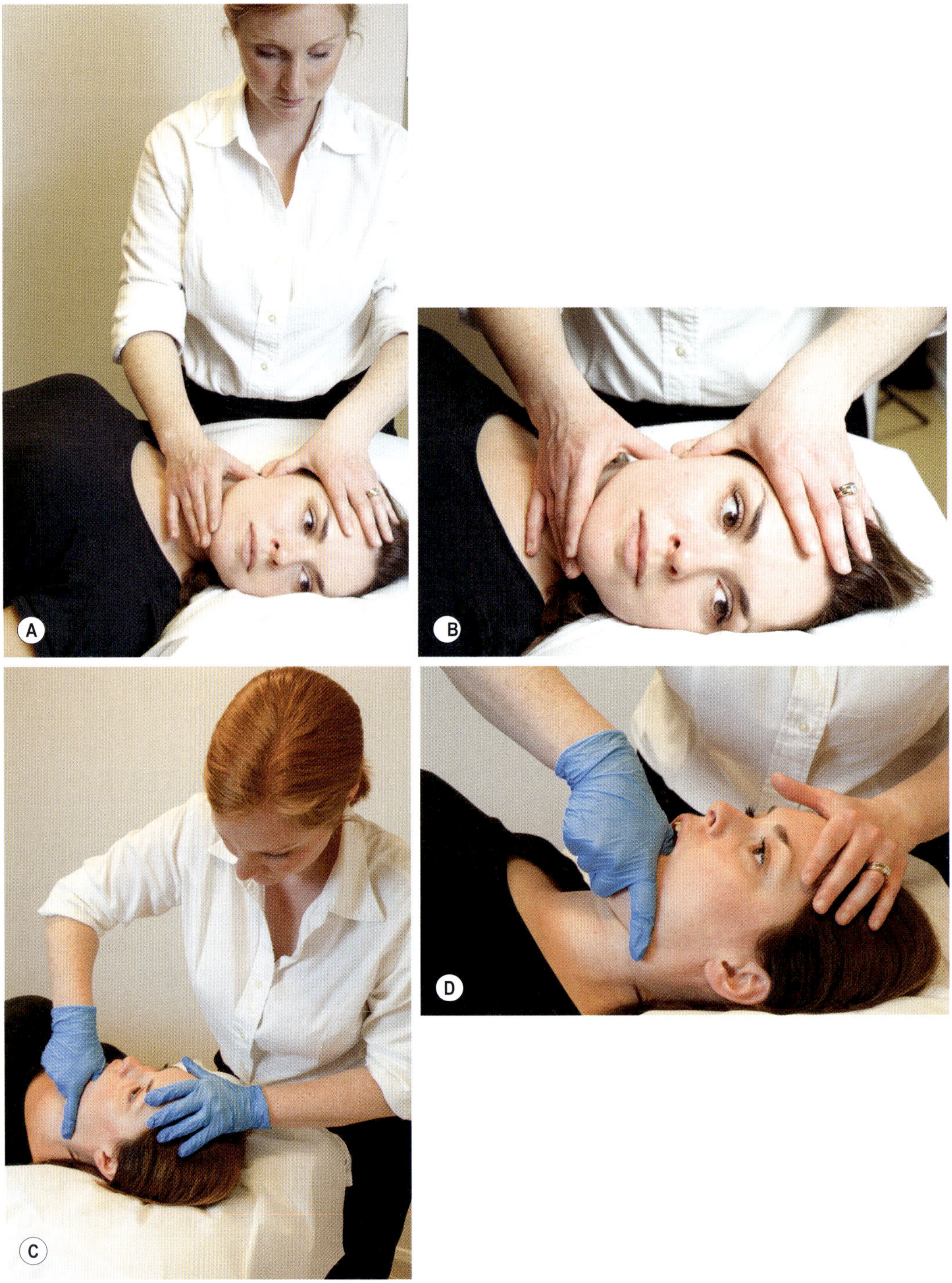

Fig. 6.11 Accessory movements to the temporomandibular joint. (A) Posteroanterior. With the patient in side-lying, thumbs apply a posteroanterior pressure to the posterior aspect of the head of the mandible. (B) Medial transverse. With the patient in side-lying, thumbs apply a medial pressure to the lateral aspect of the head of the mandible. (C) Lateral transverse. The one hand supports the head while the gloved hand is placed inside the mouth so that the thumb rests along the medial surface of the mandible (inside aspect of the lower teeth). Thumb pressure can then produce a lateral glide of the mandible. (D) Longitudinal cephalad and caudad. With the patient supine and the one hand supporting the head, the gloved hand is placed inside the mouth so that the thumb rests on the top of the lower back teeth. The thumb and outer fingers then grip the mandible and apply a downward pressure (longitudinal caudad) and an upward pressure (longitudinal cephalad).

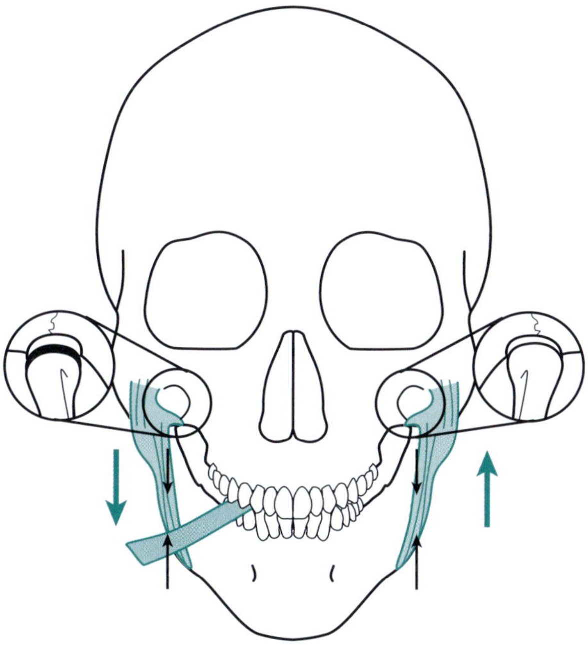

Fig. 6.12 Asking the patient to bite on a tongue depressor. When the bite is unilateral on a hard substance, the joint on the bite side has a sudden reduction in interarticular pressure, with the opposite happening to the contralateral side. This can help determine the problematic articular side. (Modified from Okeson 2013, with permission.)

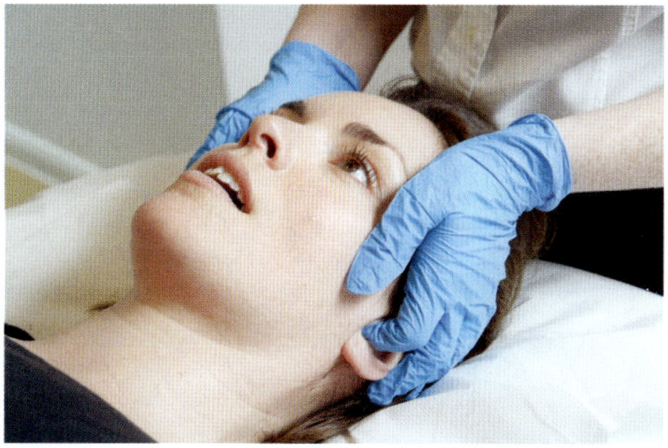

Fig. 6.13 Palpation of mandibular condyle via the auditory canal. The temporomandibular joint is palpated laterally slightly anterior to the tragus and posteriorly via the external meatus, with the mouth open or closed, and during opening and closing movements.

been shown as the most effective way to manage TMD (Medlicott & Harris, 2006; Ahmed et al., 2014).

An initially conservative approach to the management of TMD (Dimitroulis, 1998; Lyons, 2008; Wright & North, 2009) includes physiotherapy, education, drug treatment and the use of a bite guard (occlusal splint). Surgical intervention, including arthrocentesis or arthroscopy of the TMJ (Guo et al., 2009), is indicated in a limited number of patients. Manual therapy for mechanical TMJ presentations and multimodal treatment approaches have been shown to be effective in a number of studies (Cleland & Palmer, 2004; McNeely et al., 2006; Medlicott & Harris, 2006; Shin et al., 2007; Martins et al., 2016). Therefore, physiotherapists are ideally placed to provide a comprehensive assessment and effective management of patients with TMD.

REVIEW AND REVISE QUESTIONS

1. Fill in the following:
   Anterior disc displacement occurs when the ______ is sitting in an anterior position on the ______________ condyle. When the disc is sitting on the correct position on the condylar head with mouth opening this is termed anterior disc displacement _______________. If the disc does not sit on the condylar head on mouth opening this is termed anterior disc displacement _________________.
2. True or false
   An anterior disc displacement without reduction is always associated with reduced mouth opening.
3. Fill in the following:
   Symptoms in the frontal, retroorbital, temporal and occipital areas of the head can be mediated by both the _________________ and the ____ due to ______________________ in the _______________ nucleus in the _____________.
4. Due to the anatomical and biomechanical relationship with the TMJ which two other areas should be examined with a TMJ assessment?

Case Study

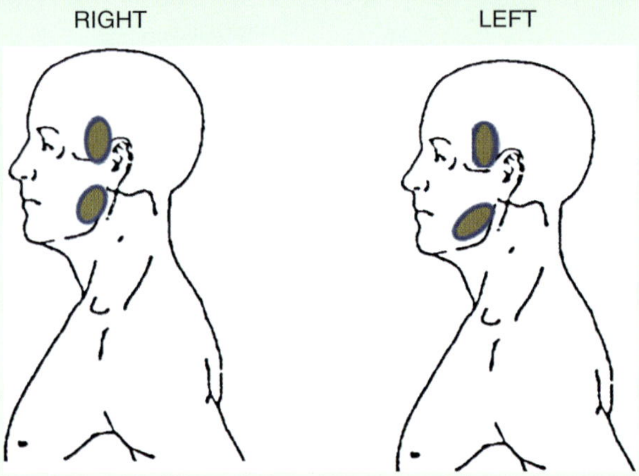

Age: 34 – female

Bilateral facial pan in the cheek and temporal area. No other reported pain on the body chart. No reported P&N or numbness within the face.

Intermittent symptoms usually coming on together and rated as 6/10 NPS.

Aggravating factors – Mouth opening, eating chewy and hard food groups

Easing factors – Eating a softer diet, avoiding talking in the evening, paracetamol

24-h pattern – AM soreness and an increase in symptoms lasting approximately 30 min. Daytime – variable depending on activities. Evening – increase in symptoms, and patient struggles to get to sleep. No unbroken sleep once asleep. Unaware of any clenching; husband has not mentioned noticing any grinding overnight.

No symptoms elsewhere

PMHx – Nil of note, 2 × C-Section – planned

DH – paracetamol PRN

Investigations – NIL

Screening Questions

No red flags associated with the cervical spine or face

No general Red flags

Clicking – patient reports clicking in both TMJs since teenage years never bothered patient

Locking – no history of locking of either TMJ

Trismus – patient feels that her mouth opening has reduced by approximately 30%; potentially this may be a red flag (Beddis et al., 2014)

Headaches – gets headaches associated with pain in the temporal region. No other headaches. Headaches have been present for 6 months and gradually worsening

Outcome Measures

NPS 6/10

GAD-7 – 7/21 suggesting mild anxiety (Ohrbach et al., 2016)

Patient Specific Functional Scale –

Opening mouth – 6

Chewing – 7

Talking – 5

HPC

Pain started approximately 6 months ago for no apparent reason. No history of trauma or injury to the area. It initially started in the morning and towards the end of the day; however, her symptoms have worsened as they are coming on more frequently and happening in the day also.

No recent dental treatment; however, she has not been able to see the dentist due to National Lockdown measures in relation to COVID-19 global pandemic.

She does recall clicking of both TMJs since her teenage years, and this has never really bothered her.

Lifestyle/Occupation/Homelife

Married with two children ages 7 and 10 (Y3 and Y6 in school) – currently homeschooling two children

Job – PA to a CEO of an IT company but currently working from home due to COVID-19. Husband works in finance and works long hours.

Enjoys Yoga/Pilates/HIT workout and attending the gym (which is currently closed due to COVID-19) so not doing as much exercise as prior to National Lockdown restrictions.

Impact on Function, Beliefs and Expectations

Feels that she is in pain which is limiting in being able to speak to family and friends and general enjoyment. She is unsure why her pain has come on but feels that she is doing a lot at the moment. She would like to be able to eat a normal diet and be pain-free.

Other questions associated with TMJ

Parafunctional habits – nail biting and lip chewing (possible microtrauma to the TMJ Okeson, 2020)

Diet – eating a very soft diet due to symptoms

SIN –

Severity – moderate 6/10 VAS, affecting ability to open mouth, eat certain food groups

Irritability – moderate – takes 30 minutes to ease

Primary diagnosis – Myalgia and headache attributed to TMD (Schiffman et al., 2014). Likely due to area of pain, agg factors of chewing using the muscles of mastication.

Also, she wakes with morning symptoms which are prevalent in those with bruxism (Kraus, 1994).

Differential diagnosis – Anterior disc displacement without reduction with limited movement (Schiffman et al., 2014). This was due to her history of clicking since a teenager so she may have been one of the population who has an anteriorly displaced disc without issue (Okeson, 2020), which has then progressed to a nonreducing anterior disc displacement. She has pain with chewing which would also load the TMJ (Okeson, 2020). Pain also with mouth opening which would stretch the retrodiscal tissue which could be a source of pain.

Need to also consider trismus and whether this is a red flag (Beddis et al., 2014) depending on the objective examination.

Potential risk factors identified for TMD – gender, likely bruxism, headache (Kumar et al., 2019).

Planning the Objective

Must – palpation, TMJ AROM, strength of the muscles of mastication, intraoral inspection, clear cervical spine. Need to be aware of the high SIN during the examination.

Informal Observation

Patient made good eye contact

Not fully articulating

Appeared to have some enlargement of the masseter bilaterally

Slight forward head posture and round shoulders bilaterally (this may affect the resting position of the mandible and muscle activity and tone) (Olivo et al., 2006)

Intraoral Observation

Linea alba and marked tongue scalloping bilaterally (signs of bruxism Okeson, 2020)

No deterioration of the wear facets on her posterior molars

Cervical spine assessment – AROM/PAIVM – NAD no reproduction of pain

AROM

Mouth opening

MCO – 28 mm (this is under 30 mm and considered trismus; Beddis et al., 2014)

MIO — 40 mm with bilateral click, no mandibular deviation but reproduction of pain; this is within the normal limits (Beddis et al., 2014); therefore would not be considered as trismus and would not be a red flag.

LD R 13 mm L 12 mm no pain

Protrusion 4 mm pain at the end of range

Palpation

Pain over the masseter bilaterally rated at 6/10 NPS, Pain on palpation of the anterior and middles fibres of temporalis with reproduction of the patient's headache 6/10 NPS

No tenderness over the TMJ bilaterally but good condylar translation with a palpable click

Pain on palpation of the deep masseter and lateral pterygoid region bilaterally 7/10 NPS

Auscultation – bilateral click both TMJ mid-opening and closing

Strength Testing

Full strength of all muscles of mastication but pain on resisted masseter and temporalis (mouth closing)

Acc movements

Distraction – springy end feel

Mouth opening – springy end feel and increased to 50 mm mouth opening (well within normal range; Beddis et al., 2014; Okeson, 2020)

Diagnosis

Accept the primary hypothesis of myalgia of myofascial pain (Schiffman et al., 2014) as the pain radiated within the boundary of the muscle on palpation. The patient also has a headache attributed to TMD (Schiffman et al., 2014). There is no clear objective sign of an anterior disc displacement without reduction as there is no limitation of movement (although you can have an anterior disc displacement without reduction without limitation of movement; Schiffman, 2014), and a click can be heard on opening and closing. It is likely that she is clenching during the night and possibly during the day due to the increased demand and stresses associated with lockdown restrictions due to the COVID-19 pandemic.

This case reflects the multifactorial nature of TMD including psychological factors (mild anxiety and stress due to the COVID-19 pandemic), physical factors (longstanding clicking) and associated risk factors such as gender and bruxism (Slade et al., 2016; Kumar et al., 2019).

REFERENCES

Ahmed, N., Poate, T., Nacher-Garcia, C., Pugh, N., Cowgill, H., Page, L., et al., 2014. Temporomandibular joint multidisciplinary team clinic. Br. J. Oral Maxillofac. Surg. 52, 827–830.

Beddis, H.P., Davies, S.J., Budenberg, A., Horner, K., Pemberton, M.N., 2014. Temporomandibular disorders, trismus and malignancy: development of a checklist to improve patient safety. Br. Dent. J. 217, 351–355.

Beltran-Alacreu, H., López-de-Uralde-Villanueva, I., Paris-Alemany, A., Angulo-Díaz-Parreño, S., La Touche, R., 2014. Intra-rater and inter-rater reliability of mandibular range of motion measures considering a neutral craniocervical position. J. Phys. Ther. Sci. 26, 915–920.

Bogduk, N., 1994. Cervical causes of headache and dizziness. In: Boyling, J.D., Palastanga, N. (Eds.), Grieve's Modern Manual Therapy, second ed. Churchill Livingstone, Edinburgh, p. 317.

Bogduk, N., Bartsch, T., 2008. Cervicogenic headache. In: Silberstein, S.D., et al. (Eds.), Wolff's Headache, eighth ed. Oxford University Press, New York, pp. 551–570.

Bogduk, N., Govind, J., 2009. Cervicogenic headache: an assessment of the evidence on clinical diagnosis, invasive tests, and treatment. Lancet Neurol. 8, 959–968.

Cairns, B.E., 2019. Trigeminal nociceptive processing. In: Fernandez-de-las-Pemas, Mesa-Jimenez (Eds.), Temporomandibular Disorders, first ed. Handspring Publishing, Edinburgh.

Chaput, È., Gross, A., Stewart, R., Nadeau, G., Goldsmith, C.H., 2012. The diagnostic validity of clinical tests in temporomandibular internal derangement: a systematic review and meta-analysis. Physiother. Can. 64, 116–134.

Cleland, J., Palmer, J., 2004. Effectiveness of manual physical therapy, therapeutic exercise, and patient education on bilateral disc displacement without reduction of the temporomandibular joint: a single case design. J. Orthop. Sports Phys. Ther. 34, 535–548.

Costa, Y.M., Alves da Costa, D.R., de Lima Ferreira, A.P., Poporatti, A.L., Svensson, P., Rodrigues Conti, P.C., et al., 2017. Headache exacerbates pain characteristics in temporomandibular disorders. J. Oral Facial Pain Headache 31, 339–345.

Cowgill, H., 2014. Physiotherapy management of temporomandibular disorders. Touch 146, 18–23.

de Wijer, A., Lobbezon-Scholte, A.M., Steenks, M.H., Bosman, F., 1995. Reliability of clinical findings in temporomandibular disorders. J. Orofac. Pain 9, 181–191.

de Wijer, A., Steenks, M.H., 2009. Clinical examination of the orofacial region in patients with headache. In: Cesar Fernandez-de-las-Penas, C., et al. (Eds.), Tension-type and Cervicogenic Headache – Physiology, Diagnosis, and Management. Jones & Bartlett, Sudbury, MA, pp. 197–206.

Dimitroulis, G., 1998. Temporomandibular disorders: a clinical update. Br. Med. J. 317, 190–194.

Dworkin, S.F., LeResche, L., DeRouen, T., Von Korff, M., 1990. Assessing clinical signs of temporo-mandibular disorders: reliability of clinical examiners. J. Prosthet. Dent. 63, 574–579.

Eriksson, P.O., Zafar, H., Nordh, E., 1998. Concomitant mandibular and head-neck movements during jaw opening-closing in man. J. Oral Rehabil. 25 (11), 859–870.

Feinstein, B., Langton, J.N.K., Jameson, R.M., Schiller, F., 1954. Experiments on pain referred from deep somatic tissues. J. Bone Joint Surg. Am. 36A, 981–997.

Franco, A.L., Goncalves, D.A.G., Castanharo, S.M., Speciali, J.G., Bigal, M.E., Camparis, C.M., 2010. Migraine is the most prevalent primary headache in individuals with temporomandibular disorders. J. Orofacial Pain 24, 287–292.

Greenhalgh, S., Selfe, J., 2010. Red Flags II: A Guide to Identifying Serious Pathology of the Spine. Elsevier, Edinburgh.

Guo, C., Shi, Z., Revington, P., 2009. Arthrocentesis and lavage for treating temporomandibular joint disorders. Cochrane Database Syst. Rev. (4), CD004973.

Hengeveld, E., Banks, K., 2014. Maitland's Peripheral Manipulation, fifth ed. Elsevier, Churchill Livingstone.

Hylander, W.L., 1979. An experimental analysis of temporomandibular joint reaction forces in macaques. Am. J. Phys. Anthropol. 51, 433.

International Classification of Headache Disorders, third edition, 2018. www.Icdh-3.org. (accessed 6.6.2021.)

International Headache Society, 2020. International Classification of Orofacial Pain, first ed. Cephalalgia 40(2), 129-221.

Julsvoll, E.H., Vøllestad, N.K., Robinson, H.S., 2016. Validation of clinical tests for patients with long-standing painful temporomandibular disorders with anterior disc displacement with reduction. Man. Ther. 21, 109–119.

Kerry, R., 2013. Examination of the temporomandibular region. In: Petty, N.J. (Ed.), Neuromusculoskeletal Examination and Assessment. Churchill Livingstone, Edinburgh, pp. 169–187.

Kerry, R., Taylor, A.J., 2006. Cervical arterial dysfunction assessment and manual therapy. Man. Ther. 11, 243–253.

Kerry, R., Taylor, A.J., 2008. Arterial pathology and cervicocranial pain – differential diagnosis for manual therapists and medical practitioners. Int. Musculoskelet. Med. 30, 70–77.

Kerry, R., Taylor, A.J., 2009. Cervical arterial dysfunction: knowledge and reasoning for manual physical therapists. J. Orthop. Sports Phys. Ther. 39, 378–387.

Taylor, A.J., Kerry, R., 2010. A 'system based approach to risk assessment of the cervical spine prior to manual therapy. Int. J. Osteopath. Med. 13 (3), 85–93.

Kraus, S., 2014. Characteristics of 511 patients with temporomandibular disorders referred to physical therapy. Oral Surg. Oral Med. Oral Pathol. Oral Radiol. 118, 432–439.

Kraus, S.L., 1994. Physical therapy management of TMD. In: Kraus, S.L. (Ed.), Temporomandibular Disorders, second ed. Churchill Livingstone, Edinburgh.

Kumar, A., Exposto, F.G., You, H., Svensson, P., 2019. Pathophysiology of temporomandibular pain. In: Fernandez-de-las-Pemas, Mesa-Jimenez (Eds.), Temporomandibular Disorders, first ed. Handspring Publishing, Edinburgh.

Lyons, M.F., 2008. Current practice in the management of temporomandibular disorders. Dent. Update 35, 314–318.

Magee, D.J., Manske, R.C., 2021. Orthopedic Physical Assessment, seventh ed. Elsevier, Saunders.

Manual for Self Manual for Self-Report Instruments. Version 29May2016. www.rdc-tmdinternational.org. (accessed on 6.6.2021.)

Martins, W.R., Blasczyk, J.C., de Oliveira, M.A.F., Gonçalves, K.F.L., Bonini-Rocha, A.C., Dugailly, P.M., et al., 2016. Efficacy of musculoskeletal manual approach in the treatment of temporomandibular disorder: a systematic review with meta-analysis. Man. Ther. 21, 10–17.

McNeely, M.L., Armijo Olivo, S., Magee, D.J., 2006. A systematic review of the effectiveness of physical therapy interventions for temporomandibular disorders. Phys. Ther. 86, 710–725.

Medlicott, M.S., Harris, S.R., 2006. A systematic review of the effectiveness of exercise, manual therapy, electrotherapy, relaxation training, and biofeedback in the management of temporomandibular disorders. Phys. Ther. 86, 955–973.

Michelotti, A., Svensson, P., 2019. Classification of temporomandibular disorders. In: Fernandez-de-las-Pemas, Mesa-Jimenez (Eds.), Temporomandibular Disorders, first ed. Handspring Publishing, Edinburgh.

Ohrbach, R., Knibbe, W., 2016. Diagnostic criteria for temporomandibular disorders: DC/TMD Scoring Manual for self-report Instruments 18.

Ohrbach, R., Gonzalez, Y., List, T., Michelotti, A., Schiffman, E., 2013. Diagnositc Criteria for Temporomandibular Disorders (DC/TMD) Clinical Examination Protocol: Version 02 June 2013. www.rdc-tmdinternational.org. (accessed 6.6.2021).

Okeson, J.P., 2020. Management of Temporomandibular Disorders and Occlusion, eighth ed. Elsevier, St Louis, MO.

Olivo, S.A., Bravo, J., Magee, D., Thie, N.M., Major, P.W., Flores-Mir, C., 2006. The association between head and cervical posture and temporomandibular disorders: a systematic review. J. Orofacial Pain 20, 9–23.

Pertes, R.A., Gross, S.G., 1995. Clinical Management of Temporomandibular Disorders and Orofacial Pain. Quintessence, Chicago.

Porto De Toledo, I., Stefani, F.M., Poporatti, A.L., Mezzono, L.A., Peres, M.A., Flores-Mir, C., et al., 2016. Prevalence of otologic signs and symptoms in adult patients with TMD: a systematic review and meta-analysis. Clin. Oral Invest. 21 (2), 597–605. https://doi.org/10.1007/s00784-016-1926-9.

Rocabado, M., 1983. Biomechanical relationship of the cranial, cervical and hyoid regions. Cranio 1, 62–66.

Rocabado, M., 2004. A university student with chronic facial pain. In: Jones, M.A., Rivett, D.A. (Eds.), Clinical Reasoning in Manual Therapy. Butterworth Heinemann, Edinburgh, pp. 243–260.

Rocabado, M., Iglarsh, A., 1991. Musculoskeletal Approach to Maxillofacial Pain. J.B. Lippincott, Philadelphia, PA.

Schiffman, E., Ohrbach, R., Truelove, E., Look, J., Anderson, G., Goulet, J.P., et al., 2014. Diagnostic criteria for temporomandibular disorders (DC/TMD): for clinical and research applications: recommendations of the international RDC/TMD consortium network and orofacial pain special interest group. J. Oral Facial Pain Headache 28, 6–27.

Schiffman, E.L., Fricton, J.R., Haley, D.P., Shapiro, B.L., 1990. The prevalence and treatment needs of subjects with temporomandibular disorders. J. Am. Dent. Assoc. 1, 295–303.

Sharma, S., Ohrbach, R., 2019. Definition, epidemiology and etiology of painful temporomandibular disorders. In: Fernandez-de-las-Pemas, Mesa-Jimenez (Eds.), Temporomandibular Disorders, first ed. Handspring Publishing, Edinburgh.

Shin, B.C., Ha, C.H., Song, Y.S., Lee, M.S., 2007. Effectiveness of combining manual therapy and acupuncture on temporomandibular dysfunction: a retrospective study. Am. J. Chin. Med. 35, 203–208.

Slade, G.D., Ohrbach, R., Greenspan, J.D., Fillingim, R.B., Bair, E., Sanders, A.E., et al., 2016. Painful temporomandibular disorder: decade of discovery from OPPERA Studies. J. Dental Res. 95, 1084–1092.

Tchivileva, I.E., Ohrbach, R., Fillingim, R.B., Greenspan, J.D., Maxiner, W., Slade, G.D., 2017. Temporal change in headache and its contributions to the risk of developing first onset temporomandibular disorders in the Orofacial Pain: Prospective Evaluation and Risk Assessment (OPPERA) Study. Pain 158, 120–129.

Walker, N., Bohannon, R.W., Cameron, D., 2000. Discriminant validity of temporomandibular joint range of motion measurements obtained with a ruler. J. Orthop. Sports Phys. Ther. 30, 484–492.

Wright, E.F., North, S.L., 2009. Management and treatment of temporomandibular disorders: a clinical perspective. J. Man. Manip. Ther. 17, 27–54.

7

Examination of the Upper Cervical Region

Neil Langridge and Gail Forrester Gale

LEARNING OUTCOMES

After studying this chapter, you should be able to:

- Describe the anatomy of the upper cervical spine (UCS).
- Recognize common symptoms associated with UCS dysfunction and pathology.
- Recognize the common headache presentations seen within a musculoskeletal clinic.
- Describe the clinical examination of the UCS.
- List the key constituents of a comprehensive subjective examination.
- Identify how clinical reasoning guides the subjective examination of those with UCS dysfunction.
- Identify how subjective data will guide the physical examination of the region.
- List the key constituents of the comprehensive physical examination of the UCS.
- Explain how physical examination findings contribute to the reasoning of common pathologies of the region.

CHAPTER CONTENTS

Introduction to the Upper Cervical Region, 197
Anatomical Overview, 197
Symptoms Associated With the Craniocervical Spine, 198
Headache, 199
Clinical Assessment in Cervicogenic Headache Disorder, 202
Upper Cervical Spine Dizziness and Proprioception, 203
Whiplash-Related Dizziness, 203
Subjective Examination/Taking the Patient's History, 204
The Patient's Perspective on their Experience, 204
Body Chart, 204
Behaviour of Symptoms, 205
Special/Red-Flag Screening Questions, 205
Cervical Arterial Dysfunction, 205
Physical Examination, 208
Observation, 208
Active Physiological Movement, 208
Neurological Testing, 208
Palpation, 211
Flexion–Rotation Test, 211
Accessory Movements, 211
Muscle Testing, 214
Cervical Arterial Dysfunction Testing, 218
Completion of the Examination, 219
Appendix 7.1 Headache Disability Index Questionnaire, 220
Appendix 7.2 Headache Disability Questionnaire, 221
Case Study, 222
References, 224

INTRODUCTION TO THE UPPER CERVICAL REGION

Anatomical Overview

The occiput, atlas (C1), axis (C2) and the surrounding soft tissues are collectively referred to as the craniocervical spine (CCS). It is an anatomically and biomechanically unique region and the most mobile area of the spine. The C1 vertebra, also known as the atlas, is located just beneath the skull and is well shaped to hold the skull's posterior curve (). The C2 vertebra known as the axis is a unique structure that enables nodding movements and with the axis allows for rotations. There are no intervertebral discs between the occiput and C1 or between C1 and C2. The C1 vertebra lacks a spinous process; it resembles a bony ring and is often referred to as a 'washer' between the occiput and C2 (Bogduk, 2002). C2 has a vertical bony growth called the odontoid peg, which provides stability and facilitates mobility. Together with C3 these vertebrae form a unique complex of joints, referred to as:

- C0–C1: the atlantooccipital joint (A-O joint)
- C1–C2: the atlantoaxial joint (A-A joint)
- C2–3 facet joints.

The A-O joint is a bicondyloid joint with long, thin congruent joint surfaces oriented in an anterior-posterior direction. This arrangement facilitates movements in the sagittal plane of upper cervical flexion and extension, also referred to as retraction and protraction, which resemble a head-on-neck nodding movement (Bogduk & Mercer, 2000; Amiri et al., 2003; Chancey et al., 2007). The A-A segment consists of three joints: a central pivot joint between the odontoid peg and the osseoligamentous ring, which is formed by the transverse ligament and the anterior arch of the atlas, and two biconvex, horizontally oriented facet joints bilaterally. This triad of articulations facilitates rotation, which is the largest movement in the CCS and indeed in the entire spine, with approximately 38–56 degree rotation occurring to each side (Ishii et al., 2004; Salem et al. 2013) (Fig. 7.1). Owing to the configuration of the occipitoatlantoaxial joint surfaces, movements of rotation and side flexion are not pure; they are coupled. Rotation in the upper cervical spine (UCS) is consistently coupled with contralateral side flexion (Salem et al., 2013).

CCS stability is provided through a combination of mechanical restraint from the ligamentous system and sensorimotor control from the neuromuscular system. The principal ligaments providing stability in this region are generally recognized as the transverse ligament (Fig. 7.2A) and the alar ligaments, with a number of other ligaments including the tectorial membrane acting as secondary stabilizers (Krakenes et al., 2001; Brolin & Halldin, 2004; Krakenes & Kaale, 2006; Tubbs et al., 2007; Osmotherly et al., 2013) (Fig. 7.2B).

Key muscle groups acting directly on the CCS and providing dynamic stability and proprioception are the craniocervical flexor (CCF) muscle group anteriorly (Fig. 7.3A) and the suboccipital muscle (SOM) group posteriorly (Fig. 7.3B) (McPartland & Brodeur, 1999; Falla, 2004; Schomacher & Falla, 2013).

The head, UCS and neck are innervated by the first four cervical spinal nerves. Nerve roots emerge at each level from C0 to C1 downwards and divide into dorsal and ventral branches called rami. The cervical plexus is formed by the anterior rami of C1–C4 and innervates the skin and somatic structures of the anterolateral neck region, occipital, auricular and lateral mastoid regions (Fig. 7.4). The dorsal rami of the C1–C4 spinal nerves innervate the skin and somatic structures of the posterior craniocervical spine.

Upper cervical spinal nerve roots and peripheral nerve trunks can be a source of pain in the head, neck and face. Referral patterns will be dermatomal in the case of nerve root disorders or within the cutaneous

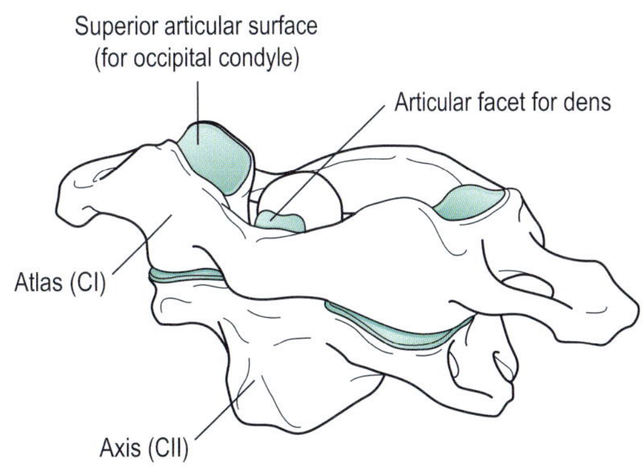

Fig. 7.1 The Atlantooccipital and Atlantoaxial Joints. (From McCarthy 2010, with permission.)

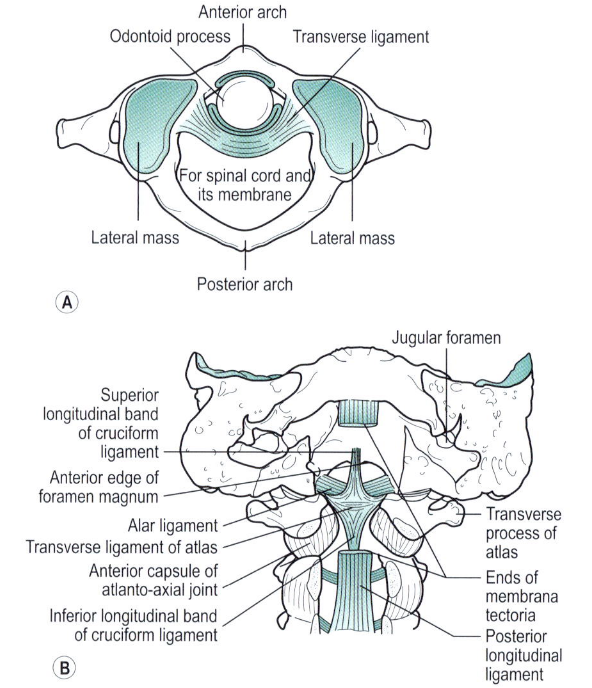

Fig. 7.2 (A) The transverse ligament. (B) The alar ligaments and tectorial membrane. (From McCarthy 2010, with permission.)

field of innervation in the case of peripheral neuropathy (fig. 4.15).

Blood is supplied to the brain and brainstem by the internal carotid arteries (ICAs) and vertebral arteries (VAs) communicating via the circle of Willis (Fig. 7.5). The ICAs and the VAs are innervated by the internal carotid plexus and the vertebral nerve respectively. These nerves communicate with the trigeminocervical nucleus (TCN) and the cervical plexus. The VAs have a close relationship to the upper cervical vertebrae which means that they are subjected to stretch and deformity on movements of the cervical spine, particularly rotation and extension (Thomas et al., 2015). As a result, the ICAs and the VAs can be a source of pain and symptoms in the upper cervical region due to either damage to the arteries themselves or due to a reduction in blood flow through the arteries to the brain or brainstem (Taylor & Kerry, 2010). The reader is referred to Chapter 8, Barnard and Ryder (2024).

KNOWLEDGE CHECK

1. Which joints make up the upper cervical spine?
2. What offers stability in the upper cervical spine?
3. What are the common referral patterns of symptoms from the upper cervical spine?

SYMPTOMS ASSOCIATED WITH THE CRANIOCERVICAL SPINE

The CCS is a common source of symptoms such as head, neck and facial pain, dizziness and nausea. These symptoms may arise due to dysfunction in musculoskeletal structures of the upper three cervical segments; however, due to the close proximity of the UCS to the brainstem, spinal cord and VAs, these structures must

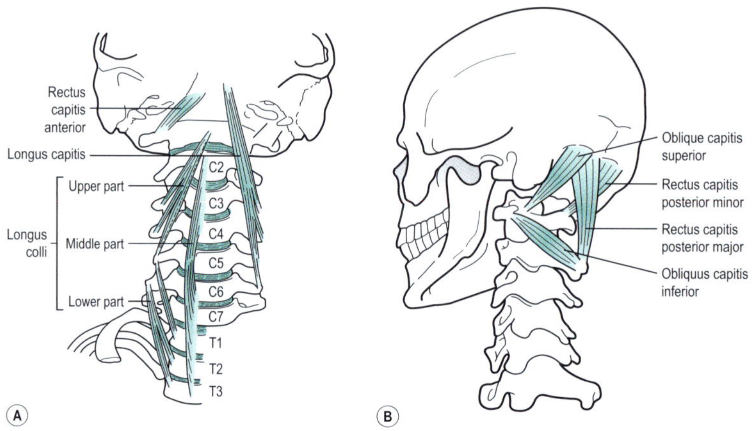

Fig. 7.3 (A) The craniocervical flexor muscle group craniocervical spine muscle group. (B) The suboccipital muscle group. (From McCarthy 2010, with permission.)

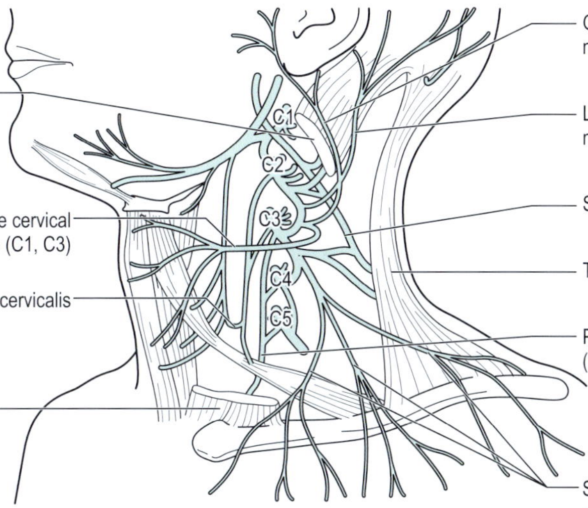

Fig. 7.4 The cervical plexus is composed of the ventral rami of the first four cervical spinal nerves (C1–C4). It innervates the anterolateral upper neck, occipital, auricular and lateral mastoid regions. (Modified from Netter 2006, with permission.)

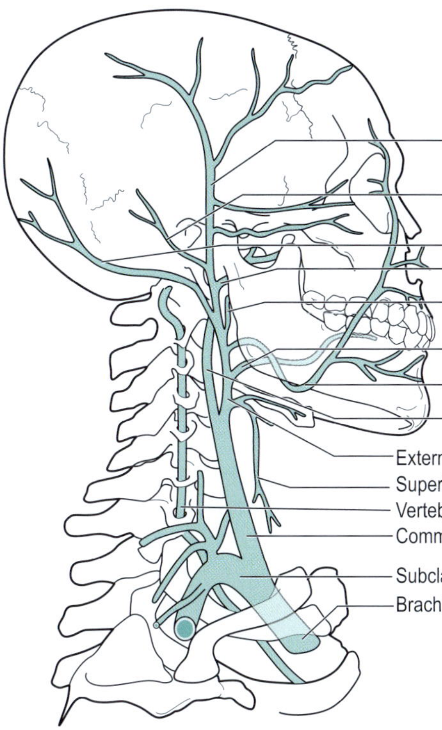

Fig. 7.5 The Cervical Arterial System. (From McCance et al., with permission.)

also be considered in the differential diagnosis of upper cervical disorders. Referral of symptoms from the UCS into the head and face is common. The mechanism of referral is thought to be through the convergence of afferent fibres from the upper three cervical segments with afferent fibres from the trigeminocervical nerve (cranial nerve V) in the TCN in the brainstem (Van Griensven, 2005; Bogduk & Bartsch, 2008; Bogduk & Govind, 2009). For further information about referred pain, see Chapter 3.

Headache

The UCS is commonly referenced as a source of headache; however, it is important to be aware that headache is complex. The International Classification for Headache Disorders (Olesen, 2018) cites over 100 different classifications; however, within musculoskeletal practice an awareness of commonly reported presentations remains important. Headache relating directly to the UCS has been cited as 0.1%–4.1% in terms of prevalence (Antonaci & Inan, 2021). The three most common headaches seen in primary care are the primary headache disorders, e.g. tension, migraine and cervicogenic. Exclusion of red flags should be the first step in any clinical reasoning. After this has been completed the clinician should be able to recognize classical signs and symptoms in order to try to develop a clinical rationale for other common headache disorders (Table 7.1).

Tension type headache (TTH) is the most commonly reported primary headache (Robbins & Lipton, 2010). People with infrequent episodic TTH are unlikely to seek medical advice and will generally self-manage. As the frequency of TTH increases so commonly does the severity of the pain and the likelihood that the patient will present for treatment; younger patients are also more likely to consult a practitioner in these cases (Holroyd et al., 2000). Usually, patients report a mild to moderate, bilateral sensation of muscle tightness or pressure lasting hours to days and not associated with constitutional or neurological symptoms. Patients may describe and indicate the location of the pain as a 'band-like feeling' around the head. Sufferers may present with bilateral tightening of the cervical spinal musculature and pericranial tenderness which can be felt by the patient and also is identified in the physical assessment (Loder & Rizzoli, 2008).

Migraine is a common disabling primary headache disorder. In the Global Burden of Disease Study 2010 (GBD, 2010), it was ranked as the third most prevalent disorder in the world. Many epidemiological studies have documented its high prevalence with socio-economic and personal impacts. Migraine has two major types:

- Migraine without aura—a clinical syndrome characterized by unilateral headache with specific features and associated symptoms, e.g. nausea, photophobia/phonophobia
- Migraine with aura—characterized by the transient focal neurological symptoms that usually precede or sometimes accompany the headache (Viana et al., 2017).

TABLE 7.1 Differential Diagnosis of Headache

	Cervicogenic Headache	Migraine	Tension-Type Headache
Onset	Usually starts in the neck or occipital region and radiates forwards	Usually starts in the head and radiates backwards	Starts in the head
Location	Occipital to frontoparietal and orbital	Frontal, periorbital, temporal	Diffuse
Lateralization	Unilateral without side shift	Mostly unilateral with side shift	Diffuse bilateral
Frequency	Chronic, episodic	1–4 per month	Episodic. 1–30 per month
Severity	Moderate to severe	Moderate to severe	Mild to moderate
Duration	1 h to weeks	4–72 h	Days to weeks
Pain characteristics	Non-throbbing, non-lancinating	Throbbing, pulsating	Dull, pressing, tightening
Triggers	Neck movement, sustained, awkward head postures	Multiple. Neck movement not typical	Multiple. Neck movement not typical
Associated signs and symptoms	Limited range of neck motion. Tender on palpation over the upper three cervical spinal segments on symptomatic side. Craniocervical flexor weakness. May have nausea, photophobia but milder than migraine	Nausea, vomiting, visual changes, photophobia, phonophobia	No nausea or vomiting. May have photophobia or phonophobia

Adapted from Haldeman and Dagenais (2001), Antonaci et al. (2006), Zito et al. (2006), Jull et al. (2008b).

Migraine without aura presents with unilateral symptoms of throbbing, of moderate intensity exacerbated with physical exertion. Clear differentials from TTH are the associated symptoms of nausea, photophobia/phonophobia and no preceding aura. Migraine with aura constitutes approximately 15%–30% of all migraines and is a headache with a transient associated neurological symptom. This is described as the aura and can be visual, motor or sensory. A visual aura is the most common and may include flashing lights, and/or zig-zag lines. The sensory aura can be numbness or paraesthesia whilst motor symptoms can be as severe as hemiplegia (Martin, 2004). The reason for the symptoms of migraine is not fully understood. Imaging has identified alterations in cerebral blood flow, cortical spreading depression (CSD) and possible neurogenic inflammation as an explanation for the symptoms experienced by the individual (De-Simone et al., 2013; Lauritzen, 2001). CSD is a slowly propagated wave of depolarization followed by suppression of brain activity a complex event that involves dramatic changes in neural and vascular function (Charles & Baca, 2013). The early authors that described this work, such as Leao (Dalkara & Moskowitz, 2017), suggested that vascular change is due to vasodilation; however, further work has suggested the vasodilation is then followed by vasoconstriction of the cerebral blood flow (Borgdorff, 2018).

Cervicogenic headache disorder (CGH) is the most common headache presentation encountered by musculoskeletal practitioners. CGH is defined as a secondary headache disorder arising from musculoskeletal dysfunction in nociceptive structures in the upper three cervical segments or occipital region. Pain originating in the neck is proposed to be referred to the head via the TCN, which descends into the spinal cord to the level of C3/4. The TCN is anatomically and functionally continuous with the dorsal grey columns of these spinal segments. The trigeminal nucleus is divided into the main sensory nucleus and spinal tract nuclei located caudally in the cervical spinal cord. Convergence forms the proposed neuro-anatomical basis for the CGH as convergence of the primary afferents of the upper three levels in the cervical spine with the TCN have been established (Choi & Sang, 2016). Hence, input via sensory afferents principally from any of the upper three cervical nerve roots will be perceived as pain in the head.

Several studies have reported the provocation of headache by stimulation of nociceptive afferents in upper cervical structures (Bogduk & Bartsch, 2008). Application of firm pressure to myofascial structures of the upper cervical segments (C0-3) stimulating a mechanical nociceptive afferent response has been shown to provoke headaches in patients with CGH, TTH, and migraine leading to challenges in differentiation (Jull & Hall, 2018; Anarte et al., 2019; Cescon et al., 2019). Painful soft tissue structures may sensitize 'wide-dynamic range cells' at the dorsal horn due to convergence leading to the experience of painful symptoms in the distributions of the TCN. Cervical musculoskeletal dysfunctions of joints and muscles have been observed in patients with cervicogenic headaches. In the context of the neurophysiological interconnection between the dorsal root of C2 (greater occipital nerve) and the TCN, it may be not surprising that in participants with headaches, most cervical musculoskeletal dysfunctions reported are present in the UCS (Zito et al., 2006; Amiri et al., 2007). Therefore, manual therapy assessment may include palpation of the sub-occipital muscles and trapezius, local assessment of restricted motion of the cervical segments C0-3 and application of load to joints in the UCS to assess whether direct palpation will reproduce the experience of the headache and therefore support a confirmatory diagnosis (Luedtke et al., 2016). An over-arching set of diagnostic criteria are set out in Table 7.2.

TABLE 7.2 Supportive Criteria in Cervicogenic Headache

	Provocation of the headache radiating from the cervical spine.
1	Loss of neck movement
2	External pressure on the occipital or higher cervical region on the symptomatic side.
3	Ipsilateral; neck, shoulder, arm pain that is non-radicular in origin.
4	Positive response to diagnostic blocks in the upper cervical spine.

Adapted from Sjaastad et al. (1998) and Arnold (2018).

Clinical Assessment in Cervicogenic Headache Disorder

Manual examination of the cervical spine structures reviewing local tone and pain responses seeking to reproduce the features of neck pain and headache are advised as part of a multi-modal assessment. Specific tests such as the cervical flexion rotation test (Ogince et al., 2007) have been validated in the presence of CGH. Further features leading to sensitization of structures and pain experiences are also vitally important to consider as part of a broad assessment. Considerations of muscular strength, general spinal mobility and sensorimotor capacity would also be advised as part of a comprehensive MSK assessment.

Initial observations of patient posture inclusive of range of motion will further inform the possible diagnosis. An association with a forward head posture with patients reporting CGH has not been supported Dumas et al. (2001) and Watson and Trott (1993) found a weak correlation with a reduction in neck angle. However, a meta-analysis conducted by Gadotti et al. (2008) identified a reduction in head range of motion in the CGH group when compared to matched controls.

The flexion-rotation test has reported validity and reliability in the assessment of CGH (Hall et al., 2010b). The flexion-rotation test is conducted with the cervical spine fully flexed to block as much rotational movement as possible above and below C1/2. The head is then rotated to the left and the right. If firm resistance is encountered and range is limited before the expected end range, then this is said to be clinically significant, with a presumptive diagnosis of limited rotation of the atlas on the axis (Hall & Robinson, 2004) (Fig 7.6). Manual examination has reported high sensitivity and specificity in detecting the presence or absence of cervical joint dysfunction (Jull et al., 1988). Moreover, Zito et al. (2006) determined upper cervical joint dysfunction detected by manual examination most clearly identified CGH sufferers, when compared to measures of posture, range of motion, cervical kinesthesia, and craniocervical muscle function. The term 'manual examination' incorporates tests of passive physiological intervertebral motion (PPIVMS), as well as passive accessory intervertebral motion (PAIVMs), e.g. posteroanterior pressures. Motion restriction and symptom responses indicate the most painful dysfunctional cervical motion segment (Jull, 1997) although the reliability of these tests has been questioned (Jonsson & Rasmussen-Barr, 2018).

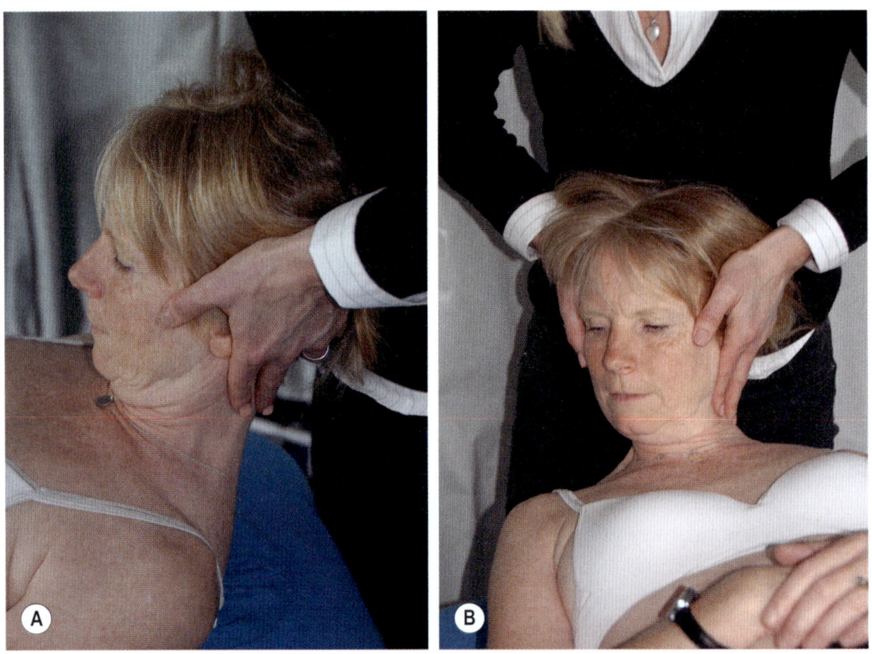

Fig. 7.6 Flexion–rotation Test. Patient in supine crook-lying and head extended beyond the end of the couch. (A) The clinician fully flexes the cervical spine to 'lock up' the subaxial spine and bias rotation to the C1–C2 level. (B) The clinician rotates the patient's head to the right and then to the left. The amount of movement is compared.

Olivier et al. (2018) found a strong correlation with pain sensitivity in the upper trapezius muscles in cervicogenic headache patients versus non-CGH. Muscular sensitivity is often associated with muscle tightness—that is, increased muscle tone (Chen & Ayata, 2016). Jull et al. (1999) investigated upper cervical muscle tightness in 15 CGH patients and 15 asymptomatic controls. They found resistance to passive muscle stretch was significantly increased in the upper trapezius muscles in the CGH group but not in any of the other muscles tested—namely, levator scapulae, scalenes (anterior, middle, and posterior divisions), and the short upper cervical extensors.

KNOWLEDGE CHECK

1. Name the common headache disorders seen in musculoskeletal practice.
2. What are the common key features of a cervicogenic headache?
3. What physical tests would be useful in the identification of a cervicogenic headache?

Upper Cervical Spine Dizziness and Proprioception

The SOMs located deep in the UCS (rectus capitis, posterior major, rectus capitis posterior minor, obliquus capitis superior and obliquus capitis inferior) have a high muscle spindle density that allows for flexible movement and sensory awareness (Kulkarni et al., 2001) The long flexors of the neck (longus colli and longus capitis) also contribute proprioceptive input to control the movement of the neck (Falla et al., 2004). Injuries such as whiplash can alter sensory feedback from the muscle groups, disrupting cervical proprioception which may present as sensations of dizziness (Sung, 2020). Cervicogenic dizziness (CGD) is a clinical syndrome without definitive tests so differentiation from other common causes of dizziness such as vestibular and vascular can be a challenge. However, the presence of neck pain should be associated with a hypothesis of CGD. Commonly CGD does not include tinnitus or hearing loss. If these symptoms are present, then the clinician should be alerted that an inner ear problem is more likely. Benign paroxysmal positional vertigo (BPPV) presenting with dizziness is a common vestibular problem associated with the attachment of inorganic material to the cupula of the posterior vertical semicircular canal (Schmidt, 1998). The cervical neck torsion test can be used to differentiate. The test is performed with the patient's head stabilized whilst their trunk is rotated; this also produces neck rotation but maintains a stationary head position (Fig 7.7). If dizziness is elicited this is more likely to be cervical in origin. Further clinical tests for CGD are highlighted below.

Whiplash-Related Dizziness

People with whiplash-associated disorders (WADs) report unsteadiness, pain and dizziness with over 50% exhibiting visual problems (Treleaven et al., 2003).

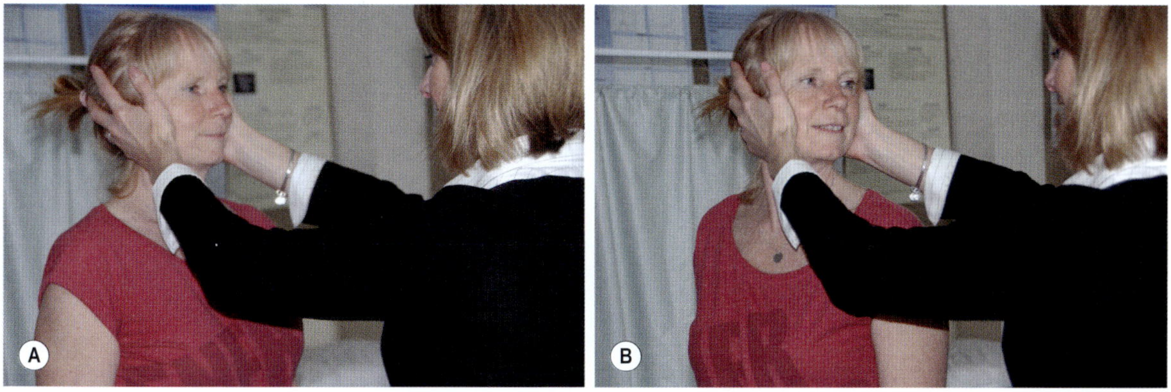

Fig. 7.7 Differential Diagnosis of Dizziness. (A) In standing, the clinician maintains the patient's head in neutral; this prevents movement within the vestibular system. (B) The patient moves the trunk to the left and then to the right in order to produce cervical rotation. Each position is held for 10 seconds, with a 10-second rest period between directions. (From Magarey et al. 2004.)

Alteration in vision can be linked to the oculomotor system which maintains the eye on a target. Eye movement is dependent on head position and on eye position within the head (Corneil, 2011). WAD disrupts cervical afferent information leading to increased cervical muscular activity, altered proprioception, and ultimately resulting in oculomotor dysfunctions, balance changes and dizziness (Fischer et al., 1997; Boo et al., 2020). Three documented reflexes serve this system. The cervico-ocular (COR), vestibulo-ocular reflex (VOR) and optokinetic reflex (OKR), with the COR receiving input from muscle spindles in the cervical spine in the deep cervical musculature and joint capsules from C1 to C3 (Ischebeck et al., 2016).

Tests for oculomotor function

1. **Gaze stability**—the patient has to keep the eyes focused on a point ahead while rotating the neck.
2. **Smooth pursuit neck torsion test** which aids in differentiating between cervical spine causes of dizziness and other causes such as vestibular. In the test eye movement is observed in either a forward-facing position or with the trunk in rotation. The patient must follow a line or moving red dot in a horizontal manner in neutral and 45 degrees cervical spine rotation (Treleaven et al., 2005). The clinician closely observes the patient's eye movements throughout both tests looking for jerky or fast movements, with reported increased effort, pain or dizziness. Tjell and Rosenhall (1998) have demonstrated that smooth pursuit changes occur in the neck rotation position in patients with a neck dysfunction and not in those with a vestibular presentation. If there is any difference noted when the neck is in rotation it may indicate a cervical contribution to impaired proprioception and dizziness.

KNOWLEDGE CHECK

1. What muscles contribute to proprioception in the upper cervical spine?
2. What reflexes are involved in the proprioception of the head on the neck?
3. What tests could you use to assess for oculomotor dysfunction and what would indicate an abnormal finding?

SUBJECTIVE EXAMINATION/TAKING THE PATIENT'S HISTORY

The Patient's Perspective on their Experience

Symptoms associated with UCS dysfunction such as pain, dizziness and visual changes can be especially worrying for the patient. How a patient interprets their symptoms will be influenced by their thoughts, beliefs, emotions and social context (Linton & Shaw, 2011). In order to treat the patient appropriately, these should be explored at the outset.

There are a number of self-reported tools that can be used to measure patient's perception of disability and help identify personal and environmental factors that may present as barriers to recovery, e.g. the Headache Disability Index Questionnaire and Headache Disability Questionnaire (Jacobson et al., 1994; Niere & Quin, 2009) (Appendices 7.1 and 7.2).

Body Chart

Firstly, the area and type of the patient's symptoms need to be carefully mapped out. Typically, patients with UCS disorders have localized pain around the occiput and pain over the head and/or face. Patients with CGH usually present with a unilateral, side-consistent headache (Bogduk & Govind, 2009).

It is also important to ask about the presence of other symptoms such as disequilibrium, dizziness and altered sensation. Patients with CGH may have associated nausea, photophobia, dizziness and blurred vision but since these are also symptoms of cervical arterial dysfunction (CAD), which can present as a headache in the early stages, careful screening of the risk factors for CAD and the signs and symptoms of brainstem ischemia needs to be carried out. (For further information the reader is directed to Rushton et al., 2020 and Chapter 8 Barnard & Ryder, 2024.) If the patient describes symptoms suggestive of CAD the clinician proceeds with a thorough assessment for potential neurovascular pathology (Kerry & Taylor, 2006; Rushton et al., 2014)

Relationship of Symptoms

Determine the relationship between the symptomatic areas—do the symptoms come on together or separately? For example, if the patient has a headache, do they also have neck pain? If so, does one pain start first? Do they both come on together or do they come on independently? Patients with CGH usually complain of a headache that starts in the suboccipital region and radiates forward into the head, face and/or eye (Hall et al., 2008b; Jull et al., 2008b; Bogduk & Govind, 2009).

Behaviour of Symptoms

Aggravating Factors

For each symptomatic area, discover what movements and/or positions aggravate the patient's symptoms and how long it takes to bring the symptoms on (or make them worse). Is the patient able to maintain this position or movement? What happens to other symptoms when this symptom is produced (or made worse)? How long does it take for symptoms to ease once the position or movement is stopped? These questions help to confirm the relationship between the symptoms and the irritability of the condition.

The clinician can also ask the patient about theoretically known aggravating factors for structures that could be a source of the symptoms. For example, repeated or sustained neck movements (e.g. rotation) or sustained, awkward head postures (e.g. chin poke position) may be a precipitating factor in CGH (Gadotti et al., 2008).

It is helpful to establish whether the patient is left- or right-handed and which is their dominant eye. Both factors may alter the stresses placed on UCS structures. It is also helpful to ascertain how the symptoms affect the patient's function; for example, what are the symptoms like during static and active postures involving the UCS, e.g. sitting, driving, reading, computer work, watching TV, sport and social activities.

Easing Factors

The clinician can ask the patient about theoretically known easing factors for structures that could be a source of the symptoms. For example, supporting the head or neck may ease symptoms from the UCS. The clinician can analyse the position or movement that eases the symptoms to help determine the structure at fault and to guide treatment selection.

Twenty-Four-Hour Behaviour of Symptoms

The clinician determines the pattern of the symptoms first thing in the morning, through the day, at the end of the day and during the night.

Night Symptoms

- What is your normal sleeping position? Do you sleep on your front?
- What is your present sleeping position?
- How many and what type of pillows do you use? Is your mattress firm or soft?
- Do your symptoms wake you at night? If so, which symptoms?
- How many times in a night/week?
- Can you get back to sleep, how long does it take and what do you have to do?

Special/Red-Flag Screening Questions

The clinician must differentiate between conditions in the UCS that are suitable for conservative management. Chapter 3 provides full details of general screening questions used to identify any precautions or contraindications to the physical exam and/or treatment. The aim of red-flag screening is to exclude serious or life-threatening pathology in the UCS, such as cranial tumours, spinal metastases, cord compression, spinal infection, inflammatory arthritis and subarachnoid haemorrhage which would require referral to a medical practitioner (Rubio-Ochoa et al., 2016). See Table 7.3 for general red-flag screening relevant to the cervical spine (Greenhalgh & Selfe, 2009). 'SNOOP' is a useful mnemonic to aid red flag screening in the cervical spine (Table 7.4).

For further information see Chapter 9, Considering serious pathology, Barnard and Ryder (2024).

Cervical Arterial Dysfunction

The close proximity of the cervical arteries to the cervical vertebrae means that movements of the UCS, particularly rotation and extension, can affect blood flow through the cervical arteries (Thomas, 2016). With an intact circle of Willis and good collateral flow, this is generally not problematic as the body can compensate for changes in flow without incident. However, manual therapy techniques and exercises directed at the UCS could have an adverse effect in patients who have abnormal cervical vessels or in whom collateral flow is inadequate. This could contribute to an 'at-risk' patient having a haemodynamic event as a result of physiotherapy treatment. Early signs and symptoms of CAD can mimic musculoskeletal dysfunction of the UCS (see Chapter 8 Barnard & Ryder, 2024; Kerry & Taylor 2006; Bogduk & Govind 2009). In the pre-ischaemic stage, CAD can present as pain in the UCS and head (Fig. 7.8).

TABLE 7.3 **General Red-Flag Screening for the Cervical Spine**

RED FLAGS		
Age of onset 20–55 years	Violent trauma	
Constant progressive pain	Systemic steroids	
Unremitting night pain	Drug abuse/human immunodeficiency virus	
Weight loss	Systemically unwell	
Widespread neurology	Past medical history of cancer	
Thoracic pain	Structural deformity	
Signs and Symptoms of Serious Spinal Pathology in the Cervical Spine		
Spinal Cancer	**Cord Compression**	**Spinal Fracture**
Age >50 Previous history of cancer Unexplained weight loss >5%–10% of body weight Failure of >1 month of conservative treatment	Clumsiness of extremities—difficulty with fine motor skills of hands Stumbling gait L'Hermitte's sign Unilateral or bilateral paraesthesias or anaesthesias Bowel or bladder dysfunction	Age >50 History of trauma History of osteoporosis History of systemic steroid use
Cluster of all four red flags provides a very high index of suspicion of spinal cancer with a diagnostic accuracy of sensitivity 1.0 + specificity 0.6		

Greenhalgh and Selfe (2009).

TABLE 7.4 **'SNOOP' Is a Useful Mnemonic to Aid Red Flag Screening in the Cervical Spine**

Sign or Symptom	Related Headache
Systemic	Headache associated with infection or nonvascular intracranial disorders
Neoplasm Neurological	Neoplasms of brain: metastasis Headache attributed to vascular and non-vascular intracranial disorders
Onset—abrupt	cervical/cranial vascular disorders
Older >50	Giant cell arteritis
Post trauma. Positional. Painkillers	Subdural hematoma. Intracranial hyper/hypotension. Medication overuse

Adapted from Do et al. (2019).

If the pathology develops, signs and symptoms of brain ischaemia may present (Table 7.5). Although CAD is a rare occurrence, care needs to be taken to differentiate vascular sources of pain from musculoskeletal sources, with the key aim being to avoid any catastrophic neurovascular event (Bogduk & Govind, 2009; Thomas, 2016).

Current evidence suggests that the most appropriate way to identify the presence of altered cervical haemodynamics or to predict the risk of a physiotherapy-induced neurovascular event is by careful assessment of the whole vascular system, checking the patient's general cardiovascular health and screening for signs and symptoms associated with CAD (Rushton et al., 2014; Thomas, 2016). These are listed in Table 7.5 and can be used by the clinician as a basis for screening questions for CAD.

Many patients present with treatable craniocervical musculoskeletal symptoms, such as neck pain, CGH

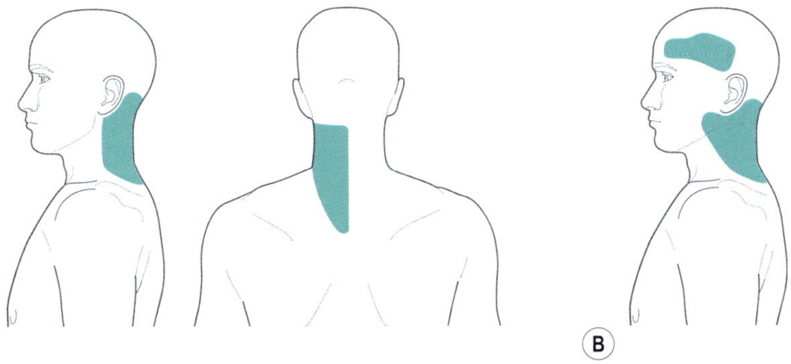

Fig. 7.8 (A) Typical pain presentation for vertebral artery dissection. (B) Typical pain presentation for internal carotid artery dissection. (From McCarthy 2010, with permission.)

TABLE 7.5 Risk Factors, Signs and Symptoms of Cervical Artery Dysfunction

	Pre-ischaemic	Ischaemic
Internal carotid artery cervical arterial dysfunction	Neck/temporal/parietal/frontal pain. Horner's syndrome, pulsatile tinnitus, cranial nerve palsies (CN IX–XII)	Transient ischaemic attack, retinal infarction, stroke
Vertebral artery cervical arterial dysfunction	Acute/recent onset of unusual ipsilateral posterior neck pain or occipital headache	5 Ds: dizziness, diplopia, dysarthria, dysphagia, drop attacks 3 Ns: facial numbness, nystagmus, nausea
Risk factors for cervical arterial dysfunction	Recent exposure to minor trauma Recent infection or viral illness Atherosclerosis risk factors Hypertension Hypercholesterolaemia Cardiac disease, vascular disease or history of cerebrovascular accident or transient ischaemic attack Diabetes mellitus Oral contraceptives Long-term use of steroids Smoking Upper cervical instability	

Kerry and Taylor, 2010), Rushton et al. (2014), Taylor and Kerry (2015), Thomas (2016).

and cervicogenic dizziness, but also with many of the risk factors identified in Table 7.5. This does not necessarily exclude them from manual therapy treatment. Careful clinical reasoning and monitoring of signs and symptoms are required in the management of these patients (Taylor & Kerry, 2010). The patient history, recognizing the potential risk factors for vascular pathology, is cited as vital to the clinical reasoning process, such as recent trauma, vascular anomalies and smoking (Hutting et al., 2021). The reader is advised to review the IFOMT Framework (Rushton et al., 2020), which offers guidance for the examination of the cervical spine for potential vascular pathologies. The framework clearly identifies the risk factors associated with vascular pathologies and treatment of the cervical spine, highlighting potential risks for dissection, non-dissection events and the reported symptoms. Headache is cited as the most commonly reported symptom for both, whilst visual changes, paraesthesia and dizziness should raise suspicion of the possibility of a vascular element. Clinical signs are described as unsteadiness, dysphagia, dysarthria, weakness, dysphasia, dizziness and alterations in cognition. If frank vascular pathology is identified, the IFOMPT Framework recommends ensuring the local policy is followed for appropriate urgent onward referral for further investigations.

KNOWLEDGE CHECK

1. What is the mnemonic for red flags in the upper cervical spine?
2. What symptoms indicate a possible cervical arterial dysfunction of the upper cervical spine?
3. What are the risk factors for cervical arterial dysfunction?

PHYSICAL EXAMINATION

An outline examination chart may be useful for some clinicians, and one is suggested in Fig. 3.8. It is important, however, that clinicians do not examine in a rigid manner. Each patient presents differently, and this should be reflected in the examination process. The tests and order of testing described below will not be appropriate or relevant to every patient with a UCS disorder. Selected tests need to be matched to the severity and irritability of the hypotheses generated. For example, if a peripheral neuropathic pain mechanism is suspected, a neurological examination will need to be included.

Observation

The clinician observes the patient in unsupported sitting or standing depending on what is relevant for that patient. One of the key elements of assessing the relevance of posture is to see whether the patient can adopt a position and whether that alters presenting symptoms. Once a patient experiences a difference in the presenting symptom, this modification can be used as a treatment guideline.

Active Physiological Movement

The clinician observes:

The range of movement and quality, e.g. where the movement is occurring:

- During full flexion can the patient perform a chin nod prior to lower cervical flexion?
- During full extension can the patient lift the chin up towards the ceiling prior to lower cervical extension?
- Does the patient return from full cervical extension in a 'chin poke' position, suggesting reliance on SCM, or can the patient tuck the chin in and curl the spine back from extension?
- During side flexion does the chin swing laterally, indicating that some side flexion has occurred in the UCS, or does the chin stay more or less in the midline, suggesting lower cervical dominance into side flexion with a potentially hypomobile UCS?
- During rotation is there a natural head-on-neck 'spinning' motion or does the patient 'carry' the head on the UCS, suggesting a more dominant mid-lower cervical spine movement with potential hypomobility at C1–C2?

Behaviour of pain and resistance through the range of movement and at the end of range of movement. Provocation of any muscle spasm.

The clinician establishes the patient's symptoms at rest and on each movement and corrects any movement deviation to determine relevance to the patient's symptoms. Overpressure is only added when a movement is full-range and pain-free to establish if active and passive ranges of motion are similar and if end of range produces pain (Fig 7.9).

Active movement testing can be used as a reassessment marker.

Differentiation Tests

Other regions may need to be examined to determine their relevance to the patient's symptoms; they may be the source of the symptoms or a contributing factor. The most likely regions are the TMJ, lower cervical spine and thoracic spine. Studies have demonstrated that movements of upper cervical protraction and retraction involve a 30% contribution from C7 to T4 and 10% from T5 to T12, suggesting that the thoracic spine and UCS are biomechanically interdependent (Persson et al., 2007). The joints within these regions can be tested fully (see relevant chapters) or partially with the use of screening tests (see Table 4.4 for further details).

Neurological Testing

A comprehensive neurological examination includes neurological integrity testing and neurodynamic tests.

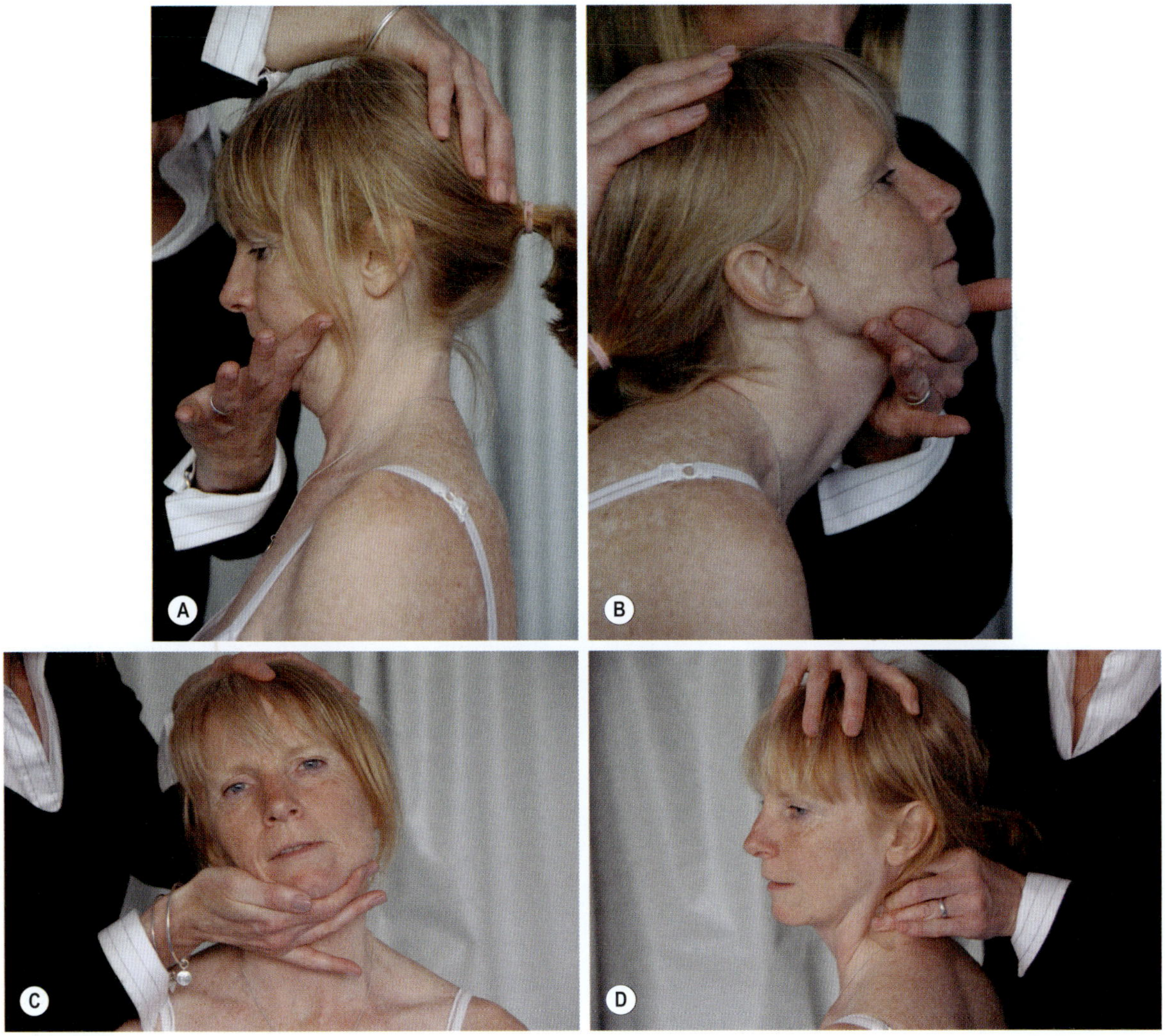

Fig. 7.9 (A) Upper cervical flexion (retraction) + overpressure. (B) Upper cervical extension (protraction) + overpressure. (C) Upper cervical side flexion + overpressure directed towards the opposite shoulder. (D) Upper cervical rotation + overpressure applied through the crown of the head with C2 stabilized using a pincer grip.

Neurological integrity testing, if indicated, is normally carried out early on in the examination process from a safety perspective.

Integrity of the Nervous System

Generally, if symptoms are localized to the UCS and head, a neurological examination can be limited to the cranial nerves and the cervical plexus (C1–C4 nerve roots) (Table 7.6).

Dermatomes/Peripheral Nerves

Light touch and pain sensation of the face, head and neck are tested using cotton wool and pinprick respectively, as described in Chapter 4 and outlined in Table 7.6. Knowledge of dermatomal patterns for the upper cervical nerve roots as well as the cutaneous field of innervation of the upper cervical peripheral nerves will enable the clinician to distinguish between any sensory loss due to a nerve root lesion from that due to

TABLE 7.6 Neurological Conductivity Testing for the Craniocervical Spine

CRANIAL NERVE TESTING

Nerve	Afferent	Efferent	Test
I. Olfactory	Smell		Smell 2–3 familiar items, eyes closed, e.g. coffee/soap/chocolate
II. Optic	Sight		Visual fields: Snellen eye chart
III. Oculomotor		Eye movement: up, down and medial gaze	Patient keeps head still and follows clinician's finger with the eyes. Clinician draws an 'H' shape in front of patient. Then clinician moves finger to patient's nose, to test patient's ability to converge the gaze
IV. Trochlear		Eye movement: down and lateral gaze	
V. Trigeminal	Skin of face	Muscles of mastication	Light touch and pinprick to forehead, cheek and lateral jaw. Clench teeth: clinician palpates masseter and temporalis bilaterally for strength of contraction. Separate jaw: clinician assesses strength of jaw opening against moderate resistance
VI. Abducens		Eye movement: lateral gaze	Tested with H movement test
VII. Facial	Taste anterior aspect of tongue (sweet)	Facial muscles	Patient asked to smile, frown, elevate eyebrows and puff out cheeks
VIII. Vestibulocochlear	Hearing and balance		Hearing: patient's eyes closed, clinician rubs pad of thumb and index finger together next to patient's ear. Determine if the patient can hear it. Test one ear at a time. Hearing should be symmetrical Balance: patient is asked to stand with eyes closed, unsupported for 30 s
IX. Glossopharyngeal	Touch and taste posterior tongue (sour)	Gag reflex Ability to swallow	Ask patient to open mouth and say 'ah': watch uvula; it should not deviate laterally Ability to swallow: ask patient to swallow, watch movement of throat and ask if there are any difficulties
X. Vagus		Muscles of pharynx and larynx	Tested above
XI. Accessory		Sternocleidomastoid and trapezius	Resisted shoulder shrug, check for symmetry and strength and observe for wasting
XII. Hypoglossal		Tongue movement	Patient asked to stick tongue out—should be straight; observe for any side-to-side deviation

Continued

CERVICAL PLEXUS		
Nerve	**Afferent (Dermatome)**	**Efferent (Myotome)**
C1		Upper cervical flexion
C2	Skin over posterior aspect of skull	Upper cervical extension
C3	Skin around posterior aspect of neck	Cervical lateral flexion
C4 and CN XI	Skin over shoulder girdle region	Shoulder girdle elevation

CN, Cranial nerve.

a peripheral nerve lesion. The UCS cutaneous nerve distribution and dermatomal areas are shown in Chapter 4, Fig. 4.16.

Myotomes/Peripheral Nerves

See Table 7.6 and Fig. 4.8 for a description of appropriate myotomal testing in the UCS for the upper cervical and cranial nerves.

Reflex Testing

There are no deep tendon reflexes for C1–C4 nerve roots. The jaw jerk (cranial nerve [CN] V) is elicited by applying a sharp downward tap on the chin with the mouth slightly open. A slight jerk is normal; excessive jerk suggests a bilateral upper motor neuron lesion.

Pathological Reflex Testing for Upper Motor Neuron Lesion

The following reflexes can be tested to check for an upper motor neuron lesion (Fuller, 1993). Both of these tests are described in Chapter 4 and are relevant for a CCS neurological examination:

- plantar response
- clonus.

Neurodynamic Tests

The following neurodynamic tests may be carried out in order to ascertain the degree to which neural tissue is responsible for the production of the patient's symptom(s) in the UCS:

- passive neck flexion
- upper-limb neurodynamic tests
- straight-leg raise
- slump.

These tests are described in detail in Chapter 4.

Palpation

PPIVMs examine the amount and quality of physiological movement available at each upper cervical level.

Flexion–extension PPIVM at C0–C1.

For application of technique, see Fig. 7.10A and B.

Side-flexion PPIVM at C0–C1.

For application of technique, see Fig. 7.10C.

Rotation PPIVM at C1–C2.

For application of technique, see Fig. 7.10D.

Flexion–Rotation Test

The flexion–rotation test can determine segmental dysfunction at C1–C2 even in the presence of a normal active range of movement. Studies have demonstrated that it has very high diagnostic utility (sensitivity = 90% and specificity = 88%) in relation to differentiating CGH of C1–C2 origin from other headache types, and it has been shown that therapists can detect these differences reliably (Ogince et al., 2007; Hall et al. 2008a, 2010a, b). The average range of C1–C2 rotation in asymptomatic subjects is between 39 and 42 degrees (Hall & Robinson, 2004).

For test application, see Fig. 7.6.

Test interpretation: the flexion–rotation test is positive if the amount of C1–C2 rotation to the side of pain is less than 32 degrees, although many subjects with CGH often have a range of around 20 degrees towards the symptomatic side (Hall & Robinson, 2004).

Accessory Movements

PAIVMs are commonly used in the UCS to gain information about the amount and quality of accessory movement available and the pain response at each upper cervical segmental level (Zito et al. 2006; Jull et al.

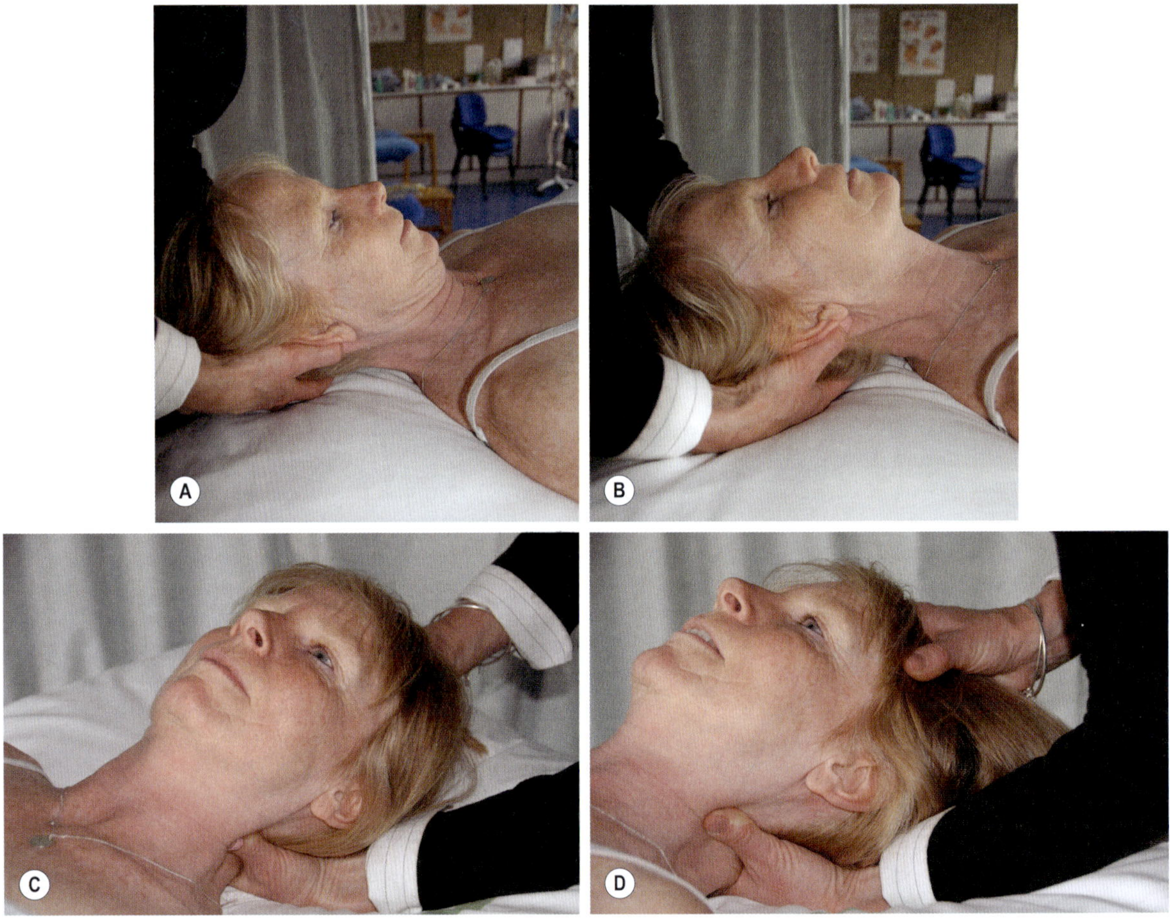

Fig. 7.10 (A and B) Flexion–extension passive physiological intervertebral movement (PPIVM) C0–C1: patient in supine, head on a pillow. Clinician cradles the patient's occiput with fingers 3–5 and palpates between the mastoid process and the lateral aspect of C1 using the tips of the thumbs. Clinician rocks the patient's head forwards and backwards in a head-on-neck nodding moment. The small amount of movement between the two bony points on each side is assessed. (C) Side-flexion PPIVM C0–C1: same starting position as for flexion-extension PPIVM. Clinician moves the patient's head into upper cervical side flexion. If the technique is performed correctly, the clinician should see a 'chin swing' to the opposite side of the side flexion being carried out (e.g. left 'chin swing' for right side flexion). The small amount of movement between the two bony points on each side is assessed. (D) Rotation PPIVM C1–C2: patient in supine, head on a pillow. Clinician grips C2 spinous process using a pincer grip with the left hand. The right hand holds the crown of the patient's head. Clinician moves the patient's head into right rotation. The point at which the C2 spinous process is felt to move to the left is assessed. The test is repeated into left rotation. It is usually more accurate to swap hands over. The amount of rotation to both sides is compared.

2007). PAIVMs can be examined with the patient's UCS in a neutral or combined position, and the techniques can be applied with a medial, lateral, cephalad or caudad bias (Maitland et al., 2005). See Box 4.3 for hints on performing accessory movements.

The accessory movements commonly tested at C1–C4 in neutral are:

- central posteroanterior
- unilateral posteroanterior
- unilateral anteroposterior.

On application of the accessory movement being tested, the clinician notes the following during early, mid and late range, taking the patient's severity and irritability into consideration:

- range and quality of movement
- resistance through the range and at the end of the range of movement
- behaviour of pain through the range
- provocation of any muscle spasm.

See Fig. 7.11. Other cervical levels are shown in Chapter 8.

It is useful to record findings on a palpation chart and/or movement diagrams (see Figs. 4.38–4.45). These are explained in detail in Chapter 4.

Accessory Movements as a Combined Technique

Accessory movements can be applied in combined positions to increase or decrease the stretch on upper cervical facet joints, joint capsules or surrounding paravertebral muscles. The different combinations can be quite confusing. Table 7.7 shows some possible combinations of starting positions and accessory movements that will increase the stretch on different aspects of the A-O and A-A joints. For a full description of upper cervical accessory movements in combined positions, see Edwards (1994, 1999).

Following accessory movements to the UCS, the clinician reassesses all the physical asterisks (movements or tests that have been found to reproduce the patient's

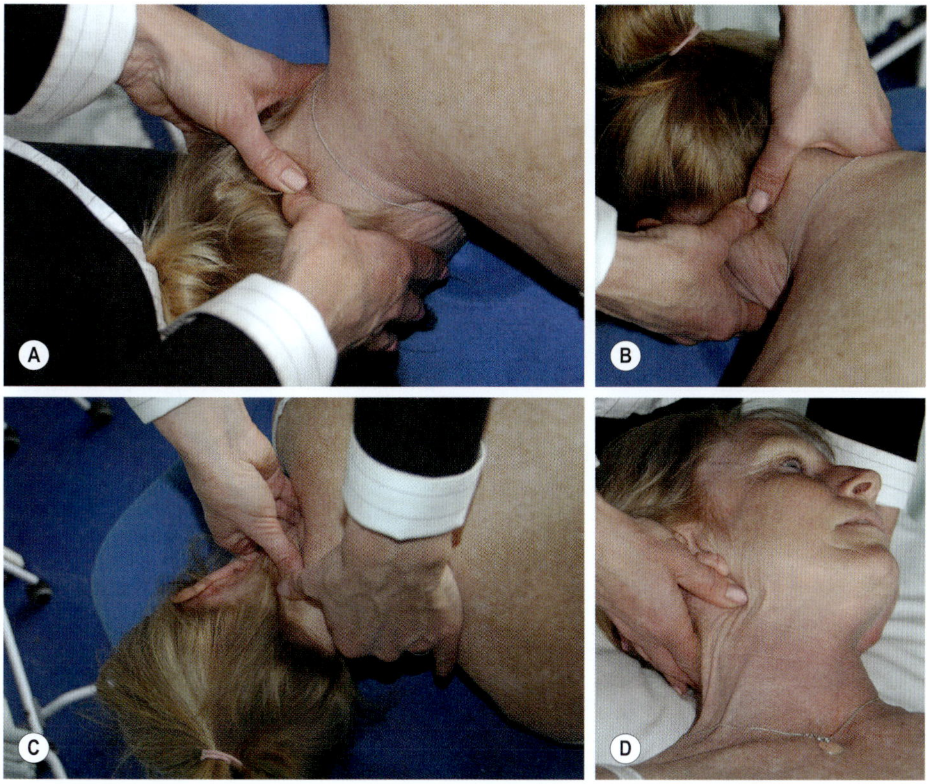

Fig. 7.11 Accessory Movement to C1. (A) Central posterior-anterior accessory movement. Pressure is applied through the thumbs onto the posterior arch of C1, directed cephaladly towards the patient's eyes. (B) Unilateral posterior–anterior accessory movement. Thumb pressure is applied laterally over the posterior arch of C1. (C) Transverse pressure. Thumb pressure is applied to the transverse process of C1. (D) Unilateral anteroposterior accessory movement. Thumb pressure is applied over the anterior aspect of the C1 transverse process.

TABLE 7.7 Passive Accessory Intervertebral Movements as a Combined Technique

Level	Combined Starting Position	Accessory	Effect
Atlantooccipital joint	In prone: flexion + right rotation (nose stays within head hole)	Unilateral posteroanterior right C1	Increase stretch posterior aspect C0–C1
	In supine: extension + left rotation	Unilateral anteroposterior on right C1	Increase stretch anterior aspect C0–C1
Atlantoaxial joint	In prone: right rotation to 30 degrees (nose rotated out of head hole) + flexion	Unilateral posteroanterior on right C2	Increase stretch posterior aspect C1–C2
	In prone: right rotation to 30 degrees (nose rotated out of head hole) + extension	Unilateral posteroanterior on right C2	Increase stretch anterior aspect C1–C2

symptoms) to establish the effect of the accessory movements on the patient's signs and symptoms.

Passive physiological and accessory movements can also be tested in other regions suspected to be a source of, or contributing to, the symptoms. Regions likely to be examined are the TMJ, lower cervical spine and upper thoracic spine.

Sustained Natural Apophyseal Glides (SNAGs)

SNAGs are indicated for peripheral nociceptive, arthrogenic and mechanical disorders. When correctly selected and applied SNAGs should:

- Decrease or relieve the patient's pain immediately
- increase the range of movement
- increase function.

For patients complaining of headaches, Mulligan (2010) describes four examination techniques:

- headache SNAGs (Fig. 7.12A)
- reverse headache SNAGs (Fig. 7.12B)
- upper cervical traction (Fig. 7.12C)
- SNAGs for restricted cervical rotation at C1–C2

For patients with upper cervical neck pain and loss of movement, suggested techniques include:

- SNAG to spinous process of C2–C4 + dysfunctional movement, e.g. rotation
- SNAG to transverse process of C2–C4 + dysfunctional movement.

For a full description of each technique, see Mulligan (2010).

Symptom Modification and Mini Treatments

In addition to gathering information throughout the physical examination about pain reproduction and movement dysfunction, the clinician may decide to perform 'mini treatments' on the symptomatic or dysfunctional spinal segment using carefully reasoned and selected techniques, for example, PPIVMs, PAIVMs, natural apophyseal glides (NAGs) and SNAGs, trigger points or hold–relax muscle techniques. Assessing the effect of the mini treatments using selected physical markers can help the clinician to confirm a working hypothesis for the patient's disorder and can also help to determine which treatment may have the biggest impact.

Muscle Testing

Muscle Strength

Changes in muscle strength, endurance and fatigability have been identified in the cervical flexors, extensors and axioscapular muscles in patients with neck pain and CGH of both insidious and traumatic onset (Jull et al., 1999, 2004, 2008a; Jull, 2000; Falla, 2004; Falla et al., 2004; O'Leary et al., 2007).

Isotonic Testing

The clinician may want to test the general strength of the cervical muscles isotonically whilst observing the quality of muscle contraction and motor recruitment patterns. This can be done in supine or prone with the head in a neutral or rotated position by asking the patient simply to lift the head off the bed. Different starting positions will bias strength testing to different muscle groups. Pillows can be used to make the test easier.

Isometric Testing

This can help to differentiate symptoms from inert structures and contractile structures. The CCS is

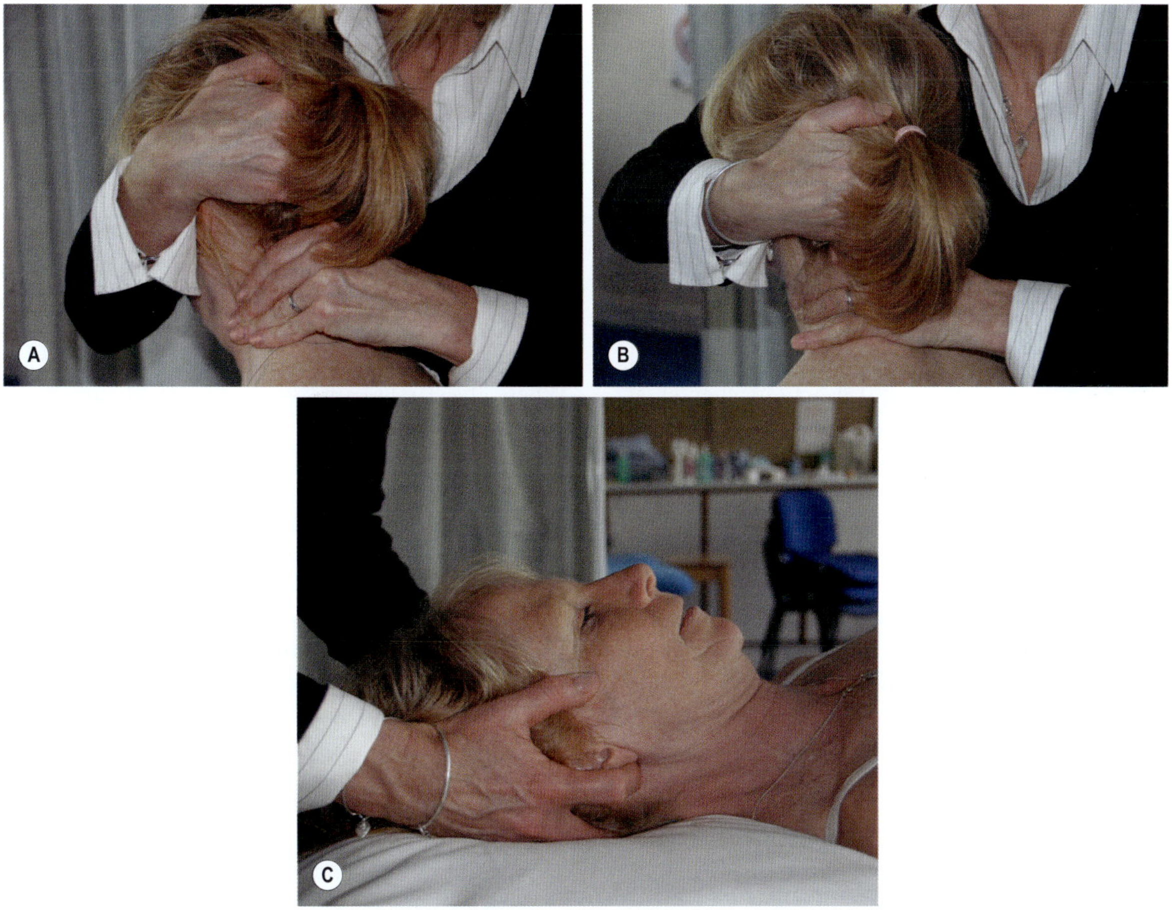

Fig. 7.12 (A) Headache sustained natural apophyseal glide (SNAG). (B) Reverse headache SNAG. (C) Cervical traction at C1–C2.

positioned in neutral and the patient is asked to hold this position against the resistance of the clinician. The clinician can provide resistance to any direction of movement and also in different parts of the range. If symptoms are reproduced on contraction this may suggest a contractile tissue disorder.

For details of these general tests, see Jull et al. (2008c). Testing the strength of these muscles is also described in Chapter 4.

Sensorimotor Control

Sensorimotor control is the integration and coordination of sensory and motor information by the central nervous system to regulate joint stability, movement acuity, coordination and balance (Roijezon et al., 2015). Afferent information from the periphery (visual, vestibular and proprioceptive systems) is combined and used to elicit an appropriate motor response from the postural muscles before and during movement (Treleaven, 2008).

Clinically, alterations in sensorimotor function in the CCS are associated with lasting pain, loss of movement, dizziness, nausea, visual disturbance, hearing disturbances and loss of postural stability (Jull et al., 2008e; Treleaven, 2008).

A growing body of evidence suggests that proprioception and motor control in the cervical spine are altered in response to pain, effusion, trauma and fatigue (Jull, 2000; Falla, 2004; Falla et al., 2004; Jull et al., 2004; Treleaven, 2011; de Vries et al., 2015; Roijezon et al., 2015). Changes include:

- increased cervical joint position sense error
- poor oculomotor function

- inhibition of the deep CCF and semispinalis
- increased activation of superficial neck muscles (scalenes, SCM, splenius capitis)
- delayed onset of CCF activation
- decreased strength and endurance capacity of the CCF and deep cervical extensors
- poor balance.

Poor muscle recruitment strategies between groups of muscles and between deep and superficial muscles along with proprioceptive deficits in the cervical region have been shown to be associated with UCS symptoms (O'Leary et al., 2007; Falla et al., 2011; Lindstrøm et al., 2011; Schomacher & Falla, 2013; Schomacher et al., 2013; de Vries et al., 2015).

Sensorimotor Testing

Sensorimotor deficits can be tested by assessment of the proprioceptive system and motor control. A range of tests can be used, including cervical joint position sense tests, postural stability tests, oculomotor function tests and motor control tests. Assessment of the proprioceptive system is described in Chapter 8. Motor control assessment is described below. For further information, see Jull et al. (2008c), Treleaven (2008), Clark et al. (2015) and Roijezon et al. (2015).

Motor control can be assessed indirectly by:

- observing posture (for example, patients with a forward head position are likely to have long, weak CCF)
- noting any changes in muscle recruitment patterns during active movements
- observing the quality of movement and where the movement is occurring
- palpating muscle activity in various positions.

In addition to this, specific muscle testing can be undertaken in the UCS.

Deep Cervical Muscle Testing

The deep cervical muscles (CCF and SOM groups) have been shown to have a high density of muscle spindles, particularly the SOMs. This suggests that, in addition to their role in controlling head-on-neck movements, they play a significant role in craniocervical proprioception (Boyd-Clark et al., 2001, 2002; O'Leary et al., 2009).

Deep Craniocervical Flexors

Assessment of the recruitment and endurance of the deep CCFs (longus colli, longus capitis, rectus capitis anterior and lateralis) is made using the low-load craniocervical flexion test (Jull et al., 2008c, 2008d). A pressure biofeedback unit (PBU: Chattanooga, Australia) is used to measure the function of the deep neck flexors.

- For starting position, see Fig. 7.13.
- The patient is then taught the correct nodding action of upper cervical flexion as if indicating 'yes'.

The patient is instructed to put their tongue on the roof of their mouth, to close their lips but not to clench their jaw. This helps to prevent substitution strategies by other muscle groups.

It is important that the head is not lifted or retracted. When the CCFs are weak, the SCM initiates the movement, causing the jaw to lead the movement, and the UCS hyperextends.

Testing is then undertaken in two stages: because pain inhibits CCF activity, testing should never induce symptoms (Arendt-Nielsen & Falla, 2009).

Stage 1–analysis of movement patterning. This is a five-level test whereby the patient attempts to increase the pressure progressively on the PBU in a correct motor strategy. Using visual feedback from the PBU, the patient attempts to hold a nod at 22, 24, 26, 28 and 30 mmHg with a few seconds rest between each stage. Ideally, subjects are able to progress through all five levels. Observation and palpation for overuse of superficial muscles (SCM, plus the scalene and hyoid groups) are made; these muscles may be active, but not dominant. A positive test is recorded when a patient is unable to achieve a level without either initiating a retraction movement and/or recruiting superficial flexors as the dominant group. A recording is made of both the level achieved and the quality of movement (Jull et al., 2008c).

Stage 2–holding capacity of deep neck flexors. This stage is only undertaken when training in stage 1 has resulted in normal patterning at all five levels. Beginning at 22 mmHg (2 mmHg above a baseline of 20 mmHg), the patient attempts to hold the test position (nod) for 10 seconds. Ten 10-second repetitions are aimed for at each level. The number of 10-second repetitions is recorded and used as the patient's baseline score. As in stage 1, a positive finding is when there is superficial muscle dominance or retraction of the neck. The clinician also observes the quality of movement, looking for jerky and poor control of the head (Jull et al., 2008c).

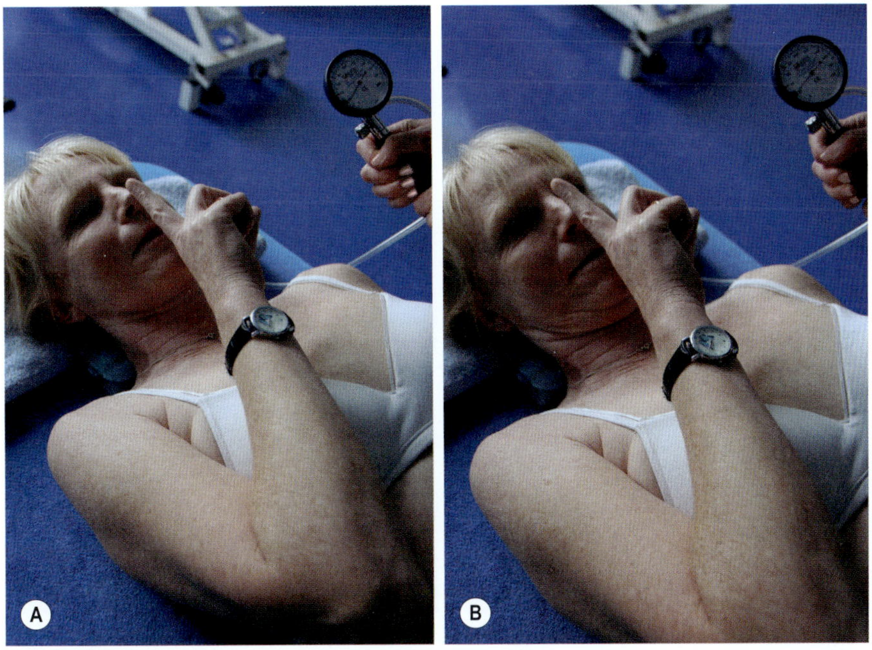

Fig. 7.13 (A and B) Craniocervical flexion test: Patient in supine crook-lying. Folded towel under occiput to ensure the head and neck are in a neutral position. A pressure biofeedback unit is placed under the cervical spine, against the occiput and inflated to 20 mmHg. Patient is asked to perform a head 'nod'. To facilitate the correct movement the patient is asked to slide her nose down her finger.

Deep Cervical Extensors

Although most clinical and research attention has been focused towards the CCF, the deep extensors also contribute towards sensorimotor control of the head on the neck. Assessment of these muscle groups is therefore justified particularly for those patients who present with a forward head position and neck pain or headaches (Schomacher et al., 2015).

For the first two tests below, the inability to perform a smooth, coordinated movement along with excessive movement in the lower cervical spine is suggestive of poor extension motor control (Jull et al., 2008c):

Craniocervical extension test (rectus capitis posterior group):

- With the patient in four-point kneeling or prone sitting, the patient performs craniocervical flexion and extension (a head-on-neck 'nodding' movement) whilst maintaining the lower cervical spine in a neutral position. The clinician can palpate this muscle group to assess for activation strategies.

Craniocervical rotation test (obliquus capitis group):

- With the patient in the same position as above, the patient performs craniocervical rotation (to less than 40 degrees), as if saying 'no' whilst maintaining the lower cervical spine in a neutral position. This muscle group is palpable, allowing the clinician to assess muscle recruitment strategies.

Deep cervical extensor test (semispinalis cervicis and multifidus muscle groups)

For test application, see Fig. 7.14.

This position will bias muscle activity towards semispinalis cervicis and discourage activity in the superficial semispinalis capitis and splenius capitis.

If there is good control between the CCF (holding the CCS in neutral) and the deep cervical extensors (producing the movement), the movement should be seen to occur around the cervicothoracic junction rather than at the craniovertebral junction or as a shearing extension movement around C5.

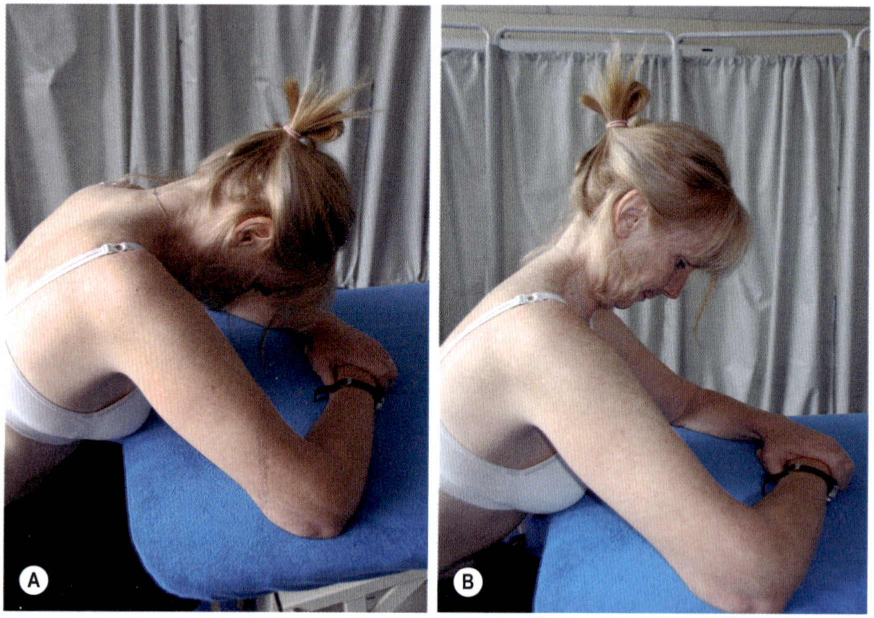

Fig. 7.14 (A and B) Deep cervical extensor test. Patient in prone propped on elbows with the craniocervical spine in neutral and lower cervical spine in full flexion. Patient performs extension of the cervical spine, around the cervicothoracic junction, returning to a head neutral position whilst maintaining the upper cervical spine in neutral.

Axioscapular Muscles

Owing to their attachments in the UCS and the occiput, activity of the upper fibres of the trapezius, levator scapulae, scalene group and SCM will influence movement patterns in the UCS. Additionally, scapular positioning and control are associated with cervical dysfunction, specifically following whiplash trauma (Jull et al., 2008c). Therefore, assessment of control and patterning of these muscle groups together with scapular control via the middle and lower fibres of trapezius and serratus muscles should be considered (see Chapters 8 and 10 for further details).

Muscle Length

The clinician tests the length of muscles, in particular, those thought prone to shortening (Janda, 2002); that is, levator scapulae, upper trapezius, SCM, pectoralis major and minor, scalenes and the deep occipital muscles. Testing the length of these muscles is described in Chapter 4 (see Table 4.9 and Fig. 4.13).

Cervical Arterial Dysfunction Testing

If vascular dysfunction is suspected following the subjective examination, further information regarding the integrity of the cervical arterial system can be gained from the following examination procedures. Further reading is recommended to support understanding of the following procedures (Chapter 8, Barnard & Ryder, 2024; Kerry & Taylor, 2010).

1. Blood pressure. In the event of acute arterial dysfunction, it is likely that there will be a systemic cardiovascular response manifesting in a dramatic change in blood pressure (usually increasing). Blood pressure can be taken using appropriate, validated procedures and equipment, in either sitting or lying.
2. Functional positional testing. In recent years there has been a shift of emphasis away from physical testing of the cervical arterial system owing to the poor reported diagnostic accuracy of these tests in detecting incompetent VA or ICA vessels (Rushton et al., 2014).

3. Pulse palpation. The VA pulses are difficult to palpate due to their size and depth. The ICA is easily accessible at the mid-cervical level, medial to the SCM. Gross pathologies, such as aneurysm formation, are characteristic in the nature of their pulse, that is, a pulsatile, expandable mass. Pain and exaggerated pulse on palpation of the temporal artery may support a hypothesis of temporal arteritis.
4. Cranial-nerve examination. Cranial nerves are peripheral nerves, which mostly arise from the brainstem. Cranial-nerve dysfunction can be a result of cervical arterial compromise; although this is rare, it tends to affect the lower cranial nerves, in particular the hypoglossal nerve (swallowing) (Thomas, 2016). Careful screening for gross asymmetries and variations from the norm in cranial nerve function is indicated if CAD is suspected (Kerry & Taylor, 2010). Table 7.6 shows a method of cranial nerve assessment (Barnard & Ryder, 2024, Chapter 8).
5. Proprioception tests. Hindbrain ischaemia associated with vertebrobasilar insufficiency can result in a gross loss of proprioceptive function. Simple proprioception testing such as tandem gait, heel-to-knee, Romberg's test and Hautant's test is undertaken to assess proprioception dysfunction.

KNOWLEDGE CHECK

1. Identify the nerves that are normally assessed in upper cervical spine disorders.
2. Name the axioscapular muscles that may influence the upper cervical spine.
3. Which joints are being tested on the flexion–rotation test, and what constitutes a positive finding?

COMPLETION OF THE EXAMINATION

Having carried out the above tests, the examination of the UCS is now complete. The subjective and physical examinations produce a large amount of information, which needs to be recorded accurately and quickly. It is vital at this stage to highlight with an asterisk (*) important findings from the examination. These findings are reassessed at, and within, subsequent treatment sessions to evaluate the effects of treatment on the patient's condition.

The physical testing procedures that specifically indicate joint, nerve or muscle tissues as a source of the patient's symptoms are summarized in Table 4.9.

On completion of the physical examination, the clinician will review and refine hypotheses developed at the end of the subjective examination (see Box 3.1). Following this the clinician will:

1. Evaluate the examination findings, formulate a clinical diagnosis and write up a problem list.
2. Determine the objectives of treatment in collaboration with the patient and devise an initial treatment plan and ongoing management strategy.
3. Explain the findings of the examination to the patient, explore any misconceptions the patient may have regarding the injury or disorder and discuss the prognosis.
4. Warn the patient of possible exacerbation up to 24–48 hours following the examination.
5. Request the patient to report details on the behaviour of the symptoms following examination at the next attendance.

For guidance on treatment and management principles, the reader is directed to the companion textbook (Barnard & Ryder, 2024).

Appendix 7.1 Headache Disability Index Questionnaire

Patient name: ______________________ Date ____________

INSTRUCTIONS: Please CIRCLE the correct response:

1. I have headache:	(1) 1 per month	(2) more than 1 but less than 4 per month	(3) more than 1 per week
2. My headache is:	(1) mild	(2) moderate	(3) severe

Please read carefully: the purpose of the scale is to identify difficulties that you may be experiencing because of your headache. Please check off 'YES', 'SOMETIMES', or 'NO' to each item. Answer each question as it pertains to your headache only.

YES	SOMETIMES	NO	
____	____	____	Because of my headaches I feel disabled.
____	____	____	Because of my headaches I feel restricted in performing my routine daily activities.
____	____	____	No one understands the effect my headaches have on my life.
____	____	____	I restrict my recreational activities (e.g. sports, hobbies) because of my headaches.
____	____	____	My headaches make me angry.
____	____	____	Sometimes I feel that I am going to lose control because of my headaches.
____	____	____	Because of my headaches I am less likely to socialize.
____	____	____	My spouse (significant other), or family and friends have no idea what I am going through because of my headaches.
____	____	____	My headaches are so bad that I feel that I am going to go insane.
____	____	____	My outlook on the world is affected by my headaches.
____	____	____	I am afraid to go outside when I feel that a headache is starting.
____	____	____	I feel desperate because of my headaches.
____	____	____	I am concerned that I am paying penalties at work or at home because of my headaches.
____	____	____	My headaches place stress on my relationships with family or friends.
____	____	____	I avoid being around people when I have a headache.
____	____	____	I believe my headaches are making it difficult for me to achieve my goals in life.
____	____	____	I am unable to think clearly because of my headaches.
____	____	____	I get tense (e.g. muscle tension) because of my headaches.
____	____	____	I do not enjoy social gatherings because of my headaches.
____	____	____	I feel irritable because of my headaches.
____	____	____	I avoid travelling because of my headaches.
____	____	____	My headaches make me feel confused.
____	____	____	My headaches make me feel frustrated.
____	____	____	I find it difficult to read because of my headaches.
____	____	____	I find it difficult to focus my attention away from my headaches and on other things.

Instructions: 1. Using this system, if 'YES' is checked on any given line, that answer is given 4 points ... a 'SOMETIMES' answer is given 2 points and a 'NO' answer is given zero. 2. Using this system, a score of 10–28% is considered to constitute mild disability; 30–48% is moderate; 50–68% is severe; 72% or more is complete.

Patient's signature: ______________________ Date: ____________

From Jacobson et al. (1994).

Appendix 7.2 Headache Disability Questionnaire

Name: ______________________ Date: ____________ Score: ________/90

Please read each question and circle the response that best applies to you

1. How would you rate the usual pain of your headache on a scale from 0 to 10?

0	1	2	3	4	5	6	7	8	9	10
No pain										Worst pain

2. When you have headaches, how often is the pain severe?

Never	1–9%	10–19%	20–29%	30–39%	40–49%	50–59%	60–69%	70–79%	80–89%	90–100% Always
0	1	2	3	4	5	6	7	8	9	10

1. On how many days in the last month did you actually lie down for an hour or more because of your headaches?

None	1–3	4–6	7–9	10–12	13–15	16–18	19–21	22–24	25–27	28–31 Every day
0	1	2	3	4	5	6	7	8	9	10

2. When you have a headache, how often do you miss work or school for all or part of the day?

Never	1–9%	10–19%	20–29%	30–39%	40–49%	50–59%	60–69%	70–79%	80–89%	90–100% Always
0	1	2	3	4	5	6	7	8	9	10

5. When you have a headache while you work (or are at school), how much is your ability to work reduced?

Not reduced	1–9%	10–19%	20–29%	30–39%	40–49%	50–59%	60–69%	70–79%	80–89%	90–100% Unable to work
0	1	2	3	4	5	6	7	8	9	10

6. How many days in the last month have you been kept from performing housework or chores for at least half of the day because of your headaches?

None	1–3	4–6	7–9	10–12	13–15	16–18	19–21	22–24	25–27	28–31 Every day
0	1	2	3	4	5	6	7	8	9	10

7. When you have a headache, how much is your ability to perform housework or chores reduced?

Not reduced	1–9%	10–19%	20–29%	30–39%	40–49%	50–59%	60–69%	70–79%	80–89%	90–100% Always
0	1	2	3	4	5	6	7	8	9	10

8. How many days in the last month have you been kept from non-work activities (family, social or recreational) because of your headaches?

None	1–3	4–6	7–9	10–12	13–15	16–18	19–21	22–24	25–27	28–31 Every day
0	1	2	3	4	5	6	7	8	9	10

9. When you have a headache, how much is your ability to engage in non-work activities (family, social or recreational) reduced?

Not reduced	1–9%	10–19%	20–29%	30–39%	40–49%	50–59%	60–69%	70–79%	80–89%	90–100% Always
0	1	2	3	4	5	6	7	8	9	10

From Niere and Quin (2009).

REVIEW AND REVISE QUESTIONS

1. Name the muscles that act on the upper cervical spine and identify their role.
2. Name the blood vessels passing through upper cervical spine that supply blood to the brain and brain stem.
3. Explain the proposed mechanism for cervicogenic headache.
4. Name the three reflexes supporting oculomotor function.
5. A 'chin poke' posture on return from full cervical extension movement suggests overuse of which neck muscle?
6. Name the nerve that supplies cutaneous sensation to the skin on the face.
7. Dizziness is common post whiplash–explain the mechanism thought to be responsible.
8. How can dizziness from a vestibular cause be differentiated from a cervicogenic cause?
9. Identify the cervical spine muscles important for proprioception and symptoms that indicate a possible dysfunction.
10. Which nerve does the jaw jerk reflex test and what would indicate an abnormal finding?

Case Study Mr G

Male, aged 48 years old

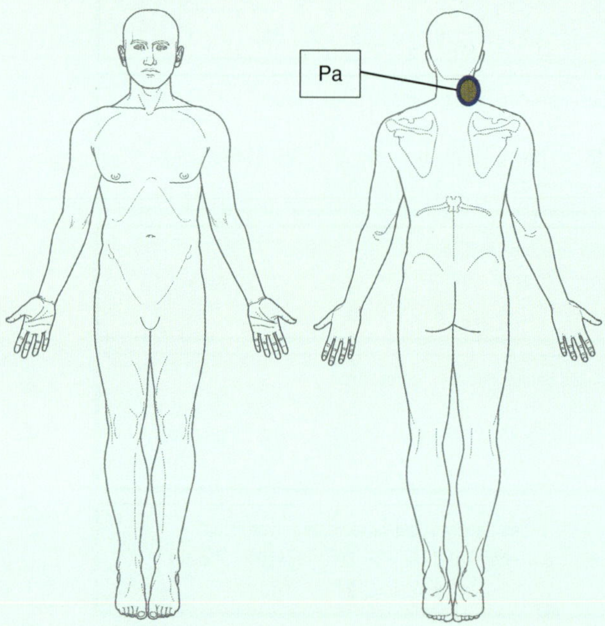

Pa—intermittent pain from base of skull/upper cervical spine that extends into the temporal region, 0/10 extending to 8/10 when pain on, reduces back after 1–2 days

Aggravating factors—when driving long distances, after sleep

Easing factors—OTC pain relief, rest, lying down, heat

24 h pattern—morning stiffness in cervical spine. Disappears after 30 min but can stay for 2 days

Sleep—Can take some time to get to sleep, can wake regularly with stiffness in neck with head turning

No symptoms anywhere else

HPC

Three years of on/off right-sided headache. No history of trauma or obvious reason. Begins in the neck and extends up towards the temporal region. Finds stiffness in neck movements. No signs of 5ds 3ns. No pain or referral into arms, legs. No aura. Occurs 3× week. No HO trauma. Pain seemed to start after a long plane journey

Lifestyle/occupation/home life

Lives with wife and 0 children. Stressful job, not exercising as much as used. Drinks a little too much in own opinion. Works in recruitment, spends all day on computer and phone talking to clients. Driving ++.

Right handed

Impact on function/beliefs and expectations

Case Study Mr G—cont'd

Can be disabling as struggles to work at a computer. Stiffness in neck can affect driving. Worried as it's not improving and does not want to use medication long term. Looking for a physical solution, keen to try exercise management. No previous therapies but wanting help as impact increasing

PMH

Mildly raised cholesterol, managed with diet. PH of gout

DH/Investigations

Occasional paracetamol

No imaging, referrals or other management.

FH nil of note

GH Good. No areas of concern re THREAD (thyroid, heart, RA, epilepsy, asthma, diabetes)

Clinical Reasoning

Mr G had an insidious onset of neck-related headache which seemed to occur after a plane journey. His episodic pain is affecting his work, home and social life and he is losing confidence in his ability to do things without triggering the symptoms. He feels it is worsening and is keen to find physical solutions.

Psychologically **(yellow flags)**—no clear diagnosis, and is worried about the future and no natural improvement

Socially **(blue/black flag)**—mildly affected with a slight reduction in social activity, remains at work

No observable **red flag** symptoms

Evaluation of Severity, Irritability and Nature

- **Severity (Pa)—moderate** (no night disturbance, regular medication, starting to affect concentration at work, NPRS of 8/10)
- **Irritability (Pa)—moderate to high** (symptoms with computer work 30 min, can take days to ease
- **Nature**—chronic neck-related headache pain with peripheral nociception of facet joint and soft tissue structures leading to sensitization of trigeminal nucleus and therefore referred pain

What are you treating? It is likely at this point we are treating a primary neck pain with associated referral pattern into the head. It is escalating with its sensitization worsening, and he is struggling to manage. It is having a negative effect on his life and social circumstances.

The mornings look a problem as does driving, and these are factors that seem to be impactful. He is generally sedentary, and this will need to be addressed. There may be some secondary factors such as thoracic stiffness, poor shoulder control, and/or loss of neck proprioception that all could be contributing.

Mr G's main **functional limitation** is being able to drive and not experience head pain and neck stiffness for long periods

Subjective markers (link to genics)

1. Driving for 2 h without neck pain and headache starting
2. Stiffness in neck when he first wakes leading to headache

Does any aspect of the history indicate caution?

Some increased levels of severity.

Can you predict the comparable signs? (Subjective marker linking with an objective sign)

Right rotation of the neck.

What is the relationship between pain and resistance?

Pa—Pain > resistance

What pain mechanisms can you identify? There is evidence peripheral sensitization and subsequent nociceptive (neck) symptoms with a secondary referral pattern.

Analysis of percentage weighting (Pain source) Myogenic 50%, Arthrogenic 50%

Analysis of percentage weighting (driver/contributing factors) Given the persistent nature of Mr Ps complaint, it is important to consider the following questions

1) Why has he developed this complaint?
2) Why has it not settled (young, fit male patient)

Based on the duration of complaint (adaptive changes and faulty movement patterns) and age (degenerative changes) proposed weighting could be: cervical spine joint hypomobility 50%, reduced neck muscle endurance capacity (30%), neck proprioception (10%), beliefs/psychological (10%).

Hypotheses to test/working diagnosis? (Differentiate between genics)

1. Reduced work capacity/endurance of neck muscles
2. Postural awareness/proprioception
3. Cervicothoracic spine active and passive movement (muscle v joint)

Planning the Physical Examination

Observation to include sitting posture (poking chin) and specifically neck posture when positioned in a car. Consider requesting an example of position at sleep and at waking.

Observe movements to assess R and L rotation and extension in lower and upper cervical spine. Observe where movement is originating from (quality, range and reproduction of any symptoms). Flexion rotation test.

Cervical spine PPIVM into R rotation to assess the passive ROM of upper cervical spine. Local pain provocation

Continued

Case Study Mr G—cont'd

palpation to see if resultant headache is reproduced, be careful to agree this due to irritability. Flexion rotation test.

Muscles

Assess neck muscle

- Endurance using deep neck flexor testing in lying or preferably sitting (to best reflect the main complaint)
- Endurance of deep cervical extensor muscles

Proprioception

Use JPE testing to examine proprioception

Main clinical findings for Mr G included

Cervicothoracic spine posture involved flexed mid thorax and cervical spine in right side flexion and head tilted to right. Partial postural correction was possible but limited by pain and loss of endurance.

When posture was corrected range of motion did not change and pain remained.

Right rotation was limited to 2/3 ROM, and a positive flexion rotation test to the right was noted. This indicated clear movement loss in the upper cervical spine.

The thoracic spine was stiff in all directions with no specific direction of loss or pain.

Other findings included reduced cervical flexor and extensor muscle endurance.

JPE inaccuracy and errors increased over repetitions (linked to muscle fatigue) and some feelings of loss of balance.

Management included

Education and advice to explain the nature of the symptom, the rationale for the loss of movement and muscular weakness. Also linking the clear loss of JPE to the condition.

Muscle strengthening 10 min 2× day

R rotation PAIVM C1/2, as management technique using Grade III/IV to reduced local joint hypomobility and resultant change in muscular tone to aid in range of motion and proprioceptive feedback (density of muscle spindles is very high in this region).

Home exercise programme

1. Range of motion exercises for neck rotation.
2. Balance and proprioceptive exercises
3. Endurance for flexors and extensors of upper cervical spine
4. General thoracic mobility exercises

Outcome

Mr G returned after 1 week and reported improvement, better range of motion, headache duration shorter and less referral into head. Could see the benefit of the exercise approach.

REFERENCES

Amiri, M., Jull, G., Bullock-Saxton, J., 2003. Measurement of upper cervical flexion and extension with the 3-space fastrak measurement system: a repeatability study. J. Man. Manip. Ther. 11, 198–203.

Amiri, M., Jull, G., Bullock-Saxton, J., Darnell, R., Lander, C., 2007. Cervical musculoskeletal impairment in frequent intermittent headache. Part 2: subjects with concurrent headache types. Cephalalgia 27 (8), 891–898.

Anarte, E., Carvalho, G.F., Schwarz, A., Luedtke, K., Falla, D., 2019. Can physical testing be used to distinguish between migraine and cervicogenic headache sufferers? A protocol for a systematic review. BMJ Open 9 (11), e031587.

Antonaci, F., Bono, G., Chimento, P., 2006. Diagnosing cervicogenic headache. J. Headache Pain 7, 145.

Antonaci, F., Inan, L.E., 2021. Headache and neck. Cephalalgia 41 (4), 438–442.

Arendt-Nielsen, L., Falla, D., 2009. Motor control adjustments in musculoskeletal pain and the implications for pain recurrence. Pain 142, 171–172.

Arnold, M., 2018. Headache classification committee of the international headache society (IHS) the international classification of headache disorders. Cephalalgia 38 (1), 1–211.

Barnard, K., Ryder, D., 2024. Principles of Musculoskeletal Treatment and Management: A Handbook for Therapists, fourth ed. Elsevier, Edinburgh.

Bogduk, N., 2002. Biomechanics of the cervical spine. In: Grant, R. (Ed.), Physical Therapy of the Cervical and Thoracic Spine, third ed. Churchill Livingstone, New York.

Bogduk, N., Bartsch, T., 2008. Cervicogenic headache. In: Silberstein, S.D., et al. (Eds.), Wolff's Headache, eighth ed. Oxford University Press, New York, pp. 551–570.

Bogduk, N., Govind, J., 2009. Cervicogenic headache: an assessment of the evidence on clinical diagnosis, invasive tests, and treatment. Lancet Neurol 8, 959–968.

Bogduk, N., Mercer, S., 2000. Biomechanics of the cervical spine. I: normal kinematics. Clin. Biomech. (Bristol, Avon) 15, 633–648.

Boo, M., Matheson, G., Lumba-Brown, A., 2020. Smooth pursuit eye-movement abnormalities associated with cervical spine whiplash: a scientific review and case report. Cureus 12 (8), e9872.

Borgdorff, P., 2018. Arguments against the role of cortical spreading depression in migraine. Neurol. Res. 40 (3), 173–181.

Boyd-Clark, L., Briggs, C.A., Galea, M.P., 2001. Comparative histochemical composition of muscle fibres in a pre and post-vertebral muscle of the cervical spine. J. Anat. 199, 709–716.

Boyd-Clark, L., Briggs, C.A., Galea, M.P., 2002. Muscle spindle distribution, morphology and density in longus colli and multifidus muscles of the cervical spine. Spine 27, 694–701.

Brolin, K., Halldin, P., 2004. Development of a finite model of the upper cervical spine in a parameter study of ligament characteristics. Spine 29, 376–385.

Calais-Germain, B., 2007. Anatomy of Movement. Revised Edition.. Eastland Press, Seattle.

Cescon, C., Barbero, M., Zuin, P., Falla, D., Palacios-Cena, M., Arendt-Nielsen, L., et al., 2019. Referred pain maps of myofascial trigger points in tension type headache. WCPT. http://repository.supsi.ch/10582/.

Chancey, V., Ottaviano, D., Myers, B.S., Nightingale, R.W., 2007. A kinematic and anthropometric study of the upper cervical spine and the occipital condyles. J. Biomech. 40, 1953–1959.

Charles, A.C., Baca, S.M., 2013. Cortical spreading depression and migraine. Nat. Rev. Neurol. 9 (11), 637.

Chen, S.P., Ayata, C., 2016. Spreading depression in primary and secondary headache disorders. Curr. Pain Headache Rep. 20 (7), 1–8.

Choi, I.L., Sang, J.R., 2016. Neuralgias of the head: occipital neuralgia. Korean Med. Sci. 31 (4), 479–488.

Clark, N., Röijezon, U., Treleaven, J., 2015. Proprioception in musculoskeletal rehabilitation. Part 2 clinical assessment and intervention. Man Ther. 20, 378–387.

Corneil, B.D., 2011. The Oxford Handbook of Eye Movements. Oxford University Press, Oxford, pp. 303–322.

Dalkara, T., Moskowitz, M.A., 2017. From cortical spreading depression to trigeminovascular activation in migraine. Neurobiol. Basis Migraine 27 (2), s86–s90.

De Simone, R., Ranieri, A., Montella, S., Bonavita, V., 2013. Cortical spreading depression and central pain networks in trigeminal nuclei modulation: time for an integrated migraine pathogenesis perspective. Neurol. Sci. 34 (1), 51–55.

de Vries, J., Ischebeck, B.K., Voogt, L.P., Van Der Geest, J.N., Janssen, M., Frens, M.A., et al., 2015. Joint position sense error in people with neck pain: a systematic review. Man. Ther. 20, 736e–744.

Do, T.P., Remmers, A., Schytz, H.W., Schankin, C., Nelson, S. E., Obermann, M., et al., 2019. Red and orange flags for secondary headaches in clinical practice: SNNOOP10 list. Neurology 92 (3), 134–144.

Dumas, J.P., Arsenault, A.B., Boudreau, G., Magnoux, E., Lepage, Y., Bellavance, A., et al., 2001. Physical impairments in cervicogenic headache: traumatic vs. non-traumatic onset. Cephalalgia 21 (9), 884–893.

Edwards, B., 1994. Examination of the high cervical spine (occiput–C2) using combined movements. In: Boyling, J. D., Palastanga, N. (Eds.), Grieve's Modern Manual Therapy, second ed. Churchill Livingstone, Edinburgh.

Edwards, B., 1999. Manual of Combined Movements: Their Use in the Examination and Treatment of Mechanical Vertebral Column Disorders, second ed. Butterworth-Heinemann, Oxford.

Falla, D., 2004. Unravelling the complexity of muscle impairment in chronic neck pain. Man. Ther. 9, 125–133.

Falla, D., Jull, G., Hodges, P.W., 2004. Feedforward activity of the cervical flexor muscles during voluntary arm movements is delayed in chronic neck pain. Exp. Brain Res. 157, 43–48.

Falla, D., O'Leary, S., Farina, D., Jull, G., 2011. Association between intensity of pain and impairment in onset and activation of deep cervical flexors in patients with persistent neck pain. Clin. J. Pain 27, 309–314.

Fischer, A.J.E.M., Verhagen, W.I.M., Huygen, P.L.M., 1997. Whiplash injury. A clinical review with emphasis on neuro-otological aspects. Clin. Otolaryngol Allied Sci. 22 (3), 192–201.

Fuller, G., 1993. Neurological Examination Made Easy. Churchill Livingstone, Edinburgh.

Gadotti, I., Olivo, S.A., Magee, D.J., 2008. Cervical musculoskeletal impairments in cervicogenic headache: a systematic review and a meta-analysis. Phys. Ther. Rev. 13, 149–166.

Global Burden of Disease, 2017. Global, regional, and national incidence, prevalence, and years lived with disability for 328 diseases and injuries for 195 countries, 1990–2016: a systematic analysis for the Global Burden of Disease Study. Lancet 390 (10100), 1211–1259. https://doi.org/10.1016/S0140-6736(17)32154-2.

Greenhalgh, S., Selfe, J., 2009. Red Flags II: A Guide to Identifying Serious Pathology of the Spine. Elsevier, Edinburgh.

Haldeman, S., Dagenais, S., 2001. Cervicogenic headaches: a critical review. Spine J. 1 (1), 31–46.

Hall, T., Briffa, K., Hopper, D., 2008b. Clinical evaluation of cervicogenic headache: a clinical perspective. J. Man. Manip. Ther. 16, 73–80.

Hall, T., Briffa, K., Hopper, D., Robinson, K., 2010a. Reliability of manual examination and frequency of symptomatic cervical motion segment dysfunction in cervicogenic headache. Man. Ther. 15, 542–546.

Hall, T., Briffa, K., Hopper, D., Robinson, K., 2010b. Comparative analysis and diagnostic accuracy of the cervical flexion rotation test. J. Headache Pain 11, 391–397.

Hall, T., Robinson, K., 2004. The flexion-rotation test and active cervical mobility: a comparative measurement study in cervicogenic headache. Man. Ther. 9, 197–202.

Hall, T., Robinson, K.W., Fujinawa, O., Akasaka, K., Pyne, E. A., 2008a. Inter-tester reliability and diagnostic validity of the cervical flexion-rotation test in cervicogenic headache. J. Manipulative Physiol. Ther. 31, 293–300.

Holroyd, K.A., Stensland, M., Lipchik, G.L., Hill, K.R., O'Donnell, F.S., Cordingley, G., 2000. Psychosocial correlates and impact of chronic tension-type headaches. Headache Head Face Pain 40 (1), 3–16.

Hutting, N., Wilbrink, W., Taylor, A., Kerry, R., 2021. Identifying vascular pathologies or flow limitations: important aspects in the clinical reasoning process. Musculoskelet. Sci. Pract. 53, 102343.

Ischebeck, B.K., de Vries, J., Van der Geest, J.N., Janssen, M., Van Wingerden, J.P., Kleinrensink, G.J., et al., 2016. Eye movements in patients with Whiplash Associated Disorders: a systematic review. BMC Musculoskelet. Disord. 17 (1), 1–11.

Ishii, T., Mukai, Y., Hosono, N., Sakaura, H., Nakajima, Y., Sato, Y., et al., 2004. Kinematics of the cervical spine in rotation in vivo three-dimensional analysis. Spine 29, E139–E144.

Jacobson, G.P., Ramadan, N.M., Aggarwal, S.K., Newman, C.W., 1994. The Henry Ford hospital headache disability inventory (HDI). Neurology 44, 837–842.

Janda, V., 2002. Muscles and motor control in cervicogenic disorders. In: Grant, R. (Ed.), Physical Therapy of the Cervical and Thoracic Spine, third ed. Churchill Livingstone, New York.

Jonsson, A., Rasmussen-Barr, E., 2018. Intra-and inter-rater reliability of movement and palpation tests in patients with neck pain: a systematic review. Physiother. Theory Pract. 34 (3), 165–180.

Jull, G., 1997. Management of cervical headache. Man. Ther. 2 (4), 182–190.

Jull, G., 2000. Deep cervical flexor dysfunction in whiplash. J. Musculoskelet. Pain 8, 143–154.

Jull, G., Amiri, M., Bullock-Saxton, J., Darnell, R., Lander, C., 2007. Cervical musculoskeletal impairment in frequent intermittent headache. Part 1: subjects with single headaches. Cephalalgia 27, 793–802.

Jull, G., Barrett, C., Magee, R., Ho, P., 1999. Further clinical clarification of the muscle dysfunction in cervical headache. Cephalalgia 19, 179–185.

Jull, G., Bogduk, N., Marsland, A., 1988. The accuracy of manual diagnosis for cervical zygapophysial joint pain syndromes. Med. J. Aust. 148 (5), 233–236.

Jull, G., Hall, T., 2018. Cervical musculoskeletal dysfunction in headache: how should it be defined. Musculoskelet. Sci. Pract. 38, 148–150.

Jull, G., Kristjansson, E., Dall'Alba, P., 2004. Impairment in the cervical flexors: a comparison of whiplash and insidious onset neck pain patients. Man. Ther. 9, 89–94.

Jull, G., O'leary, S.P., Falla, D.L., 2008d. Clinical assessment of the deep cervical muscles: the craniocervical; flexion test. J. Manipulative Physiol. Ther. 31, 525–533.

Jull, G., Sterling, M., Falla, D., Treleaven, J., O'Leary, S., 2008a. Alterations in cervical muscle function in neck pain. In: Whiplash, Headache and Neck Pain. Research Based Directions for Physical Therapists. Churchill Livingstone, Elsevier, Edinburgh (Chapter 4).

Jull, G., Sterling, M., Falla, D., Treleaven, J., O'Leary, S., 2008b. Cervicogenic headache: differential diagnosis. In: Whiplash, Headache and Neck Pain. Research Based Directions for Physical Therapists. Churchill Livingstone, Elsevier, Edinburgh (Chapter 9).

Jull, G., Sterling, M., Falla, D., Treleaven, J., O'Leary, S., 2008c. Clinical assessment: physical examination of the cervical region. In: Whiplash, Headache and Neck Pain. Research Based Directions for Physical Therapists. Churchill Livingstone, Elsevier, Edinburgh (Chapter 12).

Jull, G., Sterling, M., Falla, D., Treleaven, J., O'Leary, S., 2008e. Disturbances in postural stability, head and eye movement control in cervical disorders. In: Whiplash, Headache and Neck Pain. Research Based Directions for Physical Therapists. Churchill Livingstone, Elsevier, Edinburgh (Chapter 6).

Kerry, R., Taylor, A., 2006. Cervical arterial dysfunction assessment and manual therapy. Man. Ther. 11, 243–253.

Kerry, R., Taylor, A., 2010. Haemodynamics. In: McCarthy, C. (Ed.), Combined Movement Theory. Elsevier, London (Chapter 6).

Krakenes, J., Kaale, B., 2006. Magnetic resonance imaging assessment of craniovertebral ligaments and membranes after whiplash trauma. Spine 31, 2820–2826.

Krakenes, J., Kaale, B., Rorvik, J., Gilhus, N., 2001. MRI assessment of normal ligamentous structures in the craniovertebral junction. Neuroradiology 43, 1089–1097.

Kulkarni, V., Chandy, M.J., Babu, K.S., 2001. Quantitative study of muscle spindles in suboccipital muscles of human foetuses. Neurol India 49, 355–359.

Lauritzen, M., 2001. Relationship of spikes, synaptic activity, and local changes of cerebral blood flow. J. Cereb. Blood Flow Metab. 21 (12), 1367–1383.

Lindstrøm, R., Schomacher, J., Farina, D., Rechter, L., Falla, D., 2011. Association between neck muscle coactivation, pain, and strength in women with neck pain. Man. Ther. 16, 80–86.

Linton, S.J., Shaw, W.S., 2011. Impact of psychological factors in the experience of pain. Phys. ther. 91 (5), 700–711.

Loder, E., Rizzoli, P., 2008. Tension-type headache. BMJ 336 (7635), 88–92.

Luedtke, K., Boissonnault, W., Caspersen, N., Castien, R., Chaibi, A., Falla, D., et al., 2016. International consensus on the most useful physical examination tests used by physiotherapists for patients with headache: a Delphi study. Man. Ther. 23, 17–24.

Magarey, M., Rebbeck, T., Coughlan, B., Grimmer, K., Rivett, D.A., Refshauge, K., 2004. Pre-manipulative testing of the cervical spine review, revision and new clinical guidelines. Man. Ther. 9, 95–108.

Maitland, G., Hengeveld, E., Banks, K., English, K., 2005. Maitland's Vertebral Manipulation, seventh ed. Butterworth-Heinemann, Oxford.

Martin, V.T., 2004. Menstrual migraine: a review of prophylactic therapies. Curr. Pain Headache Rep 8 (3), 229–237.

McCarthy, C., 2010. Combined Movement Theory: Rational Mobilization and Manipulation of the Vertebral Column. Elsevier, Edinburgh.

McPartland, J., Brodeur, R., 1999. Rectus capitis posterior minor: a small but important suboccipital muscle. J. Bodyw. Mov. Ther. 3, 30–35.

Mulligan, B., 2010. Manual therapy 'nags', 'snags', 'MWMs' etc. In: Orthopaedic Physical Therapy Products, sixth ed. New Zealand.

Netter, F.H., 2006. Atlas of Human Anatomy, fourth ed. Elsevier, Philadelphia.

Niere, K., Quin, A., 2009. Development of a headache-specific disability questionnaire for patients attending physiotherapy. Man. Ther. 14, 45–51.

Ogince, M., Hall, T., Robinson, K., Blackmore, A.M., 2007. The diagnostic validity of the cervical flexion-rotation test in C1/2-related cervicogenic headache. Man. Ther. 12, 256–262.

O'Leary, S., Jull, G., Kim, M., Vicenzino, B., 2007. Craniocervical flexor muscle impairment at maximal, moderate, and low loads is a feature of neck pain. Man. Ther. 12, 34–39.

O'Leary, S., Falla, D., Elliott, J.M., Jull, G., 2009. Muscle dysfunction in cervical spine pain: implications for assessment and management. J. Orthop. Sports Phys. Ther. 39, 324–333.

Olesen, J., 2018. International classification of headache disorders. Lancet Neurol 17 (5), 396–397.

Olivier, B., Pramod, A., Maleka, D., 2018. Trigger point sensitivity is a differentiating factor between cervicogenic and non-cervicogenic headaches: a cross-sectional, descriptive study. Physiother. Canada 70 (4), 323–329.

Osmotherly, P., Rivett, D.A., Mercer, S.R., 2013. Revisiting the clinical anatomy of the alar ligaments. Eur. Spine J. 22, 6–64.

Persson, P., Hirschfeld, H., Nilsson-Wikmar, L., 2007. Associated sagittal spinal movements in performance of head pro- and retraction in healthy women: a kinematic analysis. Man. Ther. 12, 119–125.

Robbins, M.S., Lipton, R.B., 2010. The epidemiology of primary headache disorders, 30. Thieme Medical Publishers, New York, pp. 107–119. Seminars in Neurology 2.

Roijezon, U., Clark, N.C., Treleaven, J., 2015. Proprioception in musculoskeletal rehabilitation. Part 1: basic science and principles of assessment and clinical interventions. Man. Ther. 20, 368–377.

Rubio-Ochoa, J., Benítez-Martínez, J., Lluch, E., Santacruz-Zaragozá, S., Gómez-Contreras, P., Cook, C.E., 2016. Physical examination tests for screening and diagnosis of cervicogenic headache: a systematic review. Man. Ther. 21, 35–40.

Rushton, A., Carlesso, L.C., Flynn, T., Hing, W.A., Kerry, R.R., SM, V., 2020. International Framework for Examination of the cervical region for potential of vascular pathologies of the neck prior to orthopaedic manual therapy (OMT) intervention: International IFOMPT Cervical Framework. IFOMPT, Auckland.

Rushton, A., Rivett, D., Carlesso, L., Flynn, T., Hing, W., Kerry, R., 2014. International framework for examination of the cervical region for potential of cervical arterial dysfunction prior to orthopaedic manual therapy intervention. Man. Ther. 19, 222–228.

Salem, W., Lenders, C., Mathieu, J., Hermanus, N., Klein, P., 2013. In vivo three-dimensional kinematics of the cervical spine during maximal axial rotation. Man. Ther. 18, 339–344.

Schmidt, C.L., 1998 Sep. Mechanism of benign, peripheral, paroxysmal positional vertigo (BPPV). Laryngo-Rhino-Otologie. 77 (9), 485–495. https://doi.org/10.1055/s-2007-997011.

Schomacher, J., Boudreau, S.A., Petzke, F., Falla, D., 2013. Localized pressure pain sensitivity is associated with lower activation of the semispinalis cervicis muscle in patients with chronic neck pain. Clin. J. Pain 29, 898–906.

Schomacher, J., Erlenwein, J., Dieterich, A., Petzke, F., Falla, D., 2015. Can neck exercises enhance the activation of the semispinalis cervicis relative to the splenius capitis at specific spinal levels? Man. Ther. 20, 694–702.

Schomacher, J., Falla, D., 2013. Function and structure of the deep cervical extensor muscles in patients with neck pain. Man. Ther. 18, 360–366.

Sjaastad, O., Fredriksen, T.A., Pfaffenrath, V., 1998. Cervicogenic headache: diagnostic criteria. The CGHA International Study Group. Headache 38, 442–445.

Sung, Y.H., 2020. Upper cervical spine dysfunction and dizziness. J. Exer. Rehabil. 16 (5), 385.

Taylor, A., Kerry, R., 2010. A 'system based' approach to risk assessment of the cervical spine prior to manual therapy. Int. J. Osteopath. Med. 13, 85–93.

Taylor, A., Kerry, R., 2015. Haemodynamics and clinical practice. In: Jull, G., Moore, A., Falla, D., Lewis, J., McCarthy, C., Sterling, M. (Eds.), Grieve's Modern Musculoskeletal Physiotherapy, fourth ed. Elsevier, Edinburgh. Chapter 35.2).

Thomas, L.C., 2016. Cervical arterial dissection: an overview and implications for manipulative therapy practice. Man. Ther. 21, 2–9.

Thomas, L.C., McLeod, L.R., Osmotherly, P.G., Rivett, D.A., 2015. The effect of end-range cervical rotation on vertebral and internal carotid arterial blood flow and cerebral inflow: a sub analysis of an MRI study. Man. Ther. 20, 475–480.

Tjell, C., Rosenhall, U. Smooth pursuit neck torsion test: a specific test for cervical dizziness. Am, J. Otol. 19, 76–81.

Treleaven, J., 2008. Sensorimotor disturbances in neck disorders affecting postural stability, head and eye movement control. Man. Ther. 13, 2–11.

Treleaven, J., 2011. Dizziness, unsteadiness, visual disturbances and postural control implications for the transition to chronic symptoms after a whiplash trauma. Spine 36, S211–S217.

Treleaven, J., Jull, G., LowChoy, N., 2005. Smooth pursuit neck torsion test in whiplash-associated disorders: relationship to self-reports of neck pain and disability, dizziness and anxiety. J. Rehabil. Med. 37 (4), 219–223.

Treleaven, J., Jull, G., Sterling, M., 2003. Dizziness and unsteadiness following whiplash injury: characteristic features and relationship with cervical joint position error. J. Rehabil. Med. 35 (1), 36–43.

Tubbs, S., Kelly, D.R., Humphrey, E.R., Chua, G.D., Shoja, M.M., Salter, E.G., 2007. The tectorial membrane: anatomical, biomechanical, and histological analysis. Clin. Anat. 20, 382–386.

Viana, M., Sances, G., Linde, M., 2017. Clinical features of migraine aura: results from a prospective diary-aided study. Cephalalgia 37 (10), 979–989.

Van Griensven, H., 2005. Pain in Practice Theory and Treatment Strategies for Manual Therapists. Elsevier, Edinburgh.

Watson, D.H., Trott, P., 1993. Cervical headache: an investigation of natural head posture and upper cervical flexor muscle performance. Cephalalgia 13 (4), 272–284.

Zito, G., Jull, G., Story, I., 2006. Clinical tests of musculoskeletal dysfunction in the diagnosis of cervicogenic headache. Man. Ther. 11, 118–129.

8

Examination of the Cervicothoracic Region

Nicola R. Heneghan and Chris Worsfold

LEARNING OUTCOMES

After studying this chapter, you should be able to:

- Identify how clinical reasoning guides history taking in the subjective examination of people with neck pain.
- Identify the value of screening questions in relation to common presentations of the cervicothoracic spine.
- Hypothesize which structure might be at fault based on the locations of symptoms and related aggravating factors.
- Discuss the multifactorial nature of cervicothoracic spine pain and the role psychosocial factors may play in how patients may present.
- List the key constituents of a comprehensive physical examination of the cervicothoracic spine.
- Identify how subjective data will guide the physical examination of the cervicothoracic spine.
- Consider the sensitivity and specificity of key physical tests for the cervicothoracic spine.
- Discuss the value of functional testing and symptom modification when considering the aggravating factors, whilst understanding that such tests lack the validity and reliability of some physical tests.
- Explain how physical examination findings contribute to the reasoning of cervicothoracic spine pain in common clinical presentations.

CHAPTER CONTENTS

Introduction, 230
Subjective Examination/Taking the Patient's History, 230
Patient's Perspective on Their Experience, 230
Assessment Tools and Patient Reported Outcome Measures, 230
Body Chart, 230
Behaviour of Symptoms, 231
Special/Screening Questions, 232
Family History, 233
History of Current Complaint, 233
Past Medical History, 233
Plan of the Physical Examination, 234
Physical Examination, 235
Observation, 235
Active Physiological Movements, 236
Palpation, 236
Muscle Tests, 241
Neurological Tests, 243
Other Nerve Tests, 245
Sensorimotor Tests, 245
Miscellaneous Tests, 247
Completion of the Examination, 250
Case Study, 252
References, 254

INTRODUCTION

The cervical spine is the most complex articular system in the body, comprising 37 separate joints and moving over 600 times per hour (Giles & Singer, 1998), with a total sagittal plane excursion in excess of 1,000,000° per day (Sterling et al., 2008); no other part of the articular system is in such a state of constant motion. Common conditions relevant to this region include nerve root, intervertebral disc and facet joint disorders and whiplash-associated disorders. Narrowing of the spinal foramen and canal may occur (stenosis) and osseous anomalies (e.g. cervical rib) can be present (Giles & Singer, 1998). Structural changes are not strongly associated with pain, however, and are commonly found in asymptomatic subjects (Nakashima et al., 2015). The cervicothoracic region is defined here as the region between C3 and T4 and includes the joints and their surrounding soft tissues. Note that the order of subjective questioning and the physical tests described below can be altered as appropriate for the patient being examined.

SUBJECTIVE EXAMINATION/TAKING THE PATIENT'S HISTORY

Patient's Perspective on Their Experience

This includes the patient's perspectives, experience and expectations, age, employment, home situation and details of any leisure activities. In order to treat the patient appropriately, it is important that the condition is managed within the context of the patient's social and work environment.

Psychosocial factors (yellow flags) need to be assessed, as they will strongly influence recovery and treatment response. Screening for psychosocial risk factors such as a post-traumatic stress reaction is important in whiplash-associated injuries. Post-traumatic stress reactions are characterised by intrusive thoughts and flashbacks regarding the trauma (i.e. motor vehicle collision) and a state of hyperarousal that can involve feelings of irritability, difficulty concentrating and falling asleep at night (Worsfold, 2014). The reader is directed to Chapter 3 for more information.

Assessment Tools and Patient Reported Outcome Measures

The use of additional tools or patient-reported outcome measures may be used to support and guide initial assessment and/or management, examples include:

- The Neck Disability Index – the most commonly used patient-reported outcome measure for neck pain-related disability (Vernon & Mior, 1991)
- The STarT MSK screening tool – a risk stratification measure which helps to 'match' management to a patient based on the risk (low, medium and high) of developing a more persistent complaint (Dunn et al., 2021)
- Condition-specific measures (e.g. Fibromyalgia Impact Questionnaire)
- Generic domain-specific measures (e.g. Fear Avoidance Beliefs Questionnaire for fear, Patient Specific Functional Scale for self-selected functional activity) (Horn et al., 2012)

Body Chart

The following information concerning the area and type of current symptoms (e.g. pain, stiffness, paraesthesia etc.) can be recorded on a body chart (see Fig. 3.2).

Area of Current Symptoms

Be precise when mapping out the area of the symptoms. Patients may have symptoms over a large area. In addition to symptoms over the cervical spine, they may have symptoms in the form of pain (sharp, dull, deep, throbbing, burning etc.), stiffness, paraesthesia etc. over the head and face, thoracic or lumbar spine and upper limbs/hands. Ascertain which is their main complaint and record where the patient feels the symptoms are coming from.

Areas Relevant to the Region Being Examined

All other relevant areas are checked for symptoms; it is important to ask about pain or even stiffness, as this may be relevant to the patient's main symptom. Mark unaffected areas with ticks (✓) on the body chart. Check for symptoms in the head, temporomandibular joint, thoracic and lumbar spine, shoulder, elbow, wrist and hand and ascertain whether the patient has ever experienced any disequilibrium or dizziness. Co-existing and worsening symptoms (i.e. pain, paraesthesia, numbness or weakness), which may include the low back, lower limbs and gait disturbances, should not be disregarded and may be indicative of a more concerning pathology (e.g. cervical myelopathy). Dizziness and unsteadiness are commonly associated with whiplash-associated disorders and, less frequently, atraumatic neck pain and may indicate sensorimotor disturbance (Treleaven, 2008).

Head and/or neck pain can be a symptom of an underlying vascular pathology or dysfunction and can mimic presentations which are consistent with a musculoskeletal complaint. Similar risk factors exist for both including recent trauma and commonality for the presence of some symptoms (e.g. headache, neck pain, upper limb or facial paraesthesia and dizziness). See Chapter 8 in the companion text (Barnard & Ryder, 2024) for further information, and readers are recommended to review the International Federation of Orthopaedic Manipulative Physical Therapists Cervical Framework (Rushton, 2020). The clinician's aim during the patient history is to acquire sufficient high-quality information, in the form of patient data to make the best judgement on the probability of serious pathology and contraindications to treatment; furthermore, a 'risk factors' versus 'benefit of intervention' model is advocated (Rushton et al., 2014).

Quality of Pain

Establish the quality of the pain. Complaints of burning and electric shock-like pains and pains that 'have a mind of their own' are suggestive of neuropathic pain, a risk factor for poor recovery in whiplash injury (Sterling & Pedler, 2009). If the patient experiences headaches or facial symptoms, consider carrying out a full upper cervical spine examination (see Chapter 7).

Intensity of Pain

The intensity of pain can be measured using, for example, a numerical pain rating scale (NPRS), as shown in Fig. 3.4. A pain diary may be useful for patients with chronic neck pain with or without headaches to determine the pain patterns and triggering factors. The intensity of pain informs clinical reasoning severity, may provide guidance to the structures producing the symptoms and guides the scope and nature of the examination. As well as the subjective rating of NPRS, severity (low, moderate, high) is determined by questioning on analgesia use (and effectiveness), impact on activities of daily living including work and hobbies and pain disturbing sleep.

Abnormal Sensation

Check for any altered sensation (heightened sensitivity to touch, temperature) locally in the cervical and thoracic spine regions and in other relevant areas such as the upper limbs or face.

Constant or Intermittent Symptoms

Ascertain the frequency of the symptoms, whether they are constant or intermittent. If symptoms are constant, check whether there is variation in the intensity of the symptoms, as constant unremitting pain may be indicative of neoplastic disease.

Relationship of Symptoms

Determine the relationship between the symptomatic areas – do they come together or separately? For example, the patient could have shoulder, arm or wrist and hand pain or symptoms without cervical pain, or the symptoms may always be present together.

Behaviour of Symptoms

Aggravating Factors

For each symptomatic area, discover what movements and/or positions aggravate the patient's symptoms.

The clinician also asks the patient about theoretically known aggravating factors for structures that could be a source of the symptoms (e.g. looking up or neck rotation may provoke symptoms originating from structures of the facet joints). The clinician ascertains how the symptoms affect and are affected by function, such as static and active postures (e.g. sitting, standing, lying, washing, ironing, dusting, driving, reading, writing, work, sport and social activities). Note details of the training regimen for any sports activities.

Common aggravating movements and positions for the cervical spine include looking up (e.g. painting a ceiling (cervical extension), reversing the car (cervical rotation), reading or working on a laptop or personal computer (PC) (sustained flexion) and sleeping postures (cervical rotation and side flexion)). Hair washing, shaving, applying make-up, tying shoe laces and crossing the road are all potential aggravating factors, requiring a relatively large excursion of cervical range of motion (Bible, 2010). The clinician finds out if the patient is left- or right-handed.

Easing Factors

For each symptomatic area, the clinician asks what eases the patient's symptoms to help confirm the relationship between the symptoms and determine their irritability (see Chapter 3). The clinician asks the patient about theoretically known easing factors for structures that could be contributing to symptoms. For example, symptoms from the cervical spine may be eased by supporting the head or neck, whereas symptoms arising from a cervical rib may be eased by shoulder girdle elevation and/or depression. The clinician can analyse the position or movement that eases the symptoms, to help determine a possible structure at fault. For example, the patient may obtain relief from nerve root inflammation by placing her arm/hand on top of her head, thus reducing strain on sensitized neural structures (Malanga et al., 2003).

Twenty-Four-Hour Behaviour of Symptoms

The clinician determines the 24-hour behaviour of symptoms by asking questions about night, morning and evening symptoms.

Behaviour of Symptoms Over Time

The clinician determines the 24-hour behaviour of each symptomatic area by asking questions about night, morning and evening symptoms. Additional useful time points for symptom behaviour are across each week and month, considering any link to certain activities (e.g. work/leisure or hormonal influences in females).

Night symptoms. (See Chapter 3 for details of questions that must be asked.) In addition, questions specific to the positioning of the spine would be:

- What position is most comfortable/uncomfortable?
- What is your normal sleeping position (including the position of the neck, thoracic spine, arms and legs)?
- How many and what type of pillows are used?
- Is your mattress firm or soft and has it been changed recently? Have you tried sleeping in another bed and does that make any difference?
- How many times do you wake up at night? When you wake up, what do you do? How long does it take to then fall back to sleep?

Morning and evening symptoms. The clinician determines the pattern of the symptoms in the morning (on waking and on rising), through the day and at the end of the day. The status of symptoms on first waking establishes whether the patient is better with rest. Pain/stiffness on waking would suggest an inflammatory component, whereas no pain on waking but pain on rising would suggest a more mechanical pain pattern. Stiffness in the morning for the first few minutes might suggest osteoarthritis/spondylosis; stiffness and pain for a few hours may be suggestive of an inflammatory condition such as ankylosing spondylitis. If symptoms are worse after work compared with when off work, it is important to explore work-related factors (e.g. enjoyment, stress, occupational activities and other environmental factors) that may be contributing to the complaint.

Current State of the Condition

In order to determine the current state of the condition, the clinician asks whether the symptoms are getting better, getting worse or remaining unchanged since onset.

Special/Screening Questions

As detailed in Chapter 3, the clinician must differentiate between conditions that are suitable for conservative management and other systemic, neoplastic and non-musculoskeletal conditions.

Cervical Spine Fracture

Although cervical spine fracture is rare in physiotherapy practice, a high index of suspicion is indicated in patients who have sustained trauma involving dangerous mechanisms of injury (e.g. fall >1 m/5 steps), high-speed motor vehicle collisions, axial loading to the head (e.g. diving) and greater than 65 years of age, presenting with bilateral less than 45 degrees cervical rotation and paraesthesia in the extremities. This screening method is termed the 'Canadian C-spine rule' (Stiell et al., 2001). Any suspicion of cervical spine fracture requires urgent referral for medical investigation.

Vascular Pathologies of the Neck

Although rare, cervical arterial dissection has been associated with manipulation, whiplash injury and sports injuries (Hauser et al., 2010; Willett & Wachholtz, 2011). In the initial stages, cervical arterial dissection could present as stiffness and pain in the neck. Thus the clinician needs to maintain a high index of suspicion. The clinician needs to ask about symptoms that may be related to pathologies of the arterial vessels, which course through the neck, namely, the vertebral arteries and the internal carotid arteries. Pathologies of these vessels can result in neurovascular insult to the brain (stroke). These pathologies are known to produce signs and symptoms similar to musculoskeletal dysfunction of the upper cervical spine (Rushton, 2020). Care must be taken to differentiate vascular sources of pain from musculoskeletal sources. Urgent medical investigation is indicated if frank vascular pathology is identified. Many patients present with treatable musculoskeletal causes of symptoms but also have some of the reported risk factors (e.g. current or past smoker, hypertension etc.). This does not necessarily exclude them from manual therapy treatment, and careful clinical reasoning and monitoring of signs and symptoms are required in the management of these patients (Rushton, 2020). See Chapter 3 in this book and Chapter 8 in the companion text (Barnard & Ryder, 2024) for further information.

Family History

Family history relevant to the onset and progression of the patient's problem is recorded.

Presenting Condition (Reason for Referral or Current Complaint)

Symptoms, behaviour, aggravating and easing factors to determine current severity and irritability of presenting complaint.

History of Current Complaint

For each symptomatic area, the clinician needs to know how long the symptom has been present, whether there was a sudden or insidious onset and whether there was a known cause that triggered the onset of the symptom (e.g. fall, injury or change in activities). The mechanism of injury (when, where, how it happened) gives some important clues as to a potentially injured structure. If the onset was slow, the clinician finds out if there has been any change in the patient's lifestyle (e.g. a new job or hobby or a change in sporting activity), which may have affected the stresses on the cervicothoracic spine and related areas. Was there a sudden onset of pain as a result of a traumatic episode or repetitive minor trauma? Rib injuries are commonly caused by trauma (e.g. sporting injury, road traffic accident or fall). To confirm the relationship between symptoms, the clinician asks what happened to other symptoms and when each symptom began. Clarify the time course, progression and impact of the symptoms on the patient's normal function from the first onset of this episode to the present time. Find out details about any treatment/management interventions and advice given: what was it and what was the effect? How do the interventions align with patients' understanding and beliefs of their condition?

Past Medical History

The following information is obtained from the patient and/or the medical notes:

- Any history of previous similar complaints, including details pertaining to (1) duration, severity, (2) investigations (blood, imaging etc.), (3) previous management (pharmacological, conservative, surgical interventions) and importantly the results/outcome or influence of any on the complaint
- Previous injuries or accidents (e.g. sporting, road traffic accident, falls etc.), surgeries (e.g. abdominal or spinal surgery), medical conditions (e.g. cancer or endocrine) and other potentially relevant factors (e.g. diet, stress, previous management for a musculoskeletal complaint).

General Health

The clinician ascertains the state of the patient's general health to find out if the patient has other co-morbidities which may contribute to their condition or may influence management planning (e.g. any osteoporosis, respiratory disorders, cardiovascular disease, breathlessness, chest pain, malaise, fatigue, fever, stress, anxiety or depression). Some co-morbidities may be a precaution or contraindication to certain management approaches (e.g. manipulative therapy in osteoporosis). Questions relating to breathing and respiratory conditions (e.g. breathlessness, history of asthma etc.) may be appropriate owing to the potential for increased activity of accessory muscle of respiration (i.e. sternocleidomastoid, scalene muscles) and visceral referral of symptoms.

Pattern Recognition and Differential Diagnosis

Knowledge of pathological processes and symptom behaviour of some pathologies, (e.g. osteoarthritis), is applicable to all synovial joints. Table 9.1 (in Chapter 9) details pain symptom location, pattern of onset, associated symptoms and features to aid pattern recognition of a number of conditions which are relevant to the cervicothoracic spine region.

For Full Details of all Special Questions (see Chapter 3)

Drug History

If medication is taken specifically for a cervicothoracic spine complaint, is the patient taking the medication regularly? What effect does it have? How long before this appointment was the medication taken? Has the patient been prescribed long-term (6 months or more) steroids or anticonvulsants, as this may have an impact on bone density. Has the patient been prescribed hormone replacement therapy (HRT)?

Investigations, Injections and Imaging

Has the patient been referred on by their general practitioner or seen a specialist for this complaint? Is the patient under investigation for any other condition currently? Has the patient had any investigations (e.g. blood tests for systematic inflammatory conditions or infection), injections (spinal or muscular) or been radiographed or had any other investigative scans for this or any similar complaint (magnetic resonance imaging (MRI), computed tomography (CT) scan). If so what body region and any results? Has the patient had a dual-energy x-ray absorptiometry (DEXA) scan to determine bone mineral density?

Neurological Symptoms

Has the patient experienced symptoms of spinal cord compression (termed 'myelopathy' which may be secondary to trauma, degenerative disease or disc herniation), for example, numbness, tingling and/or electric shocks in the hands and feet either bilaterally or unilaterally, depending on the compression site? Also, has the patient experienced weakness or difficulty using the arms or legs, including tripping or dropping things? Sympathetic function is difficult to measure but questions about changes in swelling, sweating, skin changes (pitting oedema, shiny and inelastic skin) and circulation need to be included. Patients presenting with altered sympathetic function may report bizarre and unusual symptoms (e.g. trickling, crawling sensations).

Vascular Symptoms

The vascular supply to the upper limb passes through the thoracic outlet. Questions should include how good the patient's circulation is and whether the patient has any swelling, coldness, cyanosis, fatigability or cramping in the upper extremities. Symptoms may be indicative of complaints such as thoracic outlet syndrome.

KNOWLEDGE CHECK

1. Describe categories and types of conditions which may give rise to cervicothoracic spine pain.
2. What rheumatological conditions can cause cervicothoracic spine pain?
3. What visceral structures contribute to a complaint of cervicothoracic spine pain?
4. What may pain on coughing or sneezing indicate?

Plan of the Physical Examination

After allowing the patient an opportunity to add anything that may not have been mentioned so far, the purpose and plan for the physical examination will need to be explained and consent obtained.

A planning sheet can help guide clinicians through the clinical reasoning process and ensure the development of a working hypothesis of the most likely cause of, or contributing factors for the patient's complaint (see Appendix 3.1). A 'must, should, could' list will help prioritise your physical examination procedures to ensure that your hypothesis is supported (see Chapter 3).

The hypothesis is developed from the patient's history by identifying:

- The regions and structures that need to be examined as a possible cause for, or contributing to, the complaint. Often, it is not possible to examine fully at the first attendance, and so examination of the structures must be prioritized (must, should, could) over subsequent sessions.
- Other factors that need to be examined, e.g. working, leisure and everyday postures, breathing patterns, sensorimotor impairment and muscle weakness.
- The predominant pain mechanisms that might be driving the patient's symptoms. Pain has been classified into nociceptive (mechanical, inflammatory or ischemic), peripheral, neurogenic, central, autonomic and affective. For the clinical features of pain mechanisms, see Box 3.2.
- In what way should the physical tests be carried out? Will it be easy or hard to reproduce each symptom? Will it be necessary to use combined movements or repetitive movements to reproduce the patient's

symptoms? Are symptoms severe and/or irritable? If symptoms are severe, physical tests may be carried out to just before or to the initial onset of symptom production or in an unloaded position. No overpressures will be carried out. If symptoms are irritable, physical tests may be examined to just before or to initial symptom production, with fewer physical tests being examined.
- Are there any precautions and/or contraindications to elements of the physical examination that need to be explored further, such as neurological involvement, recent fracture, trauma, osteoporosis, steroid or anticoagulant therapy and inflammatory conditions? There may also be certain contraindications to further examination and treatment (e.g. symptoms of cord compression).

PHYSICAL EXAMINATION

The information from the patient history helps the clinician to plan an appropriate physical examination. The severity, irritability, nature and pain mechanisms of the condition are the major factors that will influence the choice and priority of physical testing procedures. The first and overarching question the clinician might ask is: 'Is this patient's condition suitable for me to manage as a clinician?' For example, a patient presenting with symptoms of spinal cord compression may only need neurological integrity testing, prior to an urgent medical referral. The nature of the patient's condition has a major impact on the physical examination. The second question the clinician might ask is: 'Does this patient have a cervicothoracic musculoskeletal dysfunction that I may be able to help?' To answer that, the clinician needs to carry out a full physical examination; however, this may not be possible if the symptoms are severe and/or irritable. The clinician would use non-provocative physical tests to support or negate their hypothesis (e.g. testing motion within a symptom-free range). If a patient's symptoms are non-severe and non-irritable, then the clinician aims to find physical tests that may reproduce each of the patient's symptoms to support or negate their hypothesis.

Each significant physical test that either provokes or eases the patient's symptoms which differ from age/gender/patient appropriate norms is highlighted in the patient's notes by an asterisk (*) for easy reference.

The order and detail of the physical tests described below need to be appropriate to the patient being examined and to the hypotheses (primary or alternatives) developed; some tests will be irrelevant, some tests will be carried out briefly, while it will be necessary to investigate others fully. It is important that readers understand that the techniques shown in this chapter are some of many; the choice depends on factors such as the relative size of the clinician and patient, as well as the clinician's preference. For this reason, novice clinicians may initially want to copy what is shown, but then quickly adapt to what suits them best.

Observation

Informal Observation

The clinician observes the patient in dynamic and static situations; the quality of movement is noted, as are the postural characteristics and facial expressions. Informal observation occurs throughout the consultation from the first point of contact (e.g. walking into the clinic).

Formal Observation

Observation of posture. Formal observation may necessitate the clinician examine the patient from the front (anterior), back (posterior) and both sides (lateral). Mirrors in a clinic setting can be useful for efficiency (reducing the amount the clinician has to move around the patient) and simultaneous observation of more than one plane. The clinician examines the patient's spinal posture in sitting and standing, noting the posture of the head and neck, thoracic spine and upper limbs. It should be noted that, in the cervicothoracic region, associations between forward head 'chin poke' posture and neck pain are poor (Richards et al., 2016) despite there being a strong tradition within physiotherapy of 'correcting posture' (Kendall & Kendall, 2015). It is important to note whilst observing patients, including symmetry and alignment that patients may present with differences or deviations from the norm which are unrelated to their complaint. All findings need to be considered as part of the clinical reasoning process when determining their potential relevance or otherwise to a patient's current complaint.

Observation of muscle form. The clinician observes the muscle bulk and tone of the patient, comparing the left and right sides. It must be remembered that handedness and level and frequency of physical activity may well explain differences in muscle bulk between sides.

Observation of soft tissues. The clinician observes the quality and colour of the patient's skin and any area of swelling or presence of scarring and takes cues for further examination.

Observation of the patient's attitudes and feelings. The age, gender and ethnicity of patients and their cultural, occupational and social backgrounds will all affect their attitudes and feelings towards themselves, their condition and the clinician. The clinician needs to be aware of and sensitive to these attitudes and to empathize and communicate appropriately so as to develop a rapport with the patient and thereby enhance the patient's compliance with the treatment.

Active Physiological Movements

For active physiological movements, the clinician notes the:

- quality of movement
- range of movement
- behaviour of pain through the range of movement
- resistance through the range of movement and at the end of the range of movement
- provocation of any muscle spasm.

The active movements with overpressure listed below and shown in Fig. 8.1 are tested with the patient sitting. Assessment can be enhanced with the use of combined movements (Edwards, 1980) (Fig. 8.2). The clinician establishes the patient's symptoms at rest and prior to each movement, and corrects any movement deviation to determine its relevance to the patient's symptoms.

For the cervical spine, the active movements and possible modifications are shown in Table 8.1. Numerous differentiation tests (Hengeveld & Banks, 2013) can be performed; the choice depends on the patient's signs and symptoms. For example, if a patient complains of pain turning to the right, the clinician can ask the patient to reproduce the movement and then de-rotate the neck to return to neutral. If symptoms reduce, this lends some support for the symptoms' source being linked to the cervical spine rather than the thoracic spine (see Chapter 9, Fig. 9.3).

It may be necessary to examine other regions to determine their relevance to the patient's symptoms; they may be the source of the symptoms, or they may be contributing to the symptoms. The most likely regions are the thoracic spine temporomandibular, shoulder, elbow, wrist and hand. The joints within these regions can be tested fully (see relevant chapter) or partially with the use of screening tests (see Table 4.4 Chapter 4 for further details).

Some functional ability has already been tested by the general observation of the patient during the subjective and physical examinations (e.g. postures adopted during the subjective examination and the ease or difficulty of undressing prior to the examination). Any further functional testing can be carried out at this point in the examination and may include sitting postures and aggravating movements of the upper limb. Clues for appropriate tests can be obtained from the subjective examination findings, particularly aggravating factors.

Palpation

The clinician palpates the cervicothoracic spine and, if appropriate, the patient's upper cervical spine, lower thoracic spine and any other relevant areas. It is useful to record palpation findings on a body chart (see Fig. 3.2) and/or palpation chart (see Fig. 4.34).

The clinician notes the following:

- the temperature of the area
- increased skin moisture
- the presence of oedema or effusion
- mobility and feel of superficial tissues (e.g. ganglions, nodules)
- the presence or elicitation of any muscle spasm
- tenderness of bone, ligaments, muscle, tendon, tendon sheath and nerve; nerves in the upper limb can be palpated at the following points:
  - the suprascapular nerve along the superior border of the scapula in the suprascapular notch
  - the brachial plexus in the posterior triangle of the neck, at the lower third of sternocleidomastoid
  - the suprascapular nerve along the superior border of the scapula in the suprascapular notch
  - the dorsal scapular nerve medial to the medial border of the scapula
  - the median nerve over the anterior elbow joint crease, medial to the biceps tendon; also at the

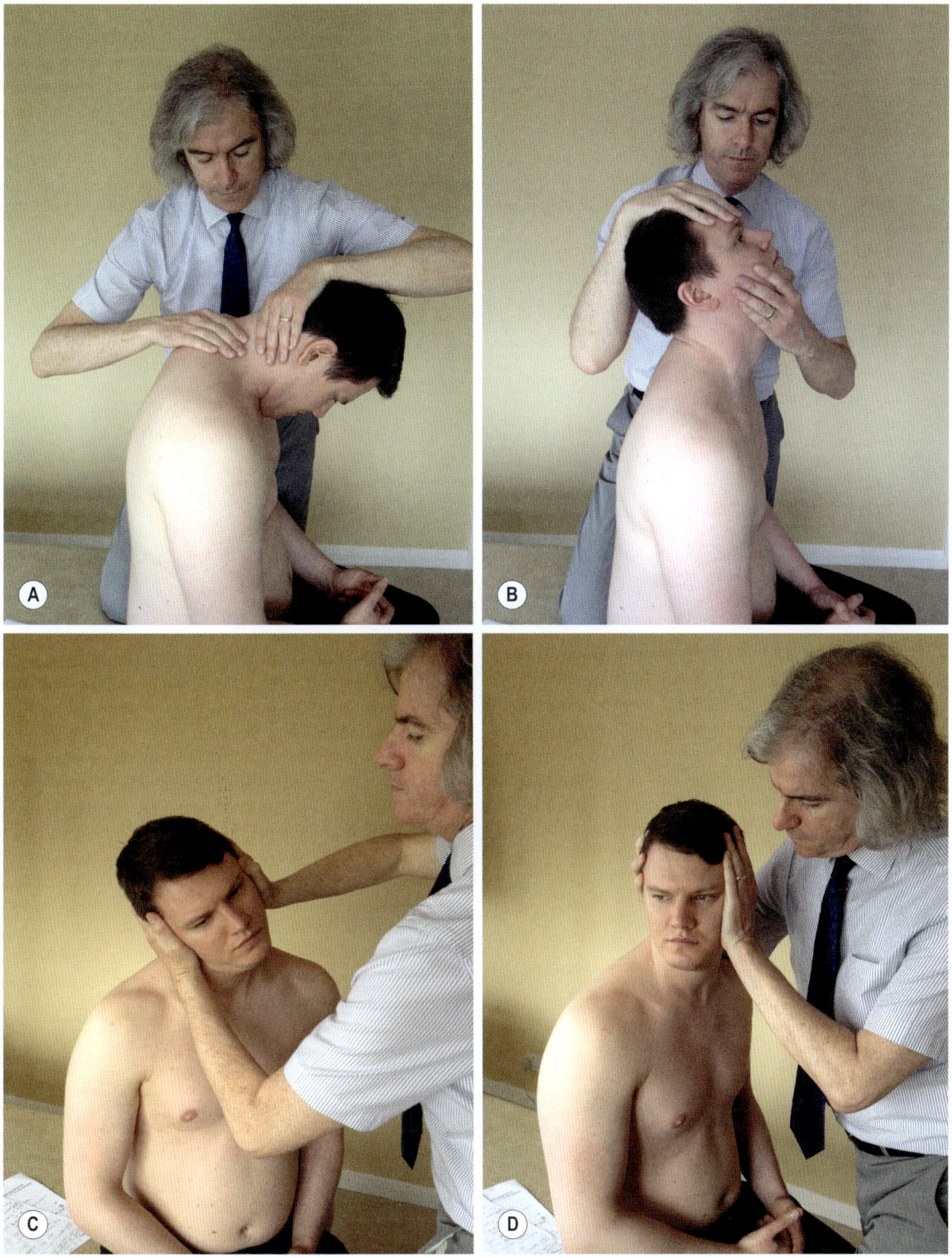

Fig. 8.1 Overpressures to the Cervical Spine. (A) Flexion. The right hand stabilizes the trunk while the left hand moves the head down so that the chin moves towards the chest. (B) Extension. The right hand rests over the head to the forehead while the left hand holds over the mandible. Both hands then apply a force to cause the head and neck to extend backwards. (C) Lateral flexion. Both hands rest over the patient's head around the ears and apply a force to cause the head and neck to tilt laterally. (D) Rotation. The left hand lies over the zygomatic arch while the right hand rests over the occiput. Both hands then apply pressure to cause the head and neck to rotate.

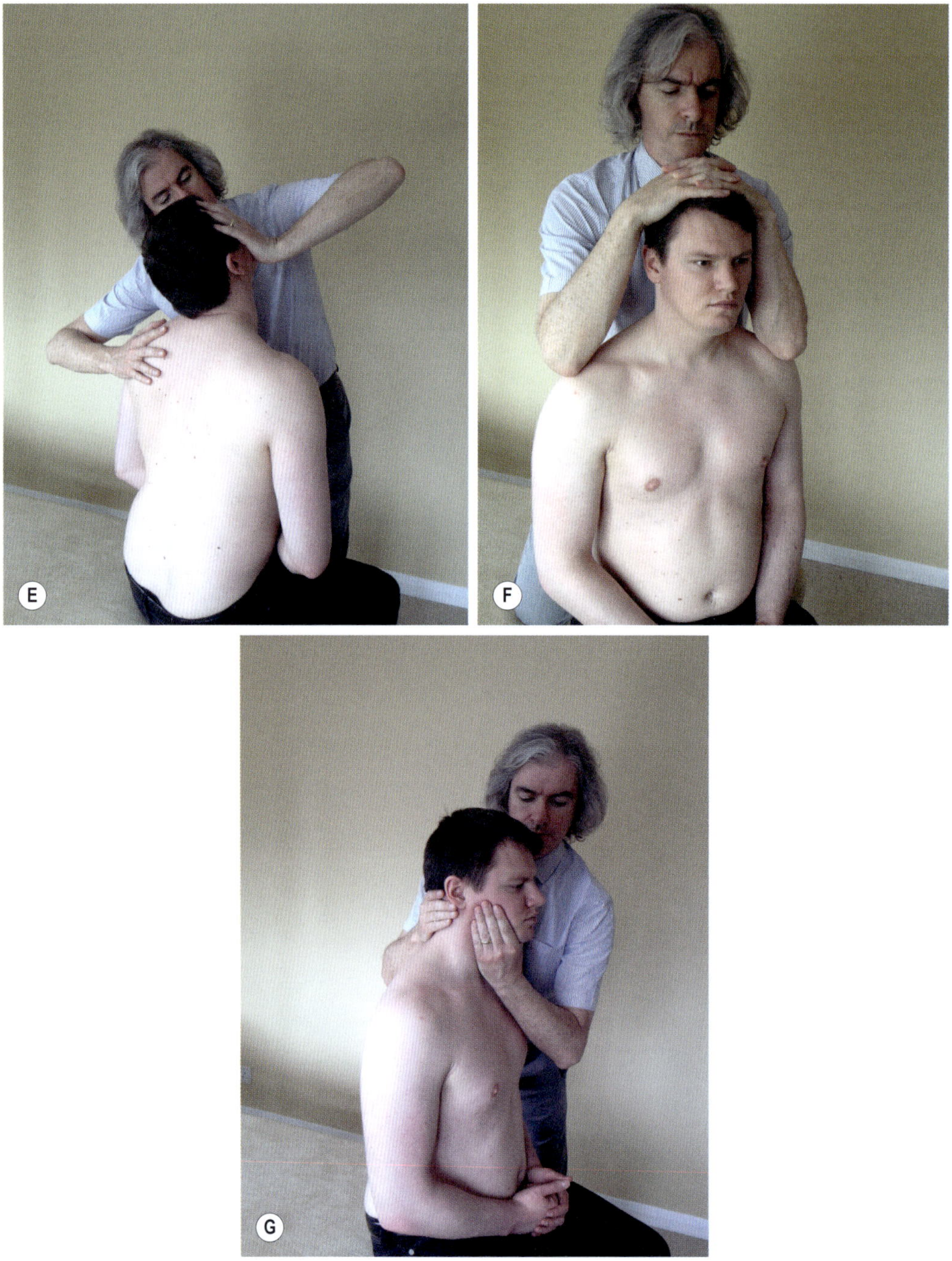

Fig. 8.1, cont'd (E) Left extension quadrant. This is a combination of extension, left rotation and left lateral flexion. The patient actively extends and, as soon as the movement is complete, the clinician passively moves the head into a left rotation and then lateral flexion by applying gentle pressure over the forehead with the left hand. (F) Compression. The hands rest over the top of the patient's head and apply a downward force. (G) Distraction. The left hand holds underneath the mandible while the right hand grasps underneath the occiput. Both hands then apply a force to lift the head upwards.

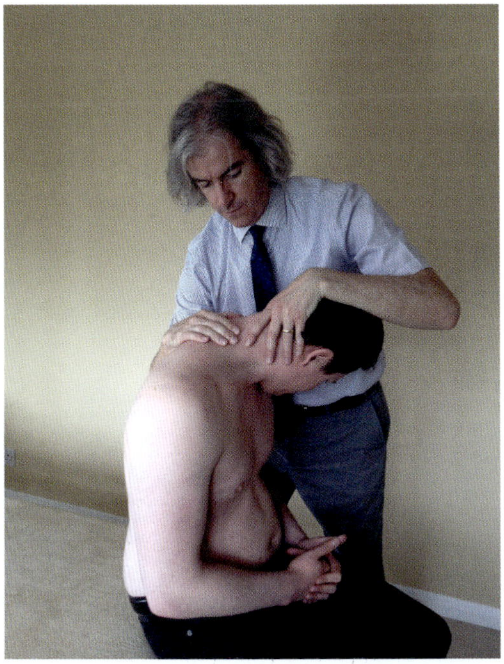

Fig. 8.2 Combined Movement to the Cervical Spine. The right hand supports the trunk while the left hand moves the head into flexion, then lateral flexion then rotation.

wrist between palmaris longus and flexor carpi radialis
- the radial nerve around the spiral groove of the humerus, between the brachioradialis and flexor carpi radialis; also in the forearm and at the wrist in the snuffbox

- increased sensitivity to light palpation (hyperalgesia/allodynia) suggests neuropathic or 'central sensitization' pain states
- increased or decreased prominence of bones
- symptoms (often pain) provoked or reduced on palpation. Posterior midline tenderness can indicate a vertebral fracture (Stiell et al., 2001).

Passive Intervertebral Examination

Passive intervertebral examination of the cervical spine is intended to produce information regarding the quantity (range) and quality (through range and end-feel) of specific motion segments and additionally to identify the source of the patient's symptoms. The validity and reliability of this concept have been challenged in recent years, demonstrating varying results (Pool et al., 2004; Piva et al., 2006). Despite this variance, there is a continuing use of these techniques, with a belief that findings from passive examination contribute towards valid diagnosis, clinical decision making and management planning (van Trijffel et al., 2005, 2009; Abbott et al., 2009). It appears that when passive intervertebral examination techniques are utilized within a cluster of tests they are useful both for diagnosing the facet joint as the source of pain and for clinical decision-making (De Hertogh et al., 2007; Schneider et al., 2014). The sensitivity and specificity of these tests are shown in Table 8.2.

Passive Physiological Intervertebral Movements

This can take the form of a passive physiological intervertebral movement (PPIVM), which examines the movement at each segmental level. A PPIVM can be a useful adjunct to passive accessory intervertebral movements (PAIVM) to identify segmental hypomobility and hypermobility. With the patient supine, the clinician palpates the gap between adjacent spinous processes and articular pillars to feel the range of intervertebral movement during flexion, extension, lateral flexion and rotation. Fig. 8.3 demonstrates a rotation PPIVM at the C4–C5 segmental level. It may be necessary to examine other regions to determine their relevance to the patient's symptoms; they may be the source of the symptoms, or they may be contributing to the symptoms. The most likely regions are the thoracic spine, temporomandibular region, shoulder, elbow, wrist and hand.

Passive Accessory Intervertebral Movements

It is useful to use the palpation chart and movement diagrams (or joint pictures) to record findings. These are explained in detail in Chapter 4.

The clinician notes the following:
- quality of movement
- range of movement
- resistance through the range and at the end of the range of movement
- behaviour of pain through the range
- provocation of any muscle spasm.

TABLE 8.1 Active Physiological Movements With Possible Modifications

Active Movements	Modifications
Cervical spine	Repeated movements
Flexion	Speed altered
Extension	Movements combined (McCarthy, 2017), e.g.
Left lateral flexion	• Extension quadrant: extension, ipsilateral rotation and lateral flexion
Right lateral flexion	• Flexion then rotation
Left rotation	• Extension then rotation
Right rotation	• Flexion then lateral flexion then rotation (see Fig. 8.2)
Compression	• Extension then lateral flexion
Distraction	Compression or distraction sustained
Upper cervical extension/protraction (pro)	Injuring movement
Repetitive protraction (rep pro)	Differentiation tests
Repetitive flexion (rep flex)	Function
Upper cervical flexion/retraction (ret)	
Repetitive retraction (rep ret)	
Repetitive retraction and extension (rep ext)	
Left repetitive lateral flexion (rep lat flex)	
Right repetitive lateral flexion (rep lat flex)	
Left repetitive rotation (rep rot)	
Right repetitive rotation (rep rot)	
Retraction and extension lying supine	
Repetitive retraction and extension lying supine	
Static (maximum of 3 min) retraction and extension lying supine or prone	
?Temporomandibular	
?Shoulder	
?Elbow	
?Wrist and hand	

TABLE 8.2 Diagnosing Facet Joint Pain: Sensitivity and Specificity of Passive Intervertebral Examination

Diagnostic Test	Sensitivity (%)	Specificity (%)
Passive intervertebral examination (PIE)	92	71
Palpation for segmental tenderness (PST)	94	73
Combined extension-rotation (ER)	83	59
PIE, PST and ER	79	84

Adapted from Schneider, 2014

The cervical and upper thoracic spine (C2–T4) accessory movements are shown in Fig. 8.4 and listed in Table 8.3.

Following accessory movements to the cervicothoracic region, the clinician reassesses all the physical asterisks (movements or tests that have been found to reproduce the patient's symptoms) in order to establish the effect of the accessory movements on the patient's signs and symptoms. Accessory movements can then be tested for other regions suspected to be a source of, or contributing to, the patient's symptoms (Fig. 8.5). Again, following accessory movements to any one region, the clinician reassesses all the asterisks. Regions likely to be examined are the upper cervical spine, lower thoracic spine, shoulder, elbow, wrist and hand (see Table 8.3).

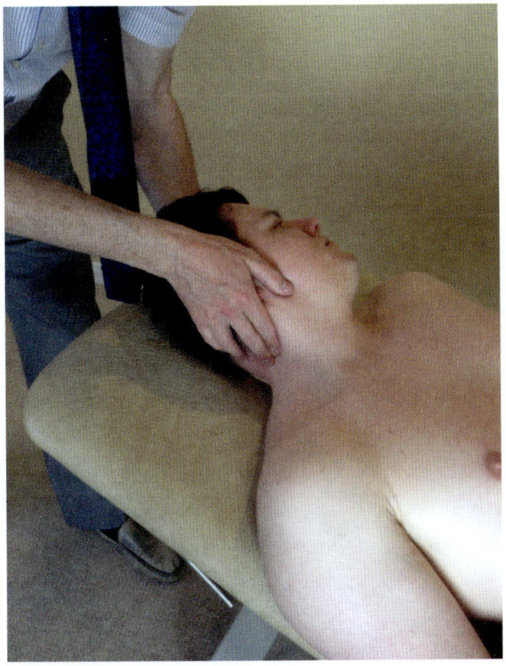

Fig. 8.3 Rotation Passive Physiological Intervertebral Movement at the C4–C5 Segmental Level. The clinician places the index finger over the right C4–C5 zygapophyseal joint region, feeling for tissue texture changes as the head is passively rotated to the left.

Natural Apophyseal Glide

These can be applied to the apophyseal joints between C2 and T3. The patient sits and the clinician supports the patient's head and neck and applies a static or oscillatory force to the spinous process or articular pillar in the direction of the facet joint plane of each vertebra (Mulligan, 2019). Fig. 8.6 demonstrates a unilateral on C5. As a treatment or mini treatment, this is repeated 6–10 times. The patient should feel no pain but may feel slight discomfort.

Reversed Natural Apophyseal Glides

The patient sits and the clinician supports the head and neck and applies a force to the articular pillars of a vertebra using the index and thumb of the hand (Fig. 8.7). A force is then applied to the pillars in the direction of the facet plane.

Sustained Natural Apophyseal Glide

The painful cervical spine movements are examined in sitting. The clinician applies a force to the spinous process and/or transverse process in the direction of the facet joint plane of each cervicothoracic vertebra as the patient moves slowly towards the pain. All cervical movements can be tested in this way. Fig. 8.8 demonstrates a C5 extension sustained natural apophyseal glide (SNAG). For further details on these techniques, see Mulligan (2019).

Muscle Tests

Muscle tests include those examining muscle strength, control, length and isometric muscle contraction.

Movement Control

A battery of tests can be used to examine movement control formally (Table 8.4). These tests have been shown to have 'substantial to excellent' intra- and interrater reliability ($k = 0.86$ and $k = 0.69$, respectively) (Segarra et al., 2015). The tests have been shown to discriminate between asymptomatic controls and individuals with neck pain (Elsig et al., 2014). The battery of tests includes cervicothoracic extension, sitting cervical retraction and protraction and quadruped cervical rotation (Fig. 8.9).

Specific muscle testing can be undertaken as follows.

Deep cervical muscle testing. Deep muscles in the cervical spine are important in the support and control of the head and neck. See Chapter 7 for testing of the deep cervical flexors and extensors.

Scapular strength. To assess gross muscle function, specific functional tests can be carried out. For example, the clinician can observe the patient performing a slow push-up from the prone position to assess the function of the serratus anterior muscle. Weakness will cause the scapula to wing (the medial border moves away from the thorax).

Isometric Muscle Testing

The cervical flexor endurance test records the length of time the supine patient can maintain her head 2 cm above the plinth before the onset of 'chin thrust', i.e. fatigue (Fig. 8.10). The clinician places his index finger on the patient's chin to identify the first onset of fatigue or 'chin thrust' (Grimmer, 1994). Normal values are 14 seconds for females and 18 seconds for males (Grimmer, 1994) and then for side flexor, endurance testing is 120 seconds and 90 seconds for males and females respectively (Swanson et al., 2020). Good intra- and inter-tester reliability of the cervical endurance test has been

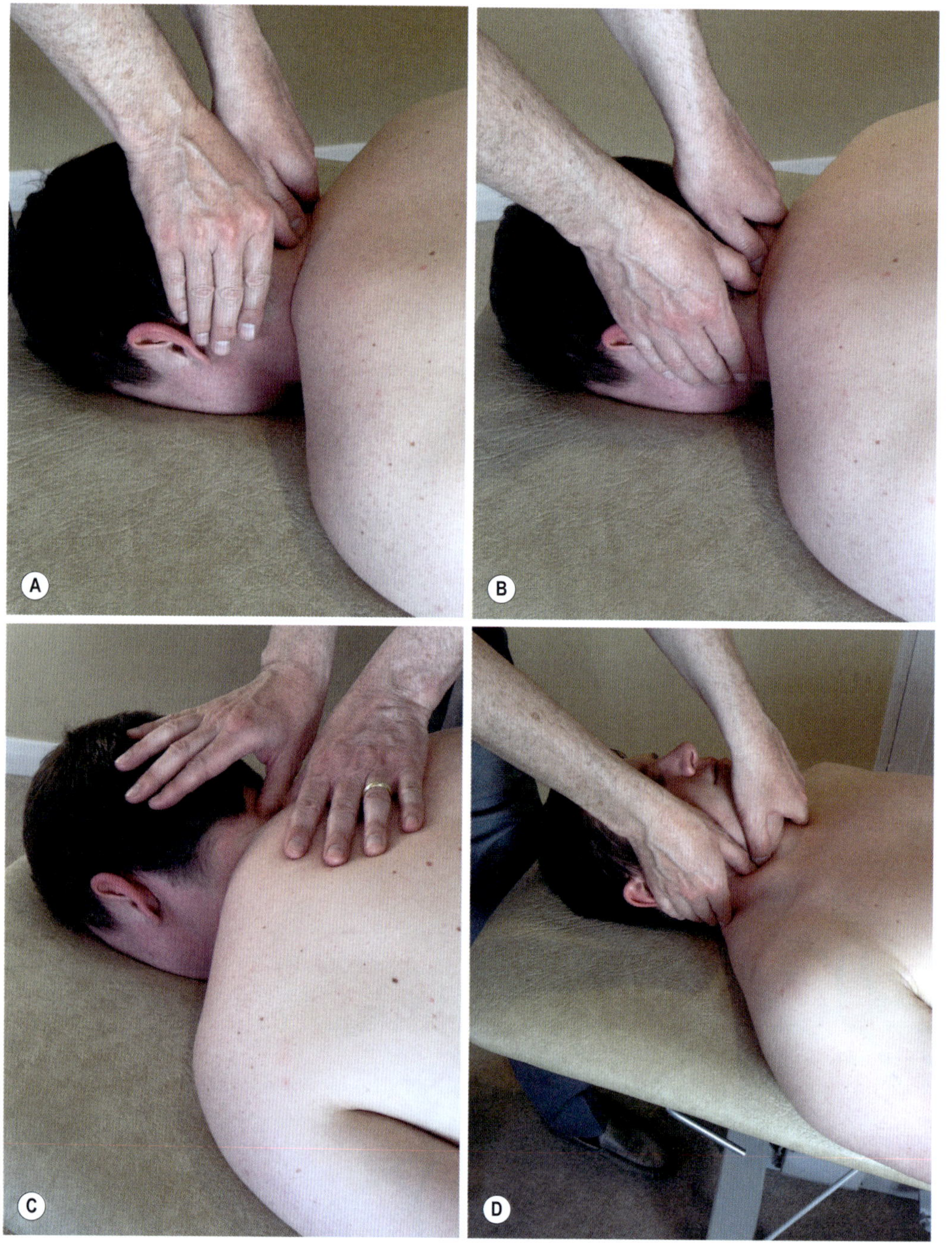

Fig. 8.4 Cervical Accessory Movements. (A) Central posteroanterior. Thumb pressure is applied to the spinous process. (B) Unilateral posteroanterior. Thumb pressure is applied to the articular pillar. (C) Transverse. Thumb pressure is applied to the lateral aspect of the spinous process. (D) Unilateral anteroposterior. In the supine position, thumb pressure is applied to the anterior aspect of the transverse process. Care is needed to avoid pressure over the carotid artery.

TABLE 8.3 Accessory Movements, Choice of Application and Reassessment of the Patient's Asterisks

Accessory Movements		Choice of Application	Identify Any Effect of Accessory Movements on Patient's Signs and Symptoms
C2–T4		Alter speed of force application	Reassess all asterisks
↕	Central posteroanterior	Start position, e.g.	
↓ ↓	Unilateral posteroanterior	• In flexion	
⇄	Transverse	• In extension	
↑ ↑	Unilateral anteroposterior (C2–T1 only)	• In lateral flexion	
Ribs 1–4			• In flexion and rotation
↔ Caud	Longitudinal caudad first rib	• In flexion and lateral flexion	
↕	Anteroposterior	• In extension and rotation	
↕	Poster anterior	• In extension and lateral flexion	
→ Med	Medial glide	Direction of the applied force	
		Point of application of applied force	
Upper cervical spine		As above	Reassess all asterisks
Lower thoracic spine		As above	Reassess all asterisks
Shoulder region		As above	Reassess all asterisks
Elbow region		As above	Reassess all asterisks
Wrist and hand		As above	Reassess all asterisks

reported (Grimmer, 1994; Olson et al., 2006; Domenech et al., 2011). The clinician can also test isometric resisted tests of neck flexor and extensor strength in the neutral head position and, if indicated, in different parts of the physiological range; testing flexion or extension in combination with rotation allows useful comparison of left- and right-side differences (Fig. 8.11). The clinician also observes the quality of the muscle activity (e.g. does there appear to be excessive effort or muscle activity?). These would suggest a lack of muscular endurance or patient fear of performing the movement. These tests should be used with caution in migraine sufferers as there is a risk of triggering a migraine episode with cervical spine endurance testing (Carvalho et al., 2021).

Muscle Length

The clinician tests the length of muscles (e.g. levator scapulae, upper trapezius, sternocleidomastoid, pectoralis minor, scalene muscles and the deep occipital muscles). Testing the length of these muscles is described in Chapter 4.

Neurological Tests

This includes neurological integrity testing, neurodynamic tests and testing of the central nervous system.

Integrity of Nervous System

As a general guide, a neurological examination is indicated if symptoms are felt below the acromion.

Dermatomes/peripheral nerves. Light touch and pain sensation of the upper limb are tested using cotton wool and pinprick, respectively, as described in Chapter 4. Knowledge of the cutaneous distribution of nerve roots (dermatomes) and peripheral nerves enables the clinician to distinguish the sensory loss due to a nerve root lesion from that due to a peripheral nerve lesion. The

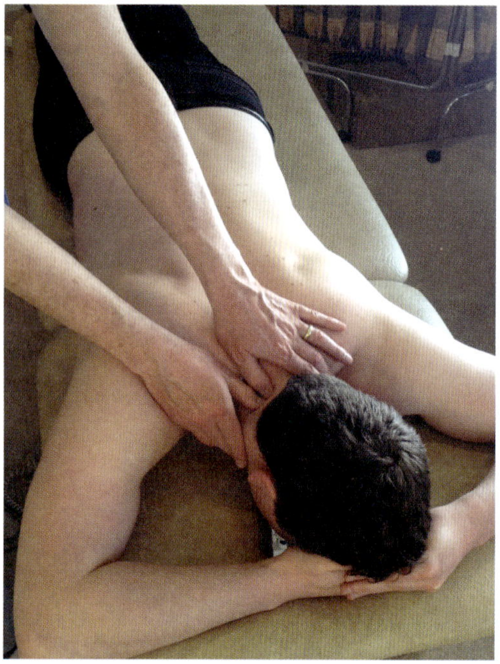

Fig. 8.5 Palpation of Accessory Movements Using a Combined Movement. Thumb pressure over the right articular pillar of C5 is carried out with the cervical spine positioned in left lateral flexion.

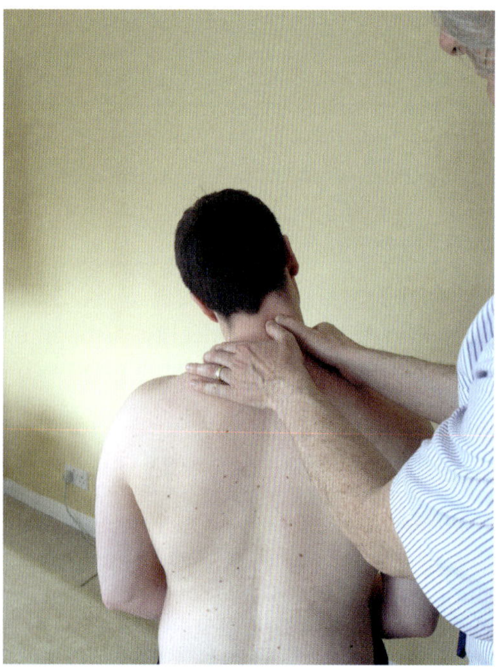

Fig. 8.6 Unilateral Natural Apophyseal Glide on C6. Thumb pressure is applied to the right articular pillar of C5 as the patient laterally flexes to the left.

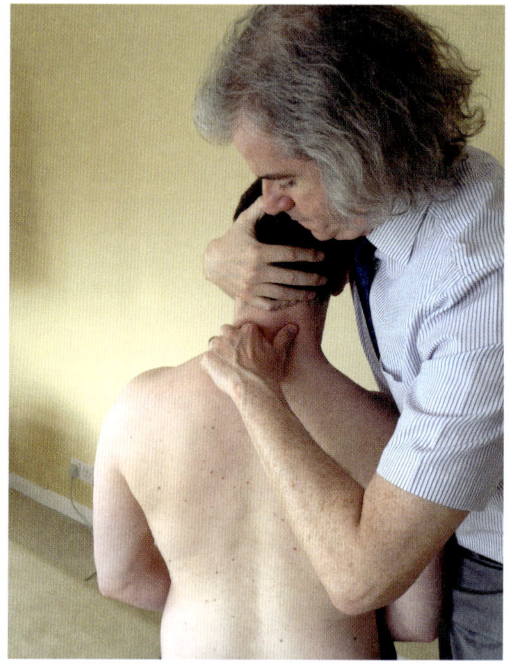

Fig. 8.7 Reversed Flexion Natural Apophyseal Glide to C5. The right hand supports the head and neck. The index and thumb of the left hand apply an anterior force to the articular pillars of C5.

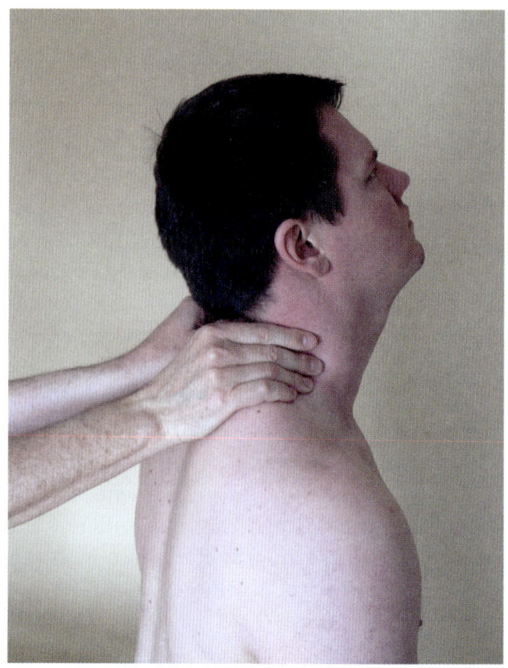

Fig. 8.8 Extension Sustained Natural Apophyseal Glide to C5. Thumb pressure is applied to the spinous process of C5 as the patient slowly extends.

TABLE 8.4 Movement Control Tests

Movement control (MC) test 1: extension cervicothoracic junction	*Instruction* Make a double chin. Then, try to look at the ceiling without losing the double-chin position and without making a hollow back *Compensatory movements* Protraction of the head Loss of the flexion in the upper cervical spine Elevation or protraction of the shoulders
MC test 2: pro- and retraction of head	*Instruction* Push the chin horizontally forward and backward *Compensatory movements* Elevation or protraction of the shoulder Excessive flexion or extension in the lower cervical spine Flexion of the thoracic spine The line between the ear and the nose cannot be held horizontally
MC test 3: quadruped cervical rotation	*Instruction* Make a straight back. Turn your head and neck slowly to the right and back to the starting position. Try to make the rotation around an axis that runs longitudinally through your head, neck and spine. Then you do the same movement to the left *Compensatory movements* Lateral flexion of the cervical spine Flexion or extension in the cervical spine Flexion, extension or lateral flexion in the thoracic spine Elevation of the shoulders

Adapted from Elsig, 2014

cutaneous nerve distribution and dermatome areas are shown in Chapter 4.

Myotomes/peripheral nerves. The following myotomes are tested and are shown in Chapter 4:

- C4: shoulder girdle elevation
- C5: shoulder abduction
- C6: elbow flexion
- C7: elbow extension
- C8: thumb extension
- T1: finger adduction.

A working knowledge of the neural innervation of muscles (myotomes) and peripheral nerves enables the clinician to distinguish motor loss due to a root lesion from that due to a peripheral nerve lesion. Peripheral nerve distributions are shown in Chapter 4.

Reflex testing. The following deep tendon reflexes are tested (see Chapter 4):

- C5–C6: biceps
- C7: triceps and brachioradialis.

Neurodynamic Tests

The following neurodynamic tests may be carried out in order to ascertain the degree to which neural tissue is responsible for the production of the patient's symptom(s):

- passive neck flexion
- upper-limb neurodynamic tests
- straight-leg raise
- long-sitting slump
- slump.

These tests are described in detail in Chapter 4.

Other Nerve Tests

Central Nervous System Testing – Upper Motor Nerve Lesions

Plantar response – Babinski's sign. Pressure applied from the heel along the lateral border of the plantar aspect of the foot produces flexion of the toes in the normal individual. Extension of the big toe with downward fanning of the other toes occurs with an upper motor neuron lesion (Fuller, 2013).

Clonus. Dorsiflex the ankle briskly, maintain the foot in that position and a rhythmic contraction may be found. More than three beats is considered abnormal.

Tinel's Sign. The clinician lightly taps the skin over the nerve to elicit a sensation of tingling or 'pins and needles' in the distribution of the nerve. Reproduction of distal pain/paraesthesia denotes a positive test indicating regeneration of an injured sensory nerve (Fuller, 2013).

Sensorimotor Tests

Sensorimotor control has been discussed in Chapter 4. Clinically, dizziness and unsteadiness are commonly associated with whiplash-associated disorders and, less

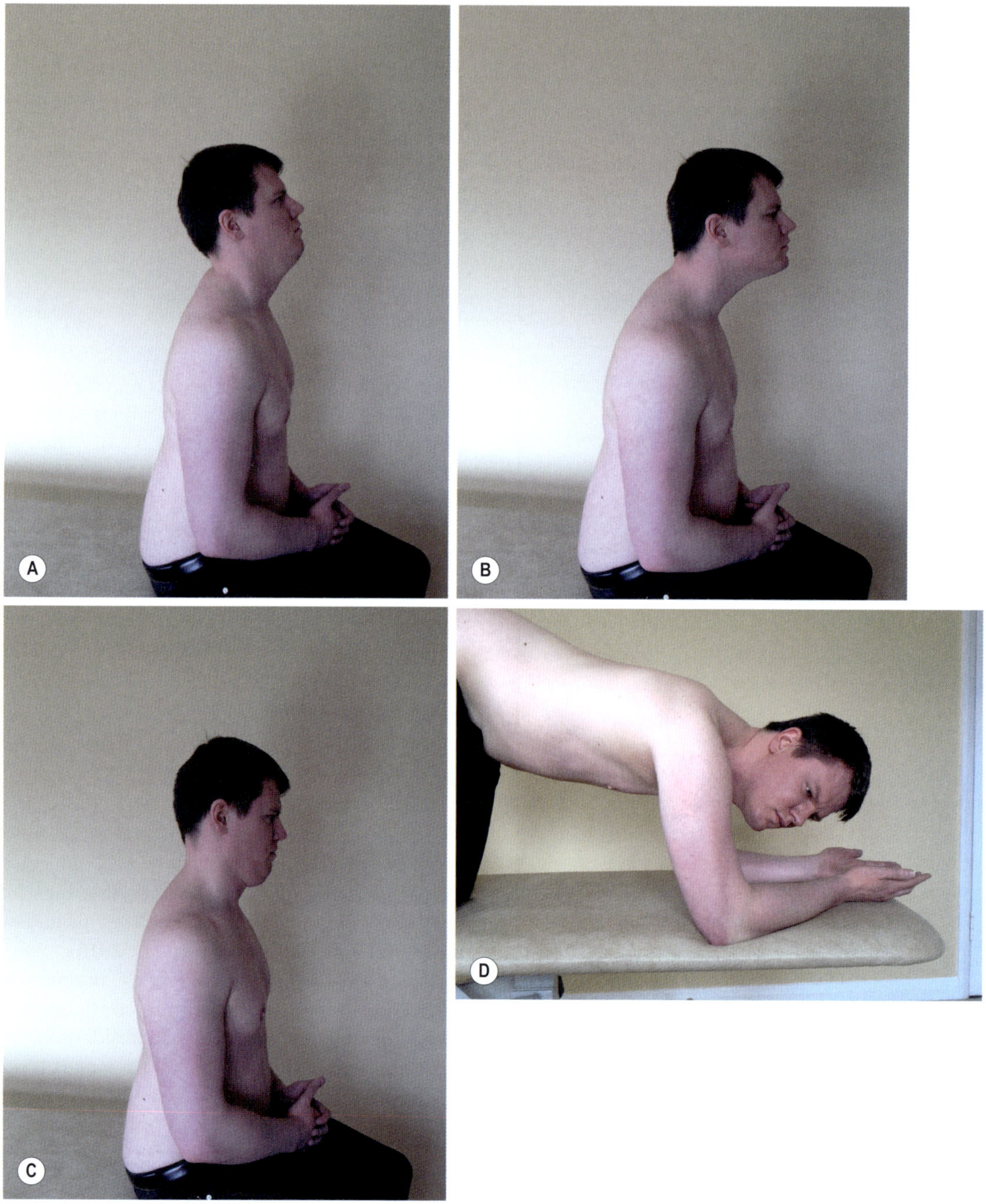

Fig. 8.9 Movement Control Tests. (A) Cervicothoracic extension. (B) Sitting cervical protraction. (C) Sitting cervical retraction. (D) Quadruped cervical rotation.

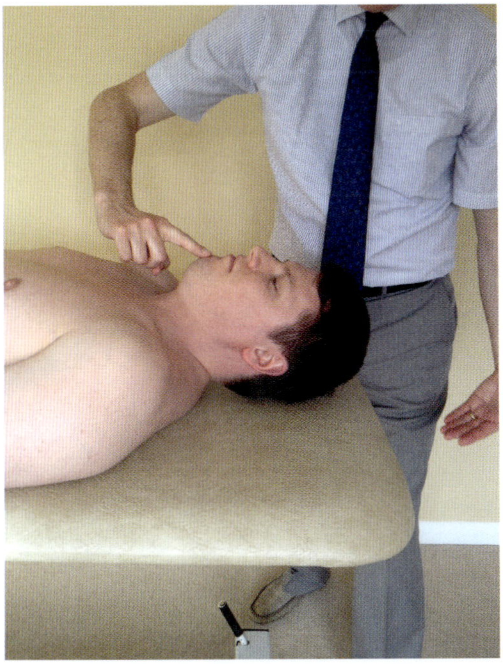

Fig. 8.10 Cervical Flexor Endurance Test. Record the length of time the supine patient can maintain the head 2 cm above the plinth, prior to the first onset of fatigue. The clinician's index finger is placed on the patient's chin to identify the onset of 'chin thrust'.

frequently, atraumatic neck pain and may indicate sensorimotor disturbance (Treleaven, 2008). It is hypothesised that afferent output from the cervical spine (e.g. from muscle spindles and/or mechanoreceptors) is impaired in neck pain and injury, and this, in turn, can lead to disruption of the reflexive balance mechanisms involving the eyes and the vestibular system, manifesting in unsteadiness and dizziness. Thus cervical proprioception, eye movement control and postural stability can all be impaired to a lesser or greater degree (Treleaven et al., 2003; Treleaven, 2008; Treleaven et al., 2011).

Sensorimotor impairment testing, therefore, involves assessing proprioception (joint position error), oculomotor control and postural stability (Fig. 8.12).

Proprioception

Cervical joint position error tests measure an individual's ability to relocate their head accurately to the same point in space with the eyes closed. Evidence suggests that cervical joint position error measured with a laser and target in the clinical setting has acceptable validity (compared with laboratory-based electromagnetic tracking (e.g. Fastrak system) and reliability (intraclass correlation coefficient >0.75)) and can discriminate between healthy controls and subjects with neck pain (Heikkilä & Aström, 1996; Heikkilä & Wenngren, 1998; Chen & Treleaven, 2013; Jørgensen et al., 2014).

Oculomotor Tests

The smooth-pursuit test involves the patient sitting and following a moving object with her eyes whilst keeping her head still. The object – usually the clinician's finger – is panned slowly, taking 5 seconds to cross an arc 30 degrees on either side of the patient's midline. The onset of pain, dizziness or increased effort suggests sensorimotor impairment. The smooth-pursuit test has good interrater reliability and has been shown to discriminate between healthy controls and subjects with chronic neck pain (Della Casa et al., 2014).

Postural Stability

Tests of postural stability include comfortable, narrow and tandem standing, tested with both eyes open and eyes closed. The test is timed for 30 seconds maximum. Patients 'fail' the test if they step or require support during the test (Field et al., 2008).

Miscellaneous Tests

Spurling's Neck Compression Test

The test is performed by extending, laterally flexing and rotating the neck to the same side and then applying downward axial pressure through the head (Fig. 8.13). The test is considered positive if radicular symptoms radiate into the limb ipsilateral to the side to which the head is laterally flexed and rotated (Malanga et al., 2003). The test appears to have high specificity and sensitivity (95% and 92%, respectively) and good to fair interrater reliability (Malanga et al., 2003; Shah & Rajshekhar, 2004).

Shoulder Abduction Test

The test is performed by actively or passively abducting the symptomatic arm and placing the patient's arm on top of her head. The test is considered positive with reduction or relief of ipsilateral cervical radicular symptoms (Malanga et al., 2003).

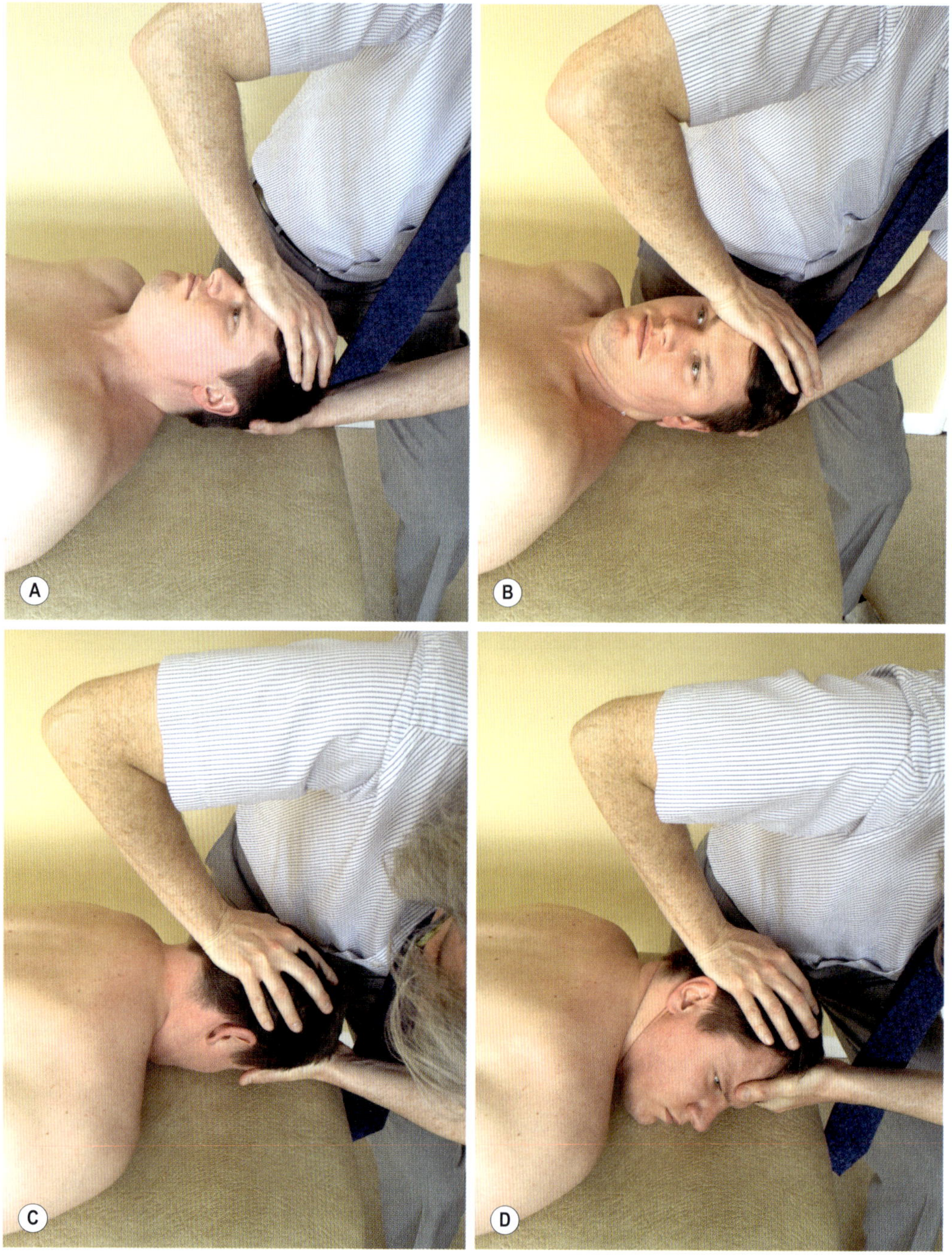

Fig. 8.11 Isometric Muscle Tests. The clinician tests isometric contractions of the neck flexors and extensors. The clinician must ensure that: (1) no movement takes place during the test; (2) the patient's head is supported firmly throughout the test; and (3) the pain response is monitored closely. (A) Flexion-neutral head position. The right hand is resisting the patient's efforts to flex the neck. (B) Flexion and left cervical rotation test. The right hand is resisting the patient's efforts to flex the neck in the sagittal plane. (C) Extension neutral head position. The right hand is resisting the patient's efforts to extend the neck. (D) Extension and right cervical rotation test. The right hand is resisting the patient's efforts to extend the neck in the sagittal plane.

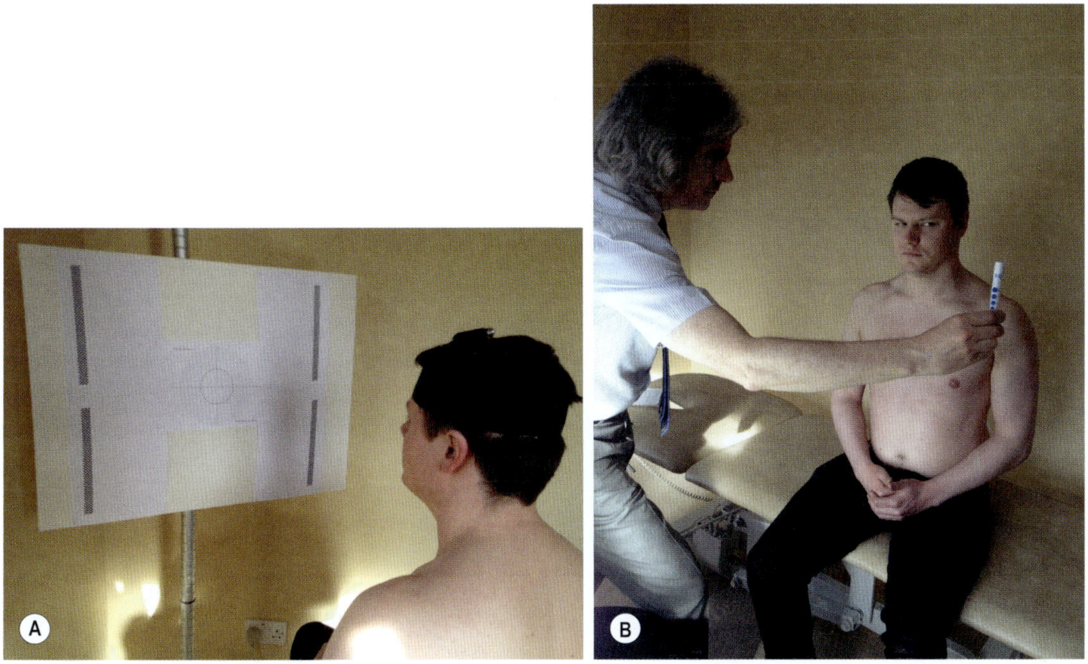

Fig. 8.12 Sensorimotor Tests. (A) Proprioception/joint position error (JPE). The patient sits 90 cm from a wall with eyes closed in a neutral head position. He moves the head in the direction being tested as far as is comfortable. He attempts to return to the precise starting position, keeping the eyes closed. The JPE between the starting point and the return point is measured in centimetres. JPE greater than 5 cm suggests impairment. (B) Oculomotor control smooth-pursuit test. The patient follows an object with his eyes moving 30 degrees on either side of the midline whilst maintaining a neutral head position.

Cervical Arterial Pathology or Dysfunction Testing

If vascular pathology or dysfunction is suspected following the subjective examination (see above), further information regarding the integrity of the vascular system can be gained from the following examination procedures. Further reading is recommended to support the understanding of these procedures.

Blood Pressure

In the event of acute arterial dysfunction, it is likely that there will be a systematic cardiovascular response, manifesting in a dramatic change in blood pressure (usually increasing). Blood pressure is taken using appropriate, validated procedures and equipment, in either sitting or lying.

Peripheral and Cranial Nerve Examination

Examination of the peripheral nerves and cranial nerves is useful to assess for an upper motor neuron lesion linked to neurovascular conditions (Fuller, 2013). See Chapter 4 for more information.

Thoracic Outlet Syndrome

There are several tests for this syndrome, which is predominantly neurogenic in nature, including:

- Roos Test (52%–84% sensitivity, 30%–100% specificity) (Fernández-de-las-Peñas et al., 2015): with the patient's arm in 90-degree abduction, the clinician places a downward pressure on the patient's scapula whilst asking the patient to repeatedly open and close their fingers. If symptoms are reproduced the test is considered positive.
- Adson's Test (79% sensitivity, 74%–100% specificity) (Fernández-de-las-Peñas et al., 2015): the patient is asked to rotate the head and lift their chin towards the affected side. If their radial pulse is absent or decreased on the symptomatic side the test is considered positive.

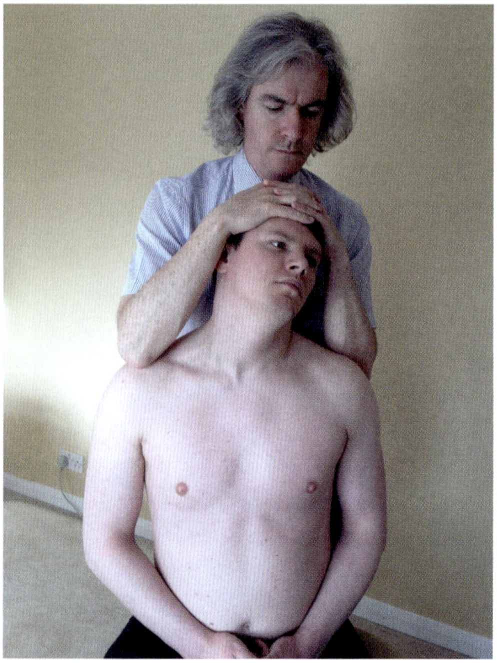

Fig. 8.13 Spurling's Neck Compression Test. Performed by extending, laterally flexing and rotating the neck to the same side and then applying downward axial pressure through the head. The test is considered positive if radicular symptoms radiate into the limb ipsilateral to the side to which the head is laterally flexed and rotated.

COMPLETION OF THE EXAMINATION

Having carried out the above tests, the examination of the cervicothoracic spine is now complete. The subjective and physical examinations produce a large amount of information, which needs to be recorded accurately and quickly. It is important, however, that the clinician does not examine in a rigid manner, simply following the suggested sequence outlined in the chart. Each patient presents differently, and this needs to be reflected in the examination process. It is vital at this stage to highlight with an asterisk (*) important findings from the examination. These findings are reassessed at, and within, subsequent treatment sessions to evaluate the effects of treatment on the patient's condition.

The physical testing procedures which specifically indicate joint, nerve or muscle tissues, as a source of the patient's symptoms, are summarized in Table 4.9. The strongest evidence that a joint is the source of the patient's symptoms is that active and passive physiological movements, passive accessory movements and joint palpation all reproduce the patient's symptoms, and that, following a treatment dose, reassessment identifies an improvement in the patient's signs and symptoms. Weaker evidence includes an alteration in range, resistance or quality of physiological and/or accessory movements and tenderness over the joint, with no alteration in signs and symptoms after treatment. One or more of these findings may indicate a dysfunction of a joint which may or may not be contributing to the patient's condition.

The strongest evidence that a muscle is the source of a patient's symptoms is if active movements, an isometric contraction, passive lengthening and palpation of a muscle all reproduce the patient's symptoms, and that, following a treatment dose, reassessment identifies an improvement in the patient's signs and symptoms. Further evidence of muscle dysfunction may be suggested by reduced strength or poor quality during the active physiological movement and the isometric contraction, reduced range and/or increased/decreased resistance, during the passive lengthening of the muscle, and tenderness on palpation, with no alteration in signs and symptoms after treatment. One or more of these findings may indicate a dysfunction of a muscle which may or may not be contributing to the patient's condition.

The strongest evidence that a nerve is the source of the patient's symptoms is when active and/or passive physiological movements reproduce the patient's symptoms, which are then increased or decreased with an additional sensitizing movement, at a distance from the patient's symptoms. In addition, there is a reproduction of the patient's symptoms on palpation of the nerve and neurodynamic testing, sufficient to be considered a treatment dose, resulting in an improvement in the above signs and symptoms. Further evidence of nerve dysfunction may be suggested by reduced range (compared with the asymptomatic side) and/or increased resistance to the various arm movements, and tenderness on nerve palpation.

On completion of the physical examination the clinician will:

- explain the findings of the physical examination and how these findings relate to the subjective assessment. An attempt should be made to clear up any

misconceptions patients may have regarding their illness or injury
- collaborate with the patient and via problem solving together devise a treatment plan and discuss the prognosis (shared decision making)
- warn the patient of possible exacerbation up to 24–48 hours following the examination
- request the patient to report details on the behaviour of the symptoms following examination at the next attendance
- evaluate the findings, formulate a clinical diagnosis and write up a problem list
- determine the objectives of treatment
- devise an initial treatment plan.

In this way, the clinician develops the following hypotheses categories (Higgs et al., 2008):
- function: abilities and restrictions
- patient's perspective on his/her experience
- source of symptoms. This includes the structure or tissue that is thought to be producing the patient's symptoms, the nature of the structure or tissues in relation to the healing process and the pain mechanisms involved
- contributing factors to the development and maintenance of the problem. There may be environmental, psychosocial, behavioural, physical or heredity factors
- precautions/contraindications to treatment and management. This includes the severity and irritability of the patient's symptoms and the nature of the patient's condition
- management strategy and treatment plan
- prognosis – this can be affected by factors such as the stage and extent of the injury as well as the patient's expectations, personality and lifestyle.

For guidance on treatment and management principles, the reader is directed to the companion textbook (Barnard & Ryder, 2024).

KNOWLEDGE CHECK

1. Describe the main types of patient observation and what you would look for in the cervicothoracic spine region.
2. Describe two tests that can be used for thoracic outlet syndrome.
3. What approaches exist to examine joints in the cervicothoracic spine?
4. What is Spurling's test, and when would you use it?
5. What is the difference between a peripheral nerve and a nerve root?

REVIEW AND REVISE QUESTIONS

1. What lifestyle and personal factors may influence neck pain?
2. List three possible outcome measures you may use for patients with a complaint of cervicothoracic pain.
3. What is the IFOMPT cervical framework and how might this assist in the assessment of patients with cervicothoracic pain?
4. How might a cervicothoracic fracture present and what is the Canadian C-spine rule?
5. What is a NAG and which of the following are true?
    - Can be applied at apophyseal joints between C1 and T4
    - The technique involves a static or oscillatory force applied to the spinous process or articular pillar in the direction of the facet joint plane
    - The technique should be pain free
    - The dosage for a treatment is three sets of 10 repetitions
6. Describe what you would include in a neurological examination.
7. Why is it important to consider sensorimotor testing in the assessment of the cervicothoracic spine?
8. Describe Spurling's test and what would constitute a positive test.

Case Study Mr P

Male, aged 38 years old

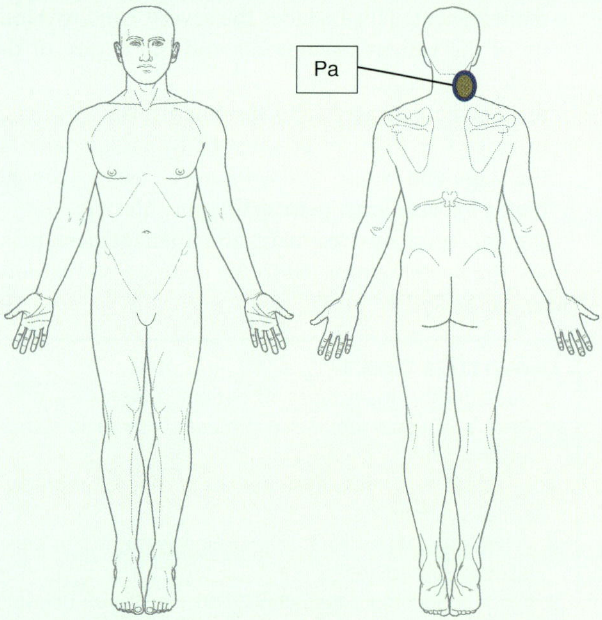

Pa – intermittent pain, with lingering ache once pain subsides

7/10, reducing to 2/10

Aggravating factors – immediate onset of pain with turning to reach for seatbelt, >1 h sitting at computer for work and driving long distances

Easing factors – immediate relief with stretching neck, warm bath

24 h pattern – bit of morning stiffness. Disappears after 20 min or so warm shower/bath. Feels weary at the end of the day especially on days where he has been sitting for more than 10/12 h.

Sleep – Can take some time to get to sleep but does not wake up with the pain.

No symptoms anywhere else

HPC

Neck pain on right side for several few months but seems to be getting worse with working at home more due to pandemic. It helps to move about and stretch periodically but never completely goes away. Finding it increasingly hard to manage symptoms and concentrate on work tasks. Additionally with staff absence at work being higher is now working much longer hours. He feels weary at the end of the day and often lies on the sofa to watch TV rather than sit.

Lifestyle/Occupation/Home Life

Lives with wife and 2 children (9 and 7 years old). Generally happy home life and no real caring responsibilities other than usual cleaning, shopping etc. Used to play 5 aside football twice a week and go to the park with kids for a kick about regularly; unable to play football currently due to the pandemic. Works in sales for an IT company, spends all day on computer and phone talking to clients.

Right handed and drives.

Impact on Function/Beliefs and Expectations

Fed up that this is affecting concentration with work tasks. Seems to be worse with doing less exercise and especially with not getting out with friends for regular 5 aside football. Feels he is too young to have a long-term problem but is unsure what he can do to help himself. Is aware that exercise makes him feel better, but not sure what to do for the best.

PMH

Has had pain for around 10 years for no particular reason. It started slowly when he was driving more for work and spending more time at a computer; the onset coincided with a new job in sales which required him to spend a lot of time driving up and down the country.

Occasional visits to a chiropractor which help with immediate relief; treatment comprised manipulation.

DH/investigations

Occasional paracetamol but other than that no other medications, no history of steroid use. No warfarin.

No imaging, referrals or other management.

FH nil of note

GH Good. No areas of concern re THREAD (thyroid, heart, RA, epilepsy, asthma, diabetes)

Clinical Reasoning

Mr P had an insidious onset of neck pain which coincided with a change in work, family life etc. Whilst the complaint has been reasonably static for the last few years, it is worse now where he is working from home, not able to get out to play his recreational sport due to government restrictions due to the pandemic.

Case Study Mr P—cont'd

psychologically **(yellow flags)** – no clear diagnosis, concerned that this is starting to affect work, frustrated he can't get out to exercise or play with kids at the park

socially **(blue/black flag)**—loss of socialization with work colleagues (and friends)

No observable **red flag** symptoms, although positively Mr P does want to exercise and spend time with his children (**pink flag**)

Evaluation of severity, irritability and nature

Severity (Pa) - moderate (no night disturbance, no regular medication, starting to affect concentration at work, NPRS of 7/10)

Irritability (Pa) - low (symptoms with sitting greater than 1 h, but eases relatively quickly with stretching and moving about)

Nature – chronic neck pain with inflammatory component and peripheral nociception of facet joint.

What are you treating? It is likely at this point we are treating a primary neck pain complaint which has moved from a sub-clinical to clinical complaint due to change in circumstances with working linked to the Covid-19 pandemic; working from home, closure of facilities (e.g. pitch where he does his football) and requirements for social distancing.

Where part of Mr P's job requires him to sit for long periods which can contribute to the thoracic spine becoming stiffer through lack of movement (adaptive changes*). (It is important to note that if tissues are not moved they will adaptively shorten).* Whilst Mr P may have some 'normal' age-related degenerative changes there is no value of additional investigations (e.g. x-ray). Mr P has not had any conservative management

Mr P's main **functional limitation** is being able to sit pain-free for long periods

Subjective markers (link to genics)

1. Sitting for 3 h without neck pain
2. Stiffness in the neck when he first wakes

Does any aspect of the history indicate caution?

No, given levels of severity and irritability and the features fit a persistent pain pattern for the neck.

Can you predict the comparable signs? (Subjective marker linking with an objective sign)

Right rotation

What is the relationship between pain and resistance?

Pa – Pain > resistance

What pain mechanisms can you identify? There is evidence of some central affective (psychology) mechanisms at play as well as peripheral inflammatory nociceptive (neck).

Analysis of percentage weighting (Pain source) Myogenic 20%, Arthrogenic 80%

Analysis of percentage weighting (driver/contributing factors) Given the persistent nature of Mr P's complaint, it is important to consider the following questions

1. why has he developed this complaint?
2. Why has it not settled (young, fit male patient)
3. What does his occupation require him to do?

Based on the duration of complaint (adaptive changes and faulty movement patterns) and age (degenerative changes) proposed weighting could be cervicothoracic spine joint hypomobility 40%, reduced neck muscle endurance capacity (40%), neck proprioception (10%), beliefs/psychological (10%).

Hypotheses to test/working diagnosis? (Differentiate between genics)

1. Reduced work capacity/endurance of neck muscles
2. Postural awareness/proprioception
3. Cervicothoracic spine active and passive movement (muscle v joint)
4. Faulty/dysfunctional movement pattern

Planning the physical examination

Observation to include sitting posture (poking chin) and specifically neck posture when positioned in front of a keyboard and observation of general appearance (e.g. affect) (request photo of work environment and sitting posture at home).

Observe movements to assess R and L rotation and extension. Observe where movement is originating from (quality, range and reproduction of any symptoms). Compare right rotation in resting/habitual sitting posture and then when corrected to a neutral posture to aid differentiation.

Cervicothoracic spine PPIVM into R rotation (C4/5 to T2/3) to assess the passive ROM (may be extended to include mid thoracic rotation PPIVM given extent of sitting); also aids differentiation between joints (level) and between muscle and joint. Thoracic spine mobility can be assessed using tests as per Chapter 9.

Muscles

Assess neck muscle

- endurance using deep neck flexor testing in lying or preferably sitting (to best reflect the main complaint)
- length of deep cervical extensor muscles, scalene muscles bilaterally, pectoralis minor and levator scapulae

Proprioception

Use JPE testing to examine proprioception.

Continued

Case Study Mr P—cont'd

Main clinical findings for Mr P included

Cervicothoracic spine posture involved fixed and flexed cervicothoracic spine and extended upper cervical spine. Partial postural correct was possible (limited by muscle shortening), and the patient was unable to maintain 'corrected' posture for more than a few minutes (proprioceptive deficits and reduced muscle endurance). Working posture involved sitting with arms unsupported, a relatively slumped posture, poking chin and concerns around height and position of desk/computer/mouse.

When posture corrected or a more neutral posture adopted, the range of right rotation increased before the onset of PA (supporting hypothesis pertaining to posture/muscle dysfunction).

PPIVM of the upper thoracic spine revealed stiff upper thoracic spine into R rotation and some resistance towards the end of right rotation cervicothoracic R rotation PPIVM.

Other findings included reduced cervical flexor muscle endurance (cervicothoracic extensors), reduced muscle length of R pectoralis minor, L scalene, L levator scapulae, L trapezius.

JPE inaccuracy and errors increased over repetitions (linked to muscle fatigue)

Management included

Education and advice Advice and education to aid understanding of the relationship between symptoms, working postures and activities. Education to contextualize complaint, with encouragement to re-introduce social physical activity over time. Using a patient-centred approach discuss approaches to ensure breaks between bouts of sitting, work postures, and alternative positioning of desk/computer/mouse.

Muscle stretching to actively lengthen shortened muscles (passively)

R rotation PPIVM C6/7, C7/T1, T1/2 as management technique using Grade III/IV to reduced local joint hypomobility

Home exercise programme

1. Development of work capacity and motor control of deep neck flexors (sitting)
2. As control returns and in the newly adopted posture add in R rotation (this can be done functionally using reaching for the seatbelt)
3. Self-stretching for R pectoralis minor, L scalene, L levator scapulae, L trapezius

Outcome

Mr P returned after 2 weeks and reported considerable improvement, no residual morning stiffness and feeling able to manage symptoms with self-stretching, adjustments to posture and work environment. Felt much more positive and whilst he had not yet started football, did feel like that this was achievable.

JPE, Joint position error; *NPRS,* numerical pain rating scale; *PPIVM,* passive physiological intervertebral movement; *ROM,* range of motion.

REFERENCES

Abbott, J.H., Flynn, T.W., Fritz, J.M., Hing, W.A., Reid, D., et al., 2009. Manual physical assessment of spinal segmental motion: intent and validity. Man. Ther. 14 (1), 36–44.

Barnard, K., Ryder, D., 2024. Principles of Musculoskeletal Treatment and Management: A Handbook for Therapists, fourth ed. Elsevier, Edinburgh.

Bible, J.E., Biswas, D., Miller, C.P., Whang, P.G., Grauer, J.N., 2010. Normal functional range of motion of the cervical spine during 15 activities of daily living. J. Spinal Disord. Tech. 23 (1), 15–21.

Carvalho, G.F., Luedtke, K., Szikszay, T.M., Bevilaqua-Grossi, D., May, A., 2021. Muscle endurance training of the neck triggers migraine attacks. Cephalalgia 41 (3), 383–391.

Chen, X., Treleaven, J., 2013. The effect of neck torsion on joint position error in subjects with chronic neck pain. Man. Ther. 18 (6), 562–567.

De Hertogh, W., Vaes, P., Duquet, W., 2007. The validity of the manual examination in the assessment of patients with neck pain. Spine (Phila Pa 1976) 7 (5), 628–629.

Della Casa, E., Affolter Helbling, J., Meichtry, A., Luomajoki, H., Kool, J., 2014. Head-eye movement control tests in patients with chronic neck pain; inter-observer reliability and discriminative validity. BMC Musculoskelet. Disord. 15 (16).

Domenech, M.A., Sizer, P.S., Dedrick, G.S., McGalliard, M.K., Brismee, J.M., 2011. The deep neck flexor endurance test: normative data scores in healthy adults. PM R 3 (2), 105–110.

Dunn, K.M., Campbell, P., Lewis, M., Hill, J.C., van der Windt, D.A., Afolabi, E., et al., 2021. Refinement and validation of a tool for stratifying patients with musculoskeletal pain. Eur. J. Pain. 25 (10), 2081–2093.

Edwards, B.C., 1980. Combined movements in the cervical spine (c2-7) their value in examination and technique choice. Aust. J. Physiother. 26 (5), 165–171.

Elsig, S., Luomajoki, H., Sattelmayer, M., Taeymans, J., Tal-Akabi, A., Hilfiker, R., 2014. Sensorimotor tests, such as movement control and laterality judgment accuracy, in persons with recurrent neck pain and controls. A case-control study. Man. Ther. 19 (6), 555–561.

Fernández-de-las-Peñas, C., Cleland, J., Dommerholt, J., 2015. 2015. Manual Therapy for Musculoskeletal Pain Syndromes: An Evidence- and Clinical-Informed Approach, first ed. Churchill Livingstone, UK.

Field, S., Treleaven, J., Jull, G., 2008. Standing balance: a comparison between idiopathic and whiplash-induced neck pain. Man. Ther. 13 (3), 183–191.

Fuller, G., 2013. Neurological Examination Made Easy, fifth ed. Churchill Livingstone, Edinburgh.

Giles, L., Singer, K., 1998. Clinical anatomy and management of cervical spine pain. Clinical anatomy and management of back pain series. Elsevier, Oxford.

Grimmer, K., 1994. Measuring the endurance capacity of the cervical short flexor muscle group. Aust. J. Physiother. 40 (4), 251–254.

Hauser, V., Zangger, P., Winter, Y., Oertel, W., Kesselring, J., 2010. Late sequelae of whiplash injury with dissection of cervical arteries. Eur. Neurol. 64 (4), 214–218.

Heikkilä, H., Aström, P.G., 1996. Cervicocephalic kinesthetic sensibility in patients with whiplash injury. Scand. J. Rehabil. Med. 28 (3), 133–138.

Heikkilä, H.V., Wenngren, B.I., 1998. Cervicocephalic kinesthetic sensibility, active range of cervical motion, and oculomotor function in patients with whiplash injury. Arch. Phys. Med. Rehabil. 79 (9), 1089–1094.

Hengeveld, E., Banks, K., 2013. Maitland's Vertebral Manipulation: Management of Neuromusculoskeletal Disorders, eighth ed., 1. Butterworth-Heinemann, Oxford.

Higgs, J., Jones, M.A., Loftus, S., Christensen, N., 2008. Clinical Decision Making and Multiple Problem Spaces: Clinical Reasoning in Health Professions. Elseveir, Amsterdam, pp. 4–19.

Horn, K.K., Jennings, S., Richardson, G., Van Vliet, D., Hefford, C., Abbott, J.H., 2012. The patient-specific functional scale: psychometrics, clinimetrics, and application as a clinical outcome measure. JOSPT 42 (1), 30–D17.

Jørgensen, R., Ris, I., Falla, D., Juul-Kristensen, B., 2014. Reliability, construct and discriminative validity of clinical testing in subjects with and without chronic neck pain. BMC Musculoskelet. Disord. 15, 408.

Kendall, F., Kendall, F.P., 2015. Muscles: Testing and Function With Posture and Pain. Lippincott Williams & Wilkins, Baltimore, MD.

Malanga, G.A., Landes, P., Nadler, S.F., 2003. Provocative tests in cervical spine examination: historical basis and scientific analyses. Pain Physician 6 (2), 199–205.

McCarthy, C., 2017. Combined Movement Theory: Rational Mobilization and Manipulation of the Vertebral Column. Elsevier, Churchill Livingstone.

Mulligan, B.R., 2019. Manual Therapy 'NAGs', 'SNAGs', 'MWMs' etc, seventh ed. Orthopedic Physical Therapy Products, New Zealand.

Nakashima, H., Yukawa, Y., Suda, K., Yamagata, M., Ueta, T., Kato, F., 2015. Abnormal findings on magnetic resonance images of the cervical spines in 1211 asymptomatic subjects. Spine (Phila Pa 1976) 40 (6), 392–328.

Olson, L.E., Millar, A.L., Dunker, J., Hicks, J., Glanz, D., 2006. Reliability of a clinical test for deep cervical flexor endurance. J. Manipulative Physiol. Ther. 29 (2), 134–138.

Piva, S.R., Erhard, R.E., Childs, J.D., Browder, D.A., 2006. Intertester reliability of passive intervertebral and active movements of the cervical spine. Man. Ther. 11 (4), 321–330.

Pool, J.J., Hoving, J.L., De Vet, H.C., Van Mameren, H., Bouter, L.M., 2004. The interexaminer reproducibility of physical examination of the cervical spine. J. Manipulative Physiol. Ther. 27 (2), 84–90.

Richards, K.V., Beales, D.J., Smith, A.J., O'Sullivan, P.B., Straker, L.M., 2016. Neck posture clusters and their association with biopsychosocial factors and neck pain in Australian adolescents. Phys. Ther. 96 (10), 1576–1587.

Rushton A, et al., International Framework for Examination of the cervical region for potential of vascular pathologies of the neck prior to Orthopaedic Manual Therapy (OMT) Intervention: International IFOMPT Cervical Framework. 2020, International Federation of Orthopaedic Manipulative Physical Therapists (IFOMPT) https://www.ifompt.org/site/ifompt/IFOMPT%20cervical%20framework%20final%202020.pd.

Rushton, A., Rivett, D., Carlesso, L., Flynn, T., Hing, W., Kerry, R., 2014. International framework for examination of the cervical region for potential of cervical arterial dysfunction prior to orthopaedic manual therapy intervention. Man. Ther. 19 (3), 222–22-8.

Schneider, G.M., Jull, G., Thomas, K., Smith, A., Emery, C., Faris, P., et al., 2014. Derivation of a clinical decision guide in the diagnosis of cervical facet joint pain. Arch. Phys. Med. Rehabil. 95 (9), 1695–1701.

Segarra, V., Duenas, L., Torres, R., Falla, D., Jull, G., Lluch, E., 2015. Inter-and intra-tester reliability of a battery of cervical movement control dysfunction tests. Man. Ther. 20 (4), 570–579.

Shah, K.C., Rajshekhar, V., 2004. Reliability of diagnosis of soft cervical disc prolapse using Spurling's test. Br. J. Neurosurg. 18, 480–483.

Sterling, A.C., Cobian, D.G., Anderson, P.A., Heiderscheit, B.C., 2008. Annual frequency and magnitude of neck motion in healthy individuals. Spine (Phila Pa 1976) 33 (17), 1882–1888.

Sterling, M., Pedler, A., 2009. A neuropathic pain component is common in acute whiplash and associated with a more complex clinical presentation. Man. Ther. 14 (2), 173–179.

Stiell, I.G., Wells, G.A., Vandemheen, K.L., Clement, C.M., Lesiuk, H., De Maio, V.J., et al., 2001. The Canadian C-spine rule for radiography in alert and stable trauma patients. JAMA 286 (15), 1841–1848.

Swanson, B.T., Bromaghin, H.M., Bubacy, N., Messick, A., Tinker, L., 2020. The lateral neck flexor endurance test: normative values in the young adult population. J. Bodyw. Mov. Ther. 24 (3), 242–245.

Treleaven, J., 2008. Sensorimotor disturbances in neck disorders affecting postural stability, head and eye movement control—Part 2: case studies. Man. Ther. 3, 266–275.

Treleaven, J., Jull, G., Grip, H., 2011. Head eye co-ordination and gaze stability in subjects with persistent whiplash associated disorders. Man. Ther. 16 (3), 252–257.

Treleaven, J., Jull, G., Sterling, M., 2003. Dizziness and unsteadiness following whiplash injury: characteristic features and relationship with cervical joint position error. J. Rehabil. Med. 35 (1), 36–43.

van Trijffel, E., Anderegg, Q., Bossuyt, P.M.M., Lucas, C., 2005. Inter-examiner reliability of passive assessment of intervertebral motion in the cervical and lumbar spine: a systematic review. Man. Ther. 10 (4), 256–269.

van Trijffel, E., Oostendorp, R.A., Lindeboom, R., Bossuyt, P.M., Lucas, C., 2009. Perceptions and use of passive intervertebral motion assessment of the spine: a survey among physiotherapists specializing in manual therapy. Man. Ther. 14 (3), 243–251.

Vernon, H., Mior, S., 1991. The neck disability index: a study of reliability and validity. J. Manip. Physiol. Ther. 14, 409–415.

Willett, G.M., Wachholtz, N.A., 2011. A patient with internal carotid artery dissection. Phys. Ther. 91 (8), 1266–1274.

Worsfold, C., 2014. When range of motion is not enough: towards an evidence-based approach to medico-legal reporting in whiplash injury. J. Forensic. Leg. Med. 25, 95–99.

9

Examination of the Thoracic Region

Nicola R. Heneghan

LEARNING OUTCOMES

After studying this chapter, you should be able to:

- Outline the key anatomical structures and biomechanical functions of the thoracic spine region.
- Describe the prevalence of, and pathologies associated with thoracic spine pain.
- Understand functional kinetic chains and thoracic spine dysfunction, specifically in relation to complaints such as neck and shoulder pain.
- Identify how clinical reasoning guides history taking in the subjective examination of people with thoracic spine pain and/or dysfunction, informed by the location, behaviour and nature of symptoms, and the value of screening questions.
- Discuss the multifactorial nature of thoracic spine pain and/or dysfunction and the role psychosocial factors may play in how people with thoracic spine pain and/or dysfunction may present.
- List the constituents of a comprehensive physical examination of the thoracic spine region, with consideration of the sensitivity and specificity of key physical tests for the thoracic spine region.
- Discuss the value of functional testing and symptom modification when considering the aggravating factors, whilst understanding that such tests lack the validity and reliability of some physical tests.
- Explain how physical examination findings contribute to the reasoning for thoracic spine pain and/or dysfunction in common clinical presentations.

CHAPTER CONTENTS

Overview of the Thoracic Spine, 258
Thoracic Spine Pain, 258
The Kinetic Chain and Thoracic Spine Dysfunction, 258
Subjective Examination/Taking the Patient's History, 259
Patient's Perspective on Their Experience, 259
Body Chart, 259
Behaviour of Symptoms, 260
Special/Screening Questions, 261
Presenting Condition (Reason for Referral or Current Complaint), 265
History of Current Complaint, 265
Past Medical History, 265
Plan of the Physical Examination, 265
Physical Examination, 266
Observation, 266
Active Physiological Movements, 267
Passive Physiological Intervertebral Movements, 271
Muscle Testing, 271
Neurological Testing, 271
Neurological Integrity, 271
Miscellaneous Tests, 273
Examination of the Ribcage, 274
Rib Mechanics During Respiration, 275
Completion of the Examination, 276
Case Study, 279
References, 282

OVERVIEW OF THE THORACIC SPINE

The thoracic spine is relatively immobile, with up to 12 separate joint articulations at each level (costovertebral, costotransverse, intervertebral and facet joints), a relatively thin intervertebral disc and lower disc to vertebral body height ratio (thoracic 1:5, cervical 2:5, lumbar 1:3). With a naturally occurring kyphosis (posterior curvature), and attachment with the 12 ribs and indirectly via costal cartilages to the sternum, the thoracic spine forms part of the thoracic or rib cage. This affords both structural protection to vital organs (heart, lungs, liver etc.) and ribcage motion for respiration. Notwithstanding the relatively small amount of motion possible at each spinal level (<5 degrees in any direction), the thoracic spine's primary functional motion, axial rotation is around 40/45 degrees, contributing 80% of total functional trunk range of motion (composite movement of the lumbar and thoracic spine). Factors which may influence the available and expected ranges of motion include age (decreasing with), activities/hobbies (individuals involved in linear activities such as cycling and running have less axial rotation) and daily activities (individuals sitting >7 hours/day exhibit considerably less axial rotation than those involved in dynamic activities such as tennis, gym etc.). As the longest and centrally situated spinal region, it is inextricably linked anatomically and biomechanically to the lumbar and cervical spines via many structures and tissues, including but not limited to joints, muscles, nerves, vascular, fascia etc. A detailed knowledge of these alongside side applied functional biomechanics and physiology is useful. Sub-dividing the thoracic spine to account for the variation in anatomy and transitional zones with the lower cervical and upper lumbar spine is helpful: upper (T1–4), middle (T4–9/10) and lower (T9/10–12).

Thoracic Spine Pain

Thoracic spine pain is often associated with specific musculoskeletal/orthopaedic complaints or rheumatology pathologies such as osteoarthritis, osteoporosis, ankylosing spondylitis, fibromyalgia and Scheuermann's disease. Unlike other spinal regions though, the 1 year and lifetime prevalence of thoracic spine pain prevalence are relatively low, at around 20% (compared to >40% in the cervical and lumbar spine (Leboeuf-Yde et al., 2009) and 13% (compared to 70% in low back pain) (Briggs et al., 2009) respectively. Thoracic spine pain often co-exists with low back and neck pain, although this is often overlooked. In the absence of a clear mechanism of onset or symptom behaviour (aggravating and easing factors) which is consistent with a musculoskeletal complaint, assessment should vitally consider indicators for 'spinal masqueraders' (visceral involvement with somatic referral e.g. liver, gall bladder) or 'red flags' where urgent onward referral may be needed (see Chapter 3).

The Kinetic Chain and Thoracic Spine Dysfunction

Whilst relatively immobile, the thoracic spine serves an important role in functional kinetic chains: a combination of successively arranged joints which constitute a *complex motor unit.* Functional movements such as looking over the shoulder when reversing a car or reaching up to a cupboard require adjunctive thoracic spine mobility to that of the cervical and shoulder joints respectively (Tsang et al., 2013; Heneghan et al., 2019). Single and bilateral arm flexion elevation (required for overhead activities, e.g. painting a ceiling, throwing a netball etc.) includes up to 8 and 15 degrees thoracic spine extension respectively (Heneghan et al., 2019); without this adjunctive mobility, structures around the shoulder may be subject to excessive tissue stress resulting in an inflammatory response and localized pain if not addressed. The thoracic spine also contributes considerably (mobility and force) to any functional movement which involves trunk rotation, e.g. golf swing or reaching for a seatbelt. Assessment of thoracic spine *dysfunction* (e.g. reduced mobility or stiffness) should be considered in patients presenting with complaints in anatomically related regions, e.g. neck or shoulder pain etc. This *dysfunction* is often 'clinically silent' (asymptomatic) or presents as a secondary clinical complaint (lower pain scores), with a patient's primary site of pain often driving clinical decision-making and management. Assessment of secondary 'pain' sites or regions of *dysfunction* may usefully direct management towards 'contributing factors' of a patient's complaint rather than a pain source in isolation (e.g. in instances where neck pain is secondary to, or co-exists with thoracic spine *dysfunction*) (Heneghan et al., 2018). The term 'regional interdependence' describes this phenomenon, where 'seemingly unrelated impairments in a remote anatomical region may contribute to, or be associated with, the patient's primary complaint' (Sueki et al., 2013).

KNOWLEDGE CHECK
1. Describe the main functions of the thoracic spine region.
2. What factors may contribute to thoracic spine dysfunction?
3. Define regional interdependence.

The order of the patient history and physical examination described below can be altered as appropriate for the patient.

SUBJECTIVE EXAMINATION/TAKING THE PATIENT'S HISTORY

Further details of questions asked during the patient history and tests carried out in the physical examination can be found in Chapters 3 and 4, respectively. Assessment and examination of the upper and lower thoracic spine may usually involve an adapted cervical and lumbar spine examination respectively (see Chapters 8 and 13).

Patient's Perspective on Their Experience

The aims of the initial assessment need to be explained to the patient and consent gained. Social and family history relevant to the onset and progression of the patient's complaint is recorded. This includes patient's thoughts, experiences and expectations, their age, employment (and all this involves in terms of physical requirements and demands), home situation and details of any leisure activities. It is vital when considering the potential involvement of the thoracic spine in any clinical complaints (neck, shoulder, low back pain etc.), that potential contributing factors to a patient's presentation are given due consideration; recognizing the relatively low prevalence of a primary pain complaint in the thoracic spine and possibility of thoracic 'dysfunction' contributing to a complaint along a functional kinetic chain. The reader is directed to Chapter 3 for further information.

Assessment Tools and Patient-Reported Outcome Measures

The use of additional tools or patient-reported outcome measures may be used to support and guide the initial assessment. The STarT MSK Tool is a risk stratification measure which helps to 'match' management to a patient based on the risk (low, medium and high) of developing a more persistent complaint (Dunn et al., 2021). Patient-reported outcome measures include condition-specific measures (e.g. Fibromyalgia Impact Questionnaire) or more generic domain-specific measures (e.g. Fear Avoidance Beliefs Questionnaire for fear, Patient Specific Functional Scale for self-selected functional activity).

Body Chart

The information concerning the type and area of current symptoms (e.g. pain, stiffness, paraesthesia etc.) can be recorded on a body chart (see Fig. 3.2).

Area of Current Symptoms

Be precise when mapping out the area of the symptoms, detailing behaviours of each and any association between areas of symptoms. Symptoms in the form of pain (sharp, dull, deep, throbbing, burning etc.), stiffness, paraesthesia etc. may be felt in the following areas: posteriorly over the thoracic spine, lateral to the spine and extending around the chest wall (including ribs) and anteriorly over the sternum. Additionally, the upper thoracic spine can refer symptoms to the upper limbs and the lower thoracic spine to the lower lumbar spine and groin region.

Areas Relevant to the Region Being Examined

All other relevant areas are checked for symptoms; it is important to ask about pain or even stiffness, as this may be relevant to the patient's main symptom. Mark unaffected areas with ticks (✓) on the body chart. Check for symptoms in the cervical spine and upper limbs if it is an upper thoracic problem or in the lumbar spine and lower limbs if it is a lower thoracic problem. If the patient has symptoms that may emanate from these areas, it may be appropriate to assess them more fully. See relevant chapters in this book.

Quality of Pain

Establish the quality of the pain (see Chapter 3).

Intensity of Pain

The intensity of pain can be measured using, for example, a numerical pain rating scale (NPRS), as shown in Fig. 3.4. The intensity of pain informs clinical reasoning severity, may provide guidance to the structures producing the symptoms and guides the scope and nature of the examination. As well as the subjective rating of NPRS, severity (low, moderate, high) is determined by questioning on analgesia use (and effectiveness), impact on activities of daily living including work and hobbies, and pain disturbing sleep.

Abnormal Sensation

Question for any altered sensation (burning, numbness, paraesthesia or heightened sensitivity to touch or temperature) over the thoracic spine, ribcage and other relevant areas.

Constant or Intermittent Symptoms

Ascertain the frequency of all the symptoms, whether they are constant, episodic or intermittent. If symptoms are constant, check whether there is variation in the intensity of the symptoms, as constant unremitting pain may be indicative of serious pathology or fracture. Symptoms may be worse during a teenage growth spurt, so exploring this is useful when considering conditions such as Scheuermann's disease. Questions relating to visceral function may be appropriate (e.g. symptoms worse with coughing, breathing, eating, drinking etc.).

Relationship of Symptoms

Determine the relationship between the symptomatic areas – do they come together or separately? For example, the patient could have shoulder pain without thoracic spine symptoms e.g. pain, stiffness or they may always be present together. If one symptomatic area becomes more severe, what happens to the other symptomatic areas?

Behaviour of Symptoms

Aggravating Factors

For each symptomatic area, explore what movements and/or positions aggravate the patient's symptoms.

The clinician ascertains how the symptoms affect function, such as static and active postures, e.g. sitting, standing, lying, performing activities of daily living, driving (and reversing the car, which requires trunk rotation), work, sports and social activities. Common aggravating factors for the thoracic spine are prolonged static positions (e.g. sitting or standing), or repetitive movements (e.g. extension and axial rotation of the trunk). Examples include desk-based occupations where work requires a semi-rotated position or leisure activities where repetitive rotation is needed (golf or racket sports). Details of ergonomics at work and the training regimes (frequency, content, intensity etc.) for any sports activities may be used to inform patient-specific and goal-orientated rehabilitation. Other aggravating factors may include breathing, coughing or sneezing, all of which affect joints, muscles and bones of the thoracic spine and connection with the ribs, costal cartilages and sternum.

Easing Factors

For each symptomatic area, the clinician asks what eases the patient's symptoms to help to confirm the relationship between the symptoms and determine their irritability (see Chapter 3). Collating the information between aggravating and easing factors helps formulate a hypothesis, plan the physical examination and inform initial advice on the modification of functional tasks. If the patient's symptoms do not fit a musculoskeletal presentation (pattern recognition), then the clinician needs to consider other possible causes, serious or otherwise.

Behaviour of Symptoms Over Time

The clinician determines the 24-hour behaviour of each symptomatic area by asking questions about night, morning and evening symptoms. Additional useful time points for symptom behaviour are across each week and month, considering any link to certain activities, e.g. work/leisure or hormonal influences in females.

Night Symptoms. (See Chapter 3 for details of questions that must be asked.) In addition, questions specific to the positioning of the spine would be:

- What position is most comfortable/uncomfortable?
- What is your normal sleeping position (including the position of the neck, thoracic spine, arms and legs)?
- How many and what type of pillows are used?
- Is your mattress firm or soft and has it been changed recently? Have you tried sleeping in another bed and does that make any difference?
- How many times do you wake up at night? When you wake up, what do you do? How long does it take to then fall back to sleep?

Morning and evening symptoms. The clinician determines the pattern of the symptoms in the morning (on waking and on rising), through the day and at the end of the day. The status of symptoms on first waking establishes whether the patient is better with rest. Pain/stiffness on waking would suggest an inflammatory component whereas no pain on waking but pain on rising would suggest a more mechanical pain pattern. Stiffness in the morning for the first few minutes might suggest osteoarthritis/spondylosis; stiffness and pain for a few hours may be suggestive of an inflammatory condition such as ankylosing spondylitis. If symptoms are worse after work compared with when off work, it is important to explore work-related factors (e.g. enjoyment, stress, occupational activities and other environmental factors) that may be contributing to the complaint.

Current State of the Condition

In order to determine the current state of the condition, the clinician asks whether the symptoms are getting better, getting worse or remaining unchanged since onset.

Special/Screening Questions

As detailed in Chapter 3, the clinician must differentiate between conditions that are suitable for conservative management and other systemic, neoplastic and non-musculoskeletal conditions.

General Health

The clinician ascertains the state of the patient's general health to find out if the patient has other co-morbidities which may contribute to their condition or may influence management planning (e.g. osteoporosis, respiratory disorders, cardiovascular disease, breathlessness, chest pain, malaise, fatigue, fever, abdominal cramps, nausea or vomiting, stress, anxiety or depression). Some co-morbidities may be a precaution or contraindication to certain management approaches (e.g. manipulative therapy in osteoporosis). Questions relating to change in visceral function may be appropriate owing to the referral pain patterns of these structures.

For full details of all special questions see Chapter 3.

Pattern Recognition and Differential Diagnosis

Knowledge of pathological processes and symptom behaviour of some pathologies, e.g. osteoarthritis, is applicable to all synovial joints. Table 9.1 details the thoracic spine pain symptom location, the pattern of onset, associated symptoms and features to aid pattern recognition of a number of conditions.

Drug History

If medication is taken specifically for a thoracic spine complaint, is the patient taking the medication regularly? What effect does it have? How long before this appointment was the medication taken? Has the patient been prescribed long-term (6 months or more) steroids or anticonvulsants, as this may have an impact on bone density. Has the patient been prescribed hormone replacement therapy (HRT)?

Investigations, Injections and Imaging

Has the patient been referred on by their GP or seen a specialist for this complaint? Is the patient under investigation for any other condition currently? Has the patient had any investigations (e.g. blood tests for systematic inflammatory conditions or infection), injections (spinal or muscular), been radiographed or had any other investigative scans for this or any similar complaint (MRI, CT scan). If so what body region and any results? Has the patient had a dual-energy x-ray absorptiometry (DEXA) scan to determine bone mineral density?

Neurological Symptoms

Has the patient experienced symptoms of spinal cord compression (termed 'myelopathy' and may be secondary to trauma, degenerative disease or disc herniation), for example, numbness, tingling and/or electric shocks in the hands and feet either bilaterally or unilaterally, depending on the compression site? Also, has the patient experienced weakness or difficulty using the arms or legs, including tripping or dropping things? Sympathetic function is difficult to measure but questions about changes in swelling, sweating, skin changes (pitting oedema, shiny and inelastic skin) and circulation need to be included. Patients presenting with altered sympathetic function may report bizarre and unusual symptoms (e.g. trickling, crawling sensations).

Vascular Symptoms

The vascular supply to the upper limb passes through the thoracic outlet. Questions should include how

TABLE 9.1 Pattern Recognition and Differentiation for Thoracic Spine Pain

	Condition	Complaint	Onset and History	Other Symptoms	Pattern Recognition
Musculoskeletal	**Thoracic disc** *Disc pathology*	*Central thoracic pain* *Severe presentations may cause signs and symptoms consistent with myelopathy (gait disturbance)*	*May be related to clear MOI or insidious onset*	*Local and referral of symptoms (including neurological symptoms) is indicative of level and extent of disc pathology*	*Young to middle-aged adult* *Mainly T8 and below* *Aggravated by coughing or straining* *FH*
	Facet joint	*Bilateral or unilateral spine pain*	*May be related to clear MOI or activity*	*Morning stiffness (inflammatory)*	*Young to middle-aged adult* *Aggravating and easing factors may be side specific*
	Osteoarthritis/ spondylosis	*Bilateral or unilateral spine pain*	*Pain – activity related*	*Morning stiffness (inflammatory)*	*Middle age to older adult*
Rheumatological	**Osteoporosis** *Low bone mineral density*	*Mid-low thoracic pain – may be localized, sharp, unremitting*	*With wedge fracture, sudden onset with minimal or no trauma, e.g. stepping off a kerb*	*Previous fractures with minimal trauma*	*Women > men* *Post-menopause* *FH* *Amenorrhea (eating disorders, following hysterectomy, in elite athletes)* *Endocrinal and metabolic diseases (diabetes and hypothyroidism)* *Drugs (steroids)* *Excessive alcohol intake* *Smoking* *Loss of height* *Poor diet (low calcium and vitamin D intake)*

	Ankylosing spondylitis *Axial spondyloarthropathy*	*Bilateral or unilateral thoracic spine pain* *>3 months*	*Young adults* *Insidious onset* *Often starts with symptoms in large proximal joints or with history of soft tissue complaints*	*Stiffness ++ (>30 min)* *Wakes up at night with pain* *Large proximal joint involvement* *Soft tissues complaints, e.g. plantar fasciitis* *Associated eye, heart, lung and bowel involvement?* *Reduced chest expansion (advanced)*	*Young adult* *Males > females* *FH* *Symptoms improve with exercise* *Low grade fever, fatigue can be reported*
	Scheuermann's disease *Condition affecting vertebral end plates*	*Central thoracic pain* *Intermittent presentation of back pain*	*Onset at puberty or later*	*Previous episodes* *Explore timing in relation to growth spurts* *Kyphosis (progressive)*	*Adolescent (12–17 years)* *Episodic complaints* *Males > females* *Long thoracic kyphosis* *Family history* *Symptomatic management and usually resolves at skeletal maturity (may present as adult)*
	Fibromyalgia syndrome *Systemic condition with multisystem abnormalities*	*Diffuse nonspecific back pain extending from upper thoracic spine down to lumbar spine* *Muscular in nature (aching or burning)* *Lasting >3 months*	*Insidious onset with a range of possible triggers*	*Sleep disorders* *Anxiety and depression* *Irritable bowel disease* *Other rheumatological conditions, e.g. AS, RA, SLE* *Symptoms easily exacerbated*	*Young to middle-aged adult* *Women > men*
Infection	**Tuberculosis leading to Pott disease** *Inflammatory infectious disease with extrapulmonary manifestation*	*Lower thoracic pain* *In advanced disease neurological complaints and signs evident*	*May have been in contact with others – travel* *Regional outbreaks*	*Pain on coughing* *Night sweats* *Fever* *Tachycardia* *Weight loss* *SOB*	*Linked to global travel* *Middle to older adult* *Foreign-born individuals mainly from Asia and sub-Saharan Africa* *Males > females* *More common in those with HIV*

Continued

TABLE 9.1 Pattern Recognition and Differentiation for Thoracic Spine Pain—cont'd

	Condition	Complaint	Onset and History	Other Symptoms	Pattern Recognition
	Shingles/Herpes zoster *Viral infection of nerves*	*Severe pain (often described burning) and usually along the course of a nerve root*	*Sudden onset of pain, often following some other life event, stress or medical management*	*Reddening of the skin and appearance of fluid filled vesicles/blisters after onset of pain – 2/3 days later*	*Patients who are* • *older* • *immunosuppressed* • *severely stressed* • *radiation treatment* *Patients should be referred without delay to their GP for pharmacological management*
	Cancer Common site for primary and metastases	*Deep back pain*	*Insidious onset* *Constant unremitting symptoms* *Previous management or investigations*	*Weight loss* *Malaise* *Night pain*	*Middle age to older adult* *Non-mechanical presentation* *Previous history of cancer* *No clear MOI*
Visceral	**Visceral complaints (Masqueraders)** Cardiovascular (MI, aortic aneurysm, heart attack) Renal (acute pyelonephritis, kidney disease) Gastrointestinal (esophagitis, peptic ulcer, acute cholecystitis, pancreatic disease, colitis) Gynaecological (disorders) Other (infection)		*Deep, diffuse, non-specific pain*	*Comorbidities evident – current or past*	*Symptoms non-mechanical in behaviour* *No obvious MSK MOI* *Symptoms vary linked to activity/involvement of system involved, e.g. eating, drinking, stress etc.*

AS, Ankylosing spondylitis, *FH*, family history; *MI*, myocardial infarction; *MOI*, mechanism of onset; *MSK*, musculoskeletal; *RA*, rheumatoid arthritis; *SLE*, systemic lupus erythematosus; *SOB*, shortness of breath.

good the patient's circulation is and whether the patient has any swelling, coldness, cyanosis, fatigability or cramping in the upper extremities. Symptoms may be indicative of complaints such as thoracic outlet syndrome (see Chapter 8 in the companion text, Barnard & Ryder, 2024).

Presenting Condition (Reason for Referral or Current Complaint)

Symptoms, behaviour, aggravating and easing factors to determine current severity and irritability of presenting complaint.

History of Current Complaint

- For each symptomatic area, the clinician needs to know how long the symptom has been present, whether there was a sudden or insidious onset and whether there was a known cause that triggered the onset of the symptom, e.g. fall, injury or change in activities. The mechanism of injury (when, where and how it happened) gives some important clues as to a potentially injured structure. If the onset was slow, the clinician finds out if there has been any change in the patient's lifestyle, e.g. a new job or hobby or a change in sporting activity, which may have affected the stresses on the thoracic spine and related areas. Was there a sudden onset of pain as a result of a traumatic episode or repetitive minor trauma? Rib injuries are commonly caused by trauma (e.g. sporting injury, road traffic accident or fall). To confirm the relationship between symptoms, the clinician asks what happened to other symptoms and when each symptom began. Clarify the time course, progression and impact of the symptoms on the patient's normal function from the first onset of this episode to the present time. Find out details about any treatment/management interventions and advice given: what was it and what was the effect? How do the interventions align with patients' understanding and beliefs of their condition?
- Where the thoracic spine is often 'clinically silent', clinicians should be minded to explore regions along functional kinetic chains when using the body chart for other presentations (e.g. neck, shoulder, low back, hips); this may reveal sub-clinical complaints or symptoms e.g. stiffness.

Past Medical History

The following information is obtained from the patient and/or the medical notes:

- Any history of previous similar complaints, including details pertaining to (1) duration, severity, (2) investigations (blood, imaging etc.), (3) previous management (pharmacological, conservative, surgical interventions) and importantly the results/outcome or influence of any on the complaints.
- Previous injuries or accidents (e.g. sporting, road traffic accident, falls etc.), surgeries (e.g. abdominal or spinal surgery), medical conditions (e.g. cancer or endocrine complaints) and other potentially relevant factors (e.g. diet, stress, previous management for a musculoskeletal complaint).

KNOWLEDGE CHECK

1. Describe categories and types of conditions which may give rise to thoracic spine pain.
2. What rheumatological conditions can cause thoracic spine pain?
3. What visceral structures might cause thoracic spine pain?
4. What may pain on coughing or sneezing indicate?

Plan of the Physical Examination

After allowing the patient an opportunity to add anything that may not have been mentioned so far, the purpose and plan for the physical examination will need to be explained and consent obtained.

A planning sheet can help guide clinicians through the clinical reasoning process and ensure the development of a working hypothesis of the most likely cause of, or contributing factors for, the patient's complaint (see Appendix 3.1). A 'must, should, could' list will help prioritize your physical examination procedures to ensure that your hypothesis is supported (see Chapter 3).

The hypothesis is developed from the patient's history by identifying:

- The regions and structures that need to be examined as a possible cause for, or contributing to, the complaint. Often, it is not possible to examine fully at the first attendance and so examination of the structures must be prioritized (must, should, could) over subsequent sessions.

- Other factors need to be examined, e.g. working, leisure and everyday postures, breathing patterns and mobility, motor control, endurance and strength.
- The predominant pain mechanisms that might be driving the patient's symptoms. Pain has been classified into nociceptive (mechanical, inflammatory or ischemic), peripheral, neurogenic, central, autonomic and affective. For the clinical features of pain mechanisms, see Box 3.2.
- In what way should the physical tests be carried out? Will it be easy or hard to reproduce each symptom? Will it be necessary to use combined movements or repetitive movements to reproduce the patient's symptoms? Are symptoms severe and/or irritable? If symptoms are severe, physical tests may be carried out to just before or to the initial onset of symptom production or in an unloaded position. No overpressures will be carried out. If symptoms are irritable, physical tests may be examined to just before or to initial symptom production, with fewer physical tests being examined.
- Are there any precautions and/or contraindications to elements of the physical examination that need to be explored further, such as neurological involvement, recent fracture, trauma, osteoporosis, steroid or anticoagulant therapy and inflammatory conditions? There may also be certain contraindications to further examination and treatment, e.g. symptoms of cord compression.

PHYSICAL EXAMINATION

The information from the patient history helps the clinician to plan an appropriate physical examination. The severity, irritability, nature and pain mechanisms of the condition are the major factors that will influence the choice and priority of physical testing procedures. The first and overarching question the clinician might ask is: 'Is this patient's condition suitable for me to manage as a clinician?' For example, a patient presenting with symptoms of spinal cord compression may only need neurological integrity testing, prior to an urgent medical referral. The nature of the patient's condition has a major impact on the physical examination. The second question the clinician might ask is: 'Does this patient have a thoracic musculoskeletal dysfunction that I may be able to help?' To answer that, the clinician needs to carry out a full physical examination; however, this may not be possible if the symptoms are severe and/or irritable. The clinician would use non-provocative physical tests to support or negate their hypothesis (e.g. testing motion within a symptom-free range). If a patient's symptoms are non-severe and non-irritable, then the clinician aims to find physical tests that may reproduce each of the patient's symptoms to support or negate their hypothesis.

Each significant physical test that either provokes or eases the patient's symptoms or with respect to asymptomatic thoracic spine dysfunction produces results which differ from age/gender/patient appropriate norms is highlighted in the patient's notes by an asterisk (*) for easy reference.

The order and detail of the physical tests described below need to be appropriate to the patient being examined and to the hypotheses (primary or alternatives) developed. It is important that readers understand that the techniques included in this chapter are a small number of the many available and used in practice.

Observation

Informal Observation

The clinician observes the patient in dynamic and static situations; the quality of movement is noted, as are the postural characteristics and facial expressions. Informal observation occurs throughout the consultation from the first point of contact (e.g. walking into the clinic).

Formal Observation

Formal observation may necessitate the clinician to examine the patient from the front (anterior), back (posterior) and both sides (lateral). Mirrors in a clinic setting can be useful for efficiency (reducing the amount the clinician has to move around the patient) and simultaneous observation of more than one plane. Common postural types which may help to describe the type and extent of thoracic spine curvature are detailed in Chapter 4. It is important to note whilst observing patients, including symmetry and alignment, that patients may present with differences or deviations from the norm which are unrelated to their

TABLE 9.2 Observation

General	• General appearance – affect (mood), signs of stress/anxiety, tension, physique, breast size, weight etc. • Postural type or deformities, e.g. kyphosis, scoliosis (curvature of the spine), pigeon or barrel chest (associated with respiratory complaints) • Scars, e.g. surgical or trauma • Skin, e.g. general condition, colour, any bruising, erythema, vesicles/blisters, swellings, lumps, moles/blemishes • Muscle wasting, symmetry of form (consideration needs to be made to side of dominance)
Posture (static)	• Standing – ability to stand still, load transferring, alignment • Sitting – ability to sit still, alignment, off-loading through arms, leg position and support • Functional postures, e.g. sitting position at work, washing up at home, sports/leisure time related posture Encourage patients to adopt/reproduce postures from their everyday life to understand possible physiological and biomechanical stressors.
Posture (dynamic)	• Sitting to standing • Lying down • Functional activity of daily living, e.g. taking off or hanging up coat, looking over shoulder, undressing for the examination etc.
Gait	• Speed, stride length, cadence, duration of stance phase and weight transfer • Arm swing and associated trunk motion • Alignment and position of head on neck and relative to the trunk • Use of any mobility aids, e.g. stick/s • Use of bag/s (e.g. rucksack, handbag) including load, position

Respiratory function	• Patient's quiet breathing pattern
	  • quality of ribcage movement and which part of the ribcage is being used primarily
	  • respiratory rate (normal is 8–14 breaths/min), rhythm and required effort to inhale and exhale
	• Observing the muscles being used by the patient will indicate the ease of breathing.
	• Note any excessive use of the accessory muscles of respiration (e.g. sternocleidomastoid, pectoralis minor, upper trapezius, scaleni muscles); common with some respiratory conditions, stress/anxiety, postural adaptations

Clinical tips	• For patients who report symptoms during a specific activity or in a specific 'environment' try to reproduce or simulate this in the clinic; this may involve a desk, keyboard, mouse, telephone where the complaint relates to a desk-based work environment or a piece of equipment for a complaint related to a sporting or leisure pursuit, e.g. golf club, tennis racquet • Where appropriate and with permission, ask patients to record (mobile phone video) postures and activities at home, in work or leisure settings to better understand what they do; this will improve the clinician's understanding and inform clinical reasoning • Job or role specifications can be useful to detail the requirements of a particular occupational post (duration, frequency, any loading, lifting, equipment, heights etc.); this may also be useful to inform planned and graded personalized rehabilitation

complaint. All findings need to be considered as part of the clinical reasoning process when determining their potential relevance or otherwise to a patient's current complaint.

Active Physiological Movements

The anatomical design of the thoracic spine offers little mobility in the sagittal plane (flexion 32 degrees, extension 25 degrees) and frontal planes (side flexion

26 degrees). The largest range of motion is that of axial rotation with a mean (standard deviation) total range (left and right rotation) of 85 ± 15 degrees. (Heneghan et al., 2016) The amount of rotation possible depends on the ability of the ribs to undergo distortion. With age the costal cartilages ossify, less distortion occurs and rotation is reduced. Rotation range is also significantly decreased in flexion when compared with neutral or extended postures (Edmondston et al., 2007). Rotation in the thoracic spine is essential for optimal functional movement; a stiff 'clinically silent' thoracic spine may create excessive loading and mobility demands in adjacent regions (e.g. shoulder, neck) which may ultimately become symptomatic. Given the complexity of the thoracic spine and its relationship with the thorax, the availability of reliable and valid measurement tools is limited with most measuring the trunk rather than being a discrete measure of the thoracic spine (Heneghan & Rushton, 2016). The active movements of the trunk (flexion, extension, axial rotation and lateral flexion) are tested with the patient sitting with feet supported (reduces muscle tone). The clinician establishes the patient's symptoms at rest prior to each movement and may try to correct any movement deviation to determine its relevance to the patient's symptoms.

For all active physiological movements, the spine will normally curve segmentally evenly and smoothly without areas of excessive or reduced movement. The clinician notes the

- influence on symptoms (pain, stiffness, paraesthesia etc.)
- range of movement
- quality of the movement through the range (e.g. leading from, segmental, any deviation, coupling)
- compensatory or adjunctive movements in adjacent regions, e.g. lifting of the pelvis during sitting trunk rotation

If indicated, it may be appropriate to repeat the movements, adding overpressures to explore the end of the available range of motion (Fig. 9.1A–D). If these movements have not reproduced symptoms, it may also be appropriate to examine 'combined movements e.g. flexion and rotation, extension and rotation, etc. Fig. 9.1E illustrates combined flexion and rotation, with the patient actively flexing the thoracic spine (primary movement) before the clinician uses their hands to maintain the flexed position and then guiding the patient into right rotation. The order in which movements are combined depends on the aggravating activities and the patient's response to the primary movement.

Table 9.3 details active physiological movements with a range of modifications suggested. Whilst not suitable for all patients, measurement of thoracic axial rotation using a smart phone or inclinometer in the sitting heel lock position is valid in young adults (Bucke et al., 2017; Heneghan et al., 2018) (see Fig. 9.2A and B).

Observation of Aggravating Functional Activities or Positions

Depending on the irritability, severity and nature of the symptoms, it is important to observe at least one key functional movement of the patient as this may be contributing to ongoing symptoms. Altering any impairments and noting the symptom response on retesting will guide further relevant testing. For example, a patient may have symptoms with left thoracic rotation; the clinician observes that this movement is performed in a flexed posture. Repeating left thoracic rotation in a more neutral posture may reduce symptoms – a form of differentiation.

Differentiation and Symptom Modification

Numerous differentiation tests can be performed to determine the nature (symptoms source or contributing factor) and origin (e.g. anatomical region or tissue) of a patient's complaint; the choice of test depends on the patient's signs and symptoms. For example, if a patient complains of pain turning to the right, the clinician can ask the patient to reproduce the movement and then de-rotate the neck to return to neutral. If symptoms reduce, this lends some support for the source of the symptoms being linked to the cervical spine rather than the thoracic spine (see Fig. 9.3).

Symptom modification with 'mini treatments' (passive or active) are applied to the thoracic vertebrae or ribs whilst the patient performs a painful active movement to aid differentiation. For example, a glide can be applied (centrally or unilaterally) over the thoracic vertebra or cutaneous stimuli in the region of the thoracic spine to facilitate movement. If there is a reduction in pain, a spinal segment may be implicated as a source of the pain or this provides evidence of

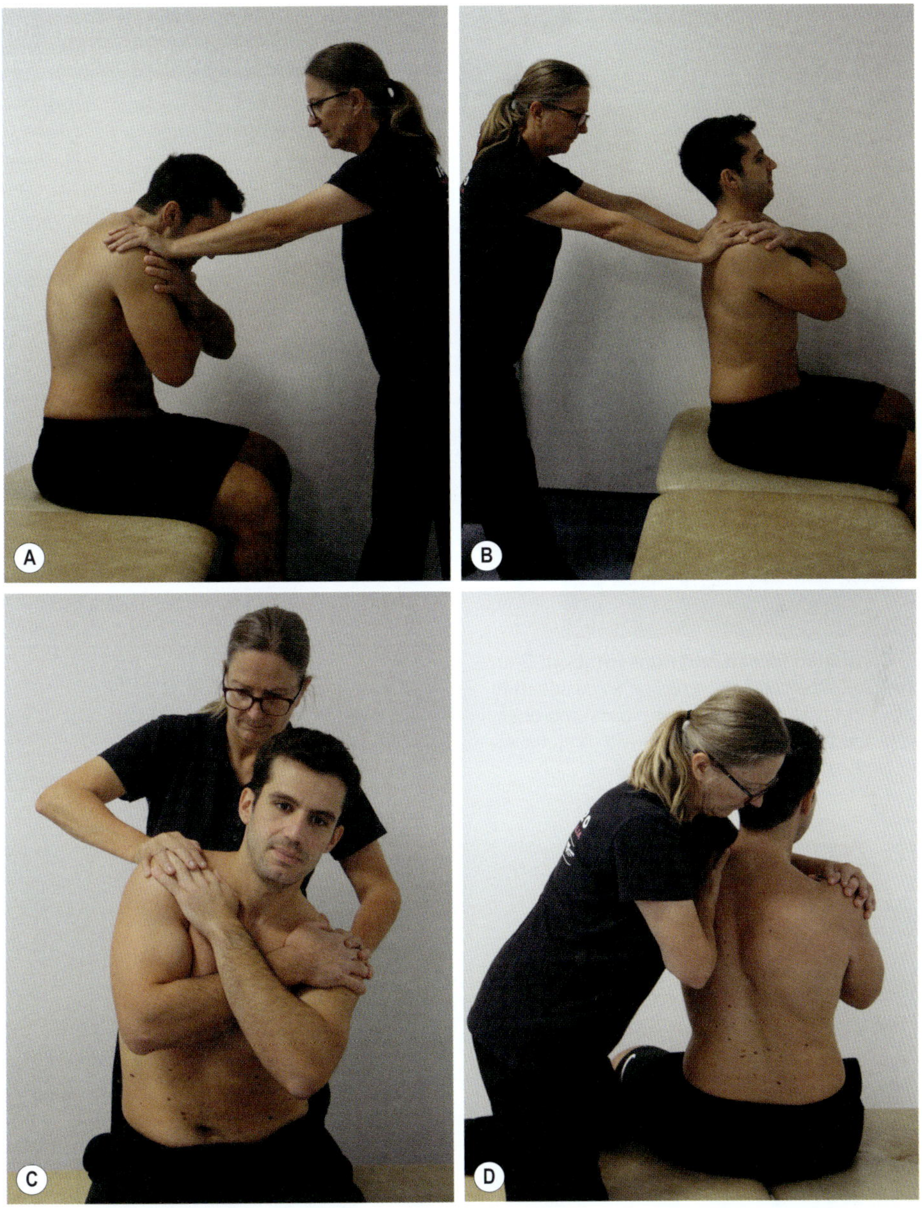

Fig. 9.1 Overpressures to the Thoracic Spine. These movements are all carried out with the patient's arms crossed. (A) **Flexion**. Both hands on top of the shoulders, angle pressure down and posteriorly through the midthoracic spine to increase thoracic flexion. (B) **Extension**. Both hands on top of shoulders, angle pressure down and anteriorly through the sternum. The pelvis may be positioned into a posterior rotation to isolate extension to the thoracic spine. (C) **Lateral flexion**. Both hands on top of the shoulders, apply a force to increase thoracic lateral flexion. (D) **Rotation**. The right hand rests behind the patient's left shoulder, and the left hand lies on the front of the right shoulder. Both hands then apply a force to increase right thoracic rotation.

thoracic dysfunction underpinning symptoms reported in another region e.g. neck or shoulder pain (see Fig. 9.4A–C and descriptions).

It may be necessary to examine other regions to determine their relevance to the patient's symptoms as they may be the source of the symptoms, or they

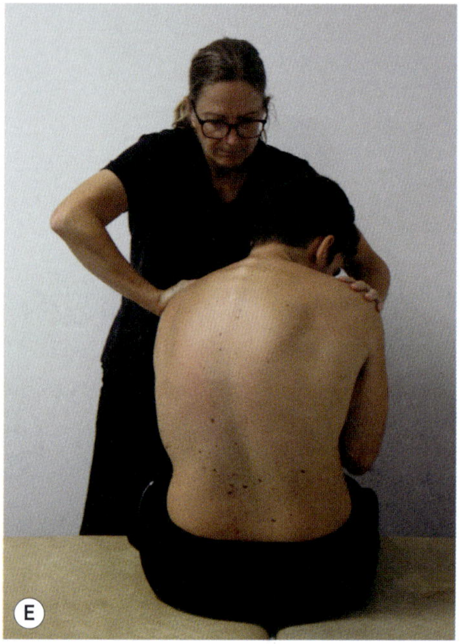

Fig. 9.1, cont'd (E) **Combined flexion and right rotation.** Both hands placed on top of the shoulders, and a flexion force added to localize to the thoracic spine. Note for any symptoms' reproduction. Maintaining the flexed position, apply a force with both hands to add right rotation. Note any change in symptoms.

TABLE 9.3 Testing of Active Physiological Movements With Modifications Suggested

Active Physiological Movement	Modifications to More Closely Reflect Function
Flexion	Overpressure
Extension	Repeated
Left lateral flexion	Speed altered/ballistic
Right lateral flexion	Combined, e.g. flexion plus rotation (see Fig. 9.1E)
Left rotation	Loaded (?with compression) or unloaded
Right rotation	Sustained
	Different starting position, e.g. forward flexed posture, adoption of functional posture
	Differentiation testing

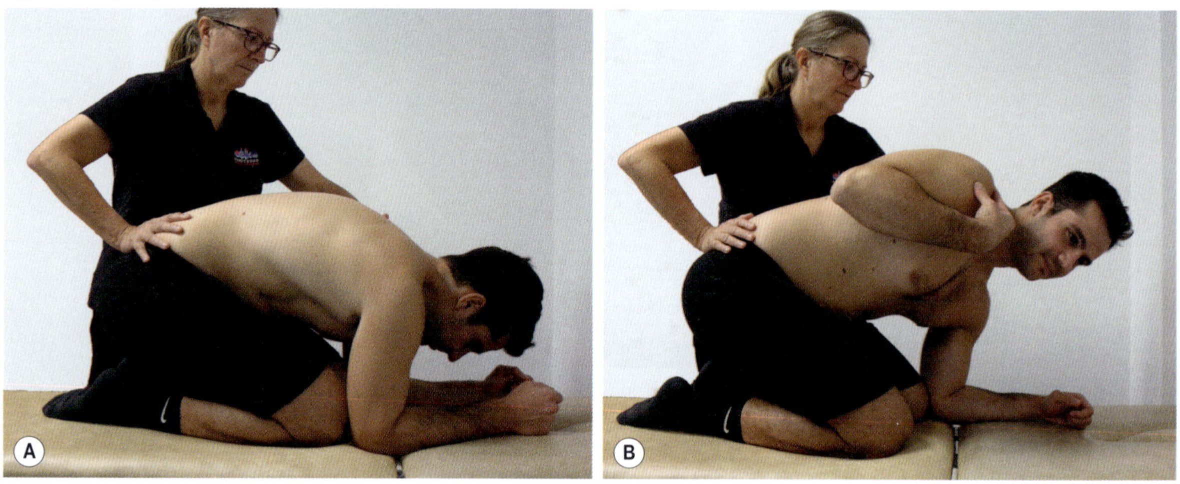

Fig. 9.2 Seated Heel Lock Position for Testing Axial Rotation. Patient sits back on heels (bed or floor) and rests elbows in front of knees and forearms in line with thighs. Using an inclinometer app, position and rest a smartphone in the C7/T1 interspinous space (reading should be near 0 to 5 degrees to account for anatomical variability), position right upper arm in line with the trunk and keep the elbow flexed, ask the individual to turn their body to the right (allowing their head to move freely); contact between the buttock and posterior thigh should be maintained throughout. Re-position the smartphone in the C7/T1 interspinous space to record active range of motion. (A) Starting position, (B) end range/position.

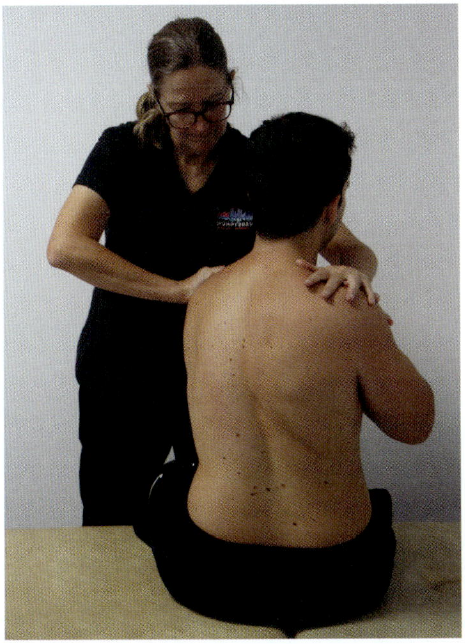

Fig. 9.3 Differentiation Testing. The clinician maintains right rotation of the thoracic spine while the patient returns the head to neutral. Any changes in symptoms are noted.

may be contributing to the symptoms (see relevant chapter).

Passive Physiological Intervertebral Movements

Passive physiological intervertebral movements (PPIVM, Fig. 9.5) enable examination of the physiological movement at each segmental level (flexion, extension, rotation, lateral flexion). Whilst they can be done in sitting, mid-thoracic PPIVM are best performed unloaded and under clinician control in a lying position. In sitting, the clinician palpates between adjacent spinous processes or transverse processes to feel the range of intervertebral movement during thoracic flexion, extension, rotation and lateral flexion. Fig. 9.5 illustrates and details a PPIVM for left rotation of the thoracic spine at T8/9.

Muscle Testing

The muscles that need to be tested will depend on hypothesis generation regarding symptom source, thoracic dysfunction and functional requirements. Because of the interdependence of this area, this may include other regions.

Muscles contribute to the integrity of the thoracic spine; mobility is influenced by muscle length, motor control by proprioception, work capacity by muscle endurance and strength with force generation. Based on a clinical reasoning framework for thoracic spine exercise prescription for rehabilitation (Heneghan et al., 2020), Box 9.1 details expert-derived definitions, relevant muscle testing and additional resources.

Neurological Testing

This includes neurological integrity testing, neurodynamic tests and testing of the central nervous system.

Neurological Integrity

The distribution of symptoms will determine the appropriate neurological examination to be carried out. Symptoms confined to the midthoracic region require dermatome/cutaneous nerve testing only since there is no myotome or reflex that can be tested. If symptoms spread proximally or distally, a neurological examination of the upper or lower limbs, respectively, is indicated (see Chapter 4).

Dermatomes/peripheral nerves. In the thoracic spine, there is a great deal of overlap of the dermatomes and the absence of one dermatome is unlikely to lead to a loss of sensation. Light touch and pain sensation are tested using cotton wool and pinprick, respectively (see Chapter 4). Knowledge of the cutaneous distribution of nerve roots (dermatomes) and peripheral nerves enables the clinician to distinguish sensory loss due to a root lesion from that due to a peripheral nerve lesion. The cutaneous nerve distribution and dermatome areas are shown in Fig. 4.13A and B.

Neurodynamic Tests

The following tests may be carried out in order to ascertain the degree to which neural tissue is responsible for the production of the patient's symptom(s):

- passive neck flexion
- upper-limb neural tests (in particular upper-limb neurodynamic test [ULNT] 3, which biases the ulnar nerve C8, T1)
- straight-leg raise
- slump (from a static seated slumped position a neural component may be implicated if symptoms

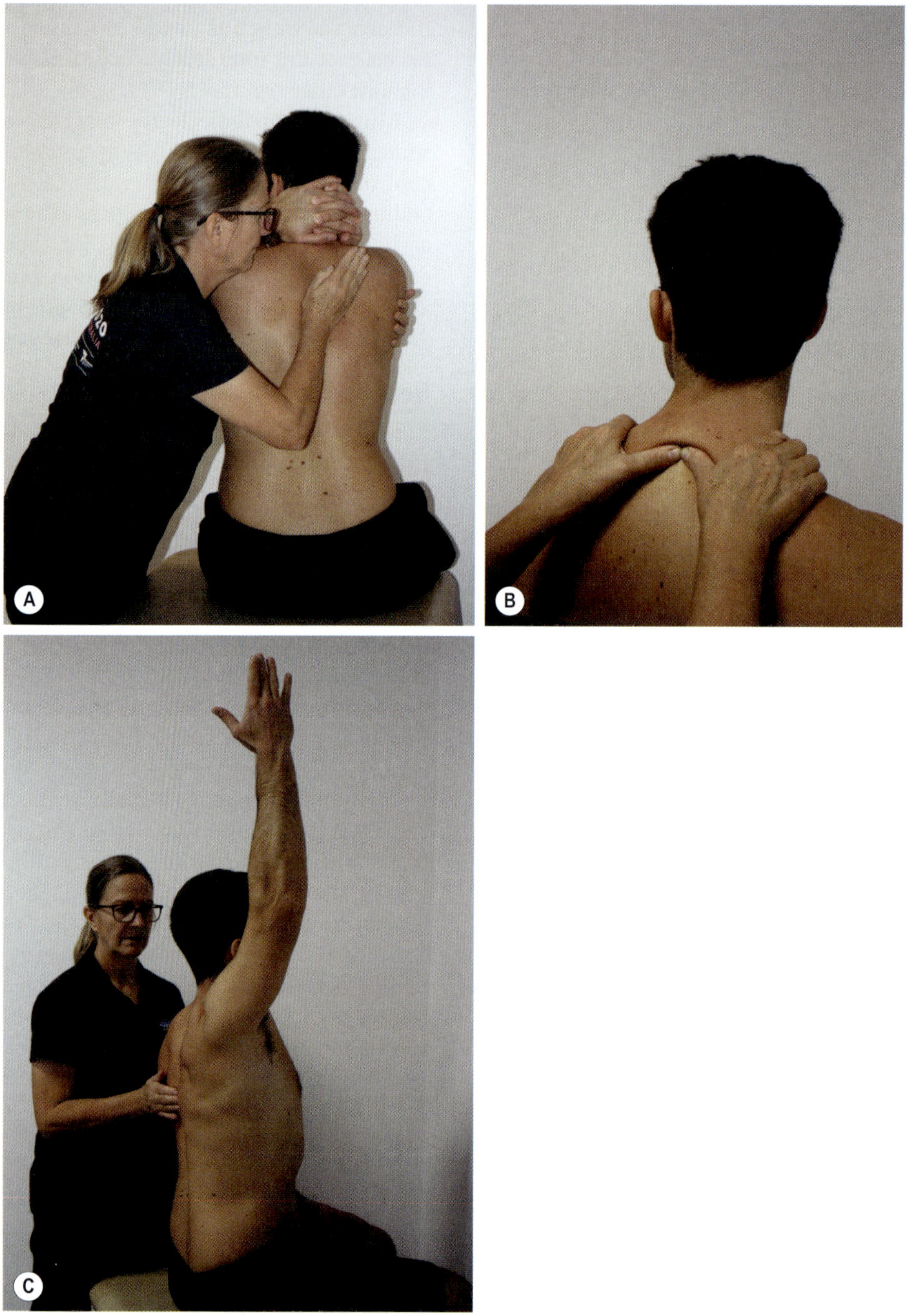

Fig. 9.4 Symptom Modification. (A) A left rotation modification procedure on the T6 transverse process. In this example, the technique aims to facilitate the glide of the right inferior facet of T6 upwards on T7. This can then be used as a treatment technique. (B) A left rotation modification procedure on the T1 spinous process. In this example, the technique aims to facilitate rotation of the T1 (hypothesis of reduced mobility between C7/T1). This can then be used as a treatment technique or repeated below the spinous process of T2, T3 to facilitate upper thoracic spine axial rotation during functional neck movement. (C) Active thoracic extension during arm elevation. In this example, the technique aims to facilitate a greater range of upper limb flexion elevation by prompting active thoracic spine extension.

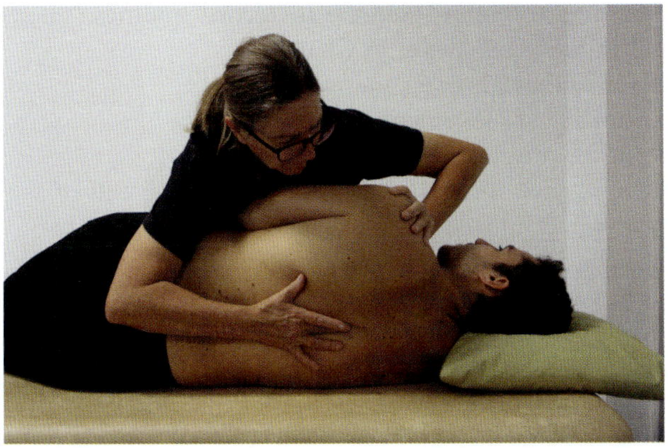

Fig. 9.5 Passive Physiological Intervertebral Movements for Rotation of the Thoracic Spine (T8/9). The clinician uses their right arm to stabilize the lumbar spine/pelvis, maintaining the lower trunk in a neutral position and uses their right hand/finger to stabilize/fix the T9 spinous process (right side of the spinous process). The patient is asked to turn their head left to look up. Placing their left hand over the pectoral region, the clinician uses their left upper arm to passively rotate the thorax posteriorly, with a force in the direction of the facet joint plane. Once the available rotation range of the upper segments is complete, tissue resistance will be felt between the T8/9 level through the left arm; the available range is very small.

diminish or are reduced with the removal of uni- or bilateral knee extension and/or ankle dorsiflexion)

These tests are described in detail in Chapter 4.

Central Nervous System Testing – Upper Motor Nerve Lesions

Plantar Response – Babinski Sign (Fuller, 2013). Pressure applied from the heel along the lateral border of the plantar aspect of the foot produces flexion of the toes in the normal individual. Extension of the big toe with downward fanning of the other toes occurs with an upper motor neuron lesion.

Clonus. Dorsiflex the ankle briskly, maintain the foot in that position and a rhythmic contraction may be found. More than three beats is considered abnormal.

Miscellaneous Tests

Respiration

There is a close relationship between the respiratory and musculoskeletal systems. Dysfunction in one can lead to dysfunction in the other (Wirth et al., 2014). The importance of breathing retraining is becoming

BOX 9.1 Expert-Derived Definitions, Relevant Muscle Testing and Examples of Tests

Muscle Testing	Outcome and Definition (Taken from Spencer et al., 2016)	Clinical Measures and Further Reading (Flexors, Extensors, Lateral Flexors and Rotators and Other Relevant Muscle Groups or Individual Muscles as Necessary)
Muscle length	**Mobility** *'develop, maintain, or restore global spinal range of movement through a specific range of motion'*	Specific muscle lengths (Kendall & Kendall, 2015) Thoracic axial rotation (smart phone inclinometer) (Bucke et al., 2017) Visual estimation of range Goniometry (Johnson et al., 2012)
Motor control linked to proprioception	**Motor control** *'the maintenance of spinal integrity during skilled movement'*	Observation of functional recruitment for muscle over- or under-activity Palpation of muscle (over- or under-activity) Quality and control of movement (Sahrmann et al., 2017; Lee et al., 2005)
Muscle endurance	**Work capacity** *'the ability to produce or tolerate variable intensities and duration of work'*	Isokinetic or handheld dynamometry Specific tests – Biering-Sorenson test, prone bridge test/prone plank
Muscle strength	***Strength*** *'the ability to produce force and maximal strength is the largest force the musculature can produce'*	Isokinetic or handheld dynamometry (Kendall & Kendall, 2015) *Testing is given in Chapter 4.*

more widely recognized. Normal breathing function relies on postural alignment, thoracic and ribcage mobility and the absence of over dominance of accessory muscles. Observation is key but costovertebral joint movement can be determined by measuring chest expansion using a cloth tape measure; measuring the difference between a maximum inhalation to exhalation (Debouche et al., 2016) Asking patients to take a deep breath and/or cough may be useful to explore symptoms reproduction.

Vascular Tests

Tests for thoracic outlet syndrome are described in Chapter 8.

Palpation. The clinician palpates the thoracic spine and, if appropriate, the cervical/lumbar spine and upper/lower limbs. It is useful to record palpation findings on a body chart and/or palpation chart (see Fig. 4.34).

The clinician notes the following:

- the temperature of the area
- bony anomalies: increased or decreased prominence of bones; deviation of the spinous process from the centre; vertebral rotation – assessed by palpating the position of the transverse processes
- mobility and feel of superficial tissues, e.g. scarring
- muscle tone
- tenderness of bone and muscle trigger points
- symptom reproduction (usually pain).

Palpation may also usefully be used to assess soft tissue extensibility, notably that of connective tissues, including but not limited to the fascia. The clinician can use different contacts (pisiform, thumbs etc.) and positions to enable this with prone lying not always being optimal, e.g. seated.

Passive Accessory Intervertebral Movements

Passive accessory intervertebral movements (PAIVM) enable examination of the component parts of a physiological movement at each segmental level. PAIVM cannot be reproduced actively by the patient (e.g. joint glide, distraction). PPIVM and PAIVM can be useful adjuncts to identify segmental hypomobility and less likely in the thoracic spine hypermobility. Given they are examining an accessory motion, PAIVM can be useful for patients with heightened severity or irritability. Further details can be found in Chapter 4. It is useful to use the palpation chart and movement diagrams (or joint pictures) to record findings. These are explained in detail in Chapter 4.

The clinician notes the following:

- quality of movement
- range of movement
- resistance through the range and at the end of the range of movement
- behaviour of pain through the range
- any provocation of muscle spasm.

The thoracic spine (T1–T12) accessory movements and rib accessory movements are shown in Figs. 9.6A–C and 9.7A–D and listed in Table 9.4. Accessory movements can then be tested in other regions suspected to be a source of, or contributing to, the patient's symptoms. Following accessory movements to the thoracic region, the clinician reassesses all the physical asterisks (movements or tests that have been found to reproduce the patient's symptoms) in order to establish the effect of the accessory movements on the patient's signs and symptoms.

EXAMINATION OF THE RIBCAGE

The ribs are strongly attached to the thoracic spine via the costovertebral and costotransverse joints and their associated ligaments. It may therefore be necessary to test these joints for mobility and pain provocation. Very few studies have been done on the biomechanics of the intact thoracic spine and ribcage. However, a model proposed by Lee (2018) is useful for clinical assessment. Lee proposes that movements of the rib joints are influenced by the mechanics of the thoracic spine. For example, flexion results in the inferior facet joint of the upper vertebra and its same-numbered rib gliding/rolling in a superior, anterior direction – a rib's mobility into flexion could therefore be palpated by applying a cephalad glide to it near the costotransverse joint (see Fig. 9.7A). The reverse occurs with extension, and the glide direction applied to the rib would be caudad. This is particularly applicable to the ribs that attach to the sternum (ribs 2–7). The lower ribs are less strongly attached to the thoracic spine and are therefore less influenced by thoracic spine movements.

A posteroanterior glide applied to the rib angle will test the anatomical structures that resist anterior translation of the rib. First, fix the contralateral transverse processes of the two vertebrae to which the rib is

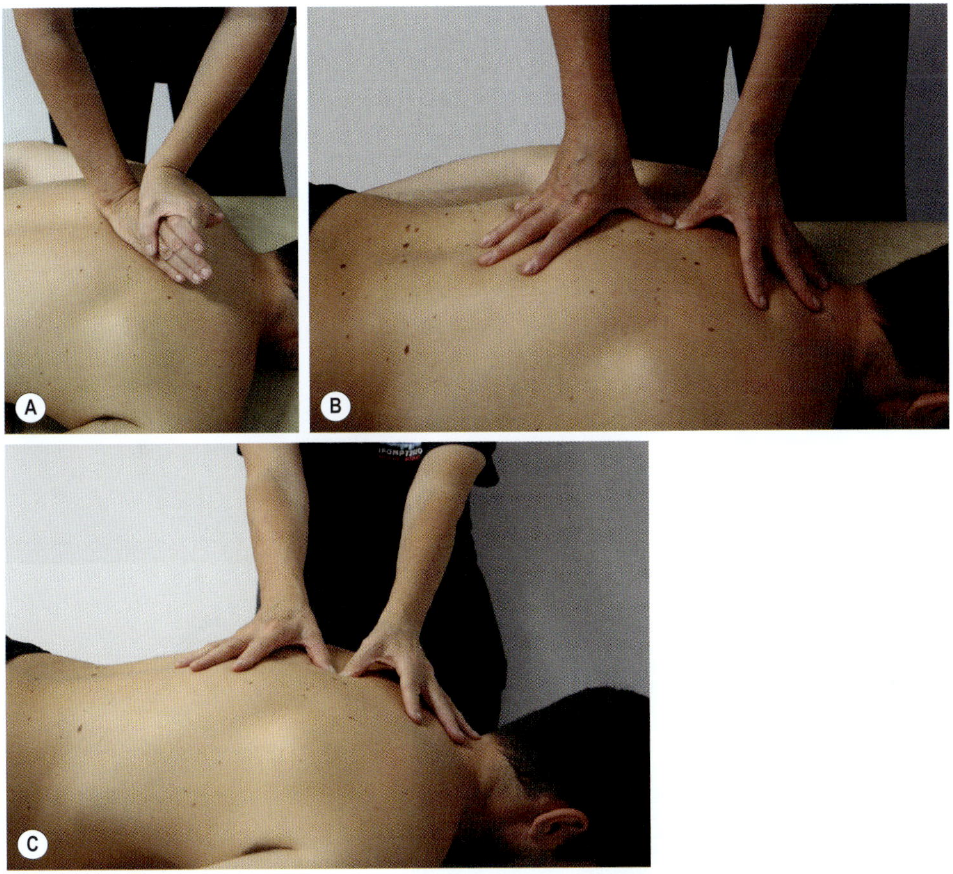

Fig. 9.6 Thoracic Spine (T1–T12) Accessory Movements. (A) Central posteroanterior. A pisiform grip is used to apply pressure to the spinous process. (B) Unilateral posteroanterior. Thumb pressure is applied to the transverse process. (C) Transverse. Thumb pressure is applied to the lateral aspect of the spinous process.

attached. For example, when applying a posteroanterior glide to the fourth rib on the right, fix T3 and T4 on the left (see Fig. 9.7B). If no movement is allowed to occur at the thoracic spine and symptoms are reproduced, the costal joints and ligaments are implicated.

Rib Mechanics During Respiration

During inspiration the first rib elevates, moving the manubrium into an anterior superior direction. A common dysfunction of the first and second ribs is when they remain in elevation. This can be caused by joint stiffness or over activity in scalene muscles. These ribs can be motion-tested by palpation with breathing and/or longitudinal caudad glides (see Fig. 9.7C).

The biomechanics of ribs and thoracic spine during inspiration are largely the same as extension, whilst expiration and flexion are similar. Rib dysfunctions can be assessed by palpating rib mobility with respiration. The mechanics of the costal joints of the ribs that attach to the sternum are oriented largely to facilitate upward and superior movement of the sternum during inspiration – pump-handle motion (Levangie & Norkin, 2011). The reverse occurs during expiration. The mobility of individual ribs can be palpated over the anterior ribcage whilst the patient is asked to breathe (see Fig. 9.7D); this is best done in a recumbent position but can be assessed in functional positions. An anteroposterior glide will assess for pain provocation and mobility. Sternocostal and costochondral junctions can be palpated for tenderness.

The lower ribs have a more upward and lateral motion and increase the transverse diameter of the

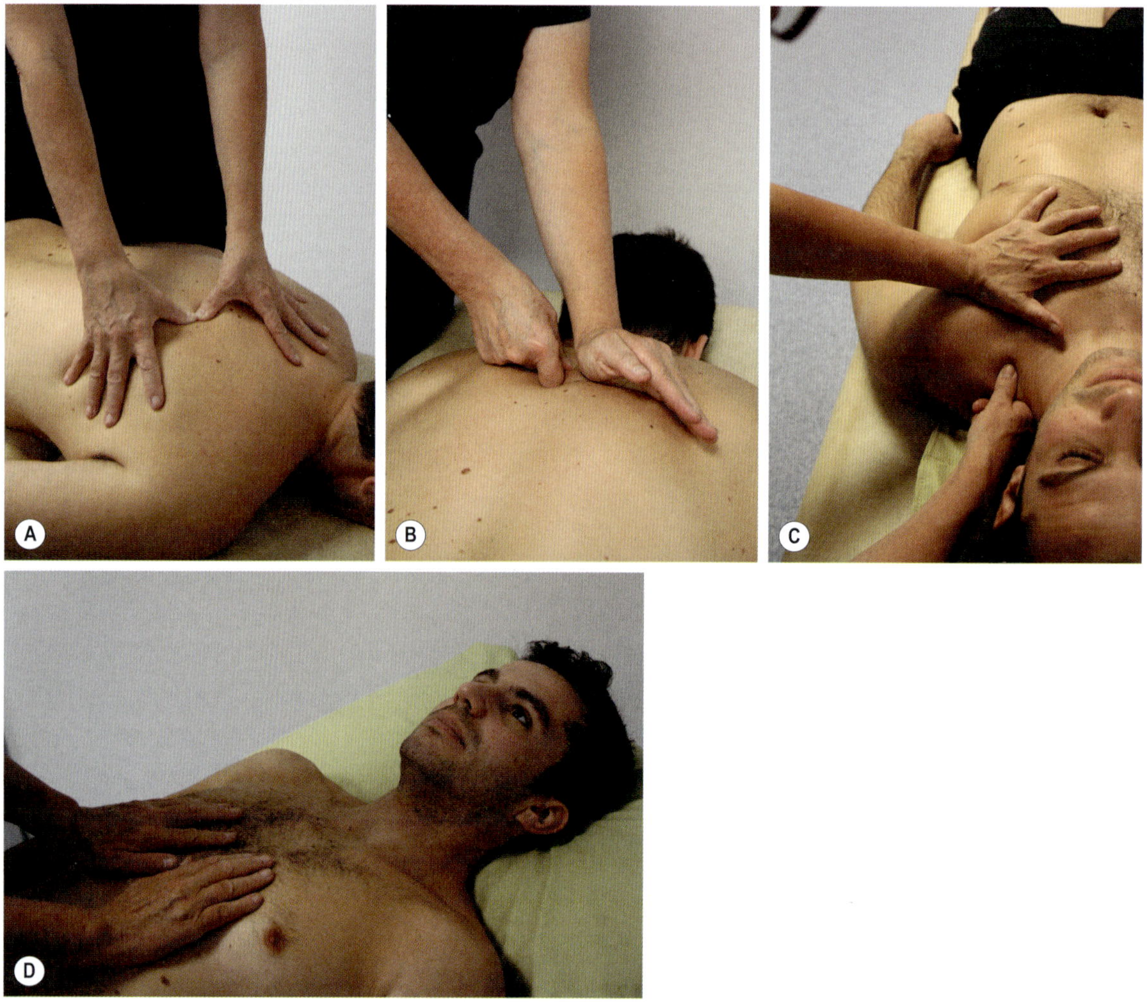

Fig. 9.7 Accessory Movements to Ribs. (A) Unilateral posteroanterior cephalad glide. Thumb pressure is applied to the rib lateral to the costotransverse joint. (B) Posteroanterior glide. Pressure with pisiform (as illustrated) or thumb is applied to the posterior aspect of the rib whilst the contralateral transverse processes of the vertebrae to which the rib is attached are fixed. (C) Longitudinal caudad glide first rib. Using key grip, pressure is applied to the superior aspect of the first rib, and pressure is applied downwards towards the feet. Pressure can be applied anywhere along the superior aspect of the rib. The rib can also be motion-tested with respiration. (D) Motion testing of the sternal ribs (2–7) with respiration. Anteroposterior pressure can also be applied to the anterior aspect of the rib, testing for symptom reproduction and stiffness.

lower thorax during inspiration – bucket-handle motion (Levangie & Norkin, 2011). Individual rib movement can be motion-tested by the clinician palpating laterally on the chest wall whilst asking the patient to do lateral costal breathing. A cephalad or caudad glide applied laterally along the rib will assess for mobility and pain provocation. This can be done with the patient in supine lying where both sides can be compared, or a more detailed assessment of the ribs laterally can be done with the patient in side-lying (Fig. 9.8).

COMPLETION OF THE EXAMINATION

- At this stage the clinician highlights with an asterisk (*) important findings from the examination. These findings need to be reassessed at, and within,

TABLE 9.4 Accessory Movements, Choice of Application and Reassessment of the Patient's Asterisks

Accessory Movements	Choice of Application	Modifications
Thoracic Spine		
↕	Central posteroanterior	In flexion, extension or lateral flexion (with various cephalad/caudad angles)
	Unilateral posteroanterior	Speed of force application
↔	Transverse	
Accessory Movements to Ribs 1–12	In flexion and rotation	
↔	Caud/ceph	In extension and rotation
↕	Anteroposterior	Speed of force application
↕	Posteroanterior	Direction of the applied force
Costochondral, Interchondral & Sternocostal Joints		
↕	Anteroposterior	In extension and rotation Speed of force application Direction of the applied force

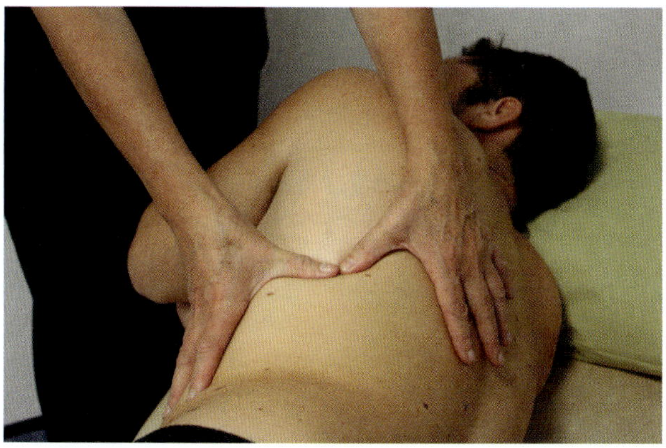

Fig. 9.8 Rib Lateral Motion Testing and Accessory Movement. A caudad glide is applied to the lateral part of the rib with the patient in side-lying. The thumb is placed along the line of the rib.

subsequent treatment sessions to evaluate the effects of treatment on the patient's condition. For full details, see Chapter 4.

- The clinician should collate the information collected, reflect on the findings and compare them with the expected clinical presentation based on the initial primary hypothesis and alternative hypotheses. Aspects of the hypotheses categories may need reviewing or refining in light of findings from the physical examination.
- What can the patient do, and what is the patient unable to do? How are the symptoms and/or dysfunction impacting on the patient's life?
- What are the patient's beliefs? Are they helpful or unhelpful in terms of driving behaviours?
- What is the symptom source? This includes the structure or tissue that is thought to be producing the patient's symptoms (e.g. arthrogenic, myogenic, neurogenic), the mechanism of the injury, the stage of the tissue-healing process and the pain mechanisms.
- What are the contributing factors that have resulted in the development and maintenance of the problem (e.g. environmental, psychosocial, behavioural, local or distant physical movement impairments or heredity factors)?
- Are there any precautions/contraindications to management? This includes the severity and irritability of the patient's symptoms and the nature of the patient's condition.
- Where will initial management be focused (advice, education, exercise, manual therapy)?
- Assessing the prognosis – this can be affected by factors such as the stage and extent of the injury as well as the patient's beliefs, expectations, personality and lifestyle. This should include an estimate of percentage improvement, the number of treatments required and the time period for this.

Before leaving the clinician needs to:

- Explain the findings of the physical examination and how these findings relate to the subjective assessment. An attempt should be made to clear up any misconceptions patients may have regarding their illness or injury.

- Allow patients sufficient opportunity to discuss their thoughts and beliefs after the examination and your explanation.
- Collaborate with the patient to plan a personalized management plan and goal setting, using evidence from the consultation to discuss the prognosis, initially offering some advice if appropriate.
- Warn the patient of possible exacerbation up to 24–48 hours following the examination.
- Request the patient to report details on the behaviour of the symptoms following examination at the next attendance; a diary may be useful to gain further precision information on symptoms behaviour.

For guidance on treatment and management principles, the reader is directed to the companion textbook (Barnard & Ryder, 2024).

KNOWLEDGE CHECK

1. Describe the main types of observation and what you would look for in the thoracic spine region.
2. List four types of muscle testing which can be used in the thoracic spine.
3. What approaches exist to examine joints in the thoracic spine?
4. What is a passive accessory intervertebral movement test, and why would you choose to use it rather than active physiological movement?
5. List five ways in which you can adapt active physiological movement testing to assist symptoms reproduction.
6. Describe the relevance of the thoracic spine to respiratory function.

REVIEW AND REVISE QUESTIONS

1. With respect to the anatomy, what characteristics of the following structures contribute to the thoracic spine being relatively stiff?
   (a) Disc
   (b) Vertebral body & joints
   (c) Ribs
2. What lifestyle and personal factors may influence thoracic mobility?
3. List three possible reasons why the thoracic spine is termed the 'Cinderella' region.
4. Complete the following
   Functional movements such as reversing the car or playing tennis require ______________ thoracic spine mobility to that of the _________ and ___________ joints respectively. Overhead activities require thoracic spine __________ ; without this, structures under excessive stress around the __________ may contribute to a patient's complaint of pain.
5. What is the relationship of the thoracic spine to the trunk, and why is this important?
6. What is osteoporosis, and which of the following are true?
   (a) Men more often present with osteoporosis than women
   (b) Endocrinal and metabolic diseases may predispose individuals to osteoporosis
   (c) Drugs (steroids) do not have any influence on bone health
   (d) Having a fracture following a mild trauma might suggest reduced bone mineral density
7. Describe three ways to differentiate involvement of the thoracic spine with a patient presenting with neck pain.
8. Complete the following and give an example of how this might be needed in everyday activities
   (a) Mobility is ______________________________
   ____
   (b) Motor control is ______________________________
   ____
   (c) Muscle endurance is ______________________________
   ____
   (d) Muscle strength is ______________________________
   ____
9. Which of the following statement is true?
   (a) PPIVMs are best done in lying because the clinician wants to examine the physiological range of motion at a single level and muscles are at rest
   (b) PPIVMs are less provocative than PAIVMs for assessment of joints in an irritable presentation
10. Describe what the role of the thoracic spine is in respiration.

Case Study Mrs J

Female, aged 48 years old

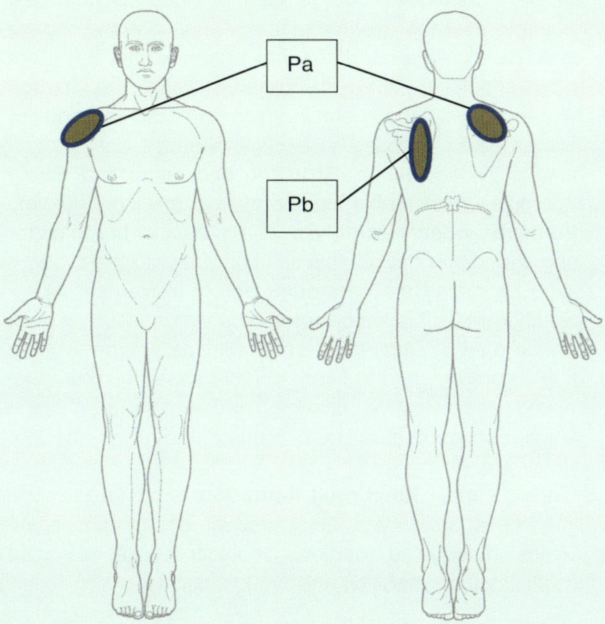

Pa – intermittent sharp pain, with lingering ache once the sharp pain subsides

8/10, reducing to 3/10

Aggravating factors – the immediate onset of pain with lifting, reaching up, drying her hair and driving long distances

Easing factors – rest, warm bath, but can take several hours to ease off

Pb – occasionally general dull and achy, feels stiff

2/10

Aggravating factors – work, prolonged sitting, forward bending

Easing factors – walking, warm bath, stretching

Relationship between Pa and Pb – unsure

24 h pattern – bit of morning stiffness around shoulder on days following her shifts. Disappears with bath or warm shower.

Sleep – does wake up turning over in bed, but can get back to sleep if she takes paracetamol. This happens several times a week.

No symptoms anywhere else

HPC

Persistent right shoulder pain following surgery 10 months ago following right shoulder surgery. Initially felt better but within weeks felt no benefit from the procedure. Now feeling really fed up as took time off work and had surgery which wasn't pleasant and feels no real benefit. Physiotherapy (6 sessions) not helped – exercises (strengthening and stretching) and mobilisation techniques to shoulder and advice. Now considering if she needs to go part time or change jobs as struggling with work, and it's affecting her relationship with work colleagues and family.

Feels she is having to take an increasing amount of medication to function and stay at work. Discharged from hospital consultant and GP just keeps offering to give her more medication (stronger pain relief and offered antidepressants – which she is reluctant to take).

Lifestyle/Occupation/Home Life

Lives with her husband and teenage son. Generally happy home life and no real caring responsibilities other than usual cleaning, shopping etc. Her husband is very helpful and has started to do more to help especially with things like vacuuming which she finds hard and very painful. Works in a supermarket, shift work, on the shop floor stacking shelves, serving at tills. Everything seems to hurt now, from working on till to stacking shelves. Previously loved work, had a great relationship with colleagues and could not imagine not working there after 20 years of service.

Right-handed and drives.

Impact on Function/Beliefs and Expectations

Trying to keep going but struggling and feeling quite down about the thought of having to live with this or change jobs. Doesn't like the idea of being disabled and not able to work (socially important). Frustrated as no one seems to know what's wrong, discharged from the hospital and GP just wants to up medication.

Tried yoga and swimming but both were too painful, so now just tries to walk every day to keep her fitness up.

PMH

- History of right shoulder pain – had several episodes of needing to take time off work over the last 3 years due to pain. Physiotherapy did not help and where each episode seemed to get worse she was then referred to a consultant. The consultant requested scans and x-rays (see below).

Continued

Case Study Mrs J—cont'd

- Right acromioplasty 10 months ago.
- Hysterectomy 8 years ago, now on HRT.

DH/Investigations

On paracetamol and NSAIDs to manage pain. Occasionally taking maximum dose to function.

Other than HRT, no other medications, no history of steroid or anticoagulant use.

Had an MRI and x-rays pre-surgery—was told arthritis in top joint shoulder (acromioclavicular joint-ACJ) and bone irritating tendons. Surgery would help by shaving bone and removing irritation on the tendon.

FH nil of note

GH Good. No areas of concern re THREAD (thyroid, heart, RA, epilepsy, asthma, diabetes)

Clinical Reasoning

Mrs J had an insidious onset of shoulder symptoms which culminated in being offered and having shoulder surgery (ACJ). Whilst generally a positive person and optimistic about surgery being the solution, she has subsequently found no improvement in her pain, and this is now affecting her in many ways

- psychologically **(yellow flags)** – feeling down, lack of a diagnosis, worries about pain getting worse with continued work
- socially **(blue flag)** – impact of relationship and socialization with work colleagues
- physically—unable to do household chores and finding increasing difficulty with requirements of work **(black flag)**

No observable **red flag** symptoms, although positively Mrs J is trying to keep going, tried swimming and yoga without success, but does walk frequently to keep up her fitness (**pink flag**)

Evaluation of Severity, Irritability and Nature

Severity (Pa) – **high** (night disturbance, taking medication, affecting function, NPRS of 8/10)

Irritability (Pa) – **high** (immediate onset of symptoms with simple activities and takes several hours to improve)

Nature – chronic inflammatory condition of the shoulder/ACJ, secondary to faulty movement patterns; developed over time due to pain and functional activities.

What are you treating? It is likely at this point we are treating a **secondary** rather than primary problem (shoulder complaint). Mrs J has been seen and managed conservatively and surgically for shoulder pain (ACJ), but without a positive outcome thus far. **Secondary problems** could be a result of altered/faulty movement patterns developed due to pain or adaptive postures/movements. Moreover, what is now a *secondary problem* could have predisposed Mrs J to a primary pain complaint in the shoulder? As we discussed earlier in the chapter, hypomobility in the thoracic spine can lead to shoulder tissues being exposed to excessive stress during overhead activities, especially at the end range and during repetitive upper limb movements, i.e. stacking shelves. Moreover, where part of Mrs J's job requires her to sit for long periods (at the till) this can contribute to the thoracic spine becoming stiffer through lack of movement (adaptive changes). *(It is important to note that if tissues are not moved they will adaptively shorten)*. Finally, where Mrs J is 48 years old, she is likely to have some 'normal' age-related degenerative changes in her thoracic spine which can contribute to a natural decline in thoracic mobility.

Mrs J's main **functional limitation** is pain-free upper limb elevation, which is a product of thoracic spine extension (coupled rotation), shoulder flexion elevation (motor control, mobility, and work capacity).

Subjective Markers (Link to genics)

1. Ability to dry hair, vacuum and work without pain in shoulder
2. Pain-free sleep, or quantify the use of medication to help get back to sleep

   Does any aspect of the history indicate caution?

   Yes, due to high levels of severity and irritability. No, as the feature fits a persistent pain pattern for the shoulder with a secondary sub clinical complaint in the thoracic spine region.

Can you predict the comparable signs? (Subjective marker linking with an objective sign)

Right shoulder flexion elevation or abduction

What is the relationship between pain and resistance?

Pa – Pain > resistance

Pb – Resistance > pain

What pain mechanisms can you identify? There is evidence of some central affective (psychology) mechanisms at play as well as peripheral inflammatory nociceptive (shoulder) and peripheral mechanical nociceptive (shoulder).

Analysis of percentage weighting (Pain source) Myogenic 25%, Arthrogenic 70%, Osteogenic 5% (all related to stress and tissue response at shoulder/AC joint)

Analysis of percentage weighting (driver/contributing factors) Given the persistent nature of Mrs J's complaint,

Case Study Mrs J—cont'd

it is important to consider the role of other systems and body regions. Questions to ask are (1) why has she developed this complaint? (2) What does her occupation require her to do? (3) Analyzing her main functional limitation, overhead activities – what are the possible contributing factors along the functional kinetic chain – shoulder joint, scapulothoracic junction, thoracic spine, lumbar spine and pelvis (a myriad of muscles, joints, and other soft tissues to consider – e.g. thoracolumbar fascia). Based on the duration of complaint (adaptive changes and faulty movement patterns) and age (degenerative changes) proposed weighting could be: thoracic spine mobility (muscle length and joint) 25%, thoracolumbar fascia (30%), faulty movement pattern (25%), reduced work capacity shoulder muscles (10%), stiffness in ACJ (5%), belief psychological (5%).

Hypotheses to Test/Working Diagnosis? (Differentiate Between Genics)

1. Faulty/dysfunctional movement pattern
2. Thoracolumbar fascia mobility/extensibility
3. Thoracic spine active and passive extension (muscle v joint)
4. Local stiffness right ACJ
5. Reduced work capacity/endurance of shoulder flexors

Planning the Physical examination ***caution re high severity and irritability Pa* (minimize and limit the use of provocative movements or control range explored, e.g. avoid end range shoulder testing)

Observation to include scars (type and location of surgery), muscle atrophy, resting position of right arm, skin condition and observation of general appearance, e.g. affect.

Observe movements (flexion and abduction through elevation) and in left upper limb to establish normal range and quality of movement. Reproduce movements and positions to reflect occupational requirements, e.g. sitting posture and using left arm to replicate movements used during tasks such as shelf stacking.

Thoracic spine (assessing for Pb resistance) Assess Mrs J's ability to *actively extend thoracic spine in sitting and standing* (looking for compensation coming from lumbar spine region and muscle motor control). Assess for hypomobility in the thoracic spine (*mid and low thoracic spine right rotation PPIVMs)* (based on movement coupling, this provides information around fact joint closing on right which reflects what is required during functional upper limb elevation).

To explore *thoracolumbar fascia mobility*, palpation of tissue extensibility (in a cephalad direction) can be assessed in a seated (loaded) position. (For more information see Holey, L.A., Dixon, J., 2014. *Connective tissue manipulation: a review of theory and clinical evidence.* J Bodyw. Mov. Ther. *18 (1), 112–118. https://doi.org/10.1016/j.jbmt.2013.08.003*).

Shoulder/ACJ Examine ACJ using passive accessory movement (less provocative than active movement)

Examine shoulder flexor and rotator cuff work capacity in mid-range flexion and/or abduction (non-provocative)

Examine active shoulder flexion elevation through to onset of pain (note range and NPRS). To examine a possible link between the thoracic spine and limited shoulder elevation, assessment could usefully include test detailed in Fig. 9.4C.

Main clinical findings for Mrs J included

Thoracic spine mobility into extension was limited due to (1) altered motor control, (2) joint hypomobility and (3) reduced tissue extensibility of the thoracolumbar fascia

Reduced work capacity of shoulder flexors and rotator cuff muscles was evident especially outer range.

When applying cutaneous stimuli over the thoracic spine region to encourage extension during mid-range shoulder elevation, Mrs J could achieve a little more range (5/10 degrees) of shoulder flexion elevation before Pa onset.

Management included

Education and advice Advice and education to aid understanding of the relationship between shoulder complaint/need for surgery and impact of age, working postures and activities on related but distant body regions (thoracic spine and connective tissues which span regions)

Deep soft tissue massage of the *tethered* thoracolumbar fascia in a seated position (directed in a cephalad direction for 10/15 min): Mrs J regained virtually full pain-free shoulder flexion elevation, improved movement quality.

Home exercise programme

1. Development of work capacity and motor control of shoulder flexors (within pain-free range) and to retain newly acquired range/mobility of the thoracolumbar fascia
2. Active mobilisation exercises for the thoracic spine (foam roller into extension – see *Heneghan, N.R., Lokhaug, S., Tyros, I., Longvastøl, S., Rushton, A., 2020. A clinical reasoning framework for thoracic spine exercise prescription in sport: a systematic review and narrative synthesis.* BMJ Open SEM *6, e000713. https://doi.org/10.1136/bmjsem-2019-000713)*

Continued

Case Study Mrs J—cont'd

Outcome

Mrs J. had four sessions of physiotherapy and a follow-up phone call. On discharge 6 weeks later she had regained full pain-free mobility (not work capacity) of her right arm, was pain-free at night, able to manage work. Mrs J understood it would take time to fully develop work capacity of relevant muscle groups, regain her fitness and be back to full function. She did report back that 4 months later she was 95% better, enjoying work and started yoga on a regular basis.

Reflections and further comments from the author

This patient really stuck in my mind and made me more analytical of patients' cases where there is a long history; the body adapts to environmental as well as personal factors, so having a comprehensive understanding from the patient's narrative of their complaint can invariably guide management in a timely manner. Tissues need movement (for biomechanical and physiology health) and without movement (which was not possible for Mrs J due to painful shoulder), inert and contractile tissues will contract, adapt or become 'tethered'.

This patient was seen in my practice before PROMs were commonplace in practice. On reflection, a generic PROM such as the Pain Self Efficacy Questionnaire might have been useful, alongside a shoulder-specific scale such as the Disabilities of the Arm, Shoulder and Hand (DASH) questionnaire.

REFERENCES

Barnard, K., Ryder, D., 2024. Principles of Musculoskeletal Treatment and Management: A Handbook for Therapists, fourth ed. Elsevier, Edinburgh.

Briggs, A.M., Smith, A.J., Straker, L.M., Bragge, P., 2009. Thoracic spine pain in the general population: prevalence, incidence and associated factors in children, adolescents and adults. A systematic review. BMC Musculoskelet. Disord. 10 (77), 1–2.

Bucke, J., Spencer, S., Fawcett, L., Sonvico, L., Rushton, A., Heneghan, N.R., 2017. Validity of the digital inclinometer and iPhone when measuring thoracic rotation. J. Athl. Train. 52 (9), 820–825.

Debouche, S., Pitance, L., Robert, A., Liistro, G., Reychler, G., 2016. Reliability and reproducibility of chest wall expansion measurement in young healthy adults. J. Manipulative Physiol. Ther. 39 (6), 443–449.

Dunn, K.M., Campbell, P., Lewis, M., Hill, J.C., van der Windt, D.A., Afolabi, E., et al., 2021. Refinement and validation of a tool for stratifying patients with musculoskeletal pain. Eur. J. Pain. 25 (10), 2081–2093.

Edmondston, S.J., Aggerholm, M., Elfving, S., Flores, N., Ng, C., Smith, R., et al., 2007. Influence of posture on the range of axial rotation and coupled lateral flexion of the thoracic spine. J. Manipulative Physiol. Ther. 30 (3), 193–199.

Fuller, G., 2013. Neurological Examination Made Easy, fifth ed. Churchill Livingstone, Edinburgh.

Heneghan, N.R., Baker, G., Thomas, K., Falla, D., Rushton, A., 2018. The influence of sedentary behaviour and physical activity on thoracic spinal mobility in young adults: an observational study. BMJ Open 8, e019371.

Heneghan, N.R., Lokhaug, S., Tyros, I., Longvastøl, S., Rushton, A., 2020. A clinical reasoning framework for thoracic spine exercise prescription in sport: a systematic review and narrative synthesis. BMJ Open SEM. 6 (1), e000713.

Heneghan, N.R., Rushton, A., 2016. Understanding why the thoracic region is the 'Cinderella' region of the spine. Man. Ther. 21, 274–276.

Heneghan, N.R., Smith, R., Tyros, I., Falla, D., Rushton, A., 2018. Thoracic dysfunction in whiplash associated disorders: a systematic review. PLoS One 13 (3), e0194235.

Heneghan, N.R., Webb, K., Mahoney, T., Rushton, A., 2019. Thoracic spine mobility, an essential link in upper limb kinetic chains in athletes: a systematic review. Transl. Sports Med. 2 (6), 301–315.

Johnson, K.D., Kim, K.M., Yu, B.K., Saliba, S.A., Grindstaff, T. L., 2012. Reliability of thoracic spine rotation range-of-motion measurements in healthy adults. J. Athl. Train. 47 (1), 52–60.

Kendall, F., Kendall, F.P., 2015. Muscles: Testing and Function With Posture and Pain. Lippincott Williams & Wilkins, Baltimore, MD.

Leboeuf-Yde, C., Nielsen, J., Kyvik, K.O., Fejer, R., Hartvigsen, J., 2009. Pain in the lumbar, thoracic or cervical regions: do age or gender matter? A population-based study of 34,902 Danish twins 20–71 years of age. BMC Musculoskelet. Disor. 10 (39), 1–12.

Lee, D., 2018. The Thorax: An Integrated Approach. Handspring Pub Ltd, Edinburgh.

Lee, L.J., Coppieters, M.W., Hodges, P.W., 2005. Differential activation of the thoracic multifidus and longissimus thoracis during trunk rotation. Spine (Phila Pa 1976) 30 (8), 870–876.

Levangie, P.K., Norkin, C.C., 2011. Joint Structure and Function. A Comprehensive Analysis, fifth ed. F.A. Davis, Philadelphia.

Sahrmann, S., Azevedo, D., Dillen, L.V., 2017. Diagnosis and treatment of movement system impairment syndromes. Braz. J. Phys. Ther. 21 (6), 391–399.

Spencer, S., Wolf, A., Rushton, A., 2016. Spinal-exercise prescription in sport: classifying physical training and rehabilitation by intention and outcome. J. Athl. Train. 51 (8), 613–628.

Sueki, D.G., Cleland, J.A., Wainner, R.S., 2013. A regional interdependence model of musculoskeletal dysfunction: research, mechanisms, and clinical implications. J. Man. Manipulative Ther. 21 (2), 90–102.

Tsang, S.M., Szeto, G.P., Lee, R.Y., 2013. Normal kinematics of the neck: the interplay between the cervical and thoracic spines. Man. Ther. 18 (5), 431–437.

Wirth, B., Amstalden, M., Perk, M., Boutellier, U., Humphreys, B.K., 2014. Respiratory dysfunction in patients with chronic neck pain – influence of thoracic spine and chest mobility. Man. Ther. 19 (5), 440–444.

10

Examination of Shoulder

Kevin Hall

LEARNING OUTCOMES

After studying this chapter, you should be able to:

- List the key constituents of a thorough subjective examination.
- Demonstrate an understanding of nonmechanical causes of shoulder pain and how these conditions might present. What questions might you ask to explore these possible nonmechanical conditions more deeply?
- Be able to generate a diagnostic hypothesis based on the subjective examination.
- List the key constituents of a thorough physical examination.
- Have an understanding of common shoulder conditions.
- Have an appreciation of which tests might be used to explore a differential diagnosis of the shoulder.

CHAPTER CONTENTS

Introduction, 284
Subjective Examination/Taking the Patients' History, 285
Serious Pathology, 285
Patients' Perspectives on Their Experience, 285
Body Chart, 285
Behaviour of Symptoms, 286
History of the Present Condition, 286
Past Medical History, 287
Plan for the Physical Examination, 287
Physical Examination, 287
Observation, 287
Active Physiological Movements, 287
Shoulder Symptom Modification Procedures, 287
Passive Physiological Movements, 289
Rotator Cuff Pathology Tests, 292
Biceps Tests, 293
Superior Labral Anterior–Posterior Tests, 293
Rotator Cuff–Related Shoulder Pain, 295
The Stiff Shoulder, 296
Glenohumeral Joint Instability, 296
Muscle Tests, 298
Neurological Examination, 301
Vascular Assessment, 301
Palpation, 302
Accessory Movements, 302
Completion of the Examination, 302
Case Study, 303
References, 304

INTRODUCTION

Understanding the biological, psychological and social factors involved in a patient's shoulder presentation and how these factors interact is important for the effective management of musculoskeletal conditions. The patient assessment provides an opportunity to gather and process this important information and collaborate with the patient in order to develop a management strategy. The general principles of the subjective and physical examination are discussed in depth in Chapters 3 and 4, respectively.

SUBJECTIVE EXAMINATION/TAKING THE PATIENTS' HISTORY

The principles of the subjective examination are described in depth in Chapter 3. Specific considerations relating to the shoulder will now be discussed.

Serious Pathology

Shoulder pain may involve local tissues or spinal structures, or be referred from nonmusculoskeletal structures. Considering serious pathology is important and is discussed in Chapter 11 of the companion textbook (Barnard & Ryder, 2024). Specific considerations relating to serious pathology for the shoulder include trauma, malignancy, infective and inflammatory conditions as well as referred pain from viscera:

1. Trauma leading to loss of rotation and abnormal shape may indicate unresolved shoulder dislocation.
2. Bilateral shoulder pain and weakness in patients over 50 with significant morning symptoms of more than 45 minutes may indicate polymyalgia rheumatica.
3. Signs of infection including shoulder pain, skin redness, fever or feeling unwell may indicate septic arthritis.
4. Identification of a shoulder mass or swelling may indicate malignancy.
5. Cardiac pathology including acute myocardial infarction, angina and pericarditis may refer into the shoulder region. Seventy percentage of patients reported shoulder pain during an acute myocardial infarction (Song et al., 2010).

Patients' Perspectives on Their Experience

Any social history that is relevant to the onset and progression of the patient's problem should be explored. This includes the patient's employment status, home situation and details of any leisure/sporting activities with a particular focus on the physical demands of the shoulder such as prolonged static postures, overhead working or a high volume of heavy lifting.

Research on prognostic indicators suggests that recovery from shoulder conditions can be affected by high levels of disability and pain at onset, duration of symptoms (Chester et al., 2013), educational background and the number of co-morbidities present (Dunn et al., 2014). Factors associated with better outcomes at 6 weeks and 6 months were lower baseline disability, patient expectation of 'complete recovery' compared to 'slight improvement', higher pain self-efficacy and lower pain severity at rest (Chester et al., 2018).

Body Chart

The following information concerning the type and area of current symptoms can be recorded on a body chart (see Fig. 3.2).

Area of Current Symptoms

It is important to be precise when mapping out the area of the symptoms. Record all symptoms that the patient is experiencing and ascertain which symptoms are the most severe. Symptoms from the glenohumeral joint are commonly felt over the anterior deltoid, often extending into the region of the distal deltoid and into the biceps. Acromioclavicular and sternoclavicular joint pain is normally felt locally around the joint.

Areas Relevant to the Region Being Examined

All other relevant areas should be checked for symptoms; it is important to ask about pain or even stiffness, as this may be relevant to the patient's main symptom. Check for symptoms in the cervical spine, thoracic spine, elbow, wrist and hand.

Quality of Pain

Establish the quality of the pain. A catching pain, or an arc of pain through elevation, is typical of some shoulder conditions. Clunking felt within the shoulder joint may be relevant to the condition occurring in some cases of labral pathology or glenohumeral joint instability.

Abnormal Sensation

Check for any altered sensation locally around the shoulder region as well as over the spine and distally in the arm. The axillary nerve supplies the area of skin in the upper region of the humerus and motor innervation to the deltoid. It is sometimes involved in shoulder dislocation and is important to consider in presentations involving trauma to the shoulder.

Relationship of Symptoms

Determine the relationship between symptomatic areas—do they present together or separately? For example, the patient may have shoulder pain without neck pain, or the pains may always be present together. This is a critical element of the examination as there is such a close relationship between the spine and shoulder region.

Behaviour of Symptoms

Aggravating Factors

Common aggravating activities for the shoulder include dressing (putting on shirts and coats), overhead activities, reaching the hand behind the back, sudden shoulder movements, lifting and lying on the shoulder. Aggravating factors for other regions, which may need to be explored if they are suspected to be a source of the symptoms, are described in Chapter 3. It is important to ask if the patient experiences any feeling of instability in the shoulder. The most notable functional restrictions should be highlighted with asterisks (*) on the body chart, explored in the physical examination and reassessed at subsequent treatment sessions. These functional movements may be integrated into the examination in the assessment of shoulder symptom modification procedures (SSMPs).

Easing Factors

For each symptomatic area a series of questions can be asked to help determine what eases the symptoms:

- What movements and/or positions ease the patient's symptoms?
- How long does it take before symptoms are eased?
- What happens to other symptoms when this symptom is eased?

Night Symptoms

Explore the impact of the condition on the patient's sleep, as described in Chapter 3, with particular focus on the patient's current sleeping position and how this differs from their normal sleeping position, e.g. are they able to lie on the affected shoulder?

Morning and Evening Symptoms

Determine the pattern of the symptoms first thing in the morning, throughout the day and at the end of the day. Morning stiffness that lasts more than 30–90 minutes may indicate an inflammatory condition such as rheumatoid arthritis or polymyalgia rheumatica; in addition, symptoms are more likely to be bilateral when these conditions are present. Stiffness lasting less than 30 minutes is more likely to be mechanical in nature.

Stage of the Condition

In order to determine the stage of the condition, ask whether the symptoms are getting better, getting worse or remaining unchanged. Some conditions such as a frozen shoulder have a more predictable natural history (1–3 years) and understanding where the patient is in their journey is important.

History of Trauma

It is important to ask if the patient has a history of trauma in relation to this current condition, but also in relation to previous traumatic incidents. If the patient has symptoms of glenohumeral joint instability or recent shoulder dislocation, care must be taken during the physical examination; e.g. for anterior dislocation, the clinician should take care when positioning the shoulder in lateral rotation and abduction.

Neurological Symptoms

Has the patient experienced symptoms of tingling in the hands or weakness or altered sensation in the arm? These symptoms may indicate involvement of the cervical spine, a peripheral entrapment neuropathy or a brachial plexopathy.

Vascular Symptoms

Does the patient complain of coldness, change in colour or loss of sensation in the arm or hands? Does the patient get symptoms when the arms are raised or if working with the arms overhead? This may indicate a vascular problem which may need further consideration (e.g. vascular thoracic outlet syndrome (TOS)).

History of the Present Condition

Ask about previous episodes of shoulder pain: how many episodes? When were they? What was the cause? What was the duration of each episode? Did the patient fully recover between episodes? If there has been no previous history of shoulder pain, has the patient had any episodes of stiffness in the cervical spine, thoracic spine, shoulder or any other relevant region? Is there a history of trauma, traumatic dislocation, spontaneous dislocation/subluxation or a history of voluntary dislocation/subluxation (party trick movements)? Ascertain the results of any past treatment for the same or a similar problem.

Past Medical History

Information relating to the past medical history is obtained from the patient and/or the medical notes as described in Chapter 3, with a particular focus on visceral structures with the capability of referring into the shoulder, such as cardiac pathology or abdominal problems relating to the stomach, liver, gallbladder, diaphragm or pancreas.

Signs that the symptoms may be referred from visceral structures include:

- Constant pain, or pain which does not change with changes in arm position or activity (nonmechanical).
- Pain which changes in relation to organ function (eating, bowel or bladder activity, or coughing or deep breathing)
- Shoulder pain which increases with exertion that does not stress the shoulder, such as walking or climbing stairs.

Symptoms that may indicate that the symptoms are referred from visceral structures include cough, breathlessness, chest pain, malaise, night sweats, fatigue, fever, nausea or vomiting (Perlow & Lucado, 2014) or the presence of indigestion, diarrhoea, constipation or rectal bleeding.

Further Investigations

Investigations may include blood tests, magnetic resonance imaging (MRI), diagnostic ultrasound, arthroscopy and arthrogram.

Plan for the Physical Examination

The information from the subjective examination helps the clinician to plan an appropriate physical examination. The severity, irritability and nature of the condition are the major factors that will influence the choice and priority of physical testing procedures. The order and detail of the physical examination need to be appropriate to the patient. The techniques described in this chapter are some of the most commonly used techniques for the assessment of the shoulder, and are by no means an exhaustive list.

PHYSICAL EXAMINATION

The principles of the physical examination are described in depth in Chapter 4. Specific considerations relating to the shoulder will now be considered.

Observation

Examine the posture of the patient, noting the posture of the shoulders, head and neck, thoracic spine and upper limbs. Note bony and soft tissue contours around the region. Examine the muscle bulk and muscle tone of the patient, comparing the left and right sides. Any atrophy in the muscles of the shoulder should be noted, ensuring observations are made from the posterior aspect as well as the front. Remember that handedness and level and frequency of physical activity may well produce differences in muscle bulk between sides.

Active Physiological Movements

For active physiological movement, note:

- quality of movement
- range of movement
- behaviour of pain through the range of movement
- resistance or apprehension at the end of the range of movement.

A movement diagram can be used to depict this information. The active movements with overpressure are shown in Fig. 10.1 and can be tested with the patient in standing and/or sitting. Movements are carried out on the left and right sides. The clinician establishes the patient's symptoms at rest, prior to each movement, and modifies any movement deviation to determine its relevance to the patient's symptoms. Physiological movements can be examined in isolation or combined to provoke symptoms in presentations that are nonsevere and nonirritable. The physiological movements that the clinician chooses to combine should be guided by the aggravating factors from the subjective examination.

Shoulder Symptom Modification Procedures

Once a symptomatic movement has been identified, SSMPs (Lewis, 2009, 2016) can be applied to the movement in an attempt to reduce the pain severity.

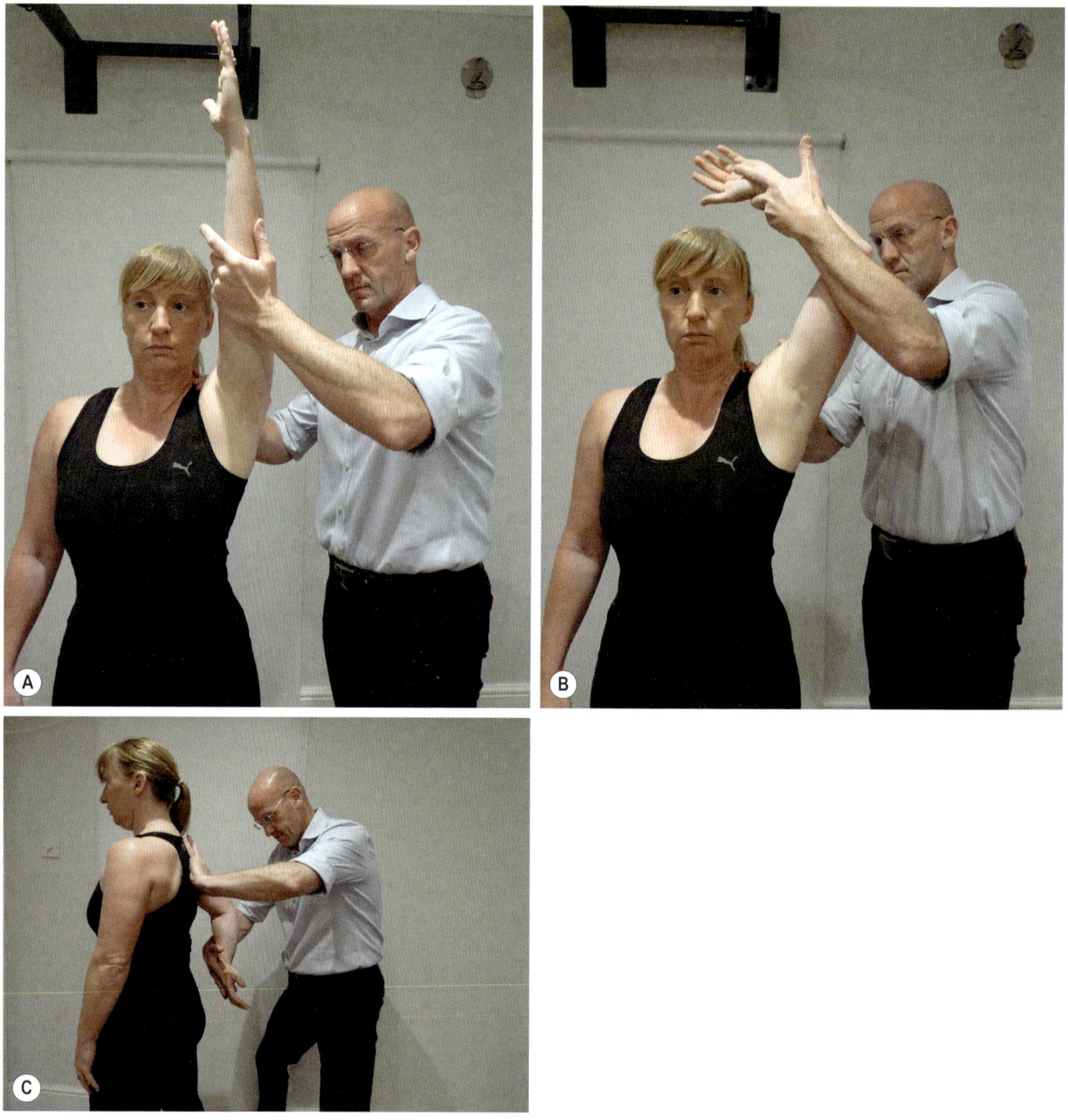

Fig. 10.1 Active Movements With Overpressure. (A) Flexion: apply pressure on the humerus into flexion whilst stabilizing the scapula. (B) Overpressure into a functional position of abduction and lateral rotation: with the patient's arm in Hand behind head (HBH) position, apply further pressure into combined flexion, abduction and lateral rotation individually to test each component of the movement. (C) Hand behind back (HBB): with the patient's arm in HBB position, apply further pressure into medial rotation, adduction and extension individually to test each component of the movement.

The symptomatic movement can be a planar physiological movement, a combined movement or any functional activity described by the patient in the subjective examination (aggravating factors). Once the pain-provoking movement has been identified, the clinician may explore the effect of applying an SSMP, to that movement. SSMPs include thoracic, scapular and humeral head procedures (Fig. 10.2). The clinician applies an SSMP and asks the patient to repeat the pain-provoking movement. If the pain is lessened by the application of the SSMP, then the clinician notes the extent of pain relief and moves on to the next SSMP, in a systematic way. For example, if active abduction reproduces 5/10 pain at 90 degrees and this is reduced to 2/10 by applying a thoracic SSMP, then this is noted by the clinician and may be incorporated into the exercise and treatment regime. The clinician then goes on to repeat abduction with scapular or humeral head procedures to see if symptoms can be reduced further or eliminated completely (see Fig. 10.2). If the symptoms improve with the addition of these assessment techniques, then the technique may become part of the treatment program. Multiple techniques can be used for a patient if indicated by the pain response. For a fuller description of SSMPs see Lewis, 2009, 2016. It is very important to consider pain severity and irritability when planning examination using SSMPs because the painful movement will be repeated several times using different modifying techniques. If the patient's pain irritability is high, symptoms may be exacerbated.

Some functional ability has already been tested by general observation of the patient during the subjective and physical examinations, e.g. the postures adopted during the subjective examination and undressing prior to the examination. Any further functional testing can be carried out at this point and may include various sitting postures or aggravating movements of the upper limb including working or sporting movements and postures. These movements may become the focus of evaluation using SSMPs.

Passive Physiological Movements

All the active movements described above can be examined passively with the patient in standing or supine lying, comparing the left and right sides. A comparison of the response of symptoms to the active and passive versions of the same movement can help to determine whether the structure at fault is noncontractile (articular) or contractile (extra-articular) (Cyriax, 1982). If the movement increases with less pain when performed passively, the contractile structures of the shoulder may be implicated.

Total rotation motion can be assessed in 90-degrees abduction by passively assessing glenohumeral joint external rotation and internal rotation. The total rotation motion is the sum of the patient's internal rotation and external rotation. A comparison can be made with the contralateral shoulder to determine if there is a deficit in range and in what direction the deficit lies. It is common for there to be asymmetry in the location of the range of shoulder rotation but the total rotation motion should be similar in both shoulders.

Posterior Shoulder Tightness

Posterior shoulder tightness (PST) has been described by many authors as a physical impairment associated with several conditions of the shoulder, including tendinopathy, labral pathology and rotator cuff—related shoulder pain (RCRSP) (Dashottar & Borstad, 2012). Theory suggests that the 'tightness' in the posterior structures alters glenohumeral joint kinematics, resulting in irritation of the related soft tissue structures causing pain and disability (Hall & Borstad, 2018). The interest in PST emerged as a result of descriptions in the literature of a deficit in internal rotation or horizontal adduction in the symptomatic shoulder compared with the asymptomatic shoulder of patients with shoulder pain (Tyler et al., 1999; Land et al., 2017).

If a correlation does exist between PST and shoulder pain, what is the meaning? It is important to remember that correlation does not imply causation, although it is a feature of causation (Anjum & Mumford, 2018). There are several possibilities that might explain an observed relationship between two entities (PST and shoulder pain):

1. PST causes shoulder pain.
2. Shoulder pain causes PST.
3. There is no causal connection between PST and shoulder pain.
4. PST and shoulder pain have no causal connection but may have a common cause.
5. PST causes shoulder pain, and shoulder pain causes PST.

These possibilities are under-represented in the literature relating to PST. It is widely acknowledged that

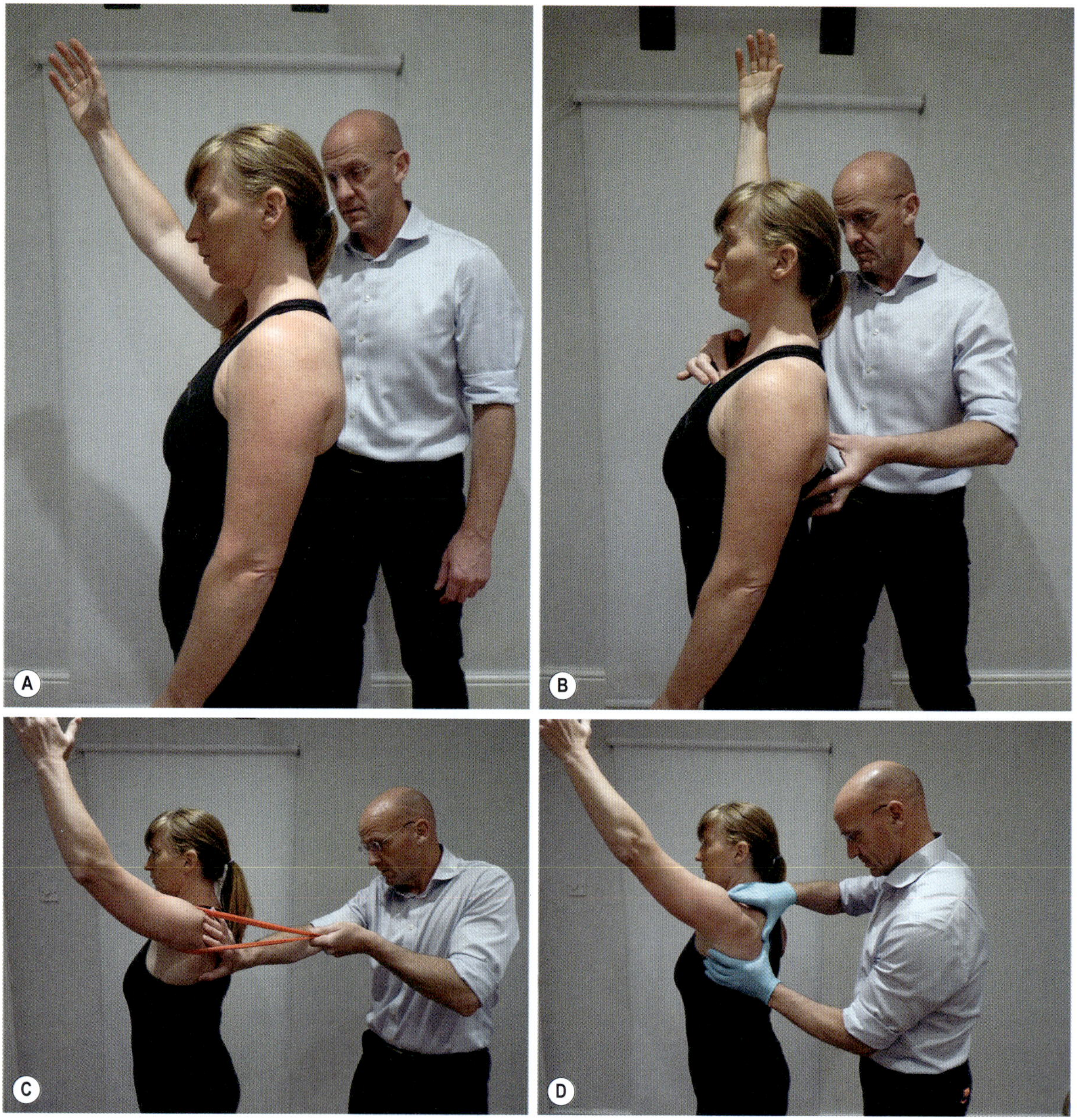

Fig. 10.2 Symptom Modification Procedure. (A) Note restriction in shoulder flexion with the thoracic spine in kyphosed position. (B) Increased shoulder flexion with change in posture. (C) Applying an anteroposterior glide to the humeral head using TheraBand. (D) Scapular facilitation.

PST might be a cause of shoulder pain, but the possibility that shoulder pain causes PST is rarely discussed (Hall & Borstad, 2018).

PST can be assessed using three clinical tests. The validity of these tests is supported by cadaveric research that has measured strain in the posterior capsule with different movements of the shoulder (Borstad & Dashottar, 2011). The three tests are:

1. Supine internal rotation in 90 degrees abduction (Fig. 10.3A). The scapula is stabilized through the coracoid process and the angle of internal rotation is measured (maintaining 90 degrees shoulder

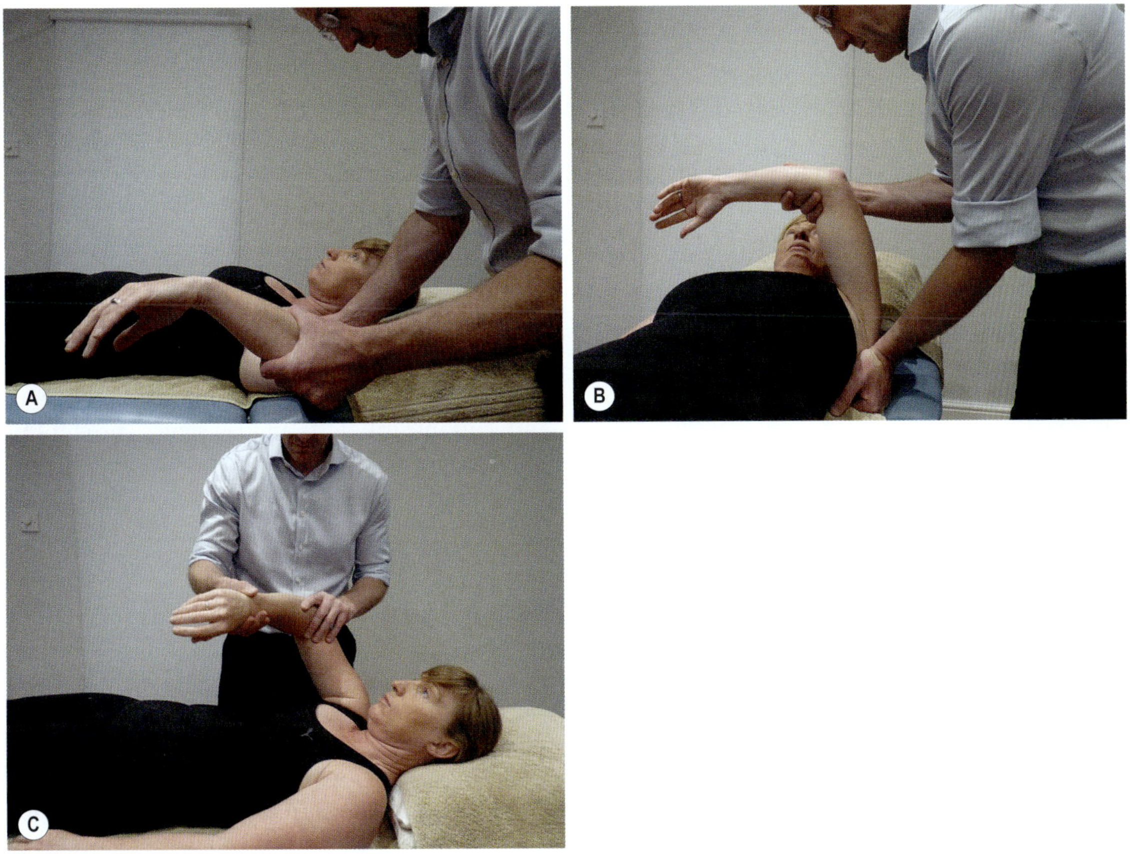

Fig. 10.3 Posterior Shoulder Tightness. (A) Supine internal rotation in 90 degrees abduction. (B) Horizontal adduction. (C) Low flexion.

abduction). Intersession reliability (intratester intraclass correlation coefficient (ICC)) of 0.87 has been reported (Hall et al., 2020).

2. Horizontal adduction (Fig. 10.3B). The lateral border of the scapula is stabilized with the clinician's caudad hand and the glenohumeral joint is moved into horizontal adduction, maintaining neutral rotation. The clinician records the angle the humerus makes with the vertical. Intersession reliability (ICC) of 0.88 has been reported (Hall et al., 2020).
3. Low flexion (Fig. 10.3C). With the patient supine and with 90 degrees of elbow flexion, the arm is elevated to 60 degrees flexion and then internally rotated to the end of range. The angle the arm makes with the horizontal is measured. Intersession reliability (ICC) of 0.86 has been reported (Hall et al., 2020).

For all three tests, the range in the symptomatic arm is compared with the range in the asymptomatic arm. The greater the difference between the contralateral shoulder and the symptomatic shoulder, the more significant the findings.

Shoulder Tests

In the next few sections, there will be a discussion regarding the clinical diagnosis of different shoulder conditions. These conditions are based on a pathoanatomical diagnosis, that is, the presence of structural pathology within the shoulder. Tests that might be performed in the physical examination to aid the diagnosis of each condition will be described, e.g. rotator cuff pathology, and the ability of these tests to identify the condition when it is present (specificity) or to exclude it when absent (sensitivity) will be discussed. It is important to remember that there is often a degree of uncertainty when making a clinical diagnosis from a pathoanatomical perspective: 'The clinical diagnostic process should be viewed through the lens of odds and probabilities' (Hegedus et al., 2015).

The diagnostic accuracy of clinical tests in identifying anatomical structures responsible for symptoms is fraught with difficulty. The result of a test (positive or negative) must be compared to a gold-standard investigation (usually ultrasound, MRI or surgical observation) that determines 'definitively' if the pathology is present. A comparison is then made with the results of the orthopaedic test to determine its accuracy. One of the problems is that these investigations/procedures are not 100% accurate at identifying the pathology in question. Further complicating the issue of the structural diagnosis is the high incidence of pathology in asymptomatic shoulders; lots of people without pain have age-related adaptations that will be identified through imaging or at surgery. Barreto et al., (2019) performed bilateral MRI imaging of 123 patients with unilateral shoulder pain. They identified a 10% increase in glenohumeral joint arthritis and full thickness rotator cuff tears in the symptomatic shoulders. All other findings were similar in the symptomatic and asymptomatic shoulders. If structural pathology is present in asymptomatic shoulders in so many cases, how do we know these changes are the cause of the patient's symptoms? This lack of certainty means that the results of these tests should be interpreted with caution, and in the context of the whole presentation.

KNOWLEDGE CHECK

1. What serious pathology might you consider when assessing a patient with shoulder pain?
2. What nerve can sometimes be injured during shoulder dislocation?
3. What are the five possible causal relationships when a correlation is identified between two variables?
4. When interpreting the results of diagnostic tests what sources if uncertainty must be considered?

Rotator Cuff Pathology Tests

Rotator cuff pathology has been described as a very common cause of shoulder pain (Lewis, 2010, 2016). There appears to be a continuum of pathology of the rotator cuff, with minor tendinopathy at one end and massive, full-thickness tears at the other end. A normal tendon is thought to develop tendinopathy, partial tears and then full-thickness tears of increasing size as pathology progresses. Many studies have demonstrated that partial and full-thickness tears of the rotator cuff are common in asymptomatic shoulders, resulting in controversy relating to the clinical relevance of rotator cuff tears (Barreto et al., 2019; Milgrom et al., 1995). Tears occur most commonly in supraspinatus. Isolated infraspinatus tears are very uncommon but can occur with supraspinatus tears. Broadly, there are two types of tests used in the physical examination of the rotator cuff: cuff integrity tests and lag signs. The cuff integrity tests (e.g. resisted lateral rotation, full/empty can) determine the force of contraction generated and monitor pain provocation. The lag signs (external rotation/drop sign/Gerber lift-off) determine if a position can be maintained and are used to identify large, full-thickness tears of the rotator cuff.

Empty- and Full-Can Tests for Supraspinatus Tear or Tendinopathy (*Fig. 10.4*)

The patient abducts the arm to 90 degrees in the scapular plane with the arm internally rotated so the thumb points downwards. The clinician applies a downward force to the distal forearm (Jobe & Moynes, 1982). Pain or weakness is a positive finding (Itoi et al., 1999). Three studies of low to moderate bias have reported sensitivity of 75%–90% and specificity of 32%–68% (Hegedus et al., 2012). The test can also be performed in external rotation with the thumb pointing up (full-can test). It was previously thought that this test can isolate activity in the supraspinatus muscle; however, electromyogram studies have demonstrated that this movement generates high levels of activity in the majority of muscles in the shoulder and therefore cannot isolate supraspinatus activity (Boettcher et al., 2009).

Gerber 'Lift-Off' for Subscapularis Tendinopathy (*Fig. 10.5*)

For patients with full internal rotation, this test can be performed by the patient placing their hand behind their back in the area of the midlumbar spine so that the dorsum of the hand is resting against the lumbar spine. The patient is asked to lift the hand away from the body. The inability to lift the hand away from the body is

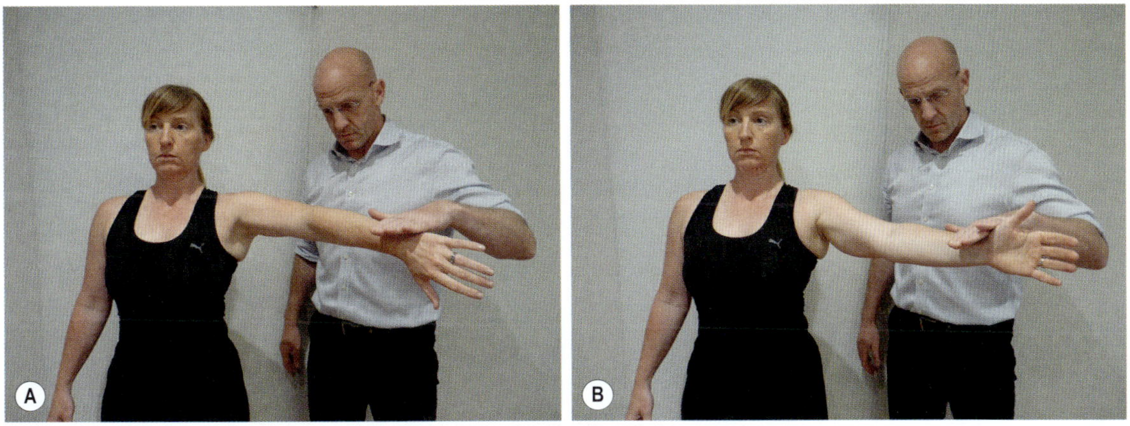

Fig. 10.4 (A) Empty-can test. (B) Full-can test.

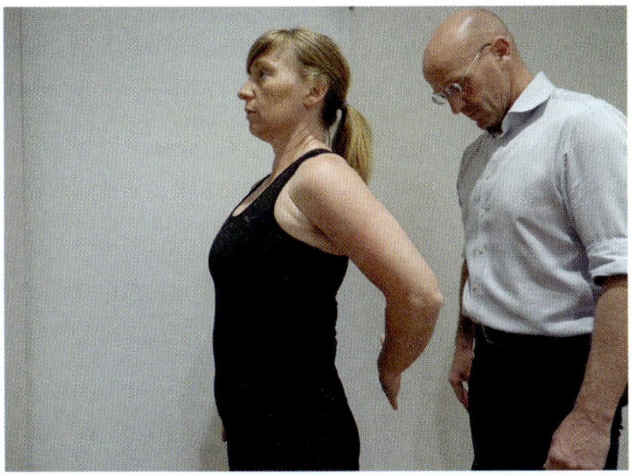

Fig. 10.5 Gerber lift-off test.

considered a positive test and is thought to indicate pathology of the subscapularis tendon. Four studies of low to moderate bias have reported sensitivity of 6%—50% and specificity of 23%—79% (Hegedus et al., 2012).

External Rotation Lag Sign for Full-Thickness Tears of the Supraspinatus and Infraspinatus (Hertel et al., 1996; Castoldi et al., 2009) (*Fig. 10.6*)

With the elbow flexed to 90 degrees, the arm is placed in 20 degrees abduction in the scapular plane and the shoulder is externally rotated to the end range (−5 degrees to reduce the effect of elastic recoil of the glenohumeral joint). The patient is asked to resist external rotation in this position. If no resistance can be provided the patient is asked to hold the arm in this position and the clinician releases the arm. If the arm drops towards the body the test is considered positive for a full-thickness tear of supraspinatus and infraspinatus (± teres minor). Two studies of low to moderate bias have reported sensitivity of 46%—100% and excellent specificity of 93%—98% (Hegedus et al., 2012).

Biceps Tests

Pathology of the long head of the biceps tendon (LHBT) may be a primary source of shoulder pain, existing in isolation or in association with other shoulder conditions. There are many clinical tests that can be used to determine the involvement of the LHBT; however, the evidence for the diagnostic accuracy of these tests is poor (Bélanger et al., 2019).

Speed's Test for Bicipital Tendinopathy (*Fig. 10.7*)

Tenderness in the bicipital groove when shoulder forward flexion is resisted (with forearm supination and elbow joint extension) indicates a positive test.

Yergason's Test (*Fig. 10.8*)

The patient has the elbow flexed to 90 degrees and the forearm in full pronation. The clinician resists supination whilst palpating in the bicipital groove. Pain or subluxation of the tendon in the groove constitutes a positive test. Holtby and Razmjou (2004) found specificity of 79% and sensitivity of 43%.

Superior Labral Anterior—Posterior Tests

A superior labral anterior-posterior (SLAP) lesion may occur either due to trauma, such as a fall on an

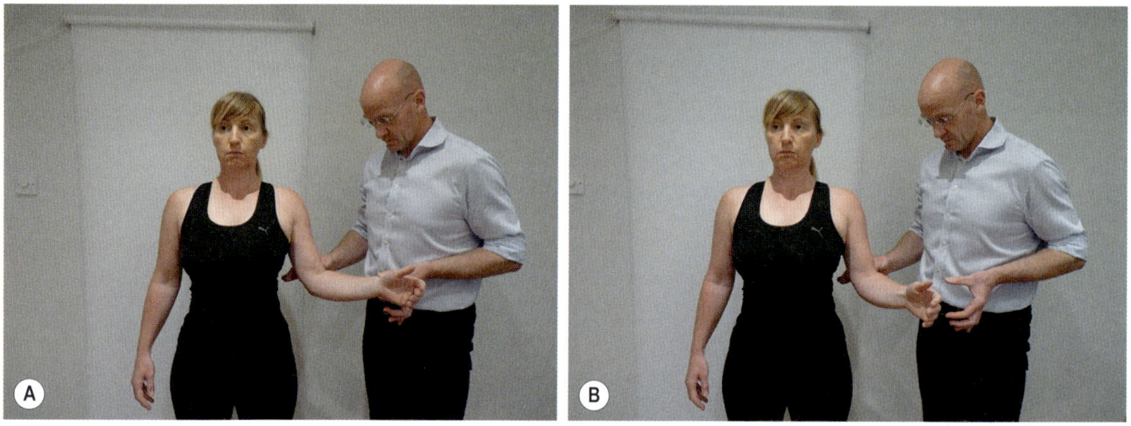

Fig. 10.6 (A and B) External rotation lag sign.

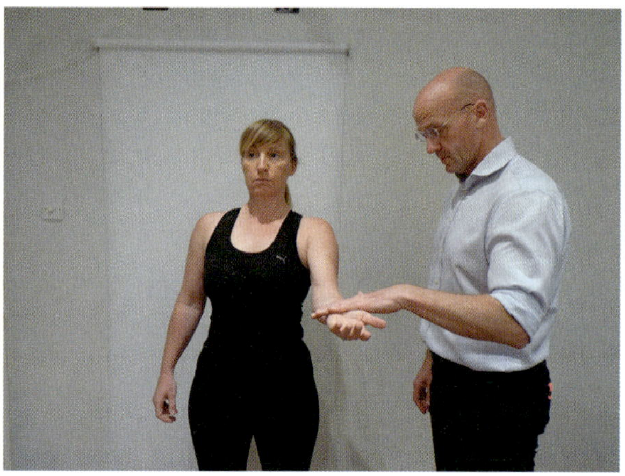

Fig. 10.7 Speed's Test.

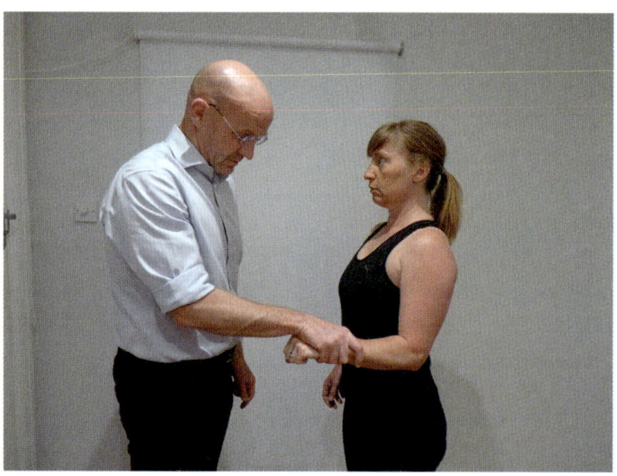

Fig. 10.8 Yergason's Test.

outstretched arm, or repeated overload of the long head of biceps, for example, in overhead athletes. Symptoms include clunking within the shoulder joint, with associated pain and loss of function, particularly in overhead positions (Powell et al., 2004). There is controversy in the literature regarding the clinical relevance of labral tears as there is a high incidence of superior labral tears in asymptomatic patients (Schwartzberg et al., 2016). Some of the common tests for SLAP lesions include:

Biceps Load Tests I and II (*Fig. 10.9*)

Biceps load test I: in 90 degrees of abduction, with the patient's elbow in 90 degrees flexion and the forearm supinated, the clinician resists elbow flexion. Pain reproduction indicates a positive test for a SLAP lesion. Improvement in pain or apprehension indicates the absence of a SLAP lesion.

- Biceps load test II is the same as test I, performed at 120 degrees of abduction. The choice of test should be guided by the range of abduction that is most provocative for the patient. Kim et al. (2001) found specificity to be 96.9% and sensitivity to be 89.7%.

Active Compression Test (O'Brien et al., 1998) (*Fig. 10.10*)

With the patient in standing, the shoulder flexed to 90 degrees, with 10–15 degrees of adduction, and medial rotation so the thumb is pointing down and the elbow in full extension. The clinician applies a downward force which the patient resists. The forearm is then supinated and the force reapplied. A positive test is

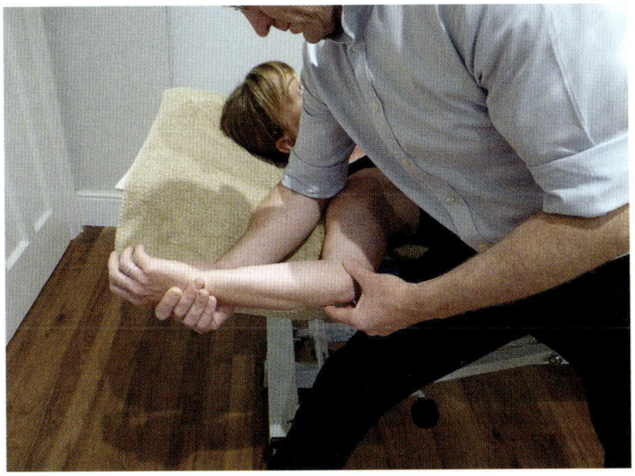

Fig. 10.9 Biceps Load Test I.

confirmed with pain and/or clicking inside the shoulder on the first part of the test, which diminishes or is relieved after the supination is applied. Schlechter et al. (2009) found that a combination of passive distraction and active compression tests resulted in a sensitivity of 70% and specificity of 90%.

Rotator Cuff—Related Shoulder Pain

The term 'rotator cuff—related shoulder pain' (RCRSP) was introduced by Lewis (2016) as an umbrella term to include conditions previously referred to as rotator cuff tendinopathy, subacromial bursitis, partial or full-thickness rotator cuff tendon tears, shoulder impingement and subacromial pain syndrome. When other causes are considered unlikely, RCRSP typically involves the experience of pain and movement impairment during elevation and external rotation (Lewis, 2016). Patients have largely full range of shoulder movement and describe pain on activities involving arm elevation and particularly under load. They may present with a painful arc of movement through elevation, particularly abduction. The term RCRSP has replaced several other terms that attempted to capture this subgroup of patients, including shoulder impingement syndrome (SIS) and sub-acromial pain syndrome (SAPS). The term SIS has lost favour following emerging evidence that it does not capture many potential mechanisms for the generation of shoulder pain and that it may induce a fear of movement due to the belief that the pain results from the impingement of soft tissue structures. The term SAPS suggests that these patients are experiencing pain solely from the sub-acromial structures, excluding possible sources from the labrum, biceps complex or glenohumeral joint. Other labels such as 'shoulder pain of unknown aetiology', are so nonspecific that they fail to achieve the goal of a label, which is to classify patients to guide treatment selection, define patients for interventional studies and to aid communication between health care professionals (Cools & Mitchener, 2017).

The terminology has been debated for many years, and it is unlikely that one label will satisfy everyone all the time (Cools & Mitchener, 2017). The mechanisms of pain generation are likely to be multifaceted and complex; they are likely to involve many biological, psychological, and social factors. No single term can capture the individual experience of each condition.

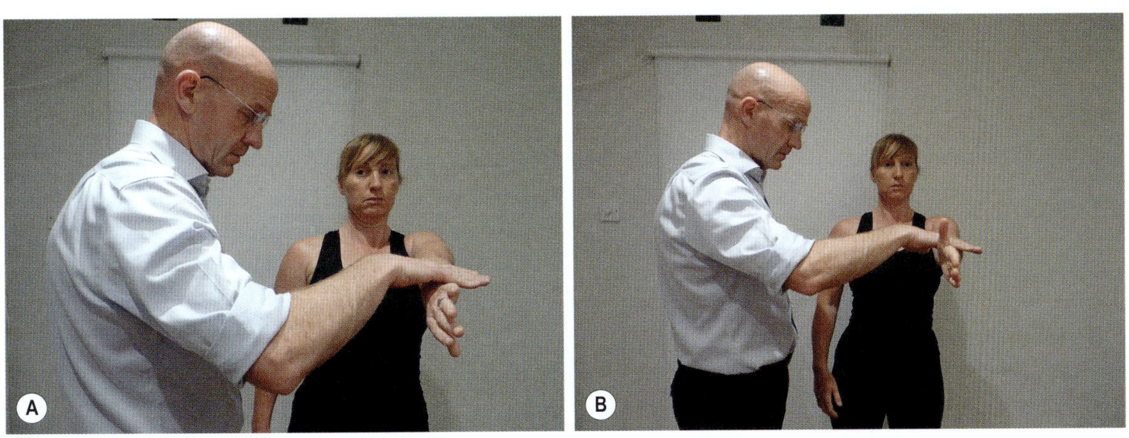

Fig. 10.10 (A and B) Active compression test.

The term RCRSP, however, is intended to communicate the concept that in many cases there is no definitive way of diagnosing a specific structure of the shoulder as definitively responsible for a patient's symptoms.

Two tests commonly used as pain provocation tests in the assessment of RCRSP are:

1. *Neer test (1983) (Fig. 10.11).* This can be performed with the patient in standing or sitting. The clinician elevates the internally rotated shoulder whilst stabilizing the scapula. Reproduction of pain is positive for this test.
2. *Hawkins–Kennedy (Hawkins & Bokor, 1990) (Fig. 10.12).* The patient is examined with 90 degrees of shoulder flexion and 90 degrees of elbow flexion. The shoulder is then internally rotated to the end range; further abduction/adduction of the shoulder can be added if the test is negative. Reproduction of pain is positive for this test.

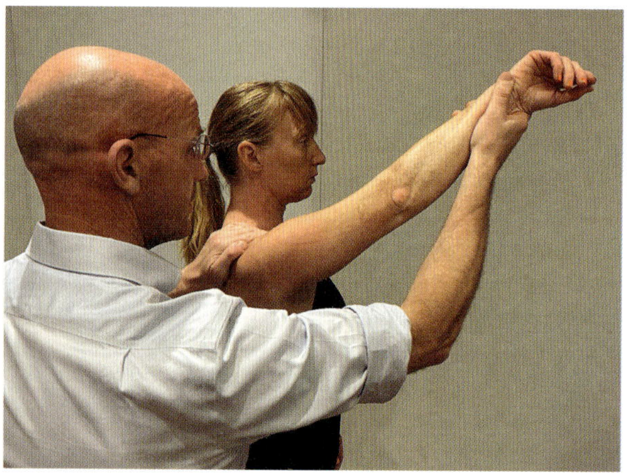

Fig. 10.11 Neer Test.

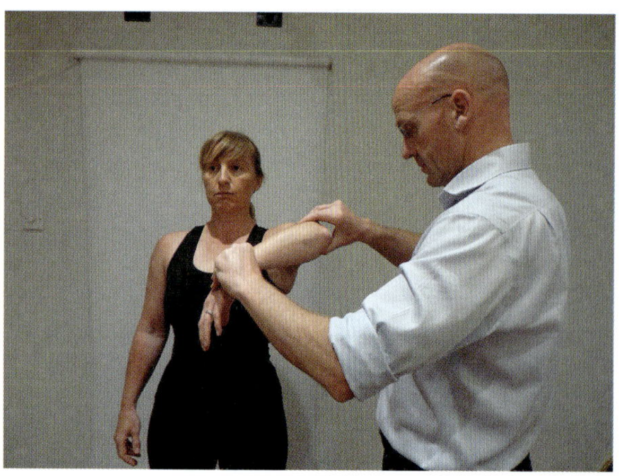

Fig. 10.12 Hawkins–Kennedy Test.

The Stiff Shoulder

Cyriax (1982) described the 'capsular pattern' of the glenohumeral joint as a limitation of lateral rotation, abduction and medial rotation. Historically the term 'capsular pattern' was used to describe conditions relating to pathology of the capsule (frozen shoulder), stiffness following immobilization and osteoarthritis of the glenohumeral joint. However, osteoarthritis is a multi-tissue pathology involving bony and soft tissue structures; for this reason, a better term to describe conditions which result in multi-directional stiffness of the glenohumeral joint is a 'stiff shoulder'. Conditions that present with multi-directional stiffness include the frozen shoulder, osteoarthritis of the glenohumeral joint, osteochondromatosis and, on very rare occasions, neoplasm. The frozen shoulder is a common condition that presents as shoulder pain and stiffness. The clinical cluster for identification of the frozen shoulder includes:

- Onset around the age of 50 years
- Active and passive movements equally restricted
- Significant loss of external rotation with power largely preserved
- X-ray imaging normal (Lewis, 2015)

External rotation in a position of 90 degrees abduction can be used to identify joint restriction, especially in the early stages, with comparisons being made with the asymptomatic shoulder. If it is difficult to assess in this position due to pain, external rotation may be assessed in standing. The use of a measuring tape from the umbilicus to the styloid process with elbows maintained at 90 degrees may ensure accurate measures of external rotation (Valentine & Lewis, 2006). X-ray imaging is not essential to diagnose a frozen shoulder; however, the advantage of x-ray imaging is to exclude other conditions that present with stiffness such as osteoarthritis, osteonecrosis, locked dislocation, osteosarcoma or osteochondromatosis. A more thorough description of the aetiology, diagnosis and management can be found in Lewis (2015).

Glenohumeral Joint Instability

Glenohumeral joint instability is a common but complex condition. Shoulder instability can occur following trauma such as dislocation (traumatic instability) or in the absence of injury (atraumatic instability).

There are several classification systems for shoulder instability (Bateman et al., 2018). One of the most popular systems is the Stanmore Triangle (Fig. 10.13) (Lewis et al., 2004), which recognizes the complexity of shoulder instability and how several causal mechanisms can be at work within the same presentation. The characteristics of the polar groups are described in Fig. 10.13. Polar type I relates to traumatic structural conditions with a predominance of structural pathology that is more likely to require surgical repair, whereas types II and III relate to common components of laxity without trauma with type II only involving components of structural pathology. The triangle allows for individuals to be considered in relation to the most predominant features of the condition, e.g. they may have had a traumatic dislocation (polar type I) but also have a muscle patterning dysfunction (polar type III). See Bateman et al. (2018) for a more thorough review of atraumatic shoulder instability.

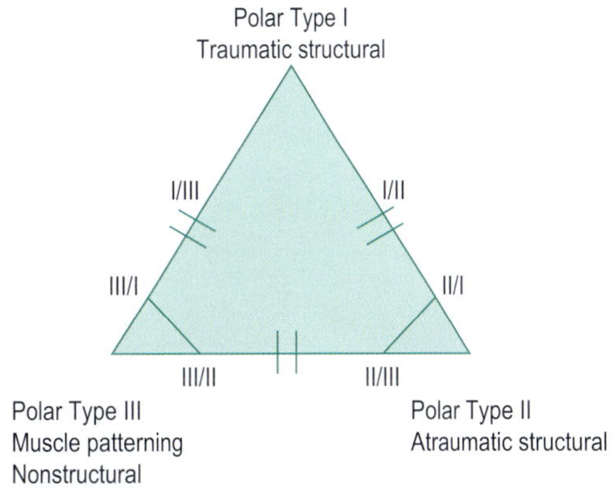

Fig. 10.13 Stanmore Triangle. (Modified from Lewis et al. 2004)

There is an important distinction between laxity and instability. Laxity is asymptomatic excessive movement in a joint with no pain and full function. Instability is a symptomatic excessive movement that may manifest as dislocation, subluxation, pain and loss of function. Laxity can be assessed in the physical examination using tests like the 'load and shift' test or the 'sulcus sign' (Figs. 10.14 and 10.15). These tests require the clinician to make a subjective judgment on what is normal or excessive. Instability provocation tests such as the 'apprehension' or 'posterior drawer' evaluate the patient's sense of apprehension relating to fear of dislocation (Figs. 10.16 and 10.17) and are therefore assessing patients' experience as opposed to just the clinician's perception in the laxity tests.

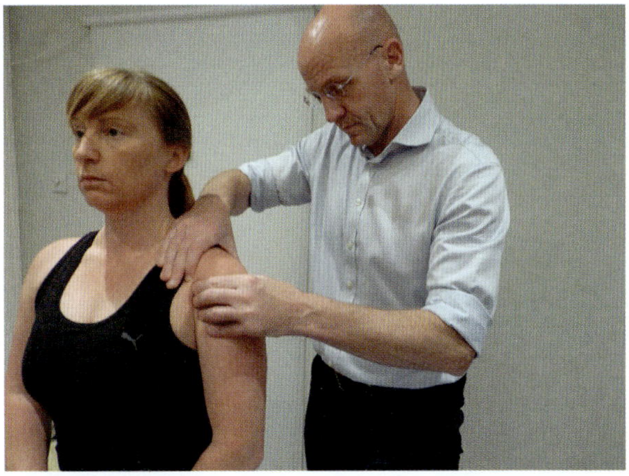

Fig. 10.14 Load and Shift Test.

Load and shift test (Fig. 10.14). With the patient in sitting or supine, the clinician stabilizes the scapula and applies a posteroanterior force to the humeral head whilst palpating the joint line to assess the amount of movement. This test can be graded from 0 to 3, with 0 being no movement and 3 being full dislocation. This can also be used as a test for posterior instability with the direction of force applied in a posterior direction. The test has been found to have a specificity of 100% and a sensitivity of 50% (Tzannes & Murrell, 2002).

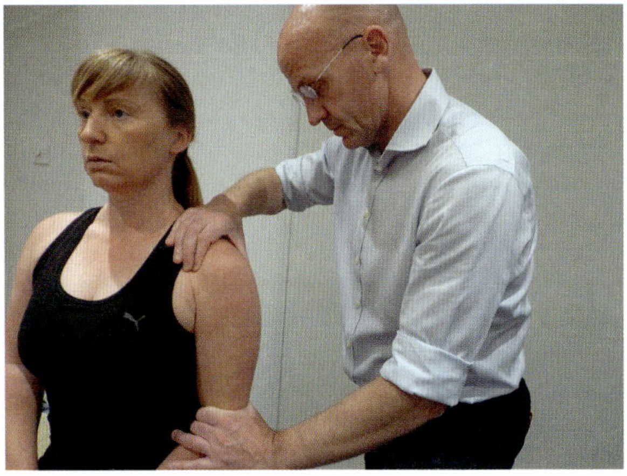

Fig. 10.15 Sulcus Sign.

Sulcus sign (Matsen et al., 1990) (Fig. 10.15). The clinician applies a longitudinal caudad force to the

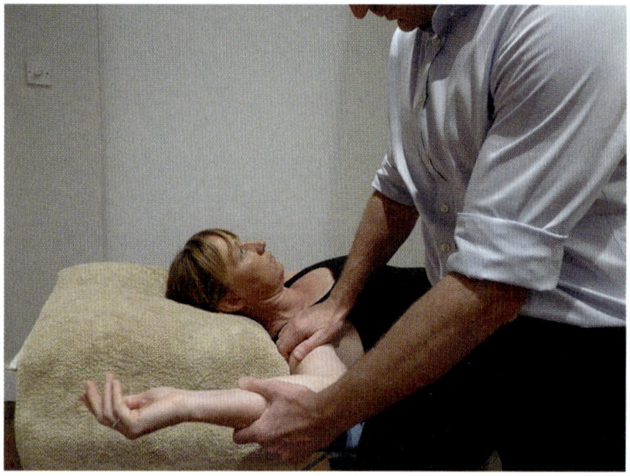

Fig. 10.16 Apprehension/Relocation Test.

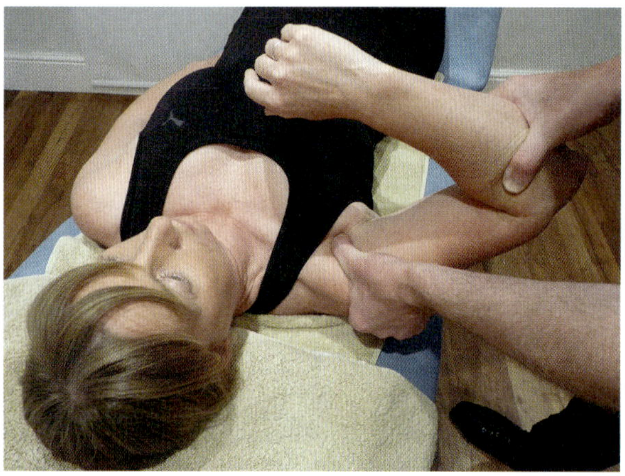

Fig. 10.17 Posterior Drawer Test.

humerus with the patient sitting and the arm relaxed in the lap to ensure the biceps muscle is not contracted. A positive test is indicated if a sulcus appears distal to the acromion, suggesting inferior instability of the shoulder. The glenohumeral joint can then be externally rotated and the test repeated. This manoeuvre causes a tightening of the middle glenohumeral ligament (Terry et al., 1991) and therefore may limit translation of the humeral head. Therefore if the test remains positive, a suspected greater amount of instability may be apparent, whereas a negative test upon application of the external rotation suggests a localized superior glenohumeral ligament or coracohumeral ligament dysfunction. The specificity of this test has been found to be 72%, and the sensitivity 85% for positive tests greater than 1 cm (Tzannes & Murrell, 2002).

Apprehension test (Fig. 10.16). With the patient supine, the clinician takes the shoulder into 90 degrees abduction and adds lateral rotation. The test is considered positive—indicating anterior instability—if the patient becomes apprehensive. Further confirmation can be achieved by using the relocation test (Jobe et al., 1989), where an anteroposterior force is applied to the head of the humerus (using the heel of the hand); apprehension is lessened, and the clinician is able to take the shoulder further into lateral rotation. It has been proposed by Lo et al. (2004) that an additional component can be added to the test—a quick release of the posteriorly directed force. This so-called surprise test, taken with the findings of the apprehension and relocation test, has been shown to have a positive predictive value of 93.6% and a negative predictive value of 71.9% (Lo et al., 2004) but will only be safe to use in a very limited number of cases. All three tests have been shown to have strong specificity. Overall, the apprehension test has the strongest diagnostic odds ratio (53.6), suggesting a good strength of association between the test and the condition (Hegedus et al., 2012).

Posterior drawer test (Fig. 10.17). With the patient lying in a supine position, the shoulder in 80–120 degrees of abduction and 20–30 degrees of flexion, the clinician controls the forearm close to the elbow whilst rotating the upper arm medially and flexing it to about 90 degrees. With the other hand, the clinician applies an AP glide to the head of the humerus feeling the amount of humeral translation. The test is often pain-free but may be associated with a degree of apprehension.

Muscle Tests

Muscle Control

Muscle control is of particular interest in the shoulder in relation to scapular function. The role of the scapula is to provide a stable base for the glenohumeral joint and to orientate the glenoid in the optimal position for glenohumeral joint function. The lack of bony articulation in the scapulothoracic region means the scapula is very mobile and reliant on well-coordinated muscle activity to control its position and function. The coordinated motion between the scapula and humerus is called scapulohumeral rhythm (McClure et al., 2009).

Scapular motion that deviates from what is considered normal is called scapular dyskinesis (Kibler et al., 2013), where 'dys' means 'alteration of' and 'kinesis' means 'motion'. In the literature, scapular dyskinesis has been linked with many types of shoulder pathology (McClure et al., 2006), although it is often unclear if dyskinesis is the cause or the result of pain and pathology in the shoulder.

The dyskinesis may result from pathology, as in the case of acromioclavicular joint strain or long thoracic nerve injury, or the presence of dyskinesis may be a causative factor in the development of pain; it is also possible that scapular dyskinesis is caused by pain. Again, it is important to consider the direction of causation.

Scapular dyskinesis is a general term and does not identify the cause of abnormal movement. Also, in order to understand what 'abnormal' movement means it is important to understand what is 'normal'. The scapula is very mobile and moves in complex three-dimensional planes, making a reliable evaluation of the nature of its movement difficult. McClure et al. (2009) describe a method of identifying scapular dyskinesis that appears to demonstrate good reliability and validity. This method involves the observation and identification of:

- winging of the inferior scapular border
- winging of the medial scapular border
- lack of smooth scapular movement during arm elevation (specifically, early elevation of the scapula during arm elevation)-or a sudden downward rotation during arm lowering.

Burn et al. (2016) identified a high prevalence of scapular dyskinesis in an asymptomatic general population with a higher prevalence in overhead athletes. In addition, scapular kinematics often do not change as pain and function improve (Clausen et al., 2018). As a result 'the exact role of the dyskinesis in creating or exacerbating shoulder dysfunction is not clearly defined' (Kibler et al., 2013), raising questions regarding the spectrum of scapular patterning that may actually be normal. Following a systematic review, Ratcliffe et al. (2014) were not able to identify a typical pattern of scapular dyskinesis in patients with RCRSP and suggested this may be due to the complex multifactorial nature of the condition; with further research, subgroups may emerge.

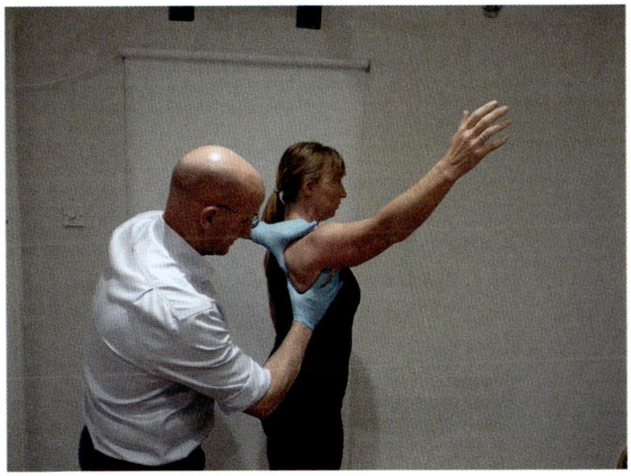

Fig. 10.18 Scapular Assistance Test.

The current recommendation is to observe and identify scapular dyskinesis and then evaluate the effect of manual correction on symptoms. In the *scapular assistance test* (Seitz et al., 2012) (Fig 10.18) the clinician assists the scapula into upwards rotation and posterior tilt as the patient elevates the arm, and the clinician evaluates the effect on the symptomatic movement (Fig. 10.19). Alternatively, using the SSMP, the clinician repositions the scapula in a new starting position, and the symptomatic movement is repeated to see if the modification improves the pain. The clinician can try protraction, retraction, elevation or depression, or any combination (Lewis, 2016) (Fig. 10.2D). If correction reduces symptoms, then it may be relevant to the presentation and intervention incorporated into the treatment strategy.

Muscle Strength

The clinician may choose to test the shoulder girdle elevators, depressors, protractors and retractors as well as the shoulder joint flexors, extensors, abductors, adductors, medial rotators and lateral rotators isometrically, through the range, or in positions of functional restriction. The clinician must consider the reason for muscle weakness if identified on examination. Possible causes include deconditioning, pain inhibition, structural pathology (e.g. massive rotator cuff tears), or peripheral nerve entrapment (e.g. suprascapular nerve). For details of these general muscle tests, readers are directed to Hislop et al. (2013) and Kendall et al. (2005).

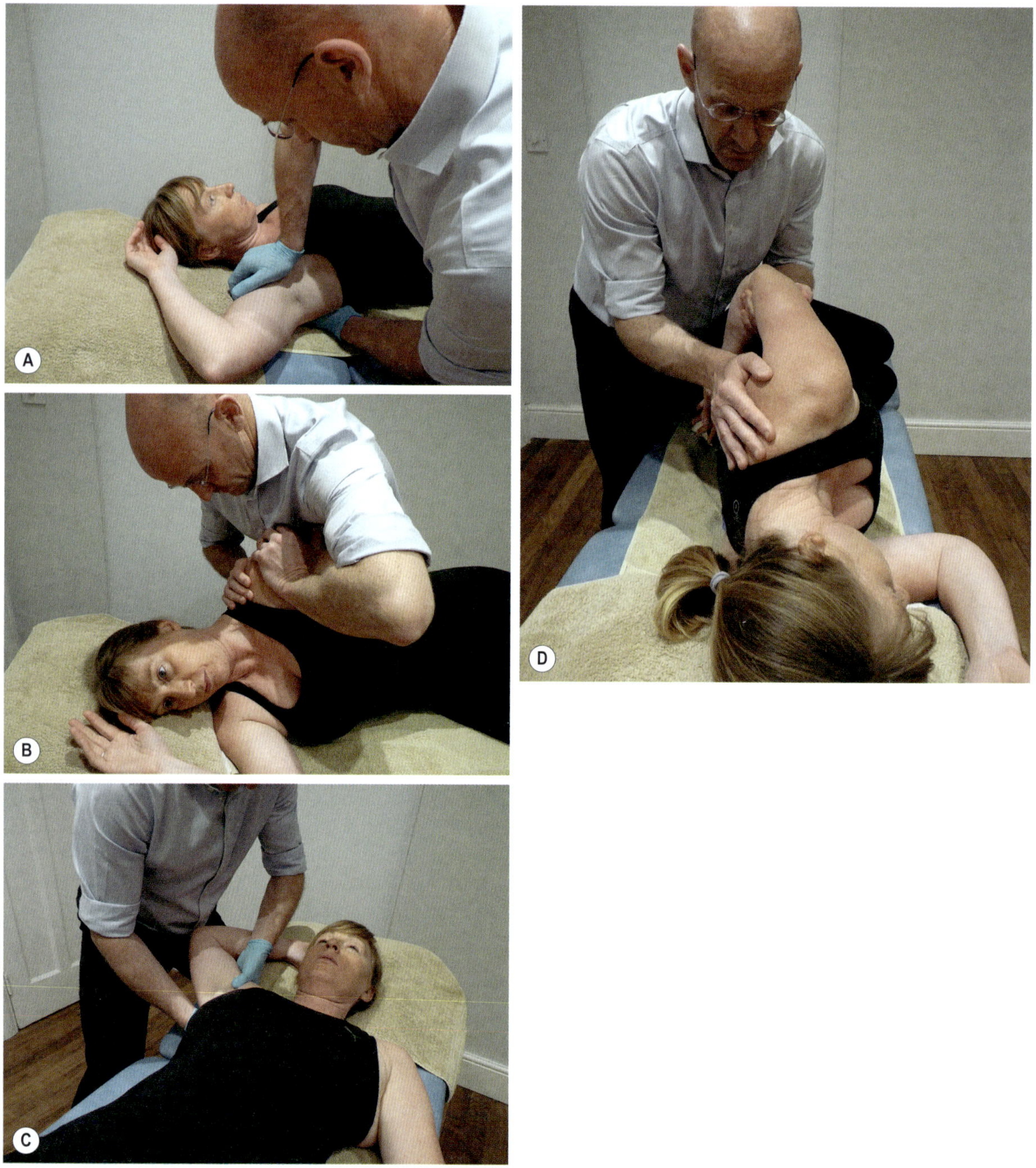

Fig. 10.19 Accessory Movements. (A) Anteroposterior glenohumeral joint in abduction/external rotation: support the patient's scapula with one hand and apply an anteroposterior force through the head of the humerus with the other hand. (B) Anteroposterior glenohumeral joint in side-lying, hand behind back position. (C) Longitudinal caudad in abduction/external rotation: support the patient's scapula with one hand and apply a force towards the patient's feet, pushing through the humeral head. (D) Longitudinal cephalad scapula with hand behind back. These techniques can be applied in different ranges of movement depending on the patient's presentation.

Neurological Examination

Neurological examination includes neurological integrity testing and neurodynamic tests. These are not routinely examined and are only indicated if the patient complains of neurological symptoms or has pain in a distribution that may indicate neurological involvement. Readers are referred to Chapter 4 for neural integrity testing of the upper limb.

Neurodynamic Tests

The upper-limb neurodynamic tests (ULNTs) may be carried out in order to ascertain the degree to which neural tissue is responsible for producing the patient's symptoms. The choice of tests should be influenced by the distribution of the patient's symptoms, e.g. if the patient has posterior upper arm and lateral elbow pain, then ULNTs with a radial nerve bias may be indicated. These tests are described in detail in Chapter 4.

Nerves may also be palpated to determine the presence of mechanosensitivity. Palpable nerves in the upper limb include:

- The suprascapular nerve, which can be palpated along the superior border of the scapula at the suprascapular notch.
- The dorsal scapular nerve, which can be palpated medial to the medial border of the scapula.
- The brachial plexus, which can be palpated in the posterior triangle of the neck; it emerges at the lower third of the sternocleidomastoid.
- The median nerve, which can be palpated over the anterior elbow joint crease, medial to the biceps tendon, and also at the wrist between palmaris longus and flexor carpi radialis.
- The radial nerve, which can be palpated around the spiral groove of the humerus, between the brachioradialis and flexor carpi radialis in the forearm, and also at the wrist in the snuffbox.

Vascular Assessment

Typically, upper limb vascular disease is less common than lower limb pathology; however, it is important to consider pathology of vascular tissues as a differential diagnosis in the upper limb. Vascular tissues can be responsible for symptoms or pain or discomfort in the arms as well as symptoms of tightness, heaviness, cramping, or weakness. Chapter 8 of *Petty's Principles of MSK Treat & Management*, 4th ed., 'Considering Vascular Tissue' provides a thorough overview of vascular considerations in the musculoskeletal context.

One specific consideration in relation to the shoulder is TOS. TOS constitutes a group of conditions of the upper limb that result in compression of the neurovascular bundle exiting the thoracic outlet. TOS classifications are based on the tissue believed to be responsible for individual symptoms: neurogenic (nTOS), venous (vTOS), and arterial (aTOS). It is believed that neurogenic TOS accounts for over 90% of the cases. Historically, TOS presents with symptom onset between the ages of 20–50 years old and is more prevalent in women (Jones et al., 2019).

Symptoms can range from mild pain and sensory changes to serious vascular or neurogenic symptoms. Patients may present with pain in the neck, face or chest, with pain in the shoulder and upper extremity common. Other symptoms may include altered or absent sensation, weakness, fatigue, or a feeling of heaviness in the arm and hand. Changes in the colouration of the skin or temperature changes may also be present.

The physical examination for the assessment of TOS is described in detail in Jones et al. (2019) and Watson et al. (2009) and may include special tests that are designed to challenge the potential sources of neurovascular compression in the neck and shoulder. These tests or provocative manoeuvres may generate false positive results in asymptomatic participants, and it is important to interpret the results in the context of the whole presentation (Young & Hardy, 1983; Swift & Nichols, 1984). The use of multiple tests in conjunction with other findings may increase diagnostic specificity. A study by Gillard et al. (2001) demonstrated that by combining the Adson and Roos tests, the specificity was increased from 76% and 30% respectively, when used alone, to 82% when both were positive.

Elevated Arm Stress Test (EAST) or Roos Test

Arms are placed in the surrender position with shoulders abducted to 90 degrees, shoulder external rotation, and elbows flexed to 90 degrees. The patient slowly opens and closes both hands for 3 minutes. A positive test is one that reproduces pain, paresthesia, heaviness or weakness.

Adson's Manoeuvre

In sitting, the patient's head is rotated towards the tested arm (Magee, 2014). The patient then extends the head while the clinician extends and laterally rotates the shoulder. The patient then takes a deep breath, and the disappearance of the radial pulse indicates a positive test.

Palpation of Pulses

The brachial pulse may be palpated on the medial aspect of the humerus in the axilla. The radial artery may be palpated medial to the radius just proximal to the wrist.

Palpation

The shoulder region may be palpated in order to identify areas with increased sensitivity to pressure. Palpatory findings are particularly useful for the identification of acromioclavicular joint pain, which is normally tender over the joint line when symptomatic. In addition, the long head of the biceps can be palpated in the bicipital groove, as can the entire clavicle, and the coracoid process where the short head of the biceps attaches. Tenderness can sometimes be identified in individuals with RCRSP distal to the anterior acromion. Tenderness can sometimes be found in individuals with SLAP lesions distal to the posterior aspect of the acromion. A more thorough description of the palpatory examination can be found in Chapter 4.

Accessory Movements

Glenohumeral, acromioclavicular and sternoclavicular joint accessory movements should be tested in provocative positions/ranges when the patient is nonsevere and nonirritable, as this is most likely to reproduce symptoms and guide treatment. Some accessory movements to the glenohumeral joint are shown in Fig. 10.19. The neutral position can be useful in severe and irritable patients or as an initial testing procedure to familiarize the patient with handling techniques.

It may be necessary to examine other regions to determine their relevance to the patient's symptoms. The most likely regions influencing the shoulder are the cervical spine, thoracic spine, sternoclavicular joint, elbow, wrist and hand. The joints within these regions can be tested fully or partially with the use of screening tests (see Chapter 4 for further details).

COMPLETION OF THE EXAMINATION

When the examination of the shoulder region is complete, the subjective and physical findings must be assimilated into a treatment plan that is generated collaboratively with the patient. Making sense of the examination findings is discussed in depth in Chapter 5. For guidance on treatment and management principles, the reader is directed to the companion textbook (Barnard & Ryder, 2024).

KNOWLEDGE CHECK

1. How would you apply the SSMPs described above to the functional movement of 'pouring a kettle'?
2. Describe the clinical cluster that can be used in the diagnosis of the frozen shoulder.
3. What clinical tests might be used in the assessment of shoulder instability?

REVIEW AND REVISE QUESTIONS

1. What are the main issues relating to the 'pathoanatomical' diagnosis of shoulder pain?
2. What features might you expect to see in the clinical examination of a patient with RCRSP?
3. Where might an individual describe pain relating to RCRSP?
4. What diagnosis might you be considering if you have chosen to use Yergason's test?
5. What are the three 'polar' types of shoulder instability described in the Stanmore triangle?
6. Describe three patterns of scapular dyskinesis often described in the literature.
7. What muscles contribute to lateral rotation of the scapular.
8. What tests might be useful in exploring a diagnosis of rotator cuff tendinopathy in the clinical examination?
9. When a 'stiff shoulder' has been identified on clinical examination what possible diagnoses should you consider?
10. What tests might you use to assess a suspected presentation of thoracic outlet syndrome?

Case Study

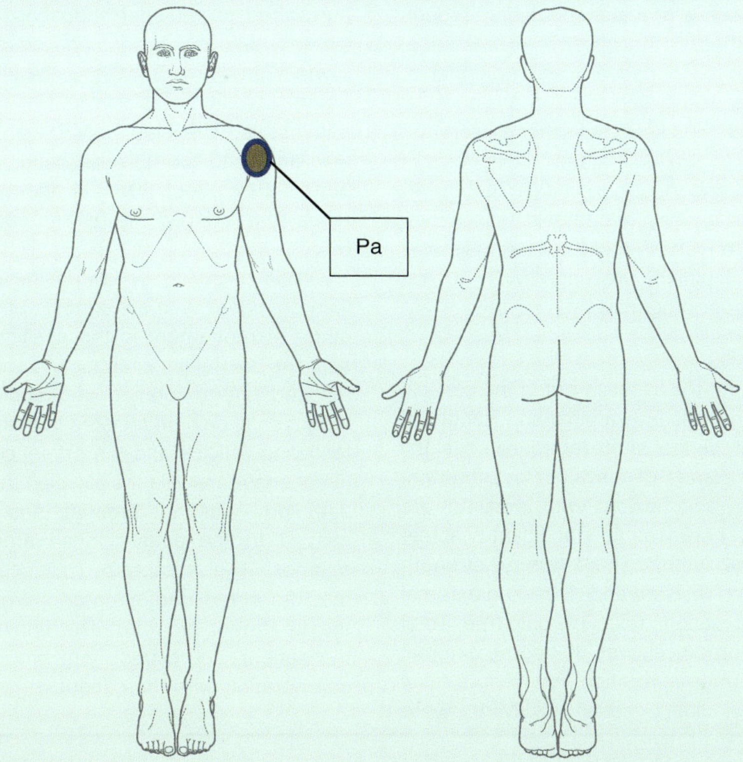

36-year-old man

Pa—intermittent aching pain with occasional catching pain.

Aggravating factors—working overhead, reaching movements. Sore by the end of the day. Unable to lie on it.

Easing factors—relative rest and avoiding aggravating factors.

24-h pattern—Sleep broken intermittently when changing position in bed at night. Unable to lie on it without being woken. Eases off by the morning and builds over the course of a working day.

PMH/DH—Fit and well. Long-standing pain in the right knee; these symptoms are stable and not causing any disability at present.

Subjective

A 36-year-old man with a 6-month history of right-sided shoulder pain, with a gradual increase in symptom severity, presented to physiotherapy. He described an insidious onset of pain located in the anterior shoulder in the region of the anterior deltoid. There was no history of trauma preceding the onset or historically. He worked as an engineer and spent a considerable amount of time working overhead, often under load in awkward positions. He described aggravating factors including elevation in all planes but worse in abduction and worse when under load and reaching and expressed concerns that his 'rotary cuff' was torn. He was able to perform all activities at work but his shoulder was often sore by the end of the day. He was able to sleep undisturbed if he avoided lying on it. He was generally pain-free at rest and at night. Over the weekend his shoulder settled, and the pain built again over the working week. He described a diurnal pattern of feeling less sore first thing in the morning with pain increasing over the working day. His past medical history was unremarkable, and he reported being otherwise fit and well.

Clinical reasoning following the subjective—The clinician was reassured that he had no pain at rest or at night, that he felt well in himself with no significant medical history and that his symptoms were nonsevere. His symptoms were mechanical and consistent in location and behaviour with a local shoulder condition. No serious pathology was suspected at this stage. The absence of recent or historical trauma to the shoulder, or a history of hypermobility, suggested that instability was unlikely. He described no

Case Study—cont'd

limitation of range suggestive of a stiff shoulder, although this needed to be clarified in the physical examination. Pain was considered to be nonsevere and nonirritable, but, again, this would be monitored through the physical examination. The clinician was keen to further explore the patient's beliefs relating to a pathoanatomical diagnosis of rotator cuff pathology during the physical examination. At this time the clinician's primary hypothesis was a presentation consistent with RCRSP, and the prognosis was considered good, as the patient presented with no dispositions predictive of poor prognosis.

Physical

There was no indication for the assessment of the cervical or thoracic spine in the initial examination. Range of movement assessment of the shoulder revealed a full range of movement in planes of elevation but through-range pain in abduction and flexion, with a painful arc from 80–120 degrees. There was no significant scapular dyskinesis in flexion or abduction. There was full strength but pain was provoked on resisted abduction and external rotation, with all other directions relatively pain-free. Total rotation motion was symmetrical, with 90-degree external rotation and 60-degree internal rotation, revealing a fairly standard range of shoulder motion. SSMPs were performed to shoulder abduction, as this was the most symptomatic movement and described as the patient's biggest problem. SSMPs were also applied to resisted external rotation as symptoms were nonsevere and nonirritable. The only SSMP that influenced symptoms was an AP to the humeral head, which reduced pain of both *'s by about 80%. In addition, the scapular assistance test reduced the pain through abduction by about 50%.

Clinical reasoning following the physical—The clinician was confident with a diagnosis of RCRSP due to the full range of movement in the position of 90-degree abduction, the painful arc in abduction and the pain provoked by resisted lateral rotation and abduction. The significant reduction in pain on resisted lateral rotation and abduction following SSMPs and the presence of full power in both directions reassured the clinician that significant structural pathology was not present, and this information was relayed to the patient in an empathic and reassuring manner. The symptom modification procedures that resulted in reduced symptoms were then integrated into the treatment program. The findings were explained to the patient, and a treatment program was developed in collaboration with the patient.

REFERENCES

Anjum, R., Mumford, S., 2018. Causation in Science and the Methods of Scientific Discovery. Oxford University Press.

Barnard, K., Ryder, D., 2024. Petty's Principles of Musculoskeletal Treatment and Management: A Handbook for Therapists, fourth ed. Elsevier, Edinburgh.

Barreto, R.P., Braman, J.P., Ludewig, P.M., Ribeiro, L.P., Camargo, P.R., 2019. Bilateral magnetic resonance imaging findings in individuals with unilateral shoulder pain. J. Shoulder Elbow Surg. 28 (9), 1699–1706. https://doi.org/10.1016/j.jse.2019.04.001.

Bateman, M., Jaiswal, A., Tambe, A.A., 2018. Diagnosis and management of atraumatic shoulder instability. J. Arthrosc. Joint Surg. 5 (2), 79–85. https://doi.org/10.1016/j.jajs.2018.05.009.

Bélanger, V., Dupuis, F., Leblond, J., Roy, J.S., 2019. Accuracy of examination of the long head of the biceps tendon in the clinical setting: a systematic review. J. Rehabil. Med. 51 (7), 479–491. https://doi.org/10.2340/16501977-2563.

Boettcher, C.E., Ginn, K.A., Cathers, I., 2009. The 'empty can' and 'full can' tests do not selectively activate supraspinatus. J. Sci. Med. Sport 12, 435–439.

Borstad, J.D., Dashottar, A.B., 2011. Quantifying strain on posterior shoulder tissues during 5 simulated clinical tests: a cadaver study. J. Orthop. Sports Phys. Ther. 41, 90–99.

Burn, M.B., McCulloch, P.C., Lintner, D.M., Liberman, S.R., Harris, J.D., 2016. Prevalence of scapular dyskinesis in overhead and nonoverhead athletes: a systematic review. Orthop. J. Sports Med. 4 (2). https://doi.org/10.1177/2325967115627608, 2325967115627608.

Castoldi, F., Blonna, D., Hertel, R., 2009. External rotation lag sign revisited: accuracy for diagnosis of full thickness supraspinatus tear. J. Shoulder Elbow Surg. 18, 529–534.

Chester, R., Jerosch-Herold, C., Lewis, J., Shepstone, L., 2018. Psychological factors are associated with the outcome of physiotherapy for people with shoulder pain: a multicentre longitudinal cohort study. Br. J. Sports Med. 52 (4), 269–275. https://doi.org/10.1136/bjsports-2016-096084.

Chester, R., Shepstone, L., Daniell, H., Sweeting, D., Lewis, J., Jerosch-Herold, C., 2013. Predicting response to physiotherapy treatment for musculoskeletal shoulder pain: a systematic review. BMC Musculoskelet. Disord. 14, 203.

Clausen, M.B., Bandholm, T., Rathleff, M.S., Christensen, K.B., Zebis, M.K., Graven-Nielsen, T., et al., 2018. The strengthening exercises in shoulder impingement trial (The SExSI-trial) investigating the effectiveness of a simple add-on shoulder strengthening exercise programme in patients with long-lasting subacromial impingement syndrome: study protocol for a pragmatic, assessor blinded, parallel-group, randomised, controlled trial. Trials 19 (1), 154. https://doi.org/10.1186/s13063-018-2509-7.

Cools, A.M., Michener, L.A., 2017. Shoulder pain: can one label satisfy everyone and everything? Br. J. Sports Med. 51 (5), 416–417. https://doi.org/10.1136/bjsports-2016-096772.

Cyriax, J., 1982. Textbook of Orthopaedic Medicine—Diagnosis of Soft Tissue Lesions, eighth ed. Baillière Tindall, London.

Dashottar, A., Borstad, J.D., 2012. Posterior glenohumeral joint capsule contracture. Shoulder Elbow 4, 230–236.

Dunn, W.R., Kuhn, J.E., Sanders, R., An, Q., Baumgarten, K.M., Bishop, J.Y., et al., 2014. Symptoms of pain do not correlate with rotator cuff tear severity: a cross-sectional study of 393 patients with a symptomatic atraumatic full-thickness rotator cuff tear. J. Bone Joint Surg. 96, 793–800.

Gillard, J., Pérez-Cousin, M., Hachulla, E., Remy, J., Hurtevent, J.F., Vinckier, L., et al., 2001. Diagnosing thoracic outlet syndrome: contribution of provocative tests, ultrasonography, electrophysiology, and helical computed tomography in 48 patients. Joint Bone Spine 68 (5), 416–424. https://doi.org/10.1016/s1297-319x(01)00298-6.

Hall, K., Borstad, J.D., 2018. Posterior shoulder tightness: to treat or not to treat? J. Orthop. Sports Phys. Ther. 48 (3), 133–136. https://doi.org/10.2519/jospt.2018.0605.

Hall, K., Lewis, J., Moore, A., Ridehalgh, C., 2020. Posterior shoulder tightness; an intersession reliability study of 3 clinical tests. Arch. Physiother. 10, 14. https://doi.org/10.1186/s40945-020-00084-w.

Hawkins, R.J., Bokor, D.J., 1990. Clinical evaluation of shoulder problems. In: Rockwood, C.A., Matsen, F.A. (Eds.), The Shoulder. W.B. Saunders, Philadelphia, p. 149.

Hegedus, E.J., Cook, C., Lewis, J., Wright, A., Park, J.Y., 2015. Combining orthopedic special tests to improve diagnosis of shoulder pathology. Phys. Ther. Sport 16 (2), 87–92. https://doi.org/10.1016/j.ptsp.2014.08.001.

Hegedus, E.J., Goode, A.P., Cook, C.E., Michener, L., Myer, C.A., Myer, D.M., et al., 2012. Which physical examination tests provide clinicians with the most value when examining the shoulder? Update of a systematic review with meta-analysis of individual tests. Br. J. Sports Med. 46, 964–978.

Hertel, R., Ballmer, F.T., Lombert, S.M., Gerber, C., 1996. Lag signs in the diagnosis of rotator cuff rupture. J. Shoulder Elbow Surg 5, 307–313.

Hislop, H., Avers, D., Brown, M., 2013. Daniels and Worthingham's Muscle Testing, Techniques of Manual Examination, ninth ed. Elsevier Saunders, St Louis.

Holtby, R., Razmjou, H., 2004. Accuracy of the Speed's and Yergason's tests in detecting biceps pathology and SLAP lesions: comparison with arthroscopic findings. Arthroscopy 20, 231–236.

Itoi, E., Kido, T., Sano, A., Urayama, M., Sato, K., 1999. Which is more useful, the 'full can test' or the 'empty can test', in detecting the torn supraspinatus tendon? Am. J. Sports Med. 27, 65–68.

Jobe, F.W., Kvitne, R.S., Giangarra, C.E., 1989. Shoulder pain in the overhand or throwing athlete. The relationship of anterior instability and rotator cuff impingement. Orthop. Rev. 18, 963–975.

Jobe, F.W., Moynes, D.R., 1982. Delineation of diagnostic criteria and a rehabilitation program for rotator cuff injuries. Am. J. Sports Med. 10, 336–339.

Jones, M.R., Prabhakar, A., Viswanath, O., Urits, I., Green, J.B., Kendrick, J.B., et al., 2019. Thoracic outlet syndrome: a comprehensive review of pathophysiology, diagnosis, and treatment. Pain Ther 8 (1), 5–18. https://doi.org/10.1007/s40122-019-0124-2.

Kendall, F.P., McCreary, E.K., Provance, P.G., Rodgers, M.M., Romani, W.A., 2005. Muscles: Testing and Function With Posture and Pain, fifth ed. Williams & Wilkins, Baltimore.

Kibler, W.B., Ludewig, P.M., McClure, P.W., Michener, L.A., Bak, K., Sciascia, A.D., 2013. Clinical implications of scapular dyskinesis in shoulder injury: the 2013 consensus statement from the 'scapular summit. Br. J. Sports Med. 47, 877–885.

Kim, S.H., Ha, K.I., Ahn, J.H., Kim, S.H., Choi, H.J., 2001. Biceps load test II: a clinical test for SLAP lesions of the shoulder. Arthroscopy 17, 160–164.

Land, H., Gordon, S., Watt, K., 2017. Clinical assessment of subacromial shoulder impingement—which factors differ from the asymptomatic population? Musculoskelet. Sci. Pract. 27, 49–56. https://doi.org/10.1016/j.msksp.2016.12.003.

Lewis, A., Kitamura, T., Bayley, J., 2004. The classification of shoulder instability: new light through old windows! Orthop. Trauma 18, 97–108.

Lewis, J., 2015. Frozen shoulder contracture syndrome—aetiology, diagnosis and management. Man. Ther. 20, 2–9.

Lewis, J., 2016. Rotator cuff related shoulder pain: assessment, management and uncertainties. Man. Ther. 23, 57–68.

Lewis, J.S., 2009. Rotator cuff tendinopathy/subacromial impingement syndrome: is it time for a new method of assessment? Br. J. Sports Med. 43, 259–264.

Lewis, J.S., 2010. Rotator cuff tendinopathy: a model for the continuum of pathology and related management. Br. J. Sports Med. 44, 918–923.

Lo, I.K., Nonweiler, B., Woolfrey, M., Litchfield, R., Kirkley, A., 2004. An evaluation of the apprehension, relocation, and surprise tests for anterior shoulder instability. Am. J. Sports Med. 32, 301–307.

Magee, D.J., 2014. Orthopedic Physical Assessment, sixth ed. Elsevier Saunders, St Louis.

Matsen, F.A., Thomas, S.C., Rockwood Jr., C.A., 1990. Anterior glenohumeral instability. In: Rockwood, C.A., Matsen, F.A. (Eds.), The Shoulder. W.B. Saunders, Philadelphia, p. 526.

McClure, P., Tate, A.R., Kareha, S., Irwin, D., Zlupko, E., 2009. A clinical method for identifying scapular dyskinesis, part 1: reliability. J. Athl. Train. 44, 160–164.

McClure, P.W., Michener, L.A., Karduna, A.R., 2006. Shoulder function and 3-dimensional scapular kinematics in people with and without shoulder impingement syndrome. Phys. Ther. 86, 1075–1090.

Milgrom, C., Schaffler, M., Gilbert, S., van Holsbeeck, M., 1995. Rotator-cuff changes in asymptomatic adults. The effect of age, hand dominance and gender. Bone Joint Surg. Br. 77-B, 296–298.

Neer, C.S., 1983. Impingement lesions. Clin. Orthop. Relat. Res. 173, 70–77.

O'Brien, S.J., Pagnani, M.J., Fealy, S., McGlynn, S.R., Wilson, J.B., 1998. The active compression test: a new and effective test for diagnosing labral tears and acromioclavicular joint abnormality. Am. J. Sports Med. 26, 610–613.

Perlow, E., Lucado, A.M., 2014. Persistent shoulder pain: possible visceral or systemic sources. Phys. Ther. Rev. 19 (2), 124–130. https://doi.org/10.1179/1743288X13Y.0000000129.

Powell, S.E., Nord, K.D., Ryu, R.K., 2004. The diagnosis, classification, and treatment of SLAP lesions. Oper. Tech. Sports Med. 12, 99–110.

Ratcliffe, E., Pickering, S., McLean, S., Lewis, J., 2014. Is there a relationship between subacromial impingement syndrome and scapular orientation? A systematic review. Br. J. Sports Med. 48, 1251–1256.

Schlechter, J.A., Summa, S., Rubin, B.D., 2009. The passive distraction test: a new diagnostic aid for clinically significant superior labral pathology. Arthroscopy 25, 1374–1379.

Schwartzberg, R., Reuss, B.L., Burkhart, B.G., Butterfield, M., Wu, J.Y., McLean, K.W., 2016. High prevalence of superior labral tears diagnosed by MRI in middle-aged patients with asymptomatic shoulders. Orthop. J. Sports Med. 4 (1), 2325967115623212.

Seitz, A.L., McClure, P.W., Lynch, S.S., Ketchum, J.M., Michener, L.A., 2012. Effects of scapular dyskinesis and scapular assistance test on subacromial space during static arm elevation. J. Shoulder Elbow Surg. 21 (5), 631–640.

Song, L., Yan, H.B., Yang, J.G., Sun, Y.H., Hu, D.Y., 2010. Impact of patients' symptom interpretation on care-seeking behaviors of patients with acute myocardial infarction. Chin. Med. J. 123 (14), 1840–1845.

Swift, T.R., Nichols, F.T., 1984. The droopy shoulder syndrome. Neurology 34, 212–215.

Terry, G.C., Hammon, D., France, P., Norwood, L.A., 1991. The stabilizing function of passive shoulder restraints. Am. J. Sports Med. 19, 26–34.

Tyler, T.F., Roy, T., Nicholas, S.J., Gleim, G.W., 1999. Reliability and validity of a new method of measuring posterior shoulder tightness. J. Orthop. Sports Phys. Ther. 29 (5), 262–269. https://doi.org/10.2519/jospt.1999.29.5.262; discussion 270–264.

Tzannes, A., Murrell, G.A.C., 2002. Clinical examination of the unstable shoulder. Sports Med 32, 447–457.

Valentine, R.E., Lewis, J.S., 2006. Intraobserver reliability of 4 physiologic movements of the shoulder in subjects with and without symptoms. Arch. Phys. Med. Rehabil. 87 (9), 1242–1249. https://doi.org/10.1016/j.apmr.2006.05.008.

Watson, L.A., Pizzari, T., Balster, S., 2009. Thoracic outlet syndrome part 1: clinical manifestations, differentiation and treatment pathways. Man. Ther. 14 (6), 586–595. https://doi.org/10.1016/j.math.2009.08.007.

Young, H.A., Hardy, D.G., 1983. Thoracic outlet syndrome. Br. J. Hosp. Med. 29, 459–461.

11

Examination of the Elbow Region

Val Jones

LEARNING OUTCOMES

After studying this chapter, you should be able to:

- Outline the key anatomical structures and biomechanical functions of the elbow joint complex.
- Discuss common pathological presentations for this region.
- Identify how clinical reasoning guides history taking in the subjective examination of people with elbow complex pain and/or dysfunction, informed by the location, behaviour and nature of symptoms, and the value of screening questions.
- Discuss the multifactorial nature of elbow pain and the role psychosocial factors may play in how people with elbow dysfunction may present.
- Identify how subjective data will guide the physical examination of the elbow complex.
- Using clinical reasoning, justify selection of tests and interpretation of findings related to common pathological presentations of the elbow complex.
- List the key constituents of a comprehensive physical examination of the elbow complex with considerations of the sensitivity and specificity of key physical tests for the elbow joint region.
- Explain how physical examination findings contribute to reasoning of common pathologies of the elbow joint.

CHAPTER CONTENTS

Introduction to the Elbow Region, 308
Subjective Examination/Taking the Patient's History, 309
Patient's Perspective on Their Experience, 309
Body Chart, 310
Behaviour of Symptoms, 310
Special/Screening Questions, 311
Special Questions—Elbow Joint Specific, 311
Drug History, 312
History of the Present Condition, 312
Gradual Symptom Onset, 313
Plan of the Physical Examination, 313
Physical Examination, 315
Observation, 315
Functional Testing, 316
Active Physiological Movements, 316
Passive Physiological Movements, 318
Joint Integrity Tests, 318
Muscle Tests, 321
Neurological Tests, 323
Vascular Considerations in Examination and Assessment, 325
Palpation, 325
Accessory Movements, 326
Completion of the Examination, 326
Case Study, 330
References, 332

INTRODUCTION TO THE ELBOW REGION

The elbow complex is composed of three bones, the humerus, ulna and radius, which together form three separate articulations: the humeroulnar joint, the humeroradial joint and the superior radioulnar joint. The joint capsule is continuous for all three joints and is reinforced by the collateral ligaments, which contribute to elbow stability. The humeroulnar joint provides most structural stability due to the tight fit between the trochlea and the trochlear notch. It is primarily involved in flexion and extension. The humeroradial joint allows flexion and extension movements as well as pronation and supination (Hengeveld & Banks, 2014). The elbow is not considered a weight-bearing joint; however, activities such as pushing and press-ups do subject the humeroradial joint to compression forces and should be considered. The superior and inferior radioulnar joints are considered as one joint; however, in this text the inferior radioulnar joint is discussed in Chapter 12. They are primarily involved in supination and pronation movements and therefore are essential in fine-tuning wrist and hand spatial positioning.

The muscles associated primarily with the elbow include three flexors (brachialis, biceps brachii and brachioradialis) and two extensors (triceps and anconeus). The role these muscles have in elbow movement depends on many factors, including functional elbow and forearm positions, type of muscle contraction and associated load. In addition, the humerus provides a stable base of attachment for many of the wrist and hand muscles via the common flexor/pronator and extensor tendon origins, which are the medial and lateral dynamic stabilizers of the elbow joint, respectively (O'Driscoll et al., 2005). These tendon origins are susceptible to overload and degenerative changes.

Anatomically the elbow forms part of the kinetic chain for the upper limb, sitting between the mobile shoulder, wrist and hand joints. The elbow's primary role is to optimize hand function by enabling an individual to place the hand in a variety of positions to perform functional activities. Normal elbow physiological ranges for flexion and extension range between −5 degrees hypertension and 145 degrees flexion, although most functional activities usually occur between 30 and 140 degrees of flexion (Sardelli et al., 2011), meaning one does not need to have full elbow range to be fully functional.

The superior radioulnar joint has on average 75 degrees of forearm pronation and 85 degrees of supination (Neumann, 2010). These physiological ranges enable a wide variety of activities. For example, elbow flexion and supination are used to bring the hand to the face and body in activities of daily living, such as eating, dressing and carrying. Similarly, elbow extension and pronation together enable the hand to be used in reaching, pushing, throwing and weight bearing, (e.g. through a walking stick). The elbow joints therefore allow transmission of forces to or from the hand such as torque as a result of twisting (e.g. using a screwdriver) or compression (e.g. pushing a heavy door). Any gross loss of flexion or extension range may significantly limit the level of functional independence for an individual (Lockard, 2006), with Søjbjerg (1996) describing a 50% loss of range, resulting in an 80% functional loss. In contrast, compensations at the elbow may arise when there are dysfunctions at the wrist or shoulder, reminding us of the importance of screening these regions too.

Elbow injuries affect people of all ages and activity levels and result in significant pain and disability (Aviles et al., 2008). Elbow pain potentially may be described as arthrogenic, myogenic, neurogenic or a combination of these, depending on the structures involved. Sports involving overhead throwing, repeated use of power grips (golf and tennis) and compression (divers, gymnasts and weightlifters) are particularly associated with acute and chronic elbow pathologies.

Particular symptoms may be indicative of certain conditions. For example, numbness and tingling in the little finger while talking on the phone may suggest ulnar neuropathy, twinges of pain on turning a key may be related to the superior radioulnar joint and an inability to extend the elbow fully may suggest synovitis or osteoarthritis (MacDermid & Michlovitz, 2006). See Table 11.1 for possible causes of pain and/or limitation of movement. Limitation of cervical or glenohumeral joint range, along with glenohumeral joint weakness, has also been linked to elbow joint pathology (Alizadehkhaiyat et al., 2007).

KNOWLEDGE CHECK

1. Which muscles are the medial and lateral dynamic stabilizers of the elbow?
2. What is the range of motion needed for function at the elbow?

TABLE 11.1 Possible Causes of Pain and/or Limitation of Movement

Trauma/defined mechanism of injury	• Fracture of humerus, radius or ulna—fall on outstretched hand • Dislocation of the head of the radius/pulled elbow (most commonly seen in young children) • Ligamentous sprain—'pop' may suggest collateral ligament injury • Elbow joint dislocation • Distal biceps rupture • Muscular strain
Inflammatory	• Inflammatory disorders: rheumatoid arthritis • Bursitis (of subcutaneous olecranon, subtendinous olecranon, radioulnar or bicipitoradial bursa)
Degenerative/repetitive conditions	• Common extensor origin dysfunction/lateral elbow tendinopathy/tennis elbow • Common flexor origin dysfunction/medial epicondylalgia/golfer's elbow • Degenerative conditions: osteoarthritis and loose bodies • Calcification of tendons or muscles (e.g. myositis ossificans)
Peripheral nerve sensitization/neuropathy entrapment	• Compression of, or injury to, the median, radial and ulnar nerve
Sinister pathologies	• Infection (e.g. tuberculosis) • Primary bone tumours
Other	• Hypermobility syndrome • Haemophilia • Referral of symptoms from the cervical spine, thoracic spine, shoulder, wrist or hand • Volkmann ischaemic contracture (e.g. supracondylar fracture of humerus)

SUBJECTIVE EXAMINATION/TAKING THE PATIENT'S HISTORY

Further details of the questions asked during the subjective examination and the tests carried out in the physical examination can be found in Chapters 3 and 4. The order of the subjective questioning and the physical tests described later should be justified through sound clinical reasoning and may depend on the type of presenting symptoms as well as the patient's expectations.

Patient's Perspective on Their Experience

To treat the patient appropriately, it is important that the condition is managed within the context of the patient's social and work environment. Social history that is relevant to the onset and progression of the patient's problem is recorded. This includes age, employment, home situation, including sleep postures, and details of any leisure and sporting activities (MacDermid & Michlovitz, 2006). It is essential to gain an understanding of the functional demands on the elbow because it may indicate direct and/or indirect mechanical influences on structures. For example, occupational activities involve sustained or repetitive activities, such as production line work, implicating the common flexor/extensor origins at the elbow. Ask specifically about details of work status and job satisfaction. In cases of athletes, ask about changes in training regimes or loads.

Identifying the patient's expectations and possible presence of unhelpful thoughts/beliefs and psychosocial factors will help to effectively plan both the subjective and physical examinations and help to guide future treatment. Following elbow fractures, fear avoidance beliefs at 2 weeks post injury predict functional outcome at 6 months, regardless of fracture severity and treatment (Jayakumar et al., 2019). Identifying psychosocial factors will also alert the perceptive clinician to investigate them early on and can impact upon outcomes of treatment (Linton et al., 2011). Patients with lateral elbow tendinopathy can exhibit psychosocial risk factors for poor treatment outcomes, such as anxiety and fear avoidance along with feelings of low job satisfaction (Alizadehkhaiyat et al., 2007; van Rijn et al., 2009). Helpful psychosocial screening questions are as follows:

- What is your main problem?
- What do you think physiotherapy can do for you?
- How do you feel about physical activity?

Patient-reported outcome measures are also recommended to measure the impact of the dysfunction on the patient's perceptions and functional limitations. Useful outcome measures include the Oxford Elbow Score (Joint-specific) Mayo Elbow Performance Score (Joint-specific), Patient-Rated Tennis Elbow Evaluation (Condition-specific) and Disabilities of the Arm, Shoulder and Hand (DASH) (The et al., 2013).

Body Chart

Information concerning the type and area of current symptoms can be recorded on a body chart (see Fig. 3.2), including hand dominance. This helps to determine the impact that symptoms in the upper limb may have on normal function. Handedness and frequency of activity may well produce physical adaptations, such as reduced range of motion and increased strength of the dominant elbow, wrist and hand, in throwing athletes (Ellenbecker et al., 2012; Wilk et al., 2012). This means comparing the left and right arm of a throwing athlete may not be adequate when restoring him or her to the preinjury status.

Area of Current Symptoms

Precisely map out the area of the symptoms. Elbow symptoms can be felt locally or may refer to the forearm and hand. Localized pain may be felt over the joint lines, including the humeroradial joint, the olecranon process, ulnar notch and medial and lateral epicondyles. Ascertain which is the worst symptom, and record where the patient feels the symptoms are coming from.

Areas Relevant to the Region Being Examined

Symptoms around the elbow complex may be referred from more proximal and distal structures, including the cervical and thoracic spine, shoulder, wrist and hand. For example, lateral elbow pain radiating symptoms distally to the forearm may arise from the common extensor tendon or more proximally from the cervical spine (C5–C6) (Neumann, 2010). Be sure to negate all possible areas that might refer or contribute to the area of pain. Mark unaffected areas with ticks (✓) on the body chart.

Quality of Pain

Establish the quality of the pain to assist in determining possible pain mechanisms; for example, sharp, catching pain may indicate an intraarticular dysfunction, whereas a deep ache localized to the lateral epicondyle with or without distal referral may be indicative of a lateral elbow tendinopathy.

Intensity of Pain

The intensity of pain can be measured as shown in Chapter 3 (see Fig. 3.4) and informs clinical reasoning of symptom severity, which may guide the extent and vigour of the physical examination.

Abnormal Sensations

Check for sensory changes such as paraesthesia, pain or hypersensitivity in the upper limb and/or hand that could indicate neural tissue source. Consider whether symptoms are likely to be peripheral (e.g. in the distribution of the median, radial and ulnar nerves of the forearm and hand or spinal nerve) in origin. Are these symptoms unilateral or bilateral? Has the patient noticed any weakness in the hand? Progressive or deteriorating neurological symptoms of nerve root compression or symptoms of cord compression would require immediate onward referral.

Constant or Intermittent Symptoms

Ascertain the frequency of symptoms, whether they are constant or intermittent. If symptoms are constant, check whether there is variation in the intensity of the symptoms, because constant unremitting pain may be indicative of a serious pathology.

Relationship of Symptoms

The relationship between symptomatic areas can be explored by careful questioning (e.g. Do the symptoms come together or separately? Can the patient experience elbow pain without shoulder or neck pain, or are pains always present together?). Understanding the relationship between symptomatic areas is invaluable in identifying order and selection of assessment and management techniques.

Behaviour of Symptoms

Aggravating Factors

For each area, identify what movements or positions aggravate the patient's symptoms (i.e. what brings them on (or makes them worse)?). Is the patient able to maintain this position or movement (severity)? What happens to other symptoms when this symptom is produced (or is made worse)? How long does it take for symptoms to ease once the position or movement is stopped (irritability)? The concepts of severity and irritability are discussed in Chapter 3.

The clinician also asks the patient about functional activities that could indicate the source of the symptoms. Common aggravating factors such as pain and stiffness when reaching or flexing the elbow may implicate the humeroulnar and humeroradial joints, whereas pain with gripping, turning a key in a lock and opening a bottle may implicate the common extensor tendon or the superior radioulnar joint. It is important to be as specific as possible when investigating aggravating factors. Where possible, break the movement or activity down into individual components because this may provide clues for what to expect during the physical examination (e.g. throwing action in athletes).

Aggravating factors for other regions may need to be considered if they are suspected to be a proximal or contributing source of the symptoms.

Easing Factors

For each symptomatic area, the clinician needs to explore the easing factors to confirm the relationship between symptoms, determine irritability and clinically reason the source of symptoms.

Painful, swollen elbows may be eased when held in a resting position of approximately 70 degrees flexion, with the hand supported, as in this position the elbow has least intracapsular pressure. It is also important to explore and confirm the relationship of symptoms when altering the position or moving proximal or distal joints. For example, symptoms from neural tissues may be relieved by shoulder girdle elevation, reducing tension on the brachial plexus and nerve roots.

The most notable functional restrictions are highlighted with asterisks (*), then explored in the physical examination and reassessed at subsequent treatment sessions to evaluate treatment intervention.

Twenty-Four-Hour Behaviour of Symptoms

The clinician determines this by asking the following:

Night symptoms. Suggested questions to establish the behaviour of symptoms at night are detailed in Chapter 3. Night pain may arise from sleep positions such as sustained elbow flexion (e.g. ulnar neuropathy).

Morning and evening symptoms. The clinician determines the pattern of the symptoms first thing in the morning, throughout and at the end of the day. The status of symptoms on first waking establishes whether the patient is better with rest. Pain/stiffness that lasts for more than 30 minutes on waking would suggest an inflammatory component to the disorder.

Special/Screening Questions

Special questions as highlighted in Chapter 3 are routinely asked because these identify certain precautions or contraindications to the physical examination and/or treatment. The clinician must differentiate between musculoskeletal conditions that are suitable for treatment and management and systemic, neoplastic and other nonmusculoskeletal conditions which require referral to a medical practitioner.

In the elbow, the following conditions and findings are particularly relevant and should be noted during the subjective assessment to determine their contribution to elbow dysfunction.

Thyroid dysfunction is associated with a higher incidence of tendinopathy (Cakir et al., 2003), and similarly, diabetes mellitus is linked with tendinopathy, delayed tissue healing and peripheral neuropathy (Boissonnault, 2011). The presence of systemic conditions, which may affect the patient's prognosis, should be taken into account during treatment planning.

Primary bone tumours around the elbow are generally rare. The suspicion of a tumour, primary or secondary, should be raised in the patient with unremitting, unexplained, nonmechanical bony elbow pain (Goodman, 2010a, 2010b) or in someone with a past medical history of carcinoma.

Special Questions—Elbow Joint Specific

The presence of bruising following injury should always be ascertained. Bruising medially or laterally may indicate a ligament tear or possible elbow dislocation, whereas anterior bruising around the elbow crease and into the forearm may indicate a distal biceps rupture, both of which requires urgent onward referral.

Locking of the joint may result from intraarticular bodies catching between joint surfaces. The age of the patient may assist the examiner, in cases of locking, because more elderly patients may have arthrosis, whereas younger patients may have osteochondritis dissecans. Any athlete in his or her second decade presenting with elbow pain should always be considered to have an osteochondral defect, unless proved otherwise, and warrants an immediate onward referral for further investigation.

In lateral elbow tendinopathy, symptoms usually occur after a period of overuse; however, if of sudden onset during one specific activity, such as a backhand during tennis, a full-thickness tear of the common extensor origin should be suspected, again requiring an onward referral.

Drug History

Previous use of medications such as steroids or the fluoroquinolone group of antibiotics has been linked with tendinopathy or complete tendon ruptures around the elbow. Smoking has also been linked to a sevenfold increased incidence of distal biceps rupture (Safran & Graham, 2002).

Past Medical and Family History

This should include details of any major or longstanding illnesses, accidents or surgery that are relevant to the patient's condition. Family history that is relevant to the onset and progression of the patient's problem is also recorded, including a family history of inflammatory arthritis, inflammatory bowel disease or psoriasis, which predisposes an individual to inflammatory arthritis. Check for a history of trauma or recurrent minor trauma. Patients with a history of elbow dislocation or fractures may be at risk of developing elbow instability secondary to the original injury (Bell, 2008) or secondary arthritis. Ascertain the results of any past treatment for the same or a similar problem. Past treatment records may be obtained for further information.

Elbow Stiffness or Arthritic Conditions

Elbow stiffness can be classified into

- degenerative (osteoarthritis),
- inflammatory, including rheumatoid arthritis and ankylosing spondylitis,
- posttraumatic arthritis—following fracture or instability
- heterotopic ossification following injury (e.g. formation of bone in extra-osseous tissues mostly in muscle or peri-articularly around capsule and ligaments).
- Postinfection (e.g. tuberculosis (TB)).

Rheumatoid arthritis commonly affects the elbow, either unilaterally or bilaterally, whereas primary degenerative arthritis is less common. Comorbid conditions with known predisposition to elbow stiffness such as haemophilia should be investigated (Nandi et al., 2009). In those with haemophilia, the elbow is prone to haemarthrosis and is cited as the second most commonly affected joint after the knee (Utukuri & Goddard, 2005).

Sudden Swelling

Sudden swelling or sudden loss of range of motion in the absence of trauma suggests infection or inflammation of the joint. Septic arthritis is uncommon in the elbow, but it may be seen in patients with a suppressed immune system or diabetes, those taking cortisone medications or intravenous drug abusers. Sudden swelling over the olecranon may indicate an olecranon bursitis.

Radiography and Medical Imaging

X-rays are the first choice following a traumatic elbow injury, because this helps to establish initial injury and any associated fractures or dislocations. Other medical tests may include blood tests, computed tomography (CT) scans, magnetic resonance imaging or nerve conduction studies.

History of the Present Condition

For each area, the clinician needs to know how long symptoms have been present and if they develop suddenly or gradually. Was there a known cause that provoked the onset of the symptoms? If the onset was traumatic (e.g. a fall), the clinician establishes how the patient fell because identifying the mechanism of injury is essential when establishing a diagnosis (Aviles et al., 2008).

Did the patient fall on the outstretched hand or on the tip of the elbow? Did the bicep contour change, indicating a possible distal biceps rupture? If associated with a throwing action and medial elbow pain, did the patient feel a 'pop', which may indicate an acute ligamentous injury (Cain et al., 2003)?

Ligamentous injuries can result from acute injuries such as a dislocation or fracture, or chronic from repetitive overloading, possibly leading to chronic recurrent instability.

Patterns of instability include:

- Posterolateral rotatory instability—is the most common and usually occurs as a consequence of previous dislocation or fracture.

- Valgus instability—due to injury of the medial ligaments, often seen in throwing athletes.
- Varus instability—due to injury of the lateral ligaments.

Patients with ligament instability may report a diffuse ache and other symptoms, such as clicking, clunking and apprehension, or giving way when moving into elbow extension during weight-bearing activities. However, with chronic medial ligamentous injuries, seen in throwers, symptoms may be present only during throwing and may be accompanied by a loss of throwing velocity or accuracy. In chronic presentations, then part of the examination should include judicious use of joint integrity and ligament tests (Aviles et al., 2008).

Gradual Symptom Onset

With gradual onset, is this associated with a change in the patient's lifestyle (e.g. a new job, leisure activity) or a change in sporting activity? What happened when symptoms first began, and how have symptoms developed or changed? Is this the first episode, or is there a history of elbow problems? If so, how many episodes? When and what duration were they? Did full recovery occur between episodes? Has the patient had any episodes of pain stiffness in the spine or other upper limb joints?

Stage of the Condition

To determine the stage of the condition, ascertain whether the symptoms are getting better or worse or remain unchanged.

When all this information has been collected, the subjective examination is complete. For ease of reference, highlight with asterisks (*) important subjective findings and one or more functional restrictions. These can be reexamined at subsequent treatment sessions to evaluate treatment intervention.

KNOWLEDGE CHECK

1. What common resting position eases painful swollen elbows and why?
2. What might locking of the elbow indicate?
3. Why is exploring patient's beliefs important in management of elbow fractures?
4. Name common systemic conditions that are linked with a higher incidence of tendinopathy.
5. What could sudden elbow swelling indicate?

Plan of the Physical Examination

During the subjective examination the clinician will begin to form hypotheses based on verbal and nonverbal communication. This information enables the clinician to plan the physical examination and provides the clinician with a clear outline of what is safe and purposeful, whilst addressing the following key questions.

Precautions and Contraindications

The clinician must first establish whether the patient has a musculoskeletal dysfunction and then identify whether this is suitable for manual and exercise therapy. Within the elbow, specific contraindications and precautions may include recent fracture, trauma, suspicion of heterotopic ossification or long-term steroid therapy. Beyond the elbow, contraindications such as neurological nerve root compression with deteriorating symptoms will also need consideration. Identifying and reviewing any precautions or contraindications will indicate if caution is needed and help the clinician decide on the sequencing, extent and suitability of clinical examination tests. The elbow extension test can be used as a screening test for suspected fractures, confirming the need for immediate onward referral/radiological evaluation (Appleboam et al., 2008). Lack of extension following trauma indicates a 95% chance of fracture, whilst full extension results in less than 5% of risk.

Developing Working and Alternative Hypotheses

Based on the subjective information the clinician's clinical reasoning will help to identify a working hypotheses and possible sources/structures that could be the cause of the patient's symptoms, including local and remote structures (e.g. joints, muscles, nerves and fascia). Remote regions which may need to be examined are the cervical and thoracic spine, shoulder, wrist and hand. In complex cases it is not always possible to examine fully all sources at the first attendance, and so, using clinical reasoning skills, the clinician will need to prioritize what 'must' be examined in the first assessment session and what 'should' or 'could' be followed up at subsequent sessions. Table 11.2 shows a suggested planning sheet for this.

What Is the Predominant Pain Mechanism?

Pain has been classified into nociceptive, peripheral neuropathic, central sensitization and autonomic

TABLE 11.2 Must, Should and Could List of Planning[a]

Must	Should	Could

• Observation (informal and formal)
• Body chart and relationship of symptoms
• Brief appraisal of cervical and thoracic spine active range
• Brief appraisal of shoulder/shoulder girdle position and relationship to elbow
• Functional demonstration
• Active range of movements, noting range, quality and symptom response
• Flexion
• Extension
• Supination
• Pronation
• Passive range of movements, noting range, quality and symptom response
• Flexion,
• Extension
• Supination
• Pronation
• Palpate elbow structures:
  • Olecranon and fossa, humeroulnar, humeroradial and superior radioulnar joint
  • Anterior capsule, collateral ligaments, annular ligament
  • Relevant nerve palpation points for ulnar, radial and median nerves
  • Common flexor and extensor tendons
• Accessory movements
• Muscle testing, including grip assessment, length and strength tests
• Ligamentous testing—only in cases of suspected instability
• Hook test—for suspected distal biceps tear only
	• Brief appraisal of shoulder, wrist and hand active movements
	• Neural and neurodynamic tests
		• Differentiation testing—neural, arthrogenic and myogenic
		• Brief appraisal of the thoracic spine active movements
		• Passive physiological and accessory intervertebral movements of cervical/ thoracic spine

[a]Tests would be selected depending on the type of dysfunction/condition and therefore would be prioritized according to the presenting patient's symptoms.

(van Griensven, 2014). The subjective examination should enable the clinician to reason clinically the symptoms' predominant pain mechanism. Clearly establishing which pain mechanisms may be causing and/or maintaining the condition will help the clinician to manage both the condition and the patient appropriately.

Sequence and Extent of Physical Tests

The severity, irritability and nature of the condition are the key factors that will influence the choice and priority of physical testing procedures. With severe or irritable symptoms, physical tests may be carried out to just before or to the initial onset of symptom production, with fewer physical tests being examined. If the patient has constant and severe and/or irritable symptoms, then the clinician aims to find physical tests that ease the symptoms. If the patient's symptoms are nonsevere and nonirritable, then physical tests that reproduce each of the patient's symptoms should be used and may include combined, sustained or repetitive movements.

PHYSICAL EXAMINATION

The clinician should have a preferred primary clinical hypothesis after the subjective examination, and the purpose of the physical examination is to confirm or refute this hypothesis. The physical planning sheet should outline what needs to be examined. The order and detail of the tests described later will need to be modified for the patient being examined; some tests will be irrelevant, some tests will be carried out briefly, others more fully. It is important to recognize that the techniques shown in this chapter are not exhaustive and that there are many modifications and variations which can be used. It is also important to understand that the reliability, sensitivity and specificity will vary between all physical tests (see Chapter 4). The diagnostic accuracy of the elbow tests which have the best available evidence to support their use has been presented and may be helpful for the clinician in appraising their clinical utility. Each significant physical test that either provokes or eases the patient's symptoms is highlighted in the patient's notes by an asterisk (*) for easy reference.

Observation

Informal Observation

Informal observation occurs throughout the consultation. The clinician should observe the patient in dynamic and static situations, assessing the patient's ability and willingness to move the upper limb, the quality of movement and any associated facial expressions.

Formal Observation

This is particularly useful in helping to determine the presence of predisposing factors such as abnormal bony alignments, preferred patterns of muscle use and observation of resting muscle lengths.

Observation of posture. The clinician assesses the bony landmarks and soft-tissue contours of the elbow region, as well as the patient's cervical spine, shoulder, wrist and hand. Careful examination of the neck and shoulder should be performed in elbow pain of insidious onset to exclude possible referral of symptoms.

Observation of bony alignment. The clinician may initially observe the relative position of the olecranon and the medial and lateral epicondyles. They should form a straight line with the elbow in extension and an isosceles triangle with the elbow in 90 degrees flexion (Fig. 11.1) (Magee & Manske, 2021). Anatomical and gender variations may alter this alignment; however, gross alterations in this positioning may indicate a fracture, dislocation, a malunion or a congenital deformity.

The clinician can assess the carrying angle of the elbow by placing the patient's arm in the anatomical position. The normal carrying angle is 5 to 10 degrees in males and 10 to 15 degrees in females; greater than 15 degrees is cubital valgus, and less than 5 to 10 degrees is cubital varus (Magee & Manske, 2021). The carrying angle should be symmetrical on each side. A fracture of the distal humerus may result in a cubital varus or a gun stock deformity. Cubital varus and valgus may also result from collateral ligament instability.

Hyperextension of up to −5/−10 degrees in the elbow, especially in females, can be normal. Increased resting elbow extension may be a result of hyperextension/lax anterior capsule and may indicate screening for generalized hypermobility should be considered (Simmonds & Keer, 2007). Decreased resting elbow flexion may suggest elbow joint stiffness or tight elbow flexor muscles.

Observation of bruising. The presence of bruising around the elbow should always be noted, with its

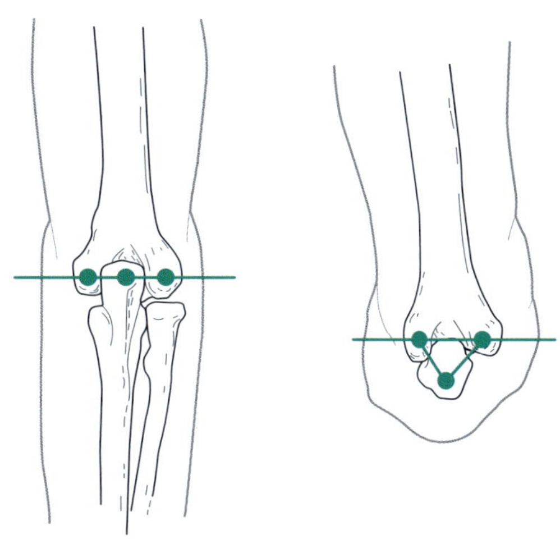

Fig. 11.1 The position of the olecranon and medial and lateral epicondyles should form a straight line with the elbow in extension and an isosceles triangle with the elbow flexed to 90 degrees. (From Magee & Manske, 2021, with permission.)

significance previously discussed in the special questions—elbow-specific section.

Observation of swelling. Swelling at the elbow can occur within the joint or be discrete. Because the elbow joints share a capsule, joint swelling will affect all three joints and the elbow may be held in a semiflexed position (approximately 70 degrees). On the lateral aspect of the elbow, intraarticular swelling may be noted as fullness in the triangular space between the lateral epicondyle, head of the radius and tip of the olecranon. Posteriorly swelling of the olecranon bursa may be observed (Magee & Manske, 2021). An infected olecranon bursa may be associated with fever and erythaema.

Observation of muscle form. The clinician examines the patient's upper limb muscle bulk and tone, comparing both sides. It must be remembered that handedness and level and frequency of physical activity may well produce differences in muscle bulk between sides. Care should be taken to note any changes in biceps contour, because a distal biceps rupture will result in a proximal biceps bulge.

Wasting in the muscles of the hand could indicate a possible peripheral nerve entrapment. Loss of muscle bulk of the intrinsics, particularly in the first dorsal interosseous space, is seen with ulna nerve lesions, along with Wartenberg sign of an abducted little finger secondary to the unopposed action of extensor digiti minimi.

Functional Testing

Informal and formal observation would already include some assessment of functional ability. Asking the patient to demonstrate a functional task such as eating will help to provide invaluable clues as to the potential structures involved. For example, eating involves elbow flexion (up to 120 degrees), supination (for positioning a spoon or fork) and shoulder flexion. Any motion deficits will quickly become apparent. Other examples of functional activities may include using the arm to rise out of a chair, throwing an object, gripping and carrying a bag.

Active Physiological Movements

Flexion and extension are the primary movements that occur at the humeroulnar and humeroradial joints. Pronation and supination are predominantly centred around the superior/inferior radioulnar joints, although there will be some contribution from the humeroradial joint (Magee & Manske, 2021). Active physiological movements of the elbow complex should be performed first, comparing sides, and be sequenced so that the most painful movements are performed last. The clinician establishes symptoms at rest prior to each movement and corrects any compensatory movement to determine its relevance to the patient's symptoms. Active physiological movements of the elbow and forearm and possible modifications are shown in Table 11.3. The clinician notes the following:

- range of movement
- quality of movement—for example, compensatory shoulder adduction and abduction can occur during supination and pronation respectively, giving the appearance of a normal range
- behaviour of pain through the range of movement
- resistance through range and at the end of movement
- provocation of any muscle spasm, guarding or apprehension which may be indicative of pain or ligament instability.

Where appropriate, active movements can be tested with overpressure with the patient lying supine or sitting (Fig. 11.2).

TABLE 11.3 Active Physiological Movements and Possible Modifications

Active Physiological Movements
Elbow flexion
Elbow extension
Forearm pronation
Forearm supination
Possible Modifications to Physiological Movements
Repeated
Speed altered
Combined movements and sequencing, e.g.
• Elbow flexion with pronation or supination
• Elbow pronation with elbow flexion or extension
Sustained
Injuring movement
Differentiation tests
Functional movements
Identify any effect of the modifications of physiological movements on patient's signs and symptoms
Reassess all *asterisks
If necessary, screen any proximal and distal regions that may refer to the area
Cervical spine
Thoracic spine
Shoulder
Wrist and hand

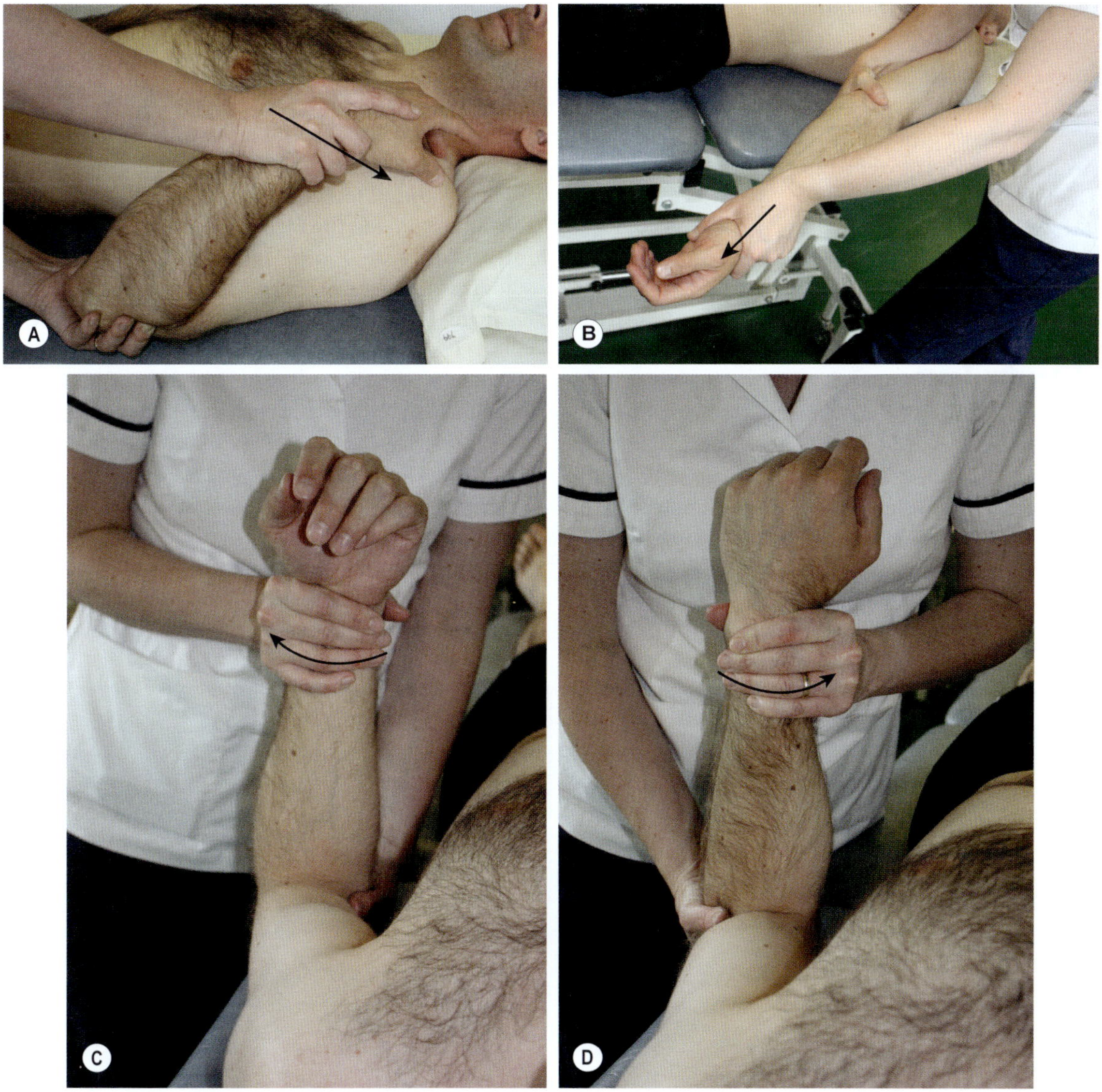

Fig. 11.2 Overpressures to the elbow complex. (A) Flexion. The left hand supports underneath the elbow while the right hand flexes the elbow. (B) Extension. The right hand supports underneath the elbow while the left hand extends the elbow. (C) Supination. (D) Pronation. The arrows represent the direction of the clinician's force.

Symptom Modification or Differentiation Testing

Various differentiation tests (Hengeveld & Banks, 2014) can be performed, and selection will depend on the patient's signs and symptoms. For example, when elbow flexion reproduces the patient's elbow pain, differentiation between the humeroradial and humeroulnar joint may be required.

The 'grip and grind' test, performed by asking the patient to rotate the loaded forearm with the elbow flexed at 90 degrees, whilst gripping the examiners hand, (like turning a door handle), will load the radiohumeral joint and confirm pathology if pain is encountered; it is positive in intraarticular conditions such as osteoarthritis, or osteochondral defects in adolescent patients.

Passive Physiological Movements

All active movements can be examined passively with the patient usually in supine, comparing sides. The clinician feels through range for restriction and/or reproduction of symptoms and assesses end-feel of the joint in the following movements (Fig. 11.3):

- elbow flexion
- elbow extension
- forearm pronation
- forearm supination
- combined movements (e.g. extension/abduction)

Joint Integrity Tests

These are included in the assessment when the history suggests a chronic instability (clicking, loss of control or throwing performance). A provocative test is used to investigate the presence of instability and therefore care should always be taken. For all of the following tests, a positive test is traditionally indicated by excessive movement relative to the unaffected side. However, 'patient apprehension' can also be considered positive with the patient requiring onward referral for further investigation.

Medial Collateral Ligament Testing

The valgus test. The integrity of the medial collateral ligament (MCL) is tested by applying an abduction force to the forearm with the elbow in 30 degrees flexion, to unlock the olecranon from the fossa, and the forearm in supination. The clinician uses one hand to stabilize the humerus in external rotation, thereby ensuring that the tension is directed at the MCL (Fig. 11.3E). Where medial elbow pain is used as the criteria for a positive test, sensitivity is 65% and specificity is 50%, but where laxity is used as the criteria for a positive test, sensitivity is 19% and specificity is 100% (O'Driscoll et al., 2005).

The moving valgus stress test examines the MCL through range (Fig. 11.4). In the seated position, the clinician externally rotates and abducts the shoulder to 90 degrees and then passively extends the elbow whilst simultaneously applying a constant valgus force. Medial

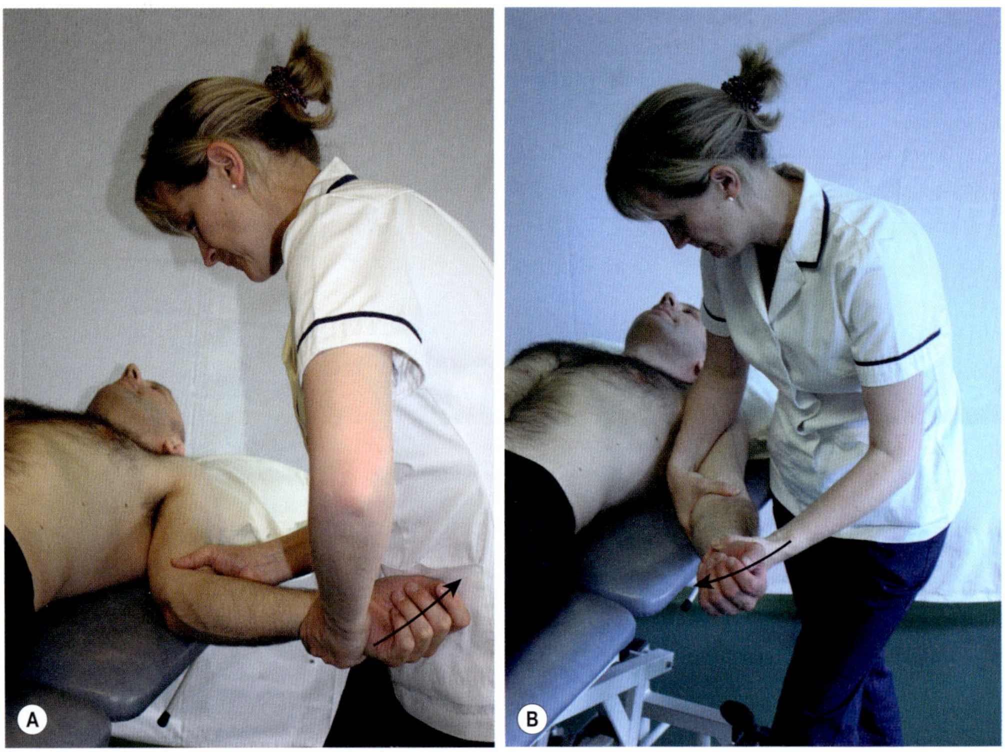

Fig. 11.3 Passive physiological movements to the elbow complex. (A) Abduction. The right hand stabilizes the humerus while the left hand abducts the forearm. (B) Adduction. The right hand stabilizes the humerus while the left hand adducts the forearm.

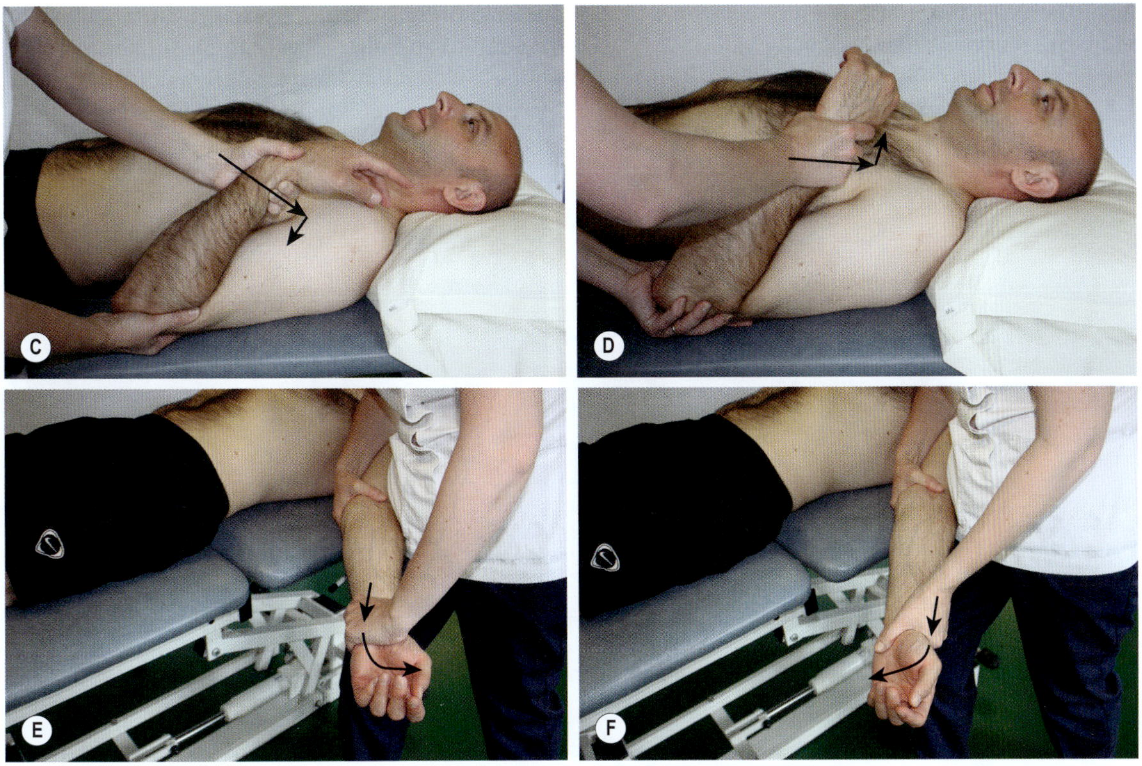

Fig. 11.3, cont'd (C) Flexion/abduction. The right hand supports underneath the upper arm while the left hand takes the arm into flexion and abduction. (D) Flexion/adduction. The left hand supports underneath the upper arm while the right hand takes the arm into flexion and adduction. (E) Extension/abduction. The right hand supports underneath the upper arm while the left hand takes the arm into extension and abduction. (F) Extension/adduction. The right hand supports underneath the upper arm while the left hand takes the forearm into extension and adduction. The arrows represent the direction of the clinician's force.

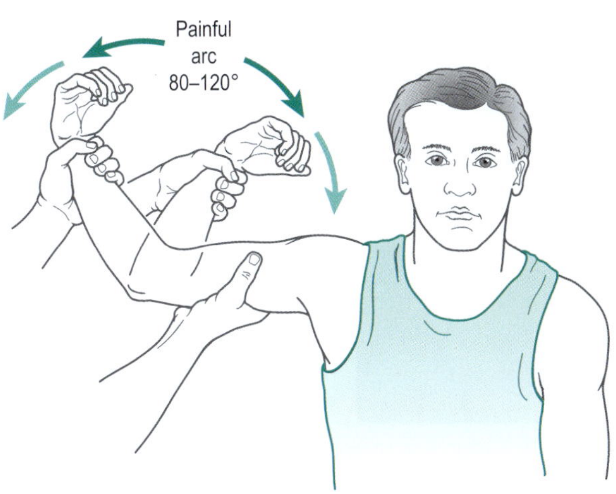

Fig. 11.4 Moving valgus stress test. (From Magee et al., 2009, with permission.)

elbow pain between an arc of 120 and 70 degrees of elbow flexion is considered a positive test (O'Driscoll et al., 2005). The moving valgus stress test for MCL tears of the elbow has been found to be sensitive (100%) and specific (75%), with likelihood ratios (LRs) of LR+ 4 and LR− 0 in a small population study by O'Driscoll et al. (2005).

Lateral Collateral Ligament Testing

The lateral collateral ligament complex is tested by applying a varus force to the forearm with the elbow in 30 degrees flexion, to unlock the olecranon from the fossa. The clinician should use one hand to stabilize the humerus in internal rotation. Quality of end-feel, excessive movement or reproduction of the patient's symptoms is a positive test and suggests instability of the elbow joint (Volz & Morrey, 1993). No diagnostic accuracy studies of this test have been performed to determine the sensitivity and specificity values.

Tests for posterolateral rotatory instability. Recurrent posterolateral instability of the elbow can be difficult to diagnose and requires a careful history and examination. It results from a rotatory subluxation of the radius and ulna relative to the humerus. The lateral ulnar collateral ligament is cited as the primary culprit in this form of elbow instability. The three tests described next should be examined sequentially, and if

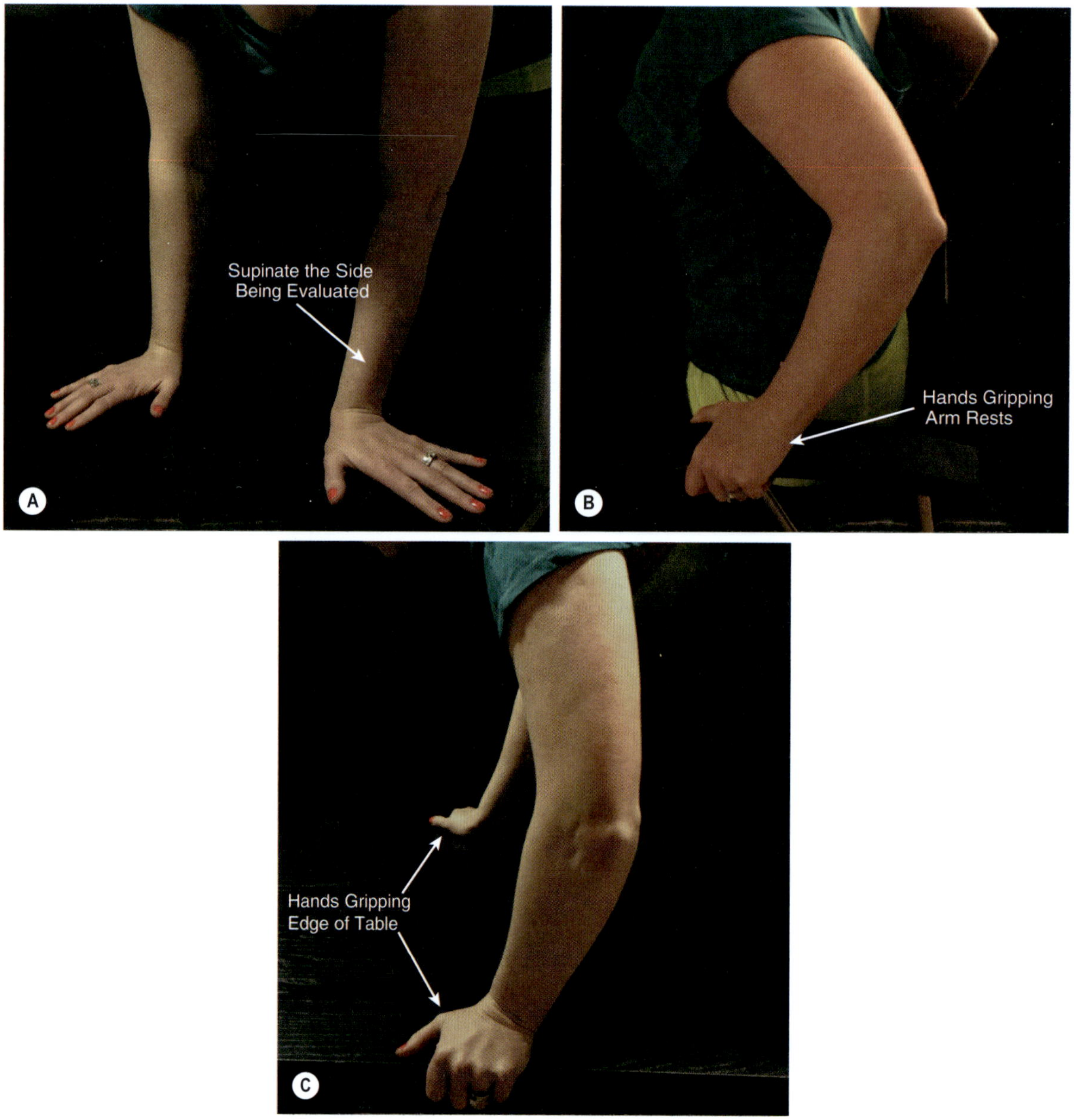

Fig. 11.5 The prone push-up test (A), the chair push-up test (B), and the tabletop relocation test (C) are additional methods for assessing posterolateral rotatory instability. In these figures, the patient's left elbow is evaluated as they push up from a flexed and supinated position into an extended position. The patient's body weight applies the necessary axial load. Each of these examinations relies on the patient pushing themselves up, which reduces apprehension because they are in control of the force and pace. A positive test is noted when the patient experiences lateral elbow pain, instability, or apprehension. (From Camp et al., 2017)

any test is positive, the remaining tests are abandoned (Fig. 11.5A–C).

Table-top relocation test. The patient stands in front of a table, hand placed over the lateral edge of a table, elbow flexed and pointing laterally, with forearm supinated. Ask patient to perform a press up with the symptomatic arm. Positive test is pain or apprehension around 40 degrees of flexion. Sensitivity for this test was reported at 100% (Arvind & Hargreaves, 2006).

Stand-up test/chair push-up test. Patient position is seated, both elbows 90 degrees flexion, holding armrests with shoulder abduction and forearm supinated. Ask the patient to arise from the chair by pushing down on both arms. A positive test is where pain increases as the elbow moves into an extended position. The sensitivity of this test is reported as 88% (Regan & Lapner, 2006; Anakwenze et al., 2014).

Push-up test. Patient lies prone with their chest on floor, elbows flexed to 90 degrees, shoulders abducted and forearms supinated. The patient is then asked to perform a push up. A positive test is apprehension, pain or radial head dislocation during the test. The sensitivity of the test is reported at 88% (Arvind & Hargreaves, 2006; Regan & Lapner, 2006).

Muscle Tests

Muscle tests include examining muscle strength, length and isometric muscle testing. The muscles that need testing will depend on the area of symptoms and functional aggravating movements.

Muscle Strength

A complete assessment of a muscle's strength would include testing the muscle isotonically through the available range. During the physical examination of the elbow, it may be appropriate to test the elbow flexors/extensors, pronators and supinators, wrist flexors, extensors, radial and ulnar deviators and any other muscle groups of relevant regions. Grip strength testing using a hand-held dynamometer is especially useful in the assessment and treatment of lateral elbow tendinopathy.

Muscle Length

To determine if the muscles of the elbow, wrist and hand are tight, passive muscle length tests are performed. The outcome of the length test may be affected by factors such as starting position of shoulder, elbow and forearm and whether the muscles are two-joint muscles. For example, passive tension in the triceps muscle may limit elbow flexion if the test starting position is in shoulder flexion or if the shoulder simultaneously moves into flexion during the test. To test triceps, the patient should be tested in sitting with the arm passively taken into full shoulder elevation while the elbow is extended. The elbow is then passively flexed, and range and end-feel of elbow flexion are noted.

Isometric Muscle Testing

The clinician tests the elbow flexors, extensors, forearm pronators, supinators, wrist flexors, extensors, radial deviators and ulnar deviators (and any other relevant muscle group), in different parts of the physiological range and, if indicated, in sustained positions with or without load. In the elbow, the greatest amount of isometric elbow flexion is found in the position of 90 to 100 degrees, with the forearm supinated. Elbow flexion ranges above or below this position significantly reduce the available isometric power (Magee & Manske, 2021). The clinician notes the strength and quality of the contraction, as well as any reproduction of the patient's symptoms. Fig. 11.6 demonstrates basic isometric elbow and wrist muscle strength tests.

Test for Muscle Integrity

A visible defect of proximal retraction of the biceps muscle belly can indicate a tendon rupture. This may be accompanied by weakness and pain in supination and, to lesser degree, weakness in elbow flexion. The hook test can be used to evaluate for the presence of an intact distal biceps tendon (O'Driscoll et al., 2007). The patient abducts the shoulder, flexes the elbow to 90 degrees and actively supinates the forearm while the examiner attempts to hook an index finger laterally under the tendon (Fig 11.7). The test is negative if the finger can be inserted 1 cm under the tendon and positive if no cord-like structure can be hooked. Sensitivity has been reported at 80% and specificity at 100% (O'Driscoll et al., 2007).

Triceps injuries are rare but may present with swelling, bruising and a palpable gap in the triceps tendon. Weakness is demonstrated by the individual being unable to extend the elbow against gravity.

Special Tests

Repeated microtrauma to the common flexor and extensor tendon origins can produce degenerative changes. Provocative tests are commonly used; however, few diagnostic accuracy studies are available to determine the clinical utility of these tests (Cook & Hegedus, 2013).

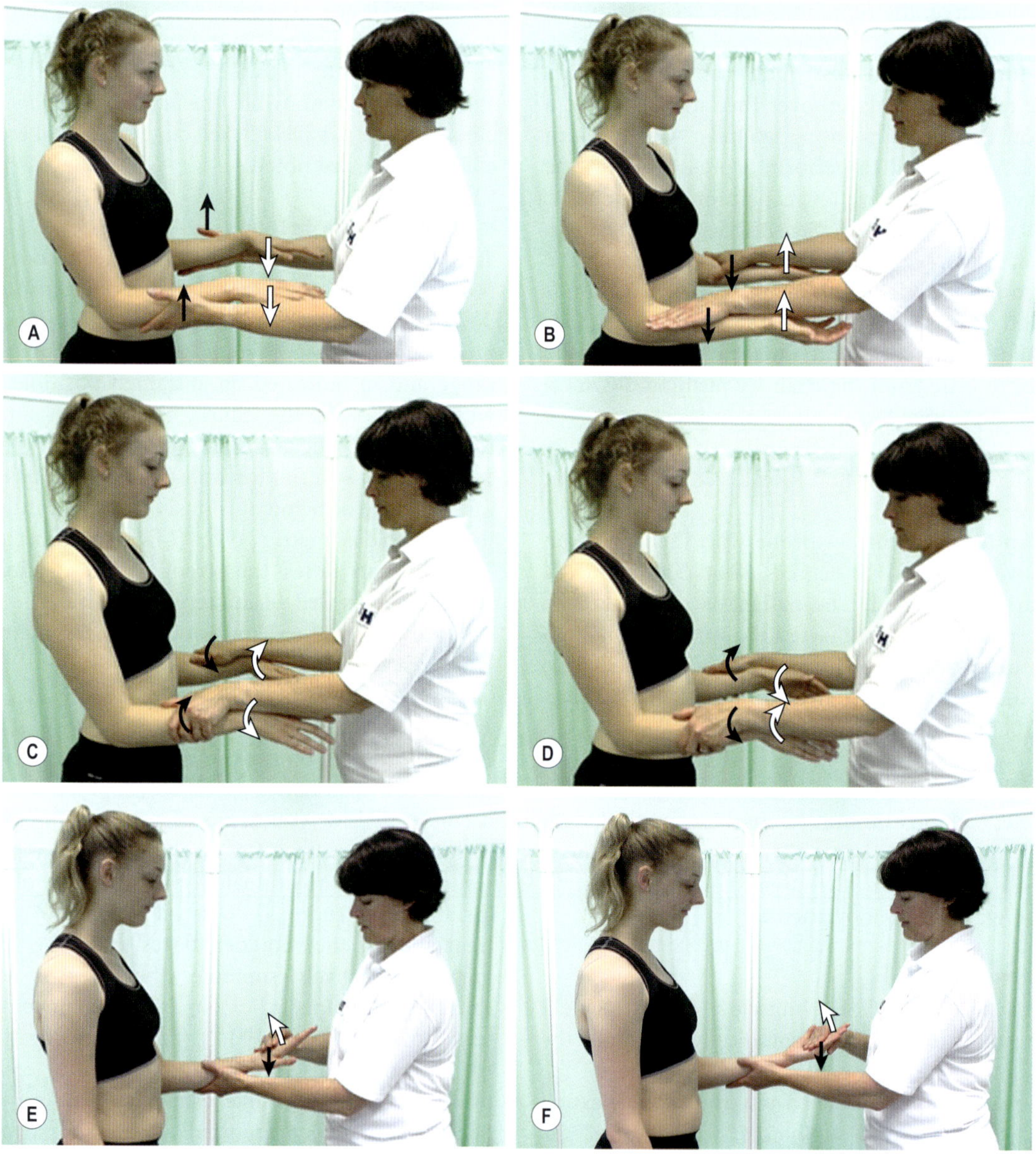

Fig. 11.6 Positioning for isometric resisted movements. Black arrows indicate clinician's direction of resistance, and white arrows represent the patient's action. (A) Elbow extension. (B) Elbow flexion. (C) Elbow/forearm supination. (D) Elbow/forearm pronation. (E) Wrist extension. (F) Wrist flexion.

Lateral elbow tendinopathy (tennis elbow tests). Pain over the lateral epicondyle accompanying gripping of the hand is generally associated with a diagnosis of tennis elbow or lateral elbow tendinopathy. Provocative clinical examination tests are used to reproduce pain and are as follows:

Cozens test—The clinician supports the patient's arm in elbow extension and then asks the patient to make a fist and resist to the wrist extensors isometrically—reproduction of pain at the lateral aspect of the elbow indicates a positive test.

Maudsley test—resisted extension of the third proximal interphalangeal joint activating extensor carpi radialis brevis—reproduction of pain or weakness over the lateral epicondyle indicates a positive test.

No data are available for the sensitivity or specificity of the Maudsley or Cozen test.

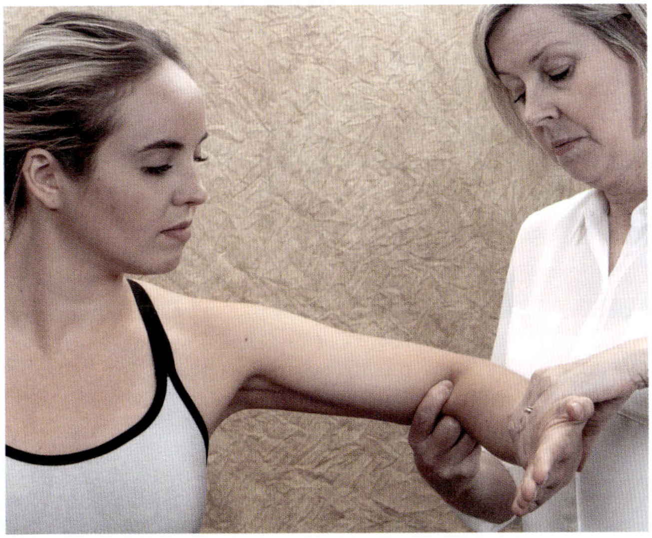

Fig 11.7 Hook test for distal biceps rupture at the elbow. It is important to do the "hook" from lateral to medial. (From Magee & Manske, 2021)

Grip strength test—The patient is seated, holding a handheld dynamometer, with the shoulder adducted and the forearm in the mid pro and supination position, wrist neutral. The patient squeezes the dynamometer as strongly as possible, firstly in 90 degrees elbow flexion and secondly in full elbow extension. A 5% or more decrease in grip strength between flexion and extension indicates lateral elbow tendinopathy, with sensitivity reported as 78% and specificity at 80% (Dorf et al., 2007).

Both sides are compared for grip strength, but variance due to hand dominance needs to be accounted for. The pain-free grip test is a reliable, valid and sensitive measure of the physical impairment of lateral elbow tendinopathy (Coombes et al., 2009). Most protocols recommend performing the pain free grip test with the elbow in relaxed extension and forearm pronation, repeating the test 3 times, at 1-minute intervals. The average of these three tests is then compared against the contralateral arm (Coombes et al., 2009; Lim, 2013). Ensure that the test position is documented, because alternative test positions can be used.

Symptom modification for lateral elbow tendinopathy. Although largely seen as treatment techniques, mobilization with movements can serve as a useful differentiation tool. In the elbow, accessory glides to the humeroulnar joint and the radial head may reduce pain during gripping activities. To test, the patient is positioned supine with the upper limb fully supported and holding a grip dynamometer. The clinician applies a lateral glide to the humeroulnar joint as the patient actively grips (Fig. 11.8). For patients with suspected tennis elbow, pain relief is a positive finding. Similarly, applying a posteroanterior glide to the radial head while the patient performs gripping may also be helpful in relieving pain. These techniques can be used to confirm and refute hypotheses of lateral elbow tendinopathy and may be helpful in guiding future management.

Medial elbow tendinopathy (golfer's elbow test). Isometric contraction of the flexor muscles of the wrist and hand can be examined for common flexor origin pain. Reproduction of pain or weakness on wrist flexion or forearm pronation over the medial epicondyle indicates a positive test. Tenderness on palpation of the area will also help to confirm a diagnosis.

Neurological Tests

Neurological examination includes neurological integrity testing, neural sensitization tests and testing for compression neuropathy. The extent of symptoms will determine the appropriate neurological examination to be carried out.

Dermatomes/Peripheral Nerves

Following trauma or compression to peripheral nerves, it is vital to assess cutaneous sensation. Knowledge of

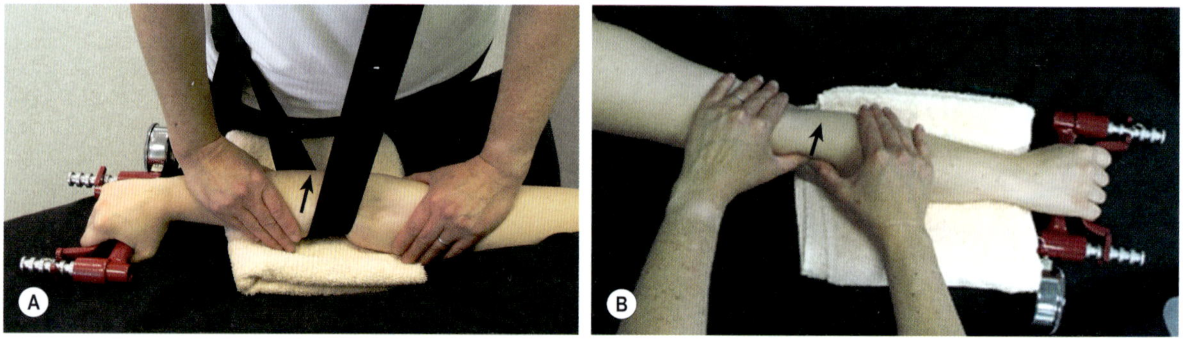

Fig. 11.8 (A) Lateral elbow mobilization with movement. The clinician applies a sustained lateral humeroulnar accessory glide while the patient grips and relaxes the dynamometer or performs the painful action. If there is significant improvement in the pain-free grip, then the clinician repeats the technique for 6 to 10 repetitions. A belt as in the example may be used to assist the accessory glide. (B) Radial head posteroanterior mobilization with movement. The clinician applies a sustained posterior–anterior accessory glide over the radial head whilst the patient grips and relaxes the dynamometer or performs the painful action. If there is significant improvement in the pain-free grip then the clinician repeats the technique for 6 to 10 repetitions. The arrows represent the direction of the clinician's force.

the cutaneous distribution of nerve roots (dermatomes) and peripheral nerves—radial (C5–T1), median (C5–T1) and ulnar (C7–T1)—enables the clinician to distinguish the sensory loss due to a nerve root lesion from that of a peripheral nerve lesion. Testing for sensory loss must therefore involve the whole upper limb and not just the elbow. The cutaneous nerve distribution and dermatome areas are shown in Chapter 4.

Myotomes/Peripheral Nerves

A working knowledge of the muscular distribution of nerve roots (myotomes) and peripheral nerves enables the clinician to distinguish motor loss due to a root lesion from that due to a peripheral nerve lesion. The peripheral nerve distributions are shown in Chapter 4.

Neurodynamic Tests

The upper-limb neurodynamic tests (1, 2a, 2b and 3) may be carried out to ascertain the degree to which neural tissue is responsible for the production of the patient's elbow symptom(s). These tests are described in detail in Chapter 4.

Testing for Ulnar Nerve Instability

Ulnar nerve instability, which has been identified in 37% of elbows, can be determined by having the patient actively extend the elbow with the forearm in supination, placing a finger at the posteromedial aspect of the medial humeral epicondyle and having the patient actively extend the elbow. The nerve dislocates if trapped anterior to the examiner's finger (Calfee et al., 2010).

Ulnar nerve compression neuropathy tests. Compression neuropathies are common in the elbow. Ulnar neuropathy of the elbow is the second most common entrapment neuropathy in the upper extremity. Ulnar neuropathy can be caused by habitual and repetitive activities (e.g. leaning on the elbows), trauma, including fractures and dislocations, rheumatic and degenerative joint disease and immobilization during surgery.

Tinel test. The clinician taps the cord-like ulnar nerve, where it lies in the groove between the olecranon and the medial epicondyle and repeats four to six times. A positive sign is indicated by paraesthesia in the distribution of the ulnar nerve (Hattam & Smeatham, 2010; Magee & Manske, 2021). Novak et al. (1994) investigated the diagnostic accuracy of this test and found values of 70% for sensitivity and 98% for specificity in a small population group; however, up to 30% of asymptomatic individuals also present with a positive test, indicating this test alone should not be used in the diagnosis of cubital tunnel syndrome.

Elbow flexion test for cubital tunnel syndrome. The cubital tunnel is formed by a tendinous arch connecting humeral and ulnar heads of flexor carpi ulnaris approximately 1 to 2 cm distal to the medial epicondyle. During elbow flexion, the cubital tunnel narrows, causing an increase in pressure on the nerve. To test for cubital tunnel syndrome the patient sits with elbow fully flexed with the forearm in supination and wrist in neutral for at least 1 minute. Variations in both the test position and the length of hold recommended do exist; however, sustained elbow flexion is common to all. A positive sign is indicated by paraesthesia or numbness in the distribution of the ulnar nerve (Buehler & Thayer, 1988). The sensitivity of elbow flexion with a hold of 30 seconds has been demonstrated by Novak et al. (1994) at just 32%, and this increases to 75% with a hold of 60 seconds. This low to moderate sensitivity suggests that the clinical examination needs to be combined with the subjective examination to aid the diagnosis of cubital tunnel syndrome. The most sensitive provocative test in the diagnosis of cubital tunnel syndrome was elbow flexion with a hold of 60 seconds when combined with pressure on the ulnar nerve (sensitivity 98% and specificity 95%; Novak et al., 1994).

Froment test. This test can be performed to assess the adductor pollicis, innervated by the ulna nerve. The examiner places the hands together with flat palms and holds a piece of paper between the thumbs and index fingers. The patient mirrors the examiner and tries to pull the paper away from the patient. If there is weakness, due to ulna nerve entrapment, the patient will instinctively flex the interphalangeal joint of the thumb using the strength of flexor pollicis longus, innervated by the anterior interosseous portion of the median nerve.

Median nerve compression neuropathy tests. Median nerve entrapment is less common in the elbow; however, proximal injury is well described, particularly around the origin of the anterior interosseous nerve (anterior interosseous syndrome), around pronator teres (pronator syndrome) or at the ligament of Struthers (supracondylar process syndrome), giving rise to symptoms similar to those seen in carpel tunnel syndrome. Common provocative tests are commonly used; however, no diagnostic accuracy studies are available to determine the sensitivity and specificity for these particular tests (Cook & Hegedus, 2013).

Pinch-grip test. This tests for anterior interosseous nerve entrapment (anterior interosseous syndrome) between the two heads of pronator teres muscle (Magee & Manske, 2021). The test is considered positive if the patient is unable actively to pinch the tips of the distal interphalangeal joints of the index finger and thumb together. The test is also known as the OK sign.

Test for pronator syndrome. With the elbow flexed to 90 degrees, the clinician resists pronation as the elbow is extended. Tingling in the distribution of the median nerve is a positive test. This involves compression of the median nerve just proximal to the formation of the anterior interosseous nerve (Magee & Manske, 2021). In addition to the anterior interosseous syndrome, with a weakened pinch grip, described previously, the flexor carpi radialis, palmaris longus and flexor digitorum muscles are affected, thus weakening grip strength; there is also sensory loss in the distribution of the median nerve.

Radial nerve compression. Radial tunnel syndrome is uncommon and often goes undiagnosed due to the relative absence of hard signs or symptoms, with pain the only finding. Compression of the proximal portion of the radial nerve in the forearm can be identified with pain approximately 2 to 3 cm distal to the common extensor origin with sustained pressure, in comparison with the contralateral elbow. There are generally no motor findings, and neurophysiology can be normal.

The posterior interosseous nerve, a branch of the radial nerve, may be injured at the elbow, as it passes through the supinator muscle (arcade of Frohse), causing posterior interosseous nerve syndrome. This presents with lateral elbow pain and weakness in the wrist extensors and ulnar deviators of the wrist. Radial deviation is intact. Symptoms can be reproduced with resisted supination.

Vascular Considerations in Examination and Assessment

Palpation of Pulses

The incidence of elbow neurovascular injury is rare but may occur following elbow dislocation and reduction. Cyanosis, pallor, lack of pulses and marked pain may suggest vascular injury or possible compartment syndrome. If compromised circulation is suspected, then palpate the brachial artery on the medial aspect of the humerus in the axilla and in the cubital fossa and check the radial artery at the wrist (Carter et al., 2010).

Palpation

The structures in the elbow region are relatively superficial and accessible to palpation. Sound knowledge of anatomy and structural relations will help the clinician to conduct a systematic and informative examination whilst noting the following:

- temperature of the area
- presence of oedema or effusion; using a tape measure and comparing sides

- mobility and feel of superficial tissues (e.g. ganglions, nodules and scar tissue)
- pain provoked or reduced on palpation; positive Tinel sign on nerve palpation
- crepitus or clicking—clicking over the radial head as the elbow moves into combined flexion and pronation, may indicate the presence of a plica.

Suggested Approach to Systematic Palpation

- Anteriorly: cubital fossa, distal biceps tendon, median nerve medial to the biceps tendon and brachial artery and head of the radius (confirmed by pronation and supination of the forearm).
- Medially: flexor pronator muscles, fan-shaped MCL and the ulnar nerve posterior to medial epicondyle.
- Laterally: wrist extensors, brachioradialis and supinator, cord-like lateral collateral ligament and annular ligament.
- Posteriorly: olecranon process, triceps and anconeus tendon insertions.

  Common palpation findings:
- Laterally, fullness in the area behind the lateral epicondyle may indicate an increase in synovial fluid. Tenderness of the lateral epicondyle/common extensor tendon is typical of lateral elbow tendinopathy
- Posteriorally, the olecranon bursa, if inflamed, may be palpable and visible. Rheumatoid nodules may be present on the posteromedial aspect of the elbow.

It is useful to record palpation findings on a body chart (see Fig. 3.2)

Accessory Movements

The clinician notes the:

- quality of movement
- range of movement
- resistance through the range and at the end of the range of movement
- behaviour of pain through the range
- provocation of any muscle spasm.

Humeroulnar joint (Fig. 11.9), humeroradial joint (Fig. 11.10), superior and inferior radioulnar joint (Figs 11.11 and 11.12) accessory movements are listed in Table 11.4. Note that each of these accessory movements will move more than one of the joints in the elbow complex—for example, a medial glide on the olecranon will cause movement at the superior radio-ulnar joint as well as the humeroulnar joint.

Following accessory movements, the clinician reassesses all the physical asterisks (movements or tests that have been found to reproduce the patient's symptoms) to establish the effect of the movements on the patient's signs and symptoms. Accessory movements can then be tested for other regions suspected to be a source of or contributing to the patient's symptoms. Regions likely to be examined are the cervical spine, thoracic spine, shoulder, wrist and hand (see Table 11.4).

KNOWLEDGE CHECK

1. What structures may be injured, seen by the presence of bruising at the elbow?
2. Which test has been shown to be sensitive and specific in the diagnosis of lateral elbow tendinopathy?
3. What device can be used to tests grip strength?
4. Identify a symptom modification identified as useful in differentiating lateral elbow tendinopathy.
5. Name and describe the tests used to examine for ulnar nerve entrapment.

COMPLETION OF THE EXAMINATION

On completion of the physical examination, the clinician will need to collate the information to evaluate and revisit how findings compare with expected findings, based on the initial working hypothesis. Throughout the physical examination the hypothesis is revisited and refined (adapted from Jones & Rivett, 2004):

- What can and can't the patient do? How are symptoms impacting on the patient's life?
- What are the mechanisms of symptoms (include anatomy, biomechanics, mechanism of injury, pain mechanism, stages of tissue healing,). Are they arthrogenic/myogenic/neurogenic?
- What are the physical impairments and associated structures/tissue sources driving the patient's symptoms?
- Does this patient's problem have any other contributing factors that may be influencing the onset or

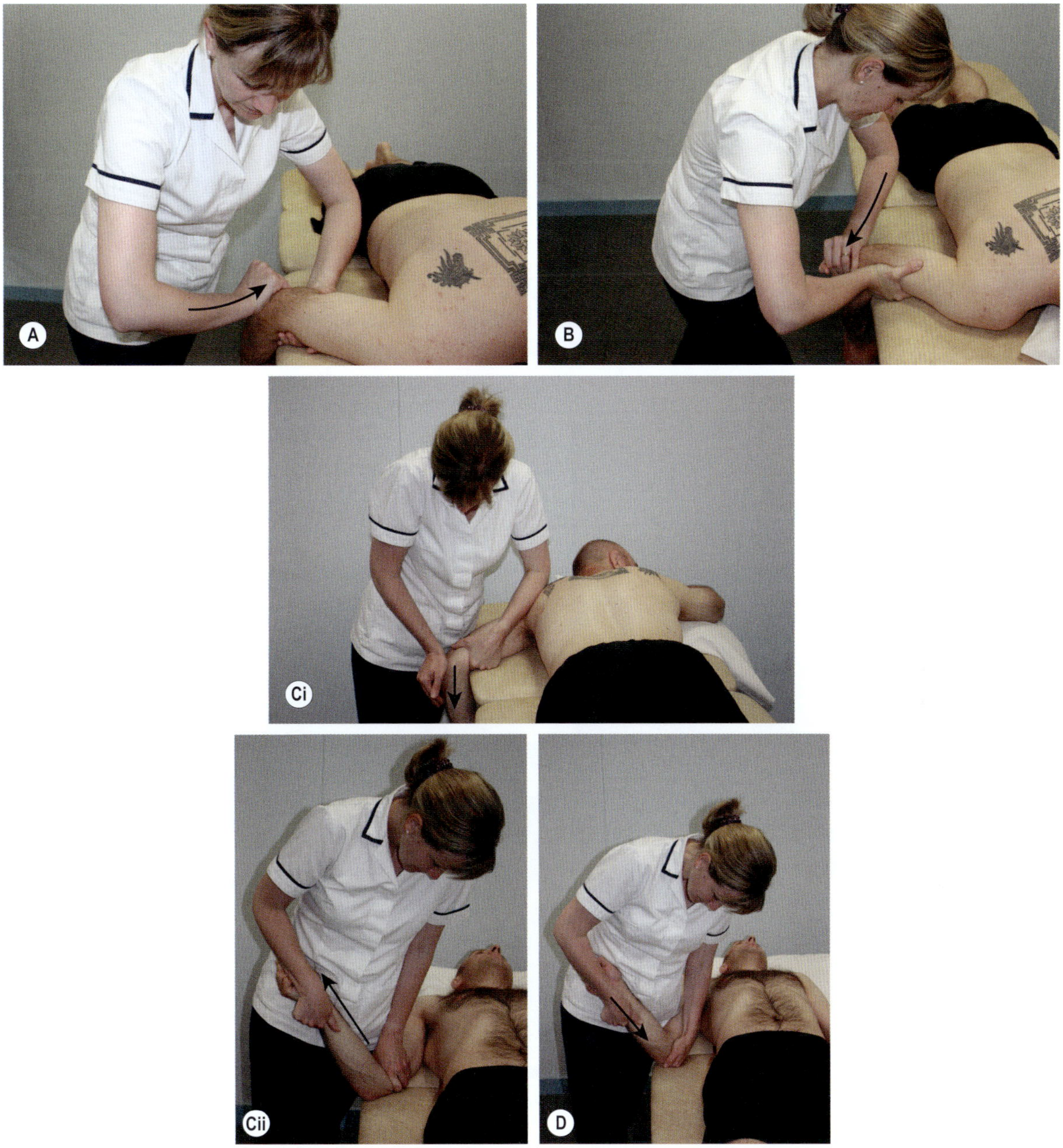

Fig. 11.9 Humeroulnar accessory movements. (A) Medial glide on the olecranon. The left hand supports underneath the upper arm, and the right heel of the hand applies a medial glide to the olecranon. (B) Lateral glide on the olecranon. The right hand supports the forearm while the left hand applies a lateral glide to the olecranon. (C) Longitudinal caudad. Longitudinal caudad can be applied directly on the olecranon; (Ci) the left hand supports underneath the upper arm and the right heel of the hand applies a longitudinal caudad glide to the olecranon or (Cii) the left hand stabilizes the upper arm and the right hand grips the shaft of the ulna and pulls the ulna upwards to produce a longitudinal caudad movement at the humeroulnar joint. (D) Compression. The left hand supports underneath the elbow while the right hand pushes down through the shaft of the ulna. The arrows represent the direction of the clinician's force.

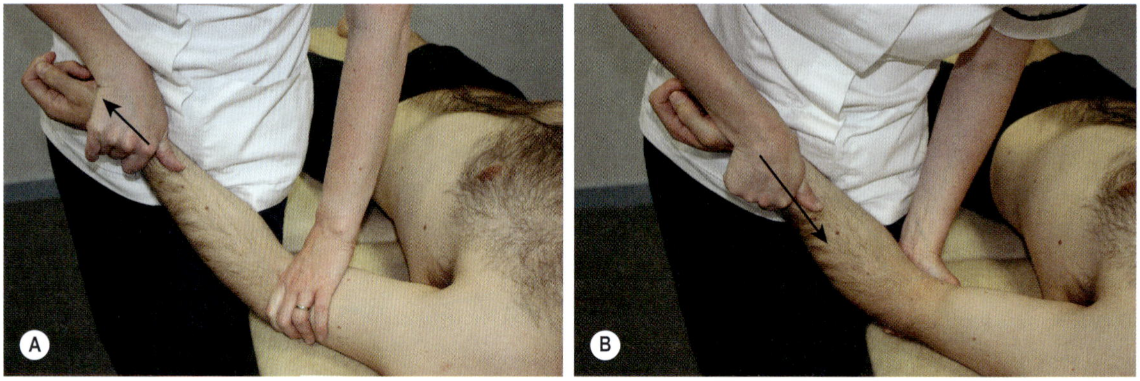

Fig. 11.10 (A and B) Humeroradial movements.

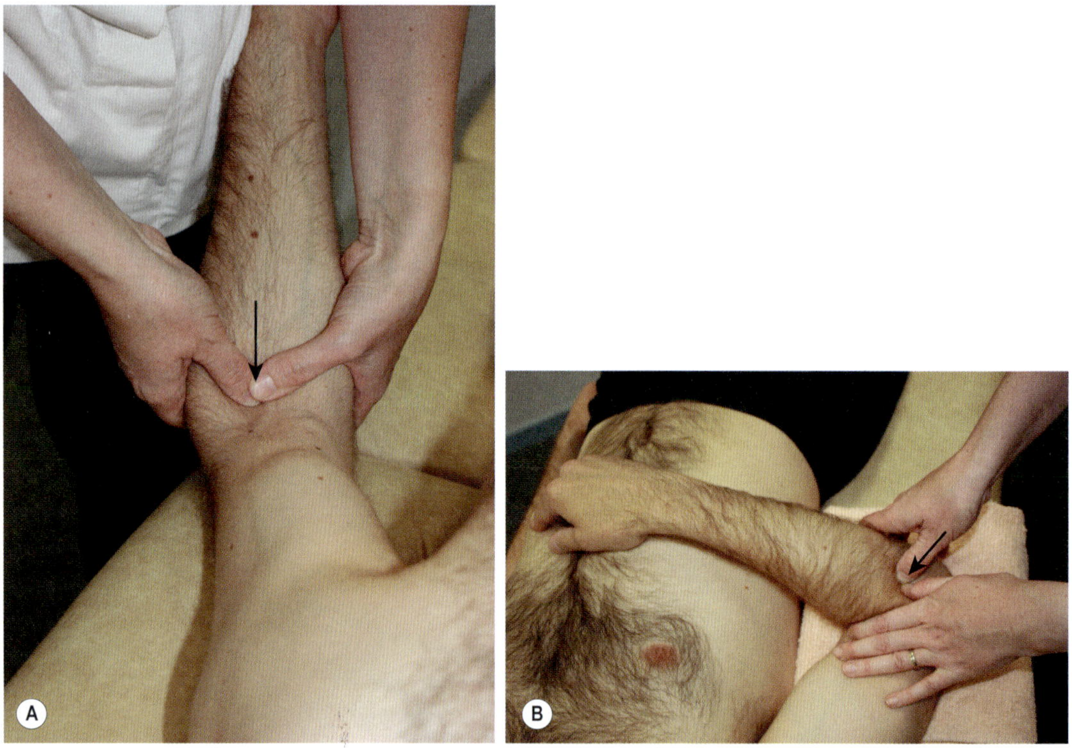

Fig. 11.11 Superior radioulnar joint accessory movements. (A) Anteroposterior. Thumb pressure is applied slowly through the soft tissue to the anterior aspect of the head of the radius. (B) Posteroanterior. Thumb pressure is applied to the posterior aspect of the head of the radius. The arrows represent the direction of the clinician's force.

maintenance of symptoms (e.g. environmental, psychosocial, behavioural, physical or heredity factors)?

- Are there any precautions/contraindications to treatment and management? This includes the severity and irritability of the patient's symptoms and the underlying cause(s) of the patient's symptoms.
- Where will initial management/treatment be focused?
- Assessing prognosis—this can be affected by factors such as the stage and cause of symptoms, patient's expectations, personality and lifestyle. Included in the prognosis should be an initial estimate of the percentage improvement for the patient, number of

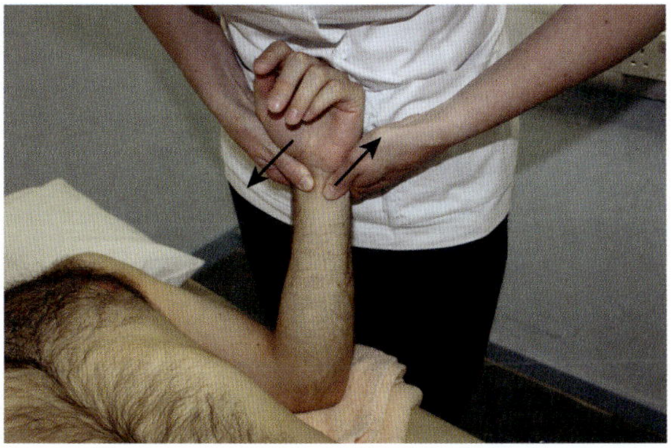

Fig. 11.12 Inferior radioulnar joint accessory movements: anteroposterior/posteroanterior glide. The left and right hands each grasp the anterior and posterior aspects of the radius and ulna. The hands then apply a force in opposite directions to produce an anteroposterior/posteroanterior glide. The arrows represent the direction of the clinician's force.

treatments required to achieve this and the time period over which it will occur.

Before the patient leaves, the clinician:

- explains the findings of the physical examination and how these relate to the subjective assessment, offering initial advice if appropriate
- allows the patient sufficient opportunity to discuss thoughts and beliefs
- revisits the patient's initial expectations, and through collaboration, identifies an agreed treatment strategy in order to achieve agreed goals
- warns the patient of possible exacerbation up to 24 to 48 hours following the examination
- requests the patient to report details on the behaviour of the symptoms following examination at the next attendance.

For guidance on treatment and management principles, the reader is directed to the companion textbook (Petty & Barnard, 2024).

TABLE 11.4 Accessory Movement, Choice of Application and Reassessment of the Patient's Asterisks

Humeroulnar Joint	Superior Radioulnar Joint	Inferior Radioulnar Joint
Med Medial glide on olecranon Lat Lateral glide on olecranon Caud Longitudinal	Anteroposterior Posteroanterior	Anteroposterior Posteroanterior

REVIEW AND REVISE QUESTIONS

Complete the following:

1. The elbow is a complex region made up of the __________, __________ and __________ joints.
2. Medial elbow pain on throwing may indicate an injury to?
3. Distal biceps ruptures are seven times more likely in smokers than nonsmokers. TRUE or FALSE
4. Name four conditions that might cause elbow joint stiffness.
5. What symptoms in the subjective history might raise a suspicion of elbow instability?
6. Name three tests for posterolateral instability, their order of application and what would be considered a positive finding
7. What medications are considered to negatively affect tendon health?
8. What common functional restrictions are reported by patients with elbow pain?
9. What might swelling over the olecranon bursa indicate?
10. How would you check that the elbow was clinically in joint and what might malalignment of the elbow indicate?

Case Study Mr. E

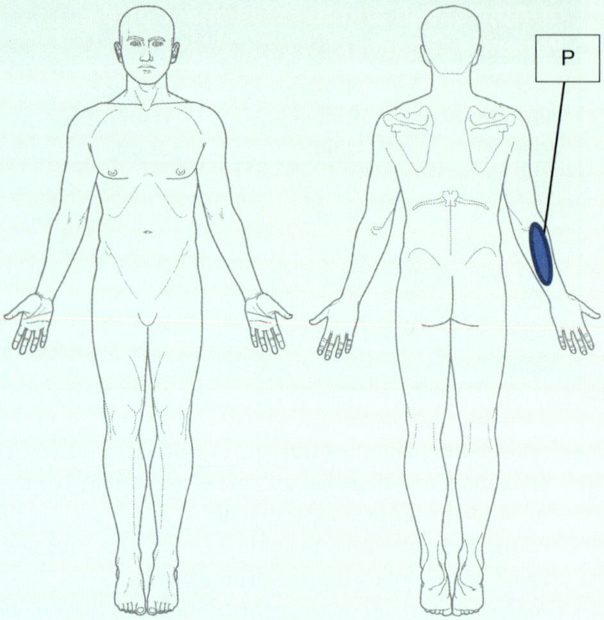

P—intermittent pain, with lingering ache once pain subsides 7/10, reducing to 0/10

Aggravating factors—immediate onset of pain with lifting, e.g. picking up a kettle, gardening and driving for long periods (over 1 h)

Easing factors—relieved after rest—30 min

24-h pattern—Morning stiffness and increased pain on rising for 15 min. Reduces after warm shower. Worse at end of day, especially after a day at work, compared with day off.

Sleep—Can take some time to get to sleep, and wakes 2–3 nights per week, if he rolls onto that side at night. Takes up to 30 min to get back to sleep again

No symptoms anywhere else

HPC

Mr. E was a 56-year-old male, right hand dominant, who presented with a 6-month history of right lateral elbow pain. He reported that his symptoms were of gradual onset after a slight jarring injury to the lateral aspect of his right elbow at work. He was working longer hours during pandemic, due to staff shortages. He feels as if pain is worsening and takes longer to settle.

Symptoms were aggravated by any repetitive use of the lower right arm, such as using a kettle, or lifting and relieved by rest. There was some residual discomfort, for 2 to 4 h following repeated use of the right wrist and hand but otherwise pain was of intermittent nature. He noticed pain got worse in cold weather.

Lifestyle/Occupation/Home Life

Lives with wife and two teenage children. Generally happy home life and no real caring responsibilities other than usual gardening, shopping, etc. Works as a bus driver, with increased workload during the pandemic. Does not take regular exercise but likes gardening in his free time.

Has recently reduced his hours at work and had been unable to participate in home activities like gardening due to the severity of his symptoms.

Impact on Function/Beliefs and Expectations

Fed up that this is affecting his ability to work but also worrying about returning to work full time because of the risks of face-to-face encounters during the pandemic. Feels that rest is his only option because activity, including previous physiotherapy exercises, flares his symptoms up. A colleague had mentioned a steroid injection, and he feels he would like to explore this option.

PMH

Type 2 diabetes and hypertension, controlled with medication. He has recently stopped smoking.

Overweight with a body mass index (BMI) of 32.

No previous history of problems.

DH/Investigations

Mr. E reported that he had been referred to a physiotherapy service early in the onset of his symptoms. He had received a course of ultrasound and stretches for the wrist extensors and been placed on an isotonic resisted wrist extensor strengthening program. He reported that during this treatment it had resulted in a significant increase in his pain and disability and his discontinuance of the treatment.

Losartan for hypertension. Metformin for diabetes.

Occasional paracetamol for pain relief, no history of steroid use. No warfarin.

X-rays following his jarring injury - nothing abnormal detected (NAD)

FH nil of note

GH Feels tired, and struggling with diabetic control

Clinical Reasoning

Mr. E had an onset of elbow pain, following a jarring injury at work, and which also coincided with a change in work

Case Study Mr. E—cont'd

life. The complaint has been worsening in the past few weeks, and he is now unable to continue with his normal occupational or recreational activities.

Psychologically **(yellow flags)**—no clear diagnosis, concerned that this is starting to affect work, frustrated that exercises made him worse, looking for a quick fix with an injection

Blue/black flag—loss of socialization with work colleagues

Red flag symptoms—symptoms followed jarring injury, although nil seen on X-ray

Evaluation of Severity, Irritability and Nature

Severity (Pa)—moderate to high (intermittent night disturbances, no regular medication, NPRS of 7/10)

Irritability (Pa)—moderate to high (symptoms with lifting a kettle immediately, and eases after 20 to 30 min of rest)

Nature—chronic lateral elbow tendinopathy with degenerative and inflammatory changes, in the same tendon

What are you treating? It is likely at this point we are treating a tendinopathy, which has moved from a subclinical to clinical complaint due to change in circumstances with working linked to the Covid-19 pandemic, with coexisting comorbidities, such as diabetes, obesity and smoking increasing his risk for developing the problem.

Mr. E's main **functional limitation** is being unable to grip and lift objects, because of pain

Subjective markers (link to genics)

1. Gripping causes immediate pain, takes 20 min to settle
2. Stiffness in elbow when he first wakes
3. Intermittent sleep disturbance 2–3 nights per week

Does any aspect of the history indicate caution?

Moderate to high levels of severity and irritability indicate caution, during physical examination process.

Can you predict the comparable signs? (Subjective marker linking with an objective sign)

Pain on gripping, worse in elbow extension, compared with elbow flexion

What is the relationship between pain and resistance?

Pa - Pain > resistance

What pain mechanisms can you identify? There is evidence of some central affective (psychology) mechanisms at play as well as peripheral nociceptive (elbow), and possibly some central sensitization due to worsening in cold weather.

Analysis of percentage weighting (Pain source) Myogenic 70%, central affective 20%, central neurogenic 10%.

Analysis of percentage weighting (driver/contributing factors) Given the persistent nature of Mr. E's complaint, it is important to consider the following questions:

1. Why has he developed this complaint?
2. Why has it not settled (comorbidities, beliefs regarding activity)
3. What does his occupation require him to do?

Based on duration of complaint and age (degenerative changes) proposed weighting could be reduced strength in wrist extensors 60%, reduced strength globally in upper limb 20%, beliefs/psychological 20%.

Hypotheses to test/working diagnosis? (Differentiate between genics)

1. Reduced strength/endurance of wrist extensors
2. Reduced strength in shoulder girdle and elbow
3. Faulty/dysfunctional movement pattern of wrist extensors—will tend to grip in wrist flexed position.

Planning the Physical Examination

Observation to include resting position of elbow and wrist, bony alignment of the elbow (Fig. 11.1), and oedema

Observe movements to assess elbow and wrist range of motion, as well as clearing shoulder and cervical spine. Observe where movement in originating from (quality, range and reproduction of any symptoms). Compare gripping in elbow extension to elbow flexion to aid differentiation.

Passive range of motion (ROM) of elbow, forearm and wrist also aids differentiation between muscle and joint.

Muscles

Assess

- Pain free grip strength using a hand-held dynamometer
- Strength in scapula, shoulder and elbow muscles

Main clinical findings for Mr. E included

Marked reduction in pain free grip strength, compared with nondominant hand, and also compared with normative grip strength data, stratified for age and gender. Adopted a wrist flexion position to grip. Reduction in grip strength worse in elbow extension, compared with elbow flexion, by 10%

Reduced strength in external rotators and flexors of ipsilateral shoulder joint

Management included

Education and advice

Advice and education to aid understanding of tendinopathy and contributing factors. Discussion regarding timescales for recovery, adoption of a graded loading programme and acceptable symptoms during exercise.

Case Study Mr. E—cont'd

Given progression and regression of exercise programme dependent on symptomatic reproduction. Advice on how systemic health including diabetic control and BMI can affect tendons, and advice on WHO advice on weekly activity guidelines. Evidence regarding detrimental effects of steroid injection examined.

Muscle strengthening to wrist extensors and supinators

Home exercise programme

1. Isometric wrist extensor loading programme
2. To start every other day, to avoid exacerbation and increase as symptoms allow
3. General cardiovascular exercise—150 min per week target of moderate intensity exercise (e.g. walking briskly).

Outcome

After 4 weeks Mr. E had an increase in pain free grip strength, but pain levels remained ISQ. Reassurance was given that functional ability was improving and tendinopathy can take weeks/months to resolve. Sleep disturbance was improved. Felt much more positive and whilst he had not yet returned to full work duties, did feel like that this was achievable.

REFERENCES

Alizadehkhaiyat, O., Fisher, A.C., Kemp, G.J., Frostick, S.P., 2007. Pain, functional disability, and psychologic status in tennis elbow. Clin. J. Pain 23, 482–489.

Anakwenze, O.A., Kancherla, V.K., Iyengar, J., Ahmad, C.S., Levine, W.N., 2014. Posterolateral rotatory instability of the elbow. Am. J. Sports Med. 42 (2), 485–491.

Appelboam, A., Reuben, A.D., Benger, J.R., Beech, F., Dutson, J., Haig, S., et al., 2008. Elbow extension test to rule out elbow fracture: multicentre, prospective validation and observational study of diagnostic accuracy in adults and children. Br. Med. J. 337, a2428.

Arvind, C.H.V., Hargreaves, D.G., 2006. Table top relocation test—new clinical test for posterolateral rotatory instability of the elbow. J. Shoulder Elbow Surg. 15 (4), 500–501.

Aviles, S., Wik, K., Safran, M., 2008. Elbow. In: Magee, D.J., Zachazewski, J.E., Quillen, W.S., Manske, R.C. (Eds.), Pathology and Intervention in Musculoskeletal Rehabilitation. Saunders, St Louis, MO.

Bell, S., 2008. Elbow instability, mechanisms and management. Curr. Orthop. 22, 90–103.

Boissonnault, W.G., 2011. Primary Care for the Physical Therapist: Examination and Triage, second ed. Elsevier Saunders, St Louis, MO.

Buehler, M.J., Thayer, D.T., 1988. The elbow flexion test. A clinical test for the cubital tunnel syndrome. Clin. Orthop. 233, 213–216.

Cain Jr., E.L., Dugas, J.R., Wolf, R.S., Andrews, J.R., 2003. Elbow injuries in throwing athletes: a current concepts review. Am. J. Sports Med. 31, 621–635.

Cakir, M., Samanci, N., Balci, N., Balci, M.K., 2003. Musculoskeletal manifestations in patients with thyroid disease. Clin. Endocrinol. 59, 162–167.

Calfee, R.P., Manske, P.R., Gelberman, R.H., Van Steyn, M. O., Steffen, J., Goldfarb, C.A., 2010. Clinical assessment of the ulnar nerve at the elbow: reliability of instability testing and the association of hypermobility with clinical symptoms. J. Bone. Joint. Surg. Am. 92 (17), 2801–2808.

Camp, L.C., Smith, J., O'Driscoll, S.W., 2017. Posterolateral Rotatory Instability of the Elbow: Part II. Supplementary Examination and Dynamic Imaging Techniques. Arthrosc. Tech. 6 (2), e407–e411.

Carter, S.J., Germann, C.A., Dacus, A.A., Sweeney, T.W., Perron, A.D., 2010. Orthopedic pitfalls in the ED: neurovascular injury associated with posterior elbow dislocations. Am. J. Emerg. Med. 28, 960–965.

Cook, C.E., Hegedus, E., 2013. Orthopedic Physical Examination Tests: An Evidence-Based Approach, second ed. Prentice Hall, Upper Saddle River, NJ.

Coombes, B.K., Bisset, L., Vicenzino, B., 2009. A new integrative model of lateral epicondylalgia. Br. J. Sports Med. 43, 252–258.

Dorf, E.R., Chhabra, A.B., Golish, S.R., McGinty, J.L., Pannunzio, M.E., 2007. Effect of elbow position on grip strength in the evaluation of lateral epicondylitis. J. Hand. Surg. Am. 32 (6), 882–886.

Ellenbecker, T.S., Kibler, W.B., Bailie, D.S., Caplinger, R., Davies, G.J., Riemann, B.L., 2012. Reliability of scapular classification in examination of professional baseball players. Clin. Orthop. Relat. Res. 470 (6), 1540–1544.

Goodman, C.C., 2010a. Screening for medical problems in patients with upper extremity signs and symptoms. J. Hand Ther. 23, 105–125.

Goodman, C.C., 2010b. Screening for gastrointestinal, hepatic/biliary, and renal/urologic disease. J. Hand Ther. 23, 140–156.

Hattam, P., Smeatham, A., 2010. Special Tests in Musculoskeletal Examination: An Evidence-Based Guide for Clinicians. Churchill Livingstone Elsevier, Edinburgh (Chapter 3).

Hengeveld, E., Banks, K., 2014. Maitland's Peripheral Manipulation: Management of Neuromusculoskeletal Disorders, fifth ed., vol. 2. Butterworth-Heinemann Elsevier, London.

Jayakumar, P., Teunis, T., Vranceanu, A.M., Moore, M.G., Williams, M., Lamb, S., et al., 2019. Psychosocial factors affecting variation in patient-reported outcomes after elbow fractures. J. Shoulder Elbow Surg. 28 (8), 1431–1440.

Jones, M.A., Rivett, D.A., 2004. Clinical Reasoning for Manual Therapists. Butterworth-Heinemann, Edinburgh.

Lim, E.C., 2013. Pain free grip strength test. J. Physiother. 59, 59.

Linton, S.J., Nicholas, M.K., MacDonald, S., et al., 2011. The role of depression and catastrophizing in musculoskeletal pain. Eur. J. Pain 15, 416–422.

Lockard, M., 2006. Clinical biomechanics of the elbow. J. Hand Ther. 19, 72–80.

MacDermid, J.C., Michlovitz, S.L., 2006. Examination of the elbow: linking diagnosis, prognosis, and outcomes as a framework for maximizing therapy interventions. J. Hand Ther. 19, 82–97.

Magee, D.J., Manske, R., 2021. Orthopedic Physical Assessment, seventh ed. Saunders Elsevier, St Louis.

Magee, D.J., Zachazewski, J.E., Quillen, W.S., 2009. Pathology and Intervention in Musculoskeletal Rehabilitation. Saunders, St Louis.

Nandi, S., Maschke, S., Evans, P.J., Lawton, J.N., 2009. The stiff elbow. Hand (NY) 4, 368–379.

Neumann, D.A., 2010. Elbow and Forearm. In: Kinesiology of the musculoskeletal system: Foundations for Rehabilitation, second ed. Mosby Elsevier, St Louis (Chapter 6).

Novak, C.B., Lee, G.W., Mackinnon, S.E., Lay, L., 1994. Provocative testing for cubital tunnel syndrome. J. Bone. Joint. Surg. Am. 19, 817–820.

O'Driscoll, S.W., Goncalves, L.B., Dietz, P., 2007. The hook test for distal biceps tendon avulsion. Am. J. Sports Med. 35 (11), 1865–1869.

O'Driscoll, S.W., Lawton, R.L., Smith, A.M., 2005. The "moving valgus stress test" for medial collateral ligament tears of the elbow. Am. J. Sports Med. 33, 231–239.

Regan, W., Lapner, P.C., 2006. Prospective evaluation of two diagnostic apprehension signs for posterolateral instability of the elbow. J. Shoulder Elbow Surg. 15 (3), 344–346.

Safran, M.R., Graham, S.M., 2002. Distal biceps tendon ruptures: incidence, demographics, and the effect of smoking. Clin. Orthop. Relat. Res. (404), 275–283.

Sardelli, M., Tashjian, R.Z., MacWilliams, B.A., 2011. Functional elbow range of motion for contemporary tasks. J. Bone. Joint. Surg. Am. 93 (5), 471–477.

Simmonds, J.V., Keer, R.J., 2007. Hypermobility and the hypermobility syndrome. Man. Ther. 12, 298–309.

Søjbjerg, J.O., 1996. The stiff elbow. Acta Orthop. Scand. 67 (6), 626–631.

The, B., Reininga, I.H., El Moumni, M., Eygendaal, D., 2013. Elbow-specific clinical rating systems: extent of established validity, reliability, and responsiveness. J. Shoulder Elbow Surg. 22, 1380–1394.

Utukuri, M.M., Goddard, N.J., 2005. Haemophilic arthropathy of the elbow. Haemophilia 11, 565–570.

van Griensven, H., 2014. Neurophysiology of pain. In: van Griensven, H., Strong, J., Unruh, A. (Eds.), Pain. A Textbook for Health Professionals, second ed. Churchill Livingstone, Edinburgh, pp. 77–90.

van Rijn, R.M., Huisstede, B.M., Koes, B.W., Burdorf, A., 2009. Associations between work-related factors and specific disorders at the elbow: a systematic literature review. Rheumatology 48, 528–536.

Volz, R.C., Morrey, B.F., 1993. The physical examination of the elbow. In: Morrey, B.F. (Ed.), The Elbow and Its Disorders, second ed. W.B. Saunders, Philadelphia.

Wilk, K.E., Macrina, L.C., Cain, E.L., Dugas, J.R., Andrews, J.R., 2012. Rehabilitation of the overhead athlete's elbow. Sports Health 4 (5), 404–414.

12

Examination of the Wrist and Hand

Dionne Ryder

LEARNING OUTCOMES

After studying this chapter, you should be able to:

- Outline the key anatomical structures and functions of the wrist and hand complex.
- Discuss common pathological presentations for this region.
- Identify how clinical reasoning guides history taking in the subjective examination of those with wrist and hand dysfunction.
- Use the information gained from the subjective examination to establish working hypotheses on to direct the physical examination.
- List the key constituents of a comprehensive physical examination of the wrist and hand complex.
- Identify how clinical reasoning of the subjective data is used to justify test selection and interpretation of findings in the physical examination.
- Have an appreciation of the sensitivity and specificity of key physical tests for the wrist and hand region.
- Use the information gained from the subjective and physical examination to establish/confirm a working hypothesis and treatment plan.

CHAPTER CONTENTS

Introduction to the Wrist and Hand Complex, 335
Anatomical Overview, 335
Function, 335
Wrist and Hand Dysfunction, 335
Subjective Examination/Taking the patient's history, 335
Patient's Perspective on Their Experience, 335
Body Chart, 336
Behaviour of Symptoms, 336
Special/Screening Questions, 337
Past Medical History, 337
History of the Present Condition, 338
Planning the Physical Examination, 338
Physical Examination, 339
Observation, 339
Functional Testing, 340
Active Physiological Movements, 340
Passive Physiological Movements, 341
Joint Integrity Tests, 341
Muscle Tests, 347
Neurological Testing, 349
Vascular Assessment, 351
Palpation, 351
Suggested Approach to Systematic Palpation, 351
Accessory Movements, 351
Completion of the Examination, 353
Case Study, 358
References, 360

INTRODUCTION TO THE WRIST AND HAND COMPLEX

Anatomical Overview

The wrist and hand is a complex comprising the ulna, radius, carpals, metacarpals and phalanges, articulating in a series of joints—the inferior radioulnar, radiocarpal (radius articulating) with proximal carpal row—scaphoid, lunate, triquetral (pisiform), midcarpal where proximal carpal row articulates with the distal row—(triquetral trapezium capitate and hamate), intercarpal, carpometacarpal (CMC), intermetacarpal, metacarpophalangeal (MCP) and interphalangeal joints, with extrinsic and intrinsic muscles plus supporting soft tissues, supplied by three peripheral nerves—the median, radial and ulnar. It is part of a kinetic chain, encompassing the cervical and thoracic spine, shoulder and elbow to allow for optimal positioning of the hand for function.

Function

The main functional requirement of the hand is prehension, which can be defined as the application of a functionally effective force, by the hand, to an object for a specific task, for example, holding a pen to write. Prehension, comprising of four major components: reach, grasp, manipulation and release, will require sufficient stability, flexibility, strength, dexterity and proprioception of the wrist and hand, the trunk and the whole upper limb (Gates et al., 2016). Prehension is fundamental to an individual's functional independence, meaning hand dysfunction can have a significant impact on all aspects of a person's life.

The hand is also a sensory organ with significant representation on sensory cortex (homunculi) (Neumann, 2010) providing kinesthetic tactile information on shape and texture, known as stereognosis.

In addition, the hand is important in communication, for example, through gesturing or sign language. Second to the face, it is the most visible part of the body, so deformity or dysfunction can have a significant psychological impact on an individual (Rumsey et al., 2003).

Wrist and Hand Dysfunction

Trauma to the wrist and hand is relatively common, for example, following a fall on an outstretched hand (FOSH), leading to fractures of the distal radius, ulna or scaphoid, as well as tears of articular disc—the triangular fibrocartilaginous complex (TFCC) and ligamentous injuries resulting in carpal instabilities. Patients can also present with tendinopathies associated with overload or degenerative changes, most commonly of the first dorsal compartment in de Quervain disease (Calveri et al., 2016). Neural tissue sensitization can result from increased pressure, for example, in the carpal tunnel, affecting median nerve function. Systemic inflammatory conditions such as rheumatoid arthritis (RA) commonly first present in the small joints of the hand, with patients often reporting early morning stiffness, pain and localized swelling (Grassi et al., 1998). Degenerative articular changes such as osteoarthritis (OA) of the CMC joint of the thumb results in pain and associated deformities that can impact significantly on normal function (Ahern et al., 2018).

An understanding of functional anatomy and biomechanics will inform clinical reasoning, guide the physical examination and ensure management strategies seek to optimize all aspects of functional restoration.

This chapter will focus on the questions asked and the tests utilized in the physical examination of the wrist and hand region. The order of the subjective questioning and the physical tests described below will be dependent on the individual patient being examined. For details on the principles of the subjective and physical examinations, the reader is directed to Chapters 3 and 4, respectively.

KNOWLEDGE CHECK

1. What is the primary function of the hand?
2. Name the bones that make up the proximal carpal row.
3. Which joints make up the wrist and hand complex?
4. What does the acronym FOSH stand for?

SUBJECTIVE EXAMINATION/TAKING THE PATIENT'S HISTORY

Patient's Perspective on Their Experience

Most patients will seek treatment because they have symptoms and/or functional limitations which are impacting on their activities of daily living (ADL), especially if their dominant hand is affected.

There are a number of region-specific valid and reliable tools that can be used to measure patients' perception of disability—useful as a prognostic indicator and essential for developing treatment goals and evaluating interventions, e.g. Michigan Hand Outcomes Questionnaire and Disabilities of the Arm, Shoulder and Hand (DASH) (Heras-Palou et al., 2003; Nolte et al., 2017).

Body Chart

An enlarged chart of the hand can be used to allow precise recording of a patient's symptoms (Fig. 12.1).

Area of Current Symptoms

Dysfunction of the wrist and hand structures produce localized symptoms. For example, pain on radial aspect of the wrist into the thumb could originate from trapezio-metacarpal joint (first CMC joint), the tendons in the first dorsal extensor compartment – abductor pollicis longus (ABPL)/extensor pollicis brevis (EPB) known as de Quervain disease or due to sensitivity of the dorsal radial sensory nerve. Pain a few centimetres more proximally may be indicative of intersection syndrome, associated with repetitive wrist flexion/extension, producing friction at the intersection of the first and second dorsal extensor compartments (Montechiarello et al., 2010).

Areas Relevant to the Region Being Examined

Symptoms in the wrist and hand may be referred from more proximal structures in the lower cervical spine, upper thoracic spine, shoulder and/or elbow.

Quality of Symptoms

The quality of the symptoms informs reasoning; a burning pain associated with altered sensation indicates a neural tissue source. Clunks/clicks with or without pain especially following trauma would suggest possible carpal instability or tears in TFCC. Patients with suspected instability may also report that their wrist feels vulnerable especially when gripping or weightbearing (Christodoulou & Bainbridge 1999).

Intensity of Pain

The intensity of pain can be measured (as explained in Chapter 3) and contributes to reasoning of severity, alongside dependence on analgesic medication, sleep disturbance and limitations in activities. Severity along with irritability will guide the extent and vigour of the physical examination.

Constant or Intermittent Symptoms

Ascertain the frequency of symptoms. Constant unremitting pain may indicate a serious pathology. Cancer is rare in the wrist and hand; however, constant pain may be suggestive of avascular necrosis (AVN), most commonly affecting the scaphoid postfracture or lunate (Kienbock disease) (Wollstein et al., 2013). If associated with other symptoms, such as sensory, motor, vasomotor and/or trophic changes, incapacitating pain could indicate the development of chronic regional pain syndrome (CRPS), which can be a complication postdistal radial fracture (Davis & Baratz, 2010).

Relationship of Symptoms

If the patient has distal and proximal symptoms, identifying if they have one without the other will aid reasoning.

Behaviour of Symptoms

Aggravating Factors

For each symptomatic area, ask whether movements and/or positions aggravate the patients' symptoms, if they are able to maintain an activity or position or do they have to stop or change position (severity)? How long does it take for symptoms to ease once the position or movement is stopped (irritability)? Irritability and severity are explained in Chapter 3.

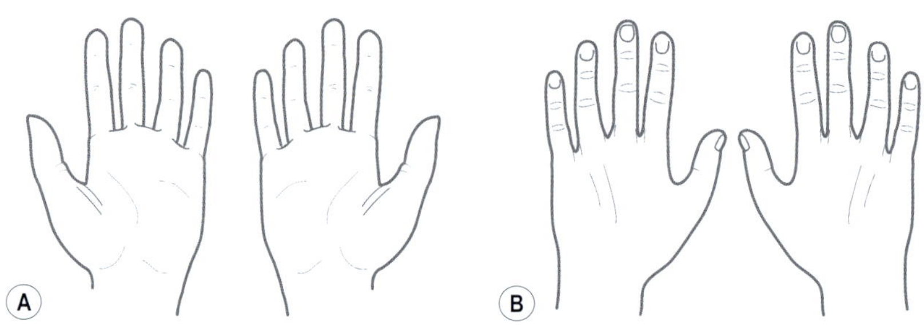

Fig. 12.1 Body chart for the hand. (A) Palmar surface. (B) Dorsal surface.

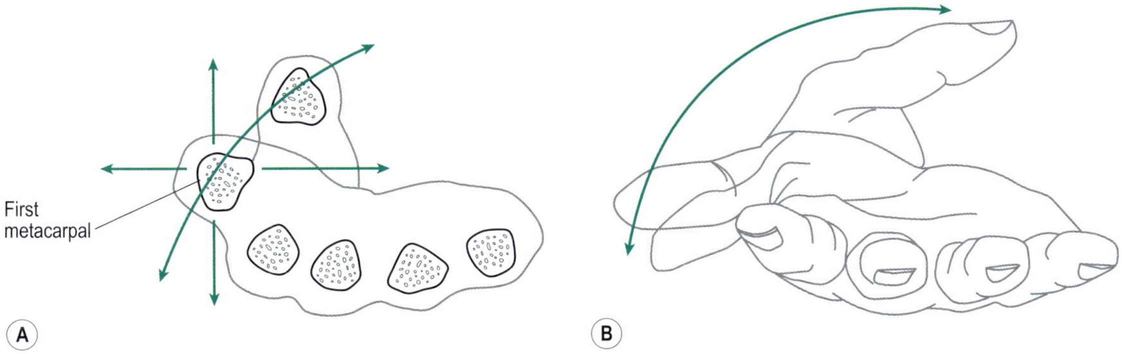

Fig. 12.2 Movement at the carpometacarpal joint of the thumb. (A) The arrows illustrate the multiple planes of movement that occur at the carpometacarpal joint of the thumb. Flexion/extension across the palm in a coronal plane about an anterior/posterior axis. Abduction/adduction away from the palm in a sagittal plane about a medial/lateral axis. (B) The arrow illustrates the movement of the thumb from reposition into opposition. Reposition is the normal anatomical position in the same plane as the second metacarpal to a position of extension and abduction into a position of full opposition – flexion and medial rotation.

The clinician should clinically reason how symptoms impact on function. For example, wrist extension, the close pack position provides a stable base for hand function, optimizing the length and tension of the long (extrinsic) flexor tendons; therefore loss of wrist extension range (20–30 degrees) will impact on grip. The thumb accounts for 50% of hand function due to its ability to oppose with the fingers (Dyer and Simmonds, 2011) (Fig. 12.2). Therefore limitation of thumb opposition/reposition and finger flexion/extension will impact most functional activities.

Easing Factors

For each symptomatic area, the clinician assesses irritability by asking what eases symptoms, how long it takes, and to what extent. For example, radiocarpal OA will be relieved by avoidance of loading and resting the wrist in a semiflexed position.

Collating information from aggravating and easing factors supports refinement of the hypothesis to further guide history taking and physical examination. If the patient's symptoms do not 'fit' a musculoskeletal pattern/presentation, then the clinician needs to consider other causes serious or otherwise and refer on.

Behaviour of Symptoms Over Time

How do symptoms behave over 24 hours?

Night symptoms. It is important to establish whether the patient has pain at night. If so, it is crucial to establish whether the pain is position-dependent indicative of a neuromusculoskeletal mechanism. For example, patients with carpal tunnel syndrome (CTS) commonly report symptoms, e.g. pain, numbness, paraesthesia waking them at night due to impaired neural microcirculation (Gelberman et al., 1981).

Morning and evening symptoms. The clinician asks about symptoms in the morning, through the day and at the end of the day. Stiffness/pain in the morning for 30 minutes or more may be suggestive of an inflammatory condition such RA. Patients with tendinopathies or neural tissue sensitivity may report worsening symptoms with increased repetition or load through the day.

Special/Screening Questions

As mentioned in Chapter 3, the clinician must differentiate between conditions that are suitable for conservative treatment and other systemic, neoplastic and nonmusculoskeletal conditions.

Past Medical History

A detailed medical history will identify contraindications or precautions to the physical examination, for example, does the patient have a history of fractures? Distal radial fracture can be indicative of low bone mineral density (BMD) along with other risk factors including age, females' menopausal status and lifestyle choices (Court-Brown & Caesar, 2006).

The state of a patient's general health will impact on their predisposition to symptoms/dysfunction and their recovery (see Chapter 3). Endocrine conditions such as thyroid dysfunction are associated with increased risk of Dupuytren contracture, trigger finger and CTS (Cakir et al., 2003). Diabetic patients also have an increased incidence of CTS (Gaston & Simpson, 2007). In poorly controlled diabetes, neuropathy affecting the hands may present with a thermal sensitivity deficit in a glove distribution, resulting in increased risk of burns due to impaired sensation (Kalk, 2005).

History of the Present Condition

For each symptomatic area, the clinician asks how long the symptoms have been present, whether there was a known cause that provoked the onset of the symptoms, such as a fall. The clinician may ask why and how the patient fell. For example, a fall on the outstretched hand can produce fractures to distal radius, commonly in older people with impaired bone density and/or scaphoid, ligamentous injury producing instability, or injury elsewhere in the kinetic chain at the elbow, shoulder or cervical spine.

In the case of lacerations, was the injury accidental or as a result of an assault with a knife or glass? Was the injury self-inflicted? Does the patient require additional psychological support?

Can the development of symptoms be associated with a change in the patient's lifestyle, e.g. a new job or leisure activity? Sustained postures or repeated movements can cause tissue impairments leading to sub-optimal movement patterns that can produce tissue injury (Caldwell & Khoo-Summers, 2010).

Is there a history of wrist and hand problems? If so, how many episodes and when were they? What was the cause? What was the duration of each episode? Did they seek treatment? Did the patient fully recover between episodes? If there have been no previous episodes, has the patient had any of symptoms elsewhere such as the cervical spine, thoracic spine, shoulder, elbow or any other relevant region? Clarifying the patient's journey can help the clinician to understand the patient's context and inform clinical reasoning.

To confirm a relationship between the symptoms, the clinician asks what happened to other symptoms when each symptom began. How symptoms have developed or changed over time will allow the clinician to stage the condition, which will inform prognosis.

Has there been any treatment to date? Has the patient seen a specialist or had any investigations, e.g. imaging, blood tests or interventions such as injections? Radiographs are commonly used to detect hand or joint fractures and dislocations. Scaphoid fractures are less easily detected on initial x-rays. Protocols recommend suspected scaphoid fractures should be re-x-rayed 10 days postinjury with a range of views recommended (Baldassarre & Hughes, 2013). Magnetic resonance imaging (MRI) or bone scans are useful in detecting subtle fractures, tears of the TFCC and scapholunate instabilities. Ultrasound is most appropriate for imaging tendons, tendon pulleys and ganglions. Other tests may include blood tests required if systemic inflammatory conditions such as RA or gout are suspected.

KNOWLEDGE CHECK

1. Which common fracture is frequently missed and can result in AVN?
2. Which tendons are implicated in de Quervain disease?
3. Which nerve is entrapped in carpal tunnel syndrome? When might symptoms be most likely reported and why?
4. In those presenting with radial fractures what additional questions should be asked and why?
5. Which modality is most useful for imaging tendons?

Planning the Physical Examination

The information from the subjective examination helps the clinician to identify an initial primary hypothesis, with alternative hypotheses as to the cause of a patient's symptoms. This will guide the physical examination and prompt the following questions.

- How extensive will the physical examination need to be? This will be guided by the assessment of severity and irritability for each symptomatic area (see Chapter 3)? If severity is judged to be high, physical testing will be limited to testing to or just short of symptom reproduction. For those with high irritability the physical examination will also be limited to avoid exacerbating symptoms, and the focus will shift to easing the patient's symptoms rather than provoking them. Alternatively, for patients with symptoms judged to be of low severity and irritability, physical testing will need to be more searching to reproduce symptoms.
- Are there any contraindications and/or precautions to the physical examination, such as bilateral symptoms indicative of spinal cord compression or an undiagnosed a recent fracture?

- What pain mechanisms are driving the patient's symptoms? What are the input mechanisms (sensory pathways)? For example, pain associated with sustained wrist and hand positions when typing may indicate ischaemic nociception. What are the processing mechanisms? What are the patient's beliefs/thoughts about their symptoms? Finally, what are the 'output mechanisms'? What is the patient's physical, psychological and behavioural response to their symptoms? Establishing the ongoing pain mechanisms causing/maintaining the patient's symptoms will inform all aspects of their care.
- What are the anatomical structures underneath the area of symptoms and those that refer into the wrist and hand region? For example, ulnar-sided pain could theoretically be referred from the cervical or thoracic spine, shoulder or elbow or could be from local structures, such as inferior radioulnar joint, TFCC, tendons such as FCU/ECU or the ulnar nerve. Based on the subjective information, the clinician decides which structures are most likely to be at fault and prioritizes physical testing accordingly. It is helpful to organize structures into ones that 'must', 'should' and 'could' be tested on day 1 and over subsequent sessions. This will develop the clinician's clinical reasoning and avoid a recipe-based assessment. A planning form can help guide the clinician's reasoning in the selection of physical examination procedures (see Appendices 3.1 and 3.2, Chapter 3). An understanding of the sensitivity and specificity (see chapter 4) of the tests applied should also be considered so that findings can be interpreted appropriately. Each significant physical test that either provokes or eases the patient's symptoms is highlighted in the patient's notes by an asterisk (*) for easy reference.

It is important that readers understand that the physical examination approaches included in this chapter are some of many and that those chosen are most clinically useful and include an indication of their level of support in the literature.

PHYSICAL EXAMINATION

Observation

Informal Observation

Throughout the subjective examination the clinician notices the patient's behaviour. Are they cradling their upper limb? Are functional limitations evident when they are undressing?

Formal Observation

Observation of posture. The clinician should observe the bony and soft-tissue contours of the spine, scapula, shoulder, elbow, wrist and hand, in a position relevant for that patient, for example, in sitting if symptoms are related to computer use (Caldwell & Khoo-Summers 2010).

When the hand is in a relaxed posture the fingers of the hand should naturally flex towards the tubercle of the scaphoid (Magee & Manske, 2021). Impaired alignment of the wrist and hand results in suboptimal movement patterns often impacting on function.

Observation of muscle form. The clinician observes muscle bulk and muscle tone comparing left and right sides; however, handedness and types of physical activity may well produce differences in muscle bulk between sides. Check for wasting of specific muscles, such as the first dorsal interosseous muscle supplied by the ulnar nerve as this may indicate a peripheral nerve problem.

Observation of soft tissues. The clinician observes the colour of the patient's limb and notes any swelling, increased hair growth on the hand, brittle fingernails, infection of the nail bed, sweating or dry palms, shiny skin, scars and bony deformities. These changes could be indicative of a range of conditions, such as peripheral nerve injury, peripheral vascular disease, diabetes mellitus, Raynaud disease or CRPS (Magee & Manske, 2021).

Common deformities of the hand include the following:

- Boutonnière deformity of fingers or thumb: the proximal interphalangeal joint (PIPJ) is flexed and the distal interphalangeal joint (DIPJ) is hyperextended (Fig. 12.3). The central slip of the extensor tendon is damaged following trauma or RA, so the lateral bands displace in a palmar direction, producing flexion of PIPJ (Eddington, 1993).
- Swan-neck deformity of fingers: the PIPJ is hyperextended due to damage to the volar plate or intrinsic muscle contracture producing flexion of the MCPJ and DIPJ (Fig. 12.4) (Eckhaus, 1993).
- Ulnar drift associated with RA results in a translocation of the carpus with deviation of the digits in an ulnar direction, increasing loading through the

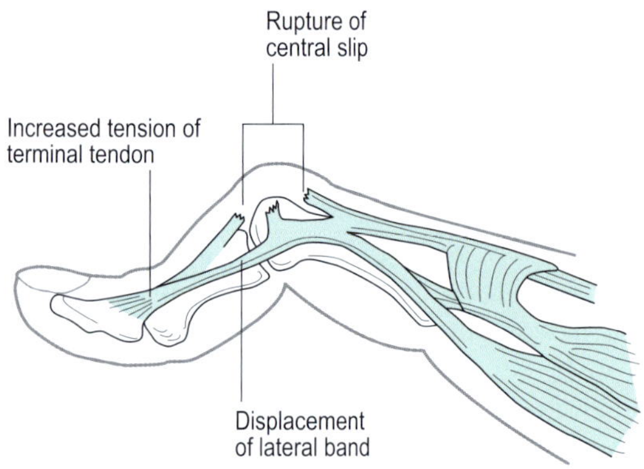

Fig. 12.3 Boutonnière deformity.

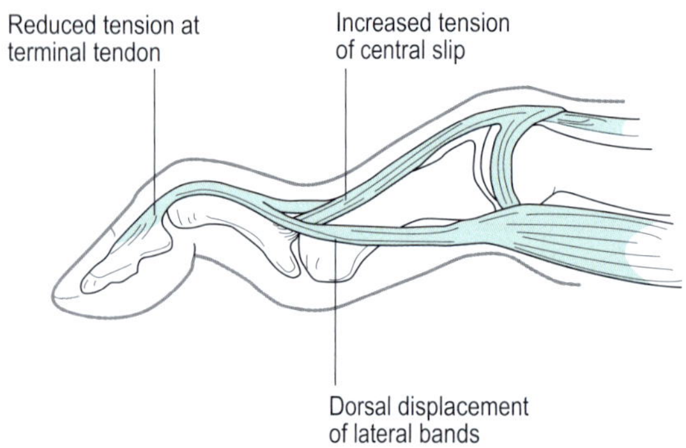

Fig. 12.4 Swan-neck deformity.

metacarpophalangeal ligaments (Morco and Bowden, 2015).

- Bouchard's nodes are calcific spurs over the dorsum of the PIPJs indicative of OA.
- Heberden's nodes are calcific spurs over the dorsum of the DIPJs and are indicative of OA.
- A pattern of deformity associated with OA of the CMC joint can produce a flexed CMC joint, failure of the deep anterior oblique ligament, resulting in hyperextension at MCPJ and reciprocal flexion at the interphalangeal joint. Unchecked ABPL pulls the thumb into an adducted position impacting on functional reposition/opposition (Batra & Kanvinde, 2007).
- Claw hand: the little and ring fingers are hyperextended at the MCPJ and flexed at the interphalangeal joints due to ulnar nerve palsy.
- Mallet finger: rupture of the terminal extensor tendon at the DIPJ is usually a result of trauma, producing a flexed distal phalanx.
- Nail health can be an indicator of underlying systemic disease, e.g. clubbing indicative of respiratory or cardiac disorders (Gollins and de Berker, 2021).
- Dupuytren's contracture of the palmar fascia produces a fixed flexion deformity of the MCPJ and PIPJ, on the ring and/or little finger, more common in males in the 50–70-year age group.

Functional Testing

Functional testing of the hand will include analysis of power and precision (or pinch) grips, required for activities, such as using a screwdriver. Is range of movement impacting on function or is there a strength deficit or a combination of factors (Gracia-Ibanez et al., 2018)?

Dexterity can be tested using the Purdue pegboard test (Blair et al., 1987), nine-hole peg test (Totten & Flinn-Wagner, 1992) and Minnesota rate of manipulation test (Totten & Flinn-Wagner, 1992).

Active Physiological Movements

The active physiological movements of the forearm, wrist and hand are shown in Table 12.1.

Movements can be tested with the patient in supine or sitting comparing right and left limbs. Range of movement for forearm and wrist can be measured using a goniometer. For finger range, a specific finger goniometer or finger flexion tip measurement to palm crease might be easier. The choice of which active movements are tested will depend on the patient's reported aggravating and easing factors and the analysis of functional tests. For example, if a patient has difficulty with pincer grip, wrist extension, index finger flexion and thumb opposition should be examined. For each active physiological movement, the clinician notes the following:

- willingness of the patient to move
- range of movement available
- quality of movement, e.g. coordination, muscle activation patterning
- behaviour of pain through the range of movement.

The clinician establishes the patient's symptoms at rest, prior to each movement, and modifies/corrects any movement deviation to reason clinically relevance to the patient's symptoms.

Symptom Modification

Modification of active movements can assist in differentiating the sources of symptoms (Hengeveld & Banks

TABLE 12.1 Active Physiological Movements
Forearm pronation Forearm supination Wrist extension Wrist flexion Radial deviation Ulnar deviation Carpometacarpal and metacarpophalangeal joints of thumb: • Flexion • Extension • Abduction • Adduction • Opposition Distal intermetacarpal joints: • Horizontal flexion • Horizontal extension Metacarpophalangeal joints (of the fingers): • Flexion • Extension • Adduction • Abduction Proximal and distal interphalangeal joints: • Flexion • Extension
Possible modifications to physiological movements
Repeated Speed altered Combined movements and sequencing Added compression or distraction Sustained Injuring movement Differentiation tests Functional movements
Identify any effect of the modifications of physiological movements on patient's signs and symptoms
Reassess all *asterisks
If necessary screen any proximal and distal regions that may refer to the area
Cervical spine Thoracic spine Shoulder Wrist and hand

et al., 2014). For example, when supination reproduces the patient's wrist symptoms, differentiation between the inferior radioulnar joint and the radiocarpal joint can be useful in refining a working hypothesis of the underlying source of symptoms. The patient actively moves the forearm into supination just to the point where symptoms are produced. The clinician applies a passive supination force to the radius and ulna; if the symptoms are coming from the inferior radioulnar joint, then pain may increase. The inferior radioulnar joint is released whilst a supination force to radiocarpal joint around the scaphoid and lunate is applied. If the symptoms are coming from the radiocarpal joint, then pain may increase. A pronation force to the scaphoid and lunate might then be expected to reduce symptoms (Fig. 12.5).

Active movements demonstrating handling for application of overpressure are shown in Fig. 12.6, and these are applied to clear the joints.

Passive Physiological Movements

All active movements can be examined passively. For the wrist and hand, the clinician needs to carefully consider the starting position to account for the long flexors and extensors of the wrist; for example, to test articular range of wrist extension the fingers will need to be flexed.

Joint Integrity Tests

When used in isolation, joint integrity tests are not sufficiently robust to diagnose an instability and must be combined with a subjective history especially of trauma, reports of clunking or weakness and demonstrate increased range/symptoms on passive movement tests or point tenderness over specific ligaments on palpation (Prosser et al., 2011; Valdes & LaStayo, 2013).

At the wrist, the most common ligamentous instabilities occur with lunate either extending dorsally on scaphoid — dorsal intercalated segment instability (DISI) or rotating in a palmar/volar direction on triquetrum — volar intercalated segment instability (VISI). Midcarpal instability (MCI) of the capitate is less common and impacts on biomechanics between proximal and distal carpal rows.

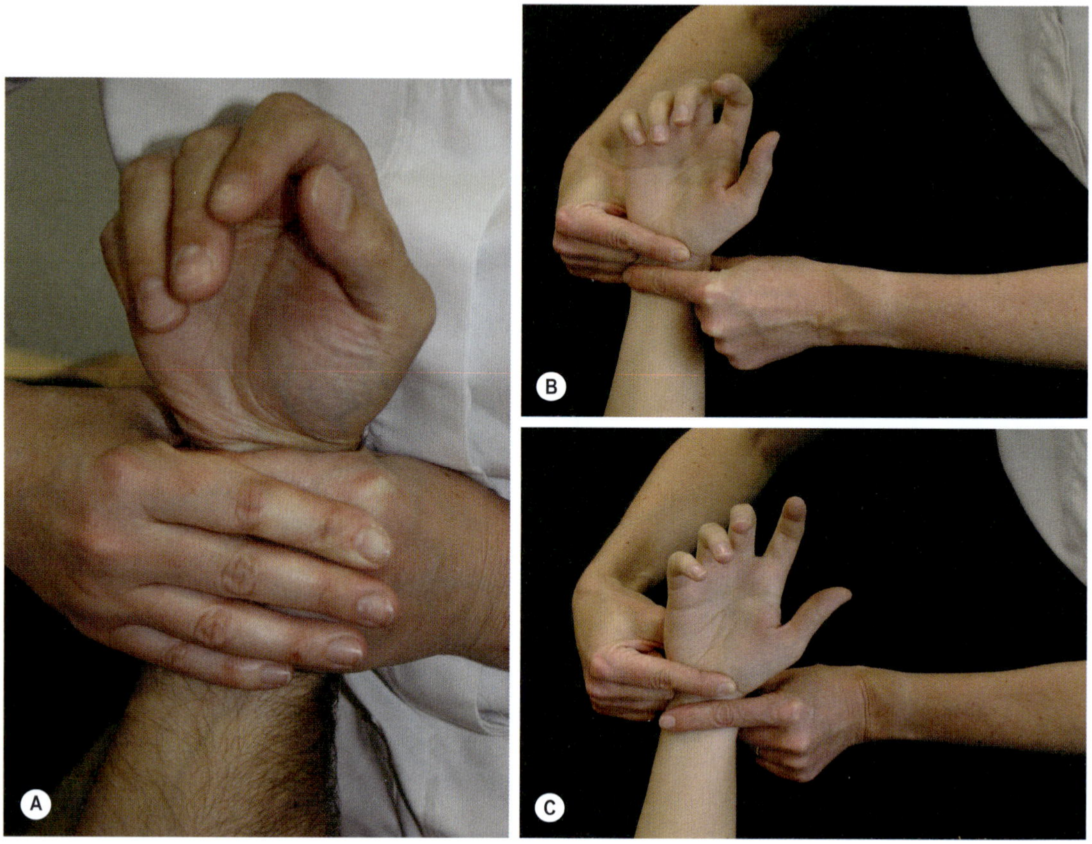

Fig. 12.5 Differentiation between the inferior radioulnar joint and radiocarpal joint. The patient supinates the forearm to the onset of symptoms. The clinician then (A) applies a supination force to the radius and ulna; (B) releases the radius and ulna and applies a supination force around the proximal row of carpal bones to affect the radiocarpal joint, and (C) supination of the radius and ulna is maintained, and a pronation force is applied to the proximal carpal row. The clinician determines the effect of each overpressure on the symptoms. The symptoms would be expected to increase when the supination force is applied to the symptomatic level; further examination of accessory movements of individual bones may then identify a symptomatic joint.

Watson (Scaphoid Shift) Test

With the patient's elbow stabilized in slight pronation on the table, the clinician maintains an anteroposterior glide on the scaphoid tubercle while passively moving the wrist from a position of ulnar deviation and slight extension to radial deviation and slight flexion (Fig. 12.7). This tests the scapholunate interosseous ligament for a suspected DISI. Posterior subluxation of the scaphoid, out of the scaphoid fossa, over the dorsal rim of the radius produces a 'clunk' on release with reproduction of the patient's pain indicating a ligamentous instability (Watson et al., 1988). A painless clunk is found in normal wrists (Wolfe et al., 1997). This test is estimated to be moderately accurate in detecting instability with sensitivity of 69% and specificity of 66% (Prosser et al., 2011). Progressive disruption of proximal row stability can lead to scapho-lunate advanced collapse (SLAC) accounting for 55% of degenerative wrist OA (Rainbow et al., 2016).

Lunotriquetral Ballottement (Reagan's) Test

This tests for instability between lunate and triquetral due to a loss of integrity of the lunotriquetral ligament (VISI). Excessive movement, crepitus or pain with anterior and posterior glide of the lunate on the triquetrum indicates a positive test (Butterfield et al.,

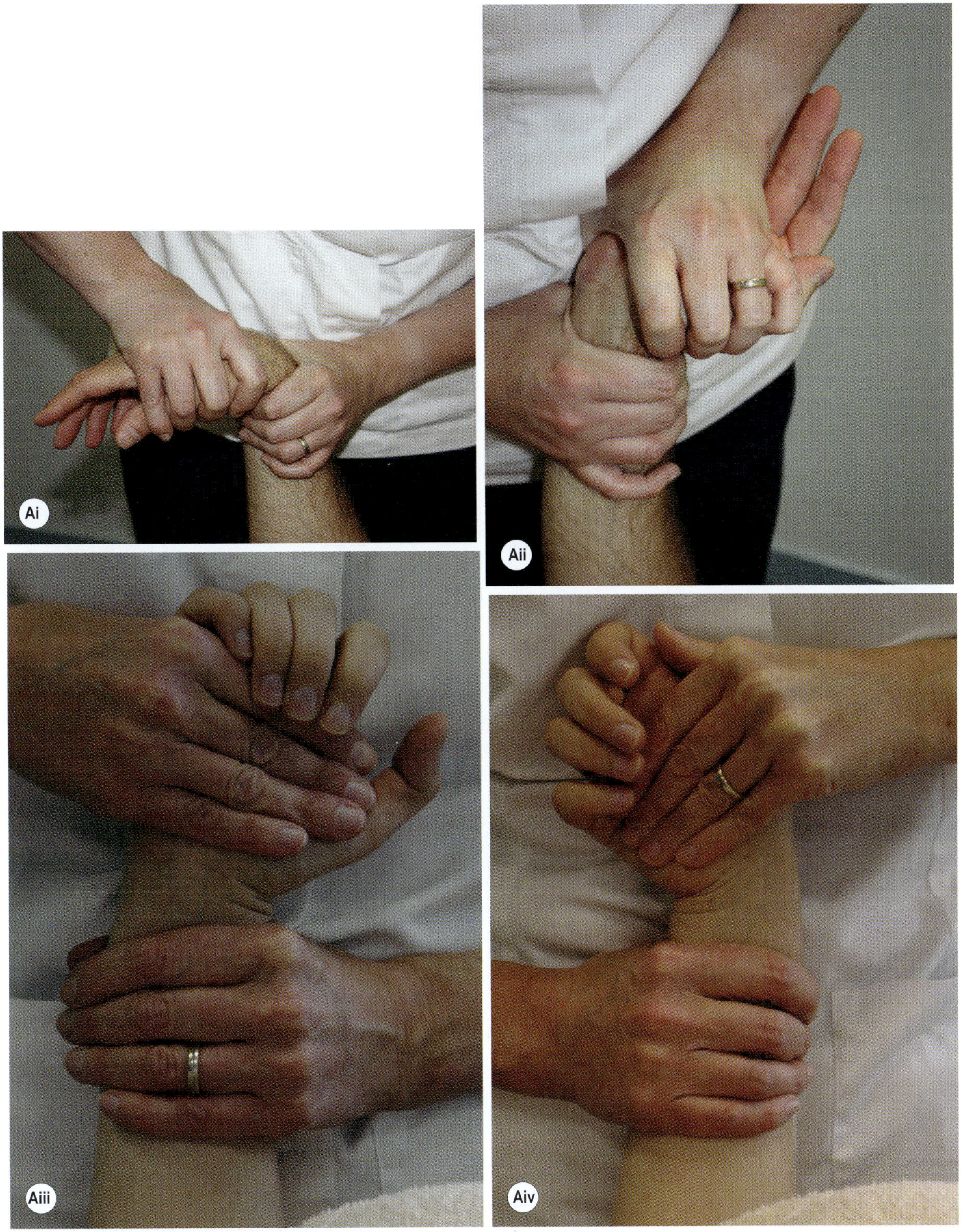

Fig. 12.6 (A) Overpressure to the wrist and hand. (Ai) Flexion. The wrist and hand are grasped by both hands and taken into flexion. (Aii) Extension. The right hand supports the patient's forearm, and the left hand takes the wrist and hand into extension. (Aiii) Radial deviation. The left hand supports just proximal to the wrist joint while the right hand moves the wrist into radial deviation. (Aiv) Ulnar deviation. The right hand supports just proximal to the wrist joint while the left hand moves the wrist into ulnar deviation.

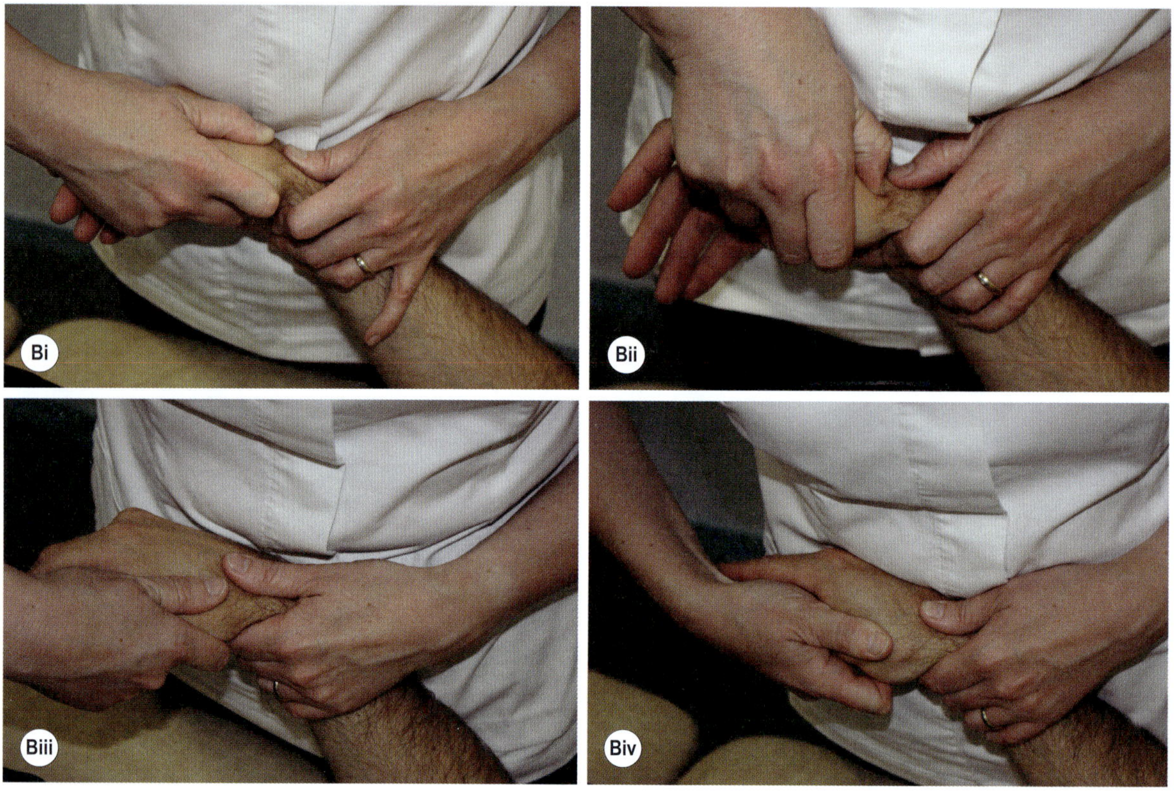

Fig. 12.6, cont'd (B) Carpometacarpal joint of thumb. For all these movements, the hands are placed immediately proximal and distal to the joint line. (Bi) Flexion. The left hand supports the trapezium while the right hand takes the first metacarpal into flexion. (Bii) Extension. The left hand supports the trapezium while the right hand takes the first metacarpal into extension. (Biii) Abduction and adduction. The left hand supports the trapezium while the right hand takes the first metacarpal into abduction and adduction. (Biv) Opposition. The right hand supports the trapezium while the left hand takes the first metacarpal across the palm into opposition.

2002). This test has limited evidence to identify robustness. This injury is often associated with TFCC tears (Hattam & Smeatham, 2010), and arthroscopy is considered gold standard for diagnosis (Lindau, 2016).

Midcarpal Shift Test

Laxity of both the dorsal radio triquetral and palmar ulnar arcuate ligaments allows the head of the capitate and hamate to sag, producing a palmar midcarpal instability (PMCI). This reduces the smooth transition of the proximal carpal row from flexion to extension during ulnar deviation of the wrist and normal translation of load from the proximal to the distal carpal rows (Lichtman & Wroten, 2006). Some patients may be hypermobile and can demonstrate clicking on ulnar deviation in the absence of trauma.

With the patient's wrist in neutral and forearm pronated, the clinician places their thumb on the dorsal distal portion of capitate applying a force in a palmar direction whilst deviating the wrist in an ulnar direction. The test is positive if a painful 'clunk' is felt and the manoeuvre reproduces the patient's symptoms (Prosser et al., 2011; Valdes & LaStayo, 2013). Comparisons should be made with the nonaffected side. Several studies have identified sensitivity as 64% and specificity 45% for this test (La Stayo & Howell, 1995; Prosser et al., 2011).

Triangular Fibrocartilaginous Complex Load Test

The TFCC, a complex stabilizing structure of the inferior radioulnar joint, is vulnerable to tearing following trauma or due to degenerative changes. This load-

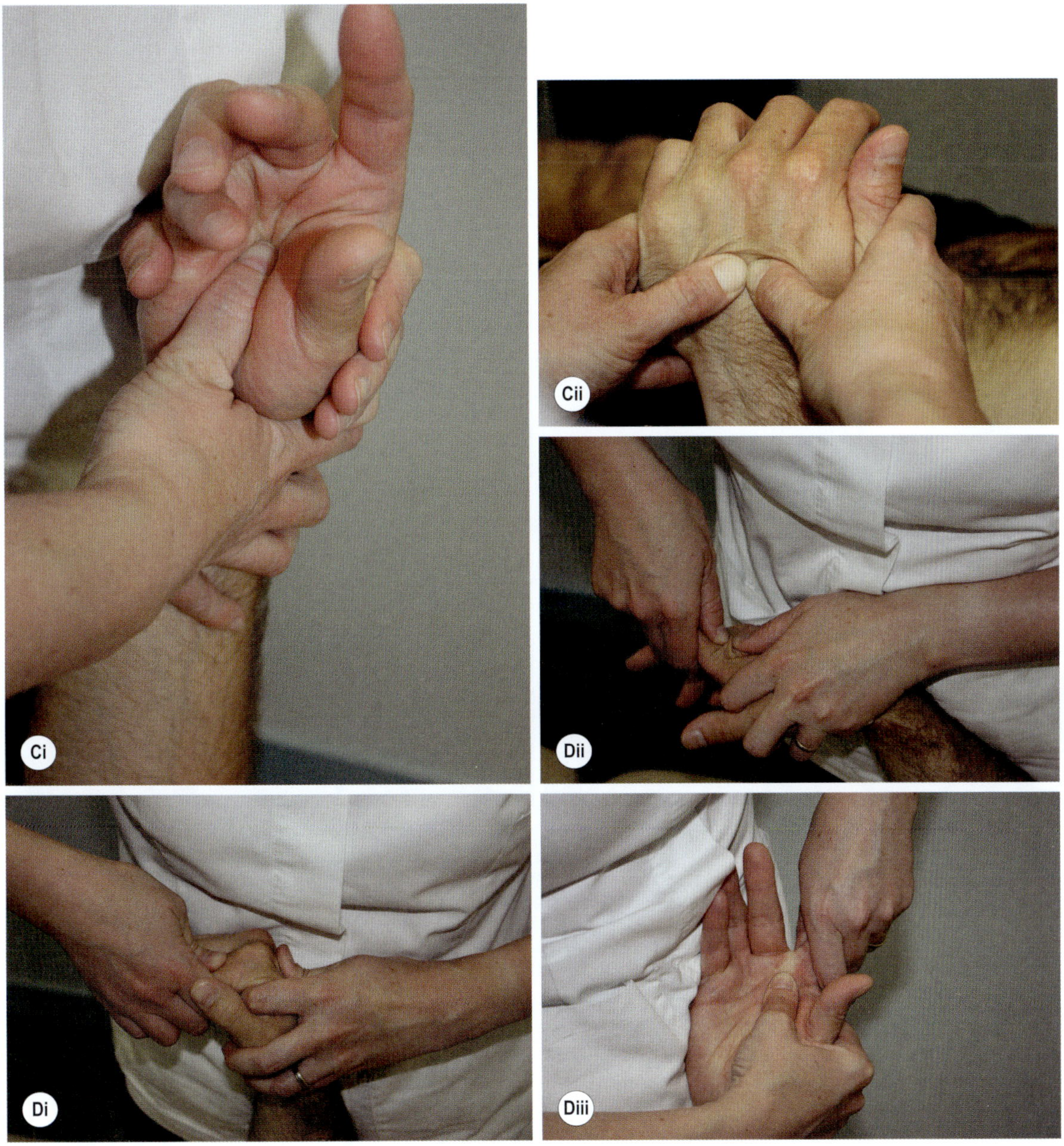

Fig. 12.6, cont'd (C) Distal intermetacarpal joints. (Ci) Horizontal flexion. The right thumb is placed in the centre of the palm at the level of the metacarpal heads. The left hand cups around the back of the metacarpal heads and moves them into horizontal flexion. (Cii) Horizontal extension. The thumbs are placed in the centre of the dorsum of the palm at the level of the metacarpal heads. The fingers wrap around the anterior aspect of the hand and pull the metacarpal heads into horizontal extension. (D) Metacarpophalangeal joints. (Di) Flexion. The left hand supports the metacarpal while the right hand takes the proximal phalanx into flexion. (Dii) Extension. The right hand supports the metacarpal while the left hand takes the proximal phalanx into extension. (Diii) Abduction and adduction. The right hand supports the metacarpal while the left hand takes the proximal phalanx into abduction as shown.

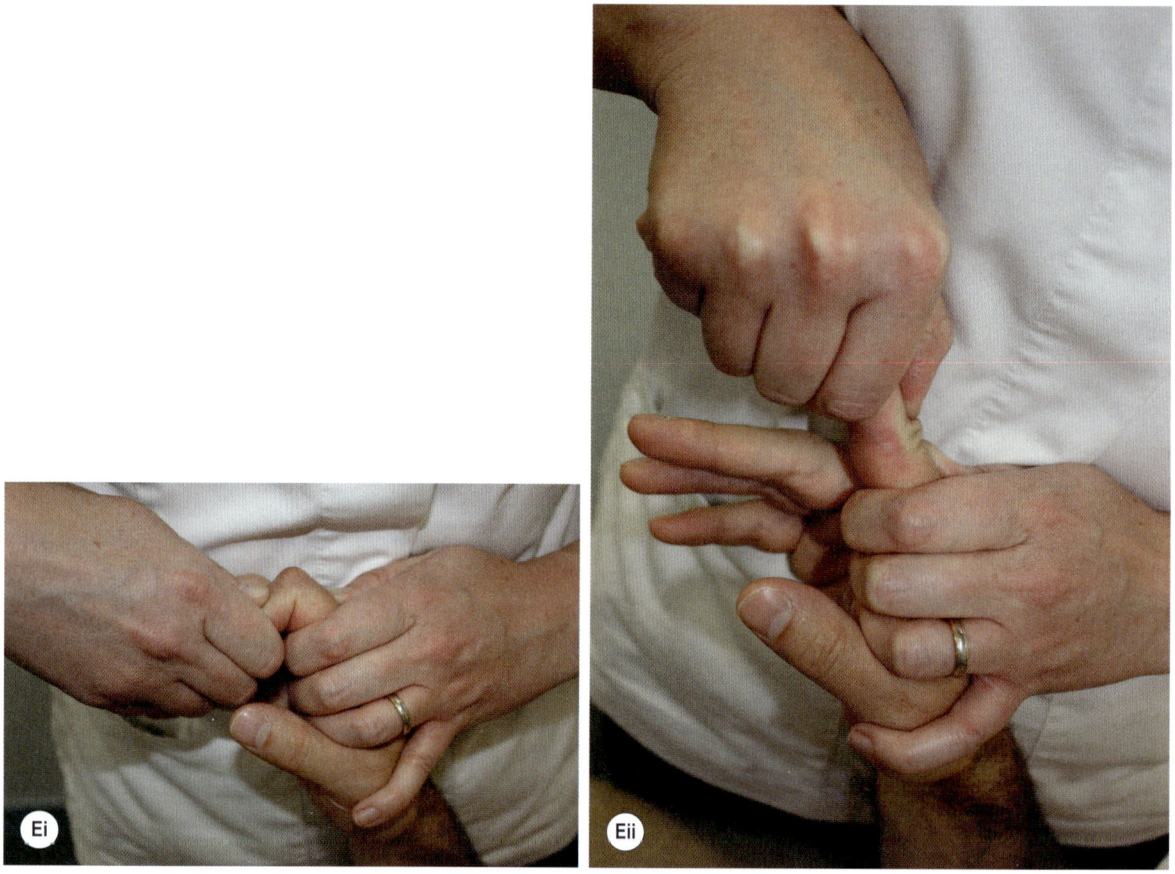

Fig. 12.6, cont'd (E) Proximal and distal interphalangeal joints. (Ei) Flexion. The left hand supports the metacarpophalangeal joint in extension while the right hand takes the proximal interphalangeal joint into flexion. (Eii) Extension. The left hand supports the metacarpophalangeal joint in extension while the right hand takes the proximal interphalangeal joint into extension.

bearing test resembles the meniscal test of the knee (Fig. 12.8). The patient's forearm is stabilized and, as if shaking hands, the clinician places her hand in the patient's palm. An axial compression load is then applied to the patient's hand while ulnar deviation is added (Hattam & Smeatham, 2010). Localized pain, apprehension and/or a click would indicate a positive test. A positive test combined with a history of pain on pronation, ulnar deviation and gripping, with crepitus and tenderness over the TFCC, would increase suspicion of a TFCC lesion (Bulstrode et al., 2002).

Ligamentous Instability Test for the Joints of the Fingers and Thumb

Excessive movement when a varus or valgus force is applied to the joint is indicative of laxity of the collateral ligaments. Most commonly affected is the ulnar collateral ligament of the thumb which can also result in an avulsion fracture. The ulnar side of the thumb will be tender on palpation, and there may be swelling and a haematoma (Mandhkani & Rhemrev, 2013).

Application of a valgus force in a 30-degree MCP flexion test will load the dorsal capsule and part of the ulnar collateral ligament. A lack of an end-feel and marked laxity in extension compared to the non-injured thumb would indicate a complete rupture of the ulnar collateral ligament (Tang, 2011).

Axial Compression Test (Grind Test)

OA of the CMC joint is the most common site of degenerative joint disease of the hand and is characterized

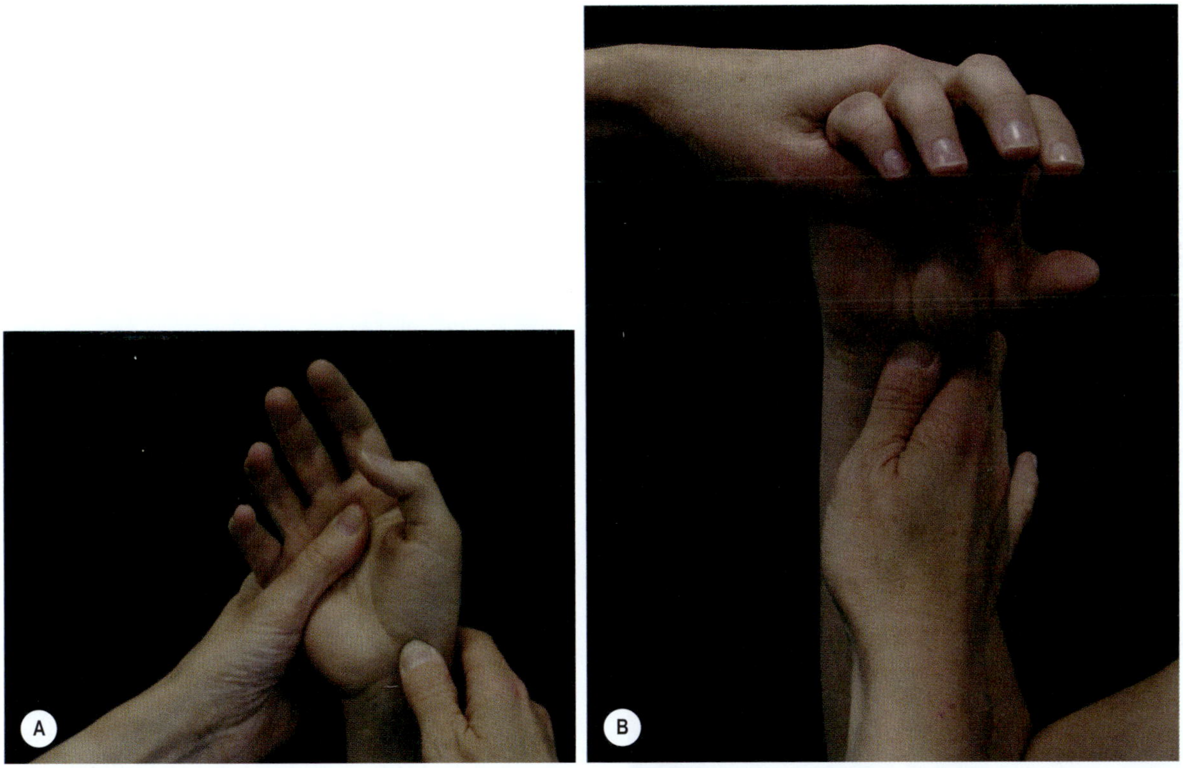

Fig. 12.7 (A and B) Watson (scaphoid shift) test. Apply a posterior glide to the scaphoid whilst moving the wrist from ulnar deviation and slight extension to radial deviation and slight flexion.

by pain on gripping activities (Gelberman et al., 2015). Diagnosis can be staged from I (mild) to IV (severe) using radiology classification (Eaton & Glickel, 1987).

The clinician stabilizes the radial side of the patient's hand with one hand whilst the other hand grips the shaft of the first metacarpal. An axial load with rotation is applied down the shaft. The test is positive if pain is elicited with reported sensitivity 64% and specificity 100%. This is a provocative test and so needs to be applied with care (Hattam & Smeatham, 2010) (Fig. 12.9).

Pressure-Shear Test

Sela et al. (2019) proposed a less provocative test with the addition of a pressure-shear force across the CMC joint with pain reproduction indicating a positive finding (sensitivity 99% and specificity 95%).

Muscle Tests

Muscle system examination is based on the patient's subjective history as well as observations of posture and movement (Kendall et al., 2010; Hislop et al., 2013). See Chapter 4 for details of muscle testing.

Muscle Strength

Manual muscle testing may be carried out for the following muscle groups:

- elbow – flexors and extensors
- forearm – pronators and supinators
- wrist joint – flexors, extensors, radial deviators and ulnar deviators
- thenar eminence – flexors, extensors, adductors, abductors and opposers
- hypothenar eminence – flexors, extensors, adductors, abductors and opposers
- finger – flexors, extensors, abductors and adductors.

Grip strength can be measured using a dynamometer to provide some baseline quantitative data on which to evaluate progress (Toemen et al., 2011). Left and right sides can be compared but variance due to hand dominance will need to be accounted for. A range

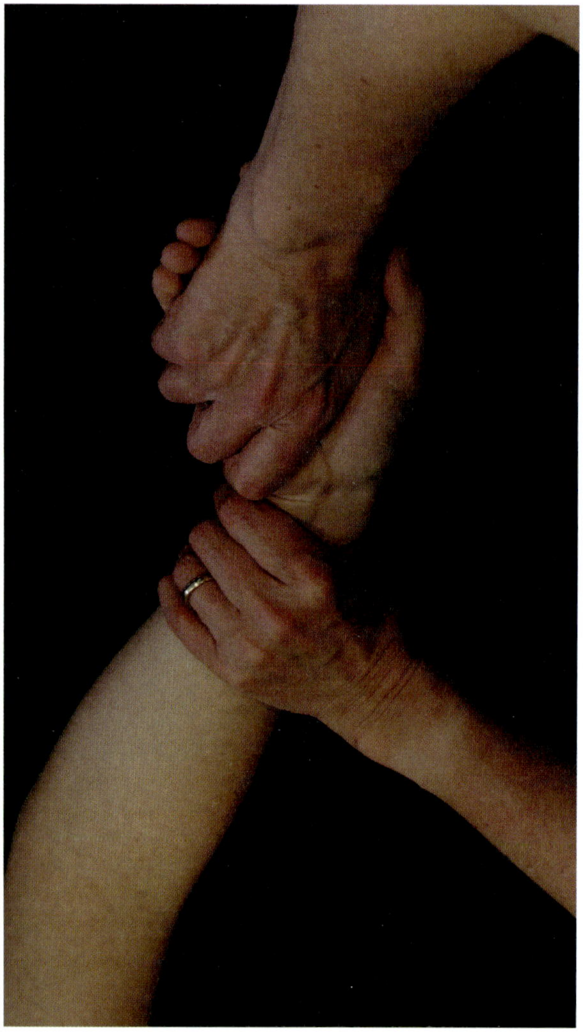

Fig. 12.8 Triangular fibrocartilaginous complex load test. The patient's forearm is stabilized and, as if shaking hands, the clinician places her hand in the patient's palm. An axial compression load is then applied to the patient's hand while ulnar deviation is added.

of pinch-grip strengths can also be measured using a pinch meter (Mathiowetz et al., 1985).

Muscle Length

Tenodesis action. To test the normal balance in the extrinsic flexor and extensor muscle length with the wrist flexed, the fingers and thumb will extend; with the wrist extended, the fingers will flex towards the palm and the thumb opposes towards the index finger (Neumann, 2010).

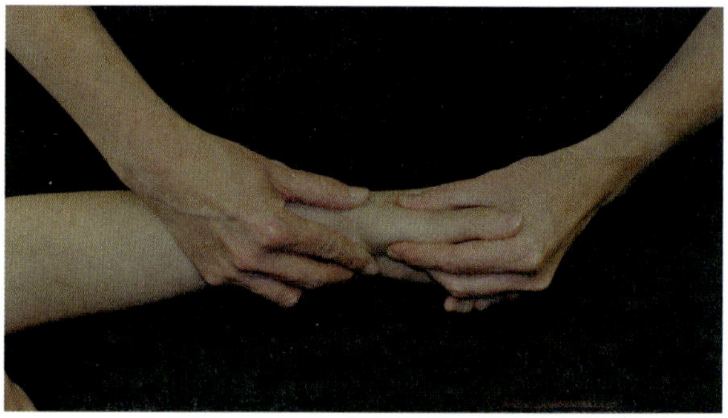

Fig. 12.9 Axial compression test (grind test). The clinician stabilizes the radial side of the patient's hand with one hand whilst the other hand grips the shaft of the first metacarpal. An axial load with rotation is applied down the shaft. The test is positive if pain is elicited. This is a provocative test and so needs to be applied with care.

Intrinsic muscle tightness. To test for muscle tightness of the intrinsics, e.g. interossei, the MCPJ is held in extension whilst the clinician passively flexes the proximal interphalangeal (PIP) joints. The test is repeated in MCP flexion. If PIP joint flexion is restricted in MCP extension but not in MCP flexion then restriction is due to the intrinsic muscle tightness. If restricted range remains unchanged, then the restriction is likely to be articular.

Extrinsic muscle tightness. With the wrist in neutral, the clinician compares the range of passive PIPJ movement with the MCPJs positioned in flexion and then in extension. If the PIPJ can be passively flexed while the MCP is extended but not when the MCPJ is flexed, this indicates extrinsic extensor tightness. Conversely, extrinsic flexor tightness is where there is a greater range of PIPJ extension with the MCPJs in flexion than with the MCPJs in extension.

The clinician may test the length of other muscles (Kendall et al., 2010; Hislop et al., 2013).

Isometric Muscle Testing

Test forearm pronation and supination, wrist flexion, extension, radial and ulnar deviation, finger and thumb flexion, extension, abduction and adduction and thumb opposition in different parts of the physiological range depending on subjective clues to provoking activities. The clinician observes the quality of the muscle contraction to hold the position, the adoption of substitution strategies as well as the reproduction of the patient's symptoms.

Other Muscle/Tendon Tests

Tests for De Quervain disease. De Quervain disease, a stenosing tenosynovitis of the ABPL and EPB tendons in the first dorsal compartment, usually presents with localized swelling and pain over the tip of the radial styloid associated with gripping activities (Batteson et al., 2008).There is some confusion regarding the two tests commonly used to assess for de Quervain disease (Goubau et al., 2014). For the Eichhoff test (often mistakenly named the Finkelstein test) patients are asked to oppose their thumb across their palm and clench their fist, whilst the clinician passively deviates their wrist into ulnar deviation (Goubau et al., 2014). This test has been associated with false positives in normal wrists. The Finkelstein test is a passive test, whereby, with the patient's thumb flexed across the palm, the clinician fixes the lower forearm with one hand and then gently passively takes the wrist into ulnar deviation (Fig. 12.10) (Elliott, 1992). These passive tests rely in pain reproduced from tendons being stressed against the radial styloid, a stretch that will also stress ligamentous structures producing false-positive results (Magee & Manske, 2021). The lack of specificity, variation in description and application may explain why findings from these tests are not supported in the literature (Valdes & LaStayo, 2013; Cheimonidou et al., 2019).

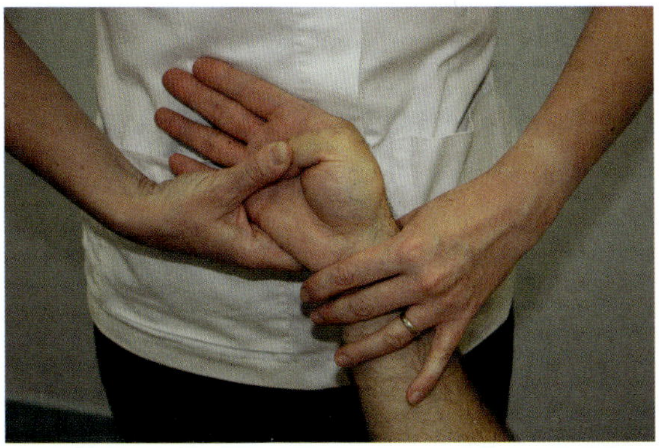

Fig. 12.10 Finkelstein test. The patient flexes the thumb and the clinician guides the patient's wrist passively into ulnar deviation of the wrist. (Handling as described by Elliott, 1992.)

Goubau et al. (2014) proposed the wrist hyperflexion and abduction of the thumb (WHAT) test as an alternative active-loading test for APL and EBP. A Sensitivity of 99% and specificity of 29% was reported for this test. The patient's wrist is positioned in hyperflexion, with the thumb abducted in full MP and IP extension, abduction is resisted against the therapist's index finger (Fig. 12.11).

Sweater finger sign test. Loss of DIPJ flexion when a fist is made is a positive test indicating a ruptured flexor digitorum profundus (FDP) tendon. The ring finger is most commonly affected (Magee & Manske, 2021).

Test for flexor digitorum superficialis. Whilst the clinician holds all of remaining fingers in extension, the patient actively flexes the free finger. Flexion produced by flexor digitorum superficialis (FDS) should occur at the MCPJ and PIPJ. The DIPJ should be flail as the FDP has been immobilized. If the FDS is inactive, the finger will flex strongly at the DIPJ as well as at the PIPJ and MCPJ, indicating activity of FDP. If the finger does not flex at all, neither flexor is active. Be aware that a proportion of the population does not have an effective FDS to the little finger, so the test is then invalidated for this digit (Townley et al., 2010).

Neurological Testing

The clinician will use clinical reasoning from reported distribution and quality of symptoms, to justify a neurological examination.

Integrity of the Nervous System

Dermatomes/peripheral nerves. Sensory testing of the upper limb can be done as described in Chapter 4. Knowledge of the cutaneous distribution of nerve roots (dermatomes) and peripheral nerves (radial [C5—T1], median [C5—T1] and ulnar [C7—T1]) enables the clinician to distinguish sensory loss due to a spinal nerve root or brachial plexus lesion from that of a peripheral nerve lesion.

Stereognosis can also be tested by placing objects in the patient's hand and recording the time taken to recognize objects by touch alone. Testing of two-point discrimination can also identify variance but has limitations (Lundborg and Rosen, 2004).

Myotomes/peripheral nerves. A working knowledge of nerve roots and peripheral nerves enables the clinician

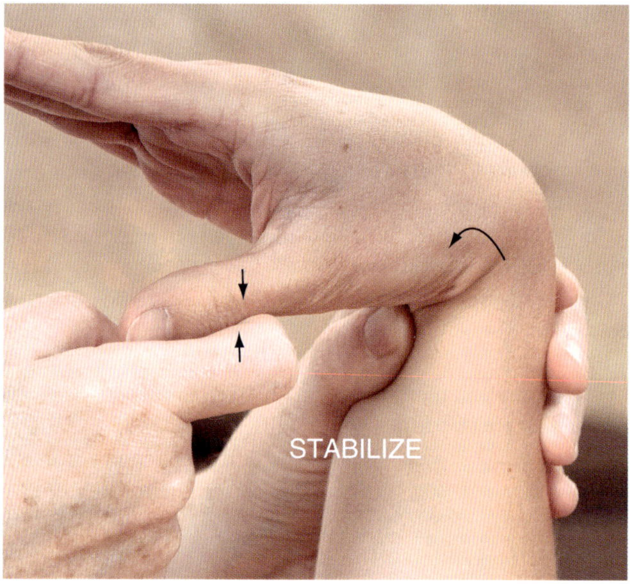

Fig 12.11 Wrist hyperflexion and abduction of the thumb (WHAT) test. (From Magee & Manske, 2021.)

to differentiate motor loss due to a root lesion from that of a peripheral nerve lesion. The distributions are shown handling for these tests in Chapter 4.

Neurodynamic Tests

The upper-limb neurodynamic tests (ULNT 1, 2a, 2b and 3) may be used to assess for a possible neural tissue contribution to the patient's wrist and hand symptom(s). Review handling for these tests in Chapter 4.

Testing for Compression Neuropathy

Median nerve. The median nerve can be palpated indirectly at the wrist between palmaris longus medially and flexor carpi radialis laterally.

Compression of the median nerve, under the flexor tendons in the retinaculum, results in CTS, the most common, peripheral, nerve entrapment neuropathy (Clark et al., 2011). Symptoms typically include burning pain, pins and needles, weakness and night pain, although no universally accepted diagnostic criteria exist. The use of Tinel's and Phalen's tests was supported in a review by Valdes and LaStayo (2013).

Tinel's sign (at the wrist). With the patient's wrist in neutral, the clinician taps firmly the midpoint of the carpal tunnel at the wrist. Paraesthesia or numbness in the sensory distribution of the median nerve would indicate a positive test. Specificity and sensitivity values vary for this test (specificity 30%—100%, sensitivity 38%—100%: Brüske et al., 2002; El Miedany et al., 2008), and so the test should be used in conjunction with other tests (Hattam & Smeatham, 2010).

Phalen's wrist flexion test. With the patient's elbow in full extension and forearm in pronation the patient's wrist is held in full flexion for 1 minute. Paraesthesia in the distribution of the median nerve indicates a positive test (Amirfeyz et al., 2005).

Modified carpal compression test. A blood pressure cuff is wrapped around the wrist and inflated to 100 mmHg for 30 seconds. An 8 cm long, 8 mm diameter wooden pencil-like object can be laid along the median nerve under the cuff to apply more direct pressure to the median nerve during the test (Tekeoglu et al. 2007). This is a useful alternative to Phalen's test, whereby the range of movement at the wrist may be restricted or painful (González del Pino et al., 1997).

Ulnar nerve. The ulnar nerve is superficial at the wrist and can be palpated in Guyon's canal between pisiform and the hook of hamate. The nerve can be injured following fractures or due to ganglions or mechanical compression when cycling or typing (Baker et al., 2007).

Froment's sign for ulnar nerve paralysis. The patient holds a piece of paper between the index finger and thumb in a lateral key grip, and the clinician attempts to pull it away. Flexion at the interphalangeal joint of the thumb due to paralysis of adductor pollicis (Froment's sign) and clawing of the little and ring fingers as a result of paralysis of the interossei and lumbrical muscles and the unopposed action of the extrinsic extensors and flexors will indicate ulnar nerve paralysis (Magee & Manske, 2021).

Radial nerve. The radial nerve is palpable at the terminal parts of the radial sensory nerve in the anatomical snuffbox at the wrist (Butler, 2000).

Vascular Assessment

If it is suspected that the patient's circulation is compromised the pulses of the radial and ulnar arteries at the wrist should be palpated.

Allen Test for the Radial and Ulnar Arteries at the Wrist

The clinician applies pressure to the radial and ulnar arteries at the wrist whilst asking the patient to open and close their hand a few times and then to keep it open. To test the patency of each artery, release the pressure over the radial artery and then repeat the process for the ulnar artery. The hand should flush within 5 seconds on release of the pressure (Magee & Manske, 2021).

Figure-of-Eight Measurement

This simple test is a reliable and valid method of measuring swelling in the hand (Pellecchia, 2003). With the patient's wrist/hand in neutral position, a measuring tape is placed on the distal ulnar styloid and brought horizontally along the palmar aspect of the wrist. The tape is brought diagonally across the dorsum of the hand and over the fifth MCPJ line, across the anterior surface of the MCPJs, then across the back of the hand to where the tape began, and the measurement is recorded in centimetres. This value can be compared to the measurement for the other hand (Magee & Manske, 2021).

Palpation

The extent of palpation will depend on the clinician's clinical reasoning and primary hypotheses. A good anatomical knowledge and systematic approach will ensure accuracy.

Suggested Approach to Systematic Palpation

- Palmar/anterior surface: palpate tendons for tenderness, crepitus: flexor carpi radialis, flexor pollicis longus, FDS, FDP, palmaris longus, flexor carpi ulnaris. Check ulnar and radial pulses, palmar fascia for thickening, thenar and hypothenar eminences for tone/bulk, flexion creases, longitudinal and transverse arches of the hand. The hook of hamate – pisohamate /Guyon's canal—a possible site of ulnar nerve compression. Assess the gap between flexor carpi ulnaris and distal ulnar styloid for TFCC tears and ulnotriquetral ligament tears.
- Dorsal/posterior surface: palpate the radial styloid, which should project more distally than the ulnar. This normal variance can be lost post-Colles fracture, resulting in excessive loading on the TFCC. Palpate ABPL/EPB and extensor pollicis longus (EPL) each side of the anatomical snuffbox; tenderness in the floor of the snuffbox can indicate scaphoid fracture, avascular necrosis or radial nerve sensitivity. Palpate the extensor tendons; check for increased or decreased prominence of carpal bones – scaphoid (through snuffbox or tubercle anteriorly), lunate, triquetral, pisiform, trapezium, trapezoid, capitate (located as a dip when the wrist is flexed) and hamate.

Accessory Movements

Wrist and hand accessory movements are shown in Fig. 12.12 and listed in Table 12.2; however, it is not necessary to test all of those listed, as selection will be based on clinical reasoning of findings so far in the physical examination. For example, if wrist extension is limited then examination will initially primarily focus on the radiocarpal joint. Accessory examination can be further refined, using the Kaltenborn tests to explore the intercarpal joints in more detail. It is not necessary to complete all 10 parts of the test. For example, if the patient's symptoms are located around the thumb, the

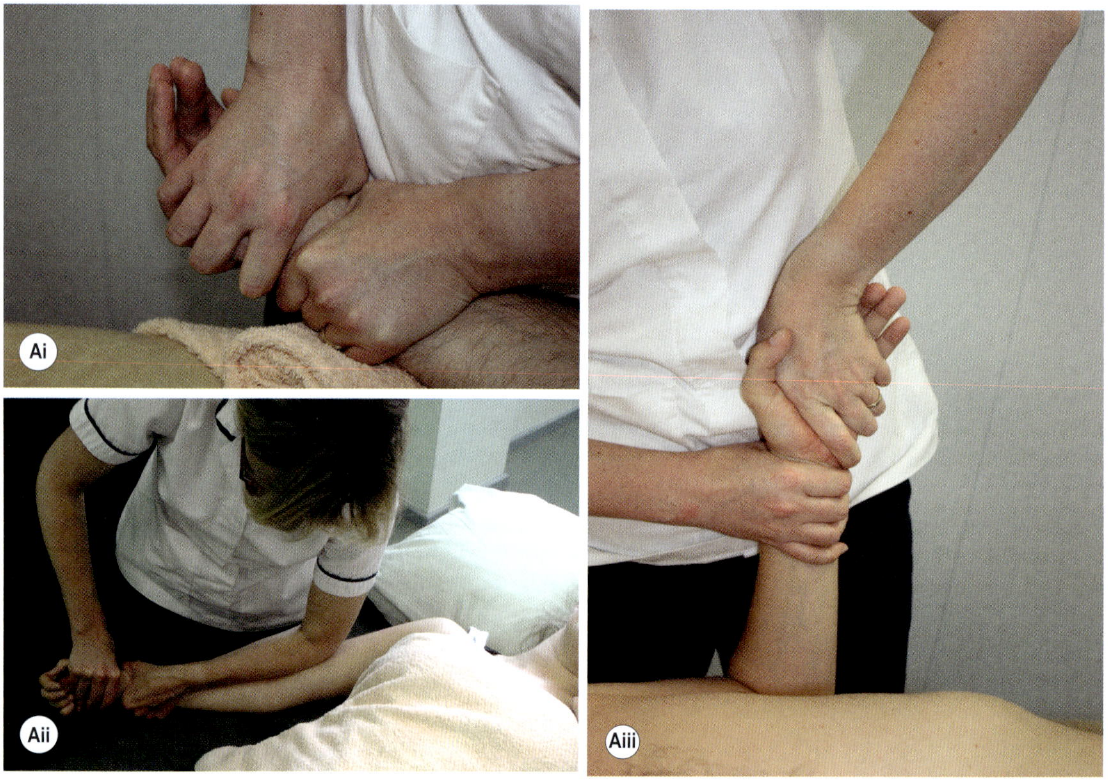

Fig. 12.12 Wrist and hand accessory movements. (Ai) Anteroposterior and posteroanterior. Anteroposterior shown: the left hand grasps around the distal end of the radius and ulna, and the right grasps the hand at the level of the proximal carpal row. The right hand then glides the patient's hand anteriorly to posteriorly. (Aii) Medial and lateral transverse. Medial shown: the left hand grasps around the distal radius and ulna, and the right hand grasps the proximal carpal row, then glides the patient's hand medially. (Aiii) Longitudinal cephalad. The right hand grasps around the distal radius and ulna, and the left hand applies a longitudinal cephalad force to the wrist through the heel of the hand. (B) Intercarpal joints. (Bi) Anteroposterior and posteroanterior. Thumb pressure can be applied to the anterior or posterior aspect of each carpal bone to produce an anteroposterior or posteroanterior movement, respectively. A posteroanterior pressure to the lunate is shown here. (Bii) Horizontal flexion. The right thumb is placed in the centre of the anterior aspect of the wrist, and the left hand cups around the carpus to produce horizontal flexion. (Biii) Horizontal extension. The thumbs are placed in the centre of the posterior aspect of the wrist, and the fingers wrap around the anterior aspect of the carpus to produce horizontal extension. (C) Pisotriquetral joint. Medial and lateral transverse, longitudinal caudad and cephalad and distraction. Shown here, the right hand stabilizes the hand, and the left hand grasps the triquetral bone and applies a medial and lateral transverse force to the bone. (D) Carpometacarpal joints. Fingers – the left hand grasps around the relevant distal carpal bone while the right hand grasps the proximal end of the metacarpal. (Di) Anteroposterior and posteroanterior. Posteroanterior shown: the right hand glides the metacarpal anteriorly. (Dii) Anteroposterior and posteroanterior. The left hand glides the thumb metacarpal anteriorly and posteriorly. (Diii) Medial and lateral rotation. The left hand rotates the thumb metacarpal medially and laterally. (E) Proximal and distal intermetacarpal joints of the fingers – anteroposterior and posteroanterior. The finger and thumb of each hand gently pinch the anterior and posterior aspects of adjacent metacarpal heads and apply a force in opposite directions to glide the heads anteriorly and posteriorly. (F) Anteroposterior and posteroanterior. The left hand glides the proximal phalanx anteriorly and posteriorly.

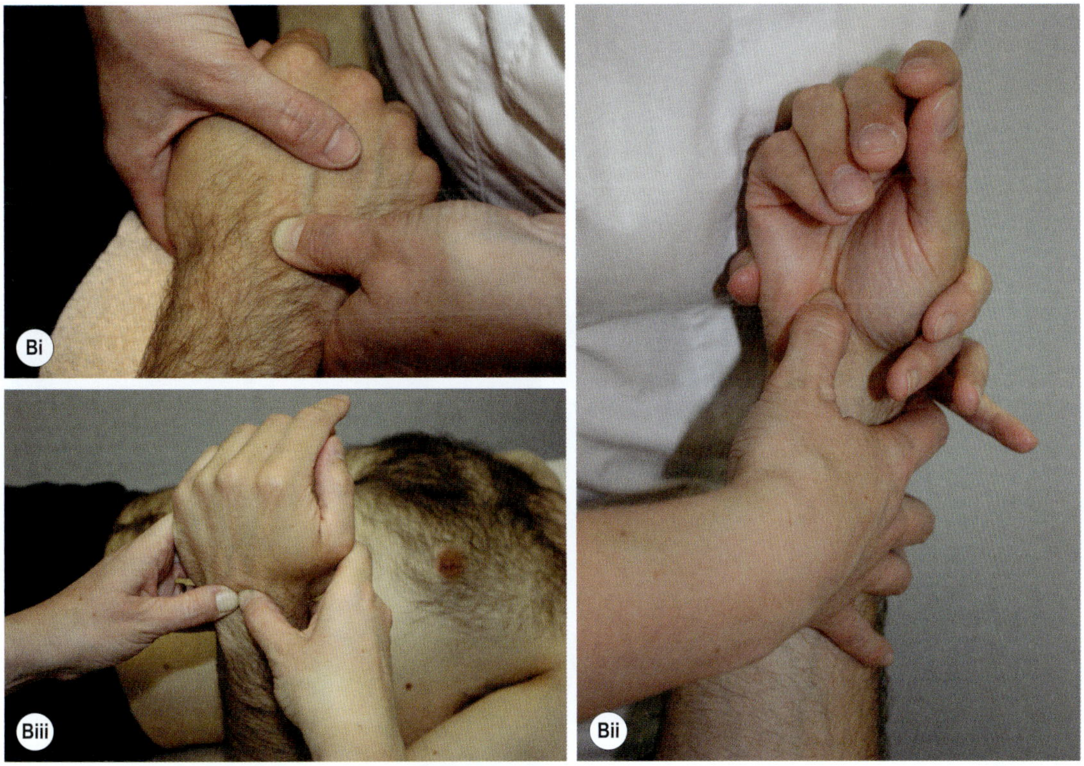

Fig. 12.12 cont'd

clinician will focus accessory testing on the radial side of the wrist and hand, exploring parts 1, 2, 5 and 6 of the Kaltenborn test (Table 12.3) in addition to the CMC joint, PIPJ and interphalangeal accessory joint, testing to identify the source of the symptoms. Although intercarpal movement is minimal, a small study comparing judgements of two experienced clinicians found there to be good intrarater reliability in identifying hyper- and hypomobile joints using the Kaltenborn test (Staes et al. 2009).

COMPLETION OF THE EXAMINATION

On completion of the physical examination, the clinician will need to collate the information to evaluate and revisit how findings compare with expected findings, based on the clinician's initial primary hypothesis and alternative hypotheses. Information needs to be accurately recorded. Significant findings from the subjective and physical examination can be highlighted with an asterisk* as reassessment markers for use within subsequent sessions to evaluate the effects of treatment on the patient's presentation.

Before the patient leaves, the clinician:

- explains the findings of the physical examination and how these relate to the subjective assessment, offering some initial advice if appropriate
- allows the patient sufficient opportunity to discuss thoughts and beliefs which may well have changed over the course of the examination
- revisits the patient's initial expectations and through collaboration with the patient identifies an agreed treatment strategy in order to achieve agreed goals
- requests the patient to report details on the behaviour of the symptoms following examination at the next attendance.

For guidance on treatment and management principles, the reader is directed to the companion textbook (Barnard & Ryder, 2024).

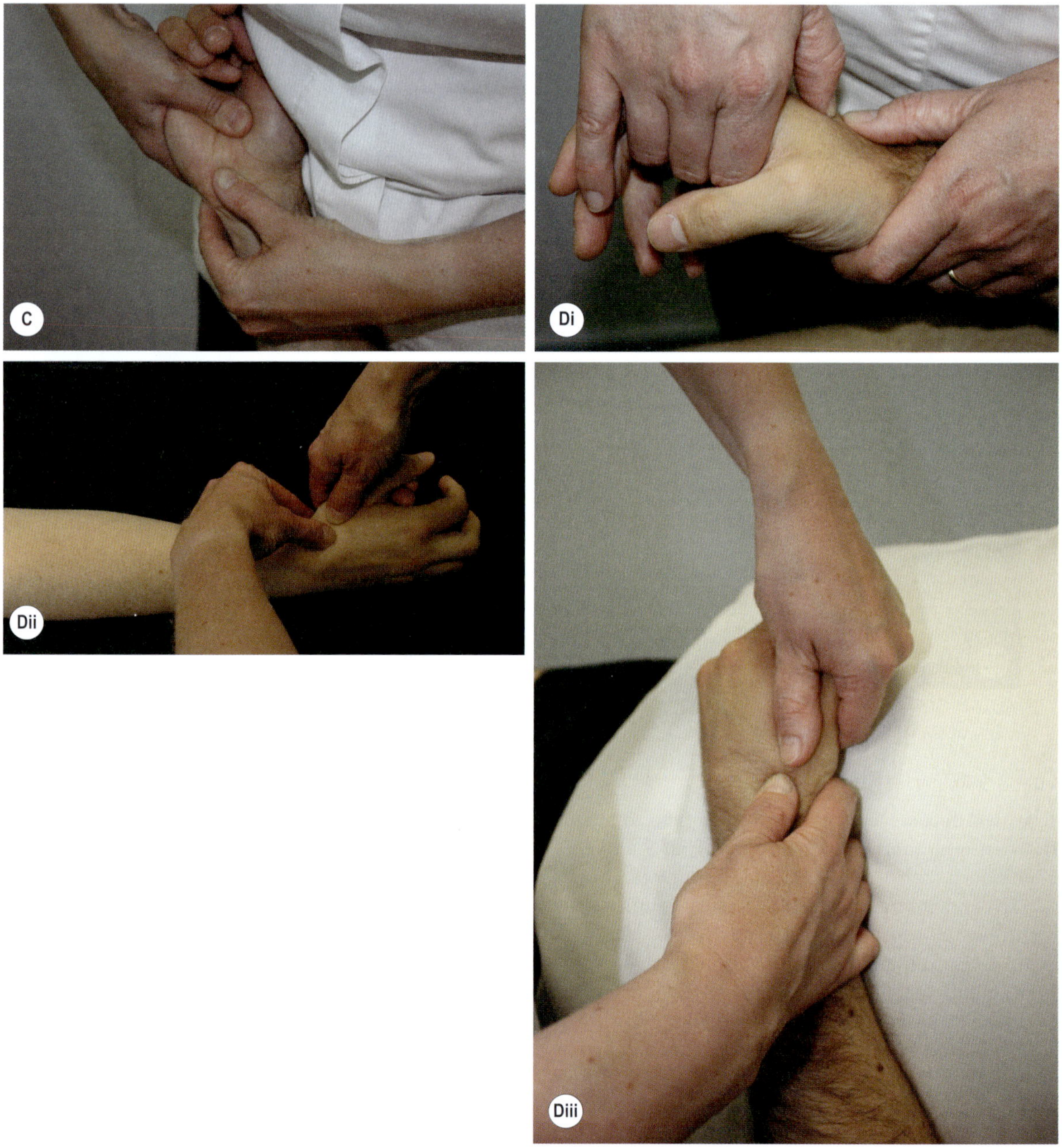

Fig. 12.12 cont'd

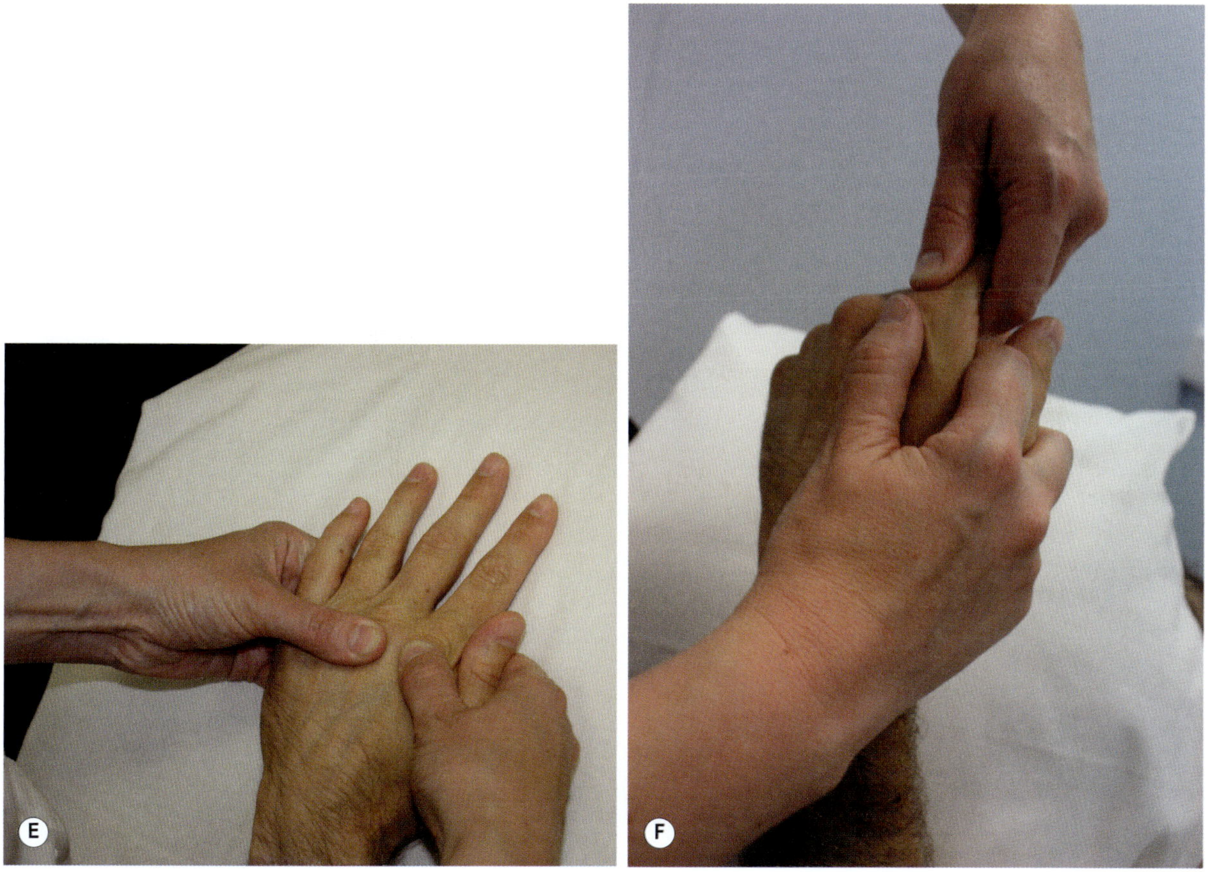

Fig. 12.12 cont'd

TABLE 12.2 Accessory Movements

Radiocarpal Joint	
↕	Anteroposterior
↕	Posteroanterior
←• Med	Medial transverse
•→ Lat	Lateral transverse
←•→ Ceph	Longitudinal cephalad
←•→ Caud	Longitudinal caudad
Intercarpal Joints	
↕	Anteroposterior
↕	Posteroanterior
↕↕	Anteroposterior/posteroanterior gliding
HF	Horizontal flexion
HE	Horizontal extension
←•→ Ceph	Longitudinal cephalad
←•→ Caud	Longitudinal caudad

Continued

Pisotriquetral Joint	
↔ Med	Medial transverse
↔ Lat	Lateral transverse
↔ Ceph	Longitudinal cephalad
↔ Caud	Longitudinal caudad
Dist	Distraction
Carpometacarpal Joints	
Fingers	
↕	Anteroposterior
↕	Posteroanterior
↔ Med	Medial transverse
↔ Lat	Lateral transverse
↶	Medial rotation
↷	Lateral rotation
Thumb	
↕	Anteroposterior
↕	Posteroanterior
↔ Med	Medial transverse
↔ Lat	Lateral transverse
↔ Ceph	Longitudinal cephalad
↔ Caud	Longitudinal caudad
↶	Medial rotation
↷	Lateral rotation
Proximal and Distal Intermetacarpal Joints	
↕	Anteroposterior
↕	Posteroanterior
HF	Horizontal flexion
HE	Horizontal extension
Metacarpophalangeal, Proximal and Distal Interphalangeal Joints of Fingers and Thumb	
↕	Anteroposterior
↕	Posteroanterior
↔ Med	Medial transverse
↔ Lat	Lateral transverse
↔ Ceph	Longitudinal cephalad
↔ Caud	Longitudinal caudad
↶	Medial rotation
↔	Lateral rotation

Choice of application and modifications to the above joints

Start position of the joint:

- Speed of force application
- Direction of the applied force
- Point of application of applied force

Identify any effect of accessory movements on patient's signs and symptoms

Reassess all *asterisks

If necessary screen any proximal and distal regions that may refer to the area

Cervical spine
Thoracic spine
Shoulder
Wrist and hand

TABLE 12.3 Ten-Point Movement Test for the Carpal Bones (Kaltenborn, 2002)

Movements Around the Capitate
1. Fix the capitate and move the trapezoid
2. Fix the capitate and move the scaphoid
3. Fix the capitate and move the lunate
4. Fix the capitate and move the hamate
Movements on the Radial Side of the Wrist
5. Fix the scaphoid and move the trapezoid and trapezium
Movements of the Radiocarpal Joint
6. Fix the radius and move the scaphoid
7. Fix the radius and move the lunate
8. Fix the ulna and move the triquetrum
Movements on the Ulnar Side of the Wrist
9. Fix the triquetrum and move the hamate
10. Fix the triquetrum and move the pisiform

KNOWLEDGE CHECK

1. Identify subjective and physical examination findings that would indicate a dysfunction in the TFCC?
2. What would constitute a positive Tinel's sign?
3. Which nerve can be palpated in Guyon's canal?
4. The WHAT test loads which tendons?
5. Watson shift test is used to examine for scapholunate instability. TRUE or FALSE?

REVIEW AND REVISE QUESTIONS

1. What is tenodesis?
2. Which test for first CMC OA has greater sensitivity and specificity?
   a. CMC grind test
   b. Shear-pressure test
3. How might a carpal instability present subjectively and on physical examination?
4. List anatomical structures that can refer into the thumb?
5. Mallet finger is a rupture of the ………….. tendon at the ………… jt.
6. What is stereognosis and how would you test it?
7. Identify two tests for carpal tunnel syndrome. What would indicate a positive test?
8. Laxity of which two ligaments produce mid carpal instability?
9. What is Froment's sign, and which nerve is being tested?
10. How would you differentially test flexor digitorum superficialis from flexor digitorum profundus?

For guidance on treatment and management principles, the reader is directed to the companion textbook (Barnard & Ryder, 2024).

Case Study

History of Present Condition

A 62-year-old female lecturer presented with a 5-month history of worsening, intermittent, sharp pain Numerical Pain Rating Scale (NPRS) 7/10 in her left thumb. Onset coincided with a period of personal stress, combined with caring for her 10-month-old granddaughter during the day, so her daughter could work from home, followed by long hours using a computer for online teaching in the evening. Due to COVID, she was no longer swimming or taking part in Tai Chi which she previously enjoyed.

Beliefs and Expectations

She was unsure what physiotherapy could offer. She believed her symptoms were never going to go, and she was feeling low in mood as a result. Her life was so different compared to pre-COVID as she was socializing less and at home more.

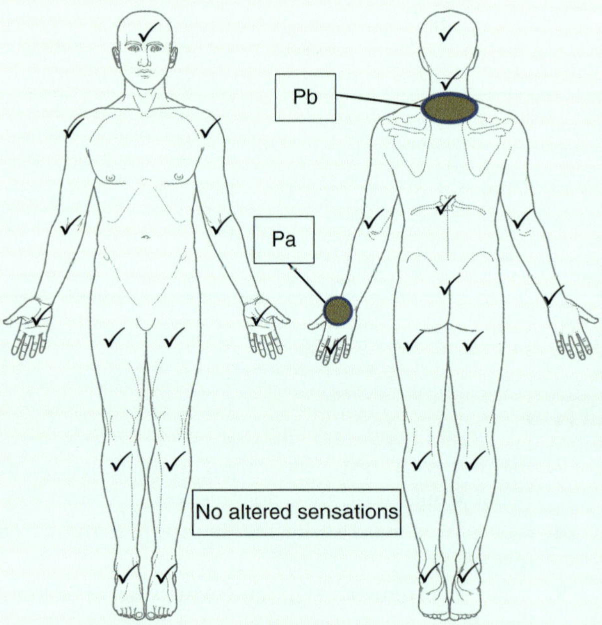

Pa – intermittent sharp pain, 7/10
Aggravating factors
Lifting her granddaughter immed
Gripping immed
Easing factors
Resting wrist completely still 10–15 min
Cradling arm across body at night
NSAID gel
Pb intermittent tension
Aggravating factors
Stress
Easing factors
Relaxing
24 h pattern – worse with activity esp lifting
Sleep – disturbance due to pain 2–3× a night esp after days when she has been caring for her granddaughter. She could fall asleep again while lying with left hand cradled across chest.

Aggravating and Easing Factors

She is right hand dominant so can manage most ADL. Her main concern was thumb pain aggravated immediately on lifting her granddaughter. She feared dropping her as she had no strength in her left wrist. Symptoms eased with holding her wrist completely still for 10–15 min and taking oral NSAIDs, although she had stopped taking tablets due to gastric symptoms and had switched to topical NSAID gel. She also reported a 3-month history of tension across her cervicothoracic region more noticeable in the left upper trapezius area when stressed but not coinciding with her thumb pain. Thumb pain is worse with use of her left hand to lift or grip and so she avoids using her left hand whenever possible. Her sleep was disturbed – two to three times at night, usually on the days she had been looking after her granddaughter.

Past Medical History

Modified radical mastectomy 12 years previously for left Ca breast followed by chemotherapy – no reconstruction, advised not to lift due to residual lymphoedema in left arm.

A year ago had right glut medius tendinopathy managed successfully with physiotherapy.

Clinical Reasoning After the Subjective

Symptoms in the thumb and upper trapezius tension are not directly related; however, altered posture and movement patterns due to thumb pain could provide an indirect relationship. Alternatively, thumb symptoms could be related to a reduction in left limb strength with a change in lifestyle demands precipitating symptoms. Increased upper trapezius muscle tone secondary to a neural driver is possible but less likely as there is no altered sensation reported, but generalized weakness is described. Due to previous chemotherapy, surgery and increased key board work nerve sensitivity especially of the radial nerve based on distribution would need to be excluded.

A primary hypothesis of de Quervain due to location and description of symptoms, aggravated by mechanical

Case Study—cont'd

loading and linked to an increase in loading is typical of tendinopathies – commonly affecting postmenopausal women. Chemotherapy will have induced a more rapid transition to menopause, and this patient has not been treated with hormone replacement therapy as a result of her breast cancer history. A decline in oestrogen has been linked to increased incidence of tendinopathies and is known to impact on bone density. Secondary to mastectomy and lymphoedema increased weight of her left upper limb and a strength deficit/deconditioning may result in increasing distal loading through the wrist to compensate. Differential diagnosis with first CMC jt OA as this joint is also susceptible to pain on loading in this specific age group of postmenopausal women.

The pain mechanism is of mechanical nociception with an inflammatory component as evidenced by symptoms easing with rest and NSAID gel. She is displaying some catastrophization and understandable fear avoidant behaviours which will impact on her pain perception and level of threat. In addition, she reports a personal increase in stress which could produce upregulation of her sympathetic nervous system through release of proinflammatory sympathetic catecholamines. Resulting impaired antiinflammatory function of cortisol may be contributing to the on-going inflammatory process. She is missing her social network and is less physically active which will reduce the resilience of her tissues and impact on her overall wellbeing.

Evaluation of Severity, Irritability and Nature

Severity (Pa) – High (night disturbance, medication helpful, affecting mood, NPRS of 7/10).

Severity (Pb) – Low (does not limit activities, minimal impact describes as a tension, not a pain).

Irritability (Pa) – Yes (symptoms reproduced immediately, easing takes 10–15 min with rest and holding wrist still, can settle back to sleep quite quickly.)

Irritability (Pb) – No (no specific agg/ease – related to stress).

Nature (Pa) – Persistent thumb pain peripheral nociception of tendons in first dorsal space with ongoing inflammatory component.

Nature (Pb) – Altered tension in upper trapezius due to change in lifestyle, altered posture due to thumb pain, increase demands on left upper limb with poor conditioning.

Physical Examination

Observation

On observation of posture, upper cervical spine in extension with low cervical flexion, left shoulder girdle depressed and protracted compared to right. Left arm cradled on lap. Minimal lymphoedema in left upper limb. Reduced muscle tone compared with right dominant upper limb.

Functional testing

Thumb pain reproduced on pincer and power grips. Also reproduced on lifting a weight especially in mid position of forearm.

Range of Movement

Right cervical lateral flexion reproduced left upper trapezius tension which was eased with scapula elevation. Glenohumeral and elbow joint clear with overpressure.

End of range ulnar deviation reproduced thumb pain – symptom modification – no change in symptoms with the addition of elbow extension, or shoulder girdle elevation/depression reducing the likelihood of a neural component.

Thumb flexion, extension and abduction reproduced localized pain. Due to pain on active thumb reposition there was some passive restriction of the left thumb web.

Muscle testing

Reduced strength in left lower traps, serratus anterior, biceps and triceps – nondominant limb and deconditioning secondary to previous breast surgery. Related to sensation of tension in upper trapezius muscles.

Palpation

Key palpation findings – prominent radial styloid, with local tenderness in first dorsal compartment, no evidence of thickening. Local tenderness in adductor pollicis. First CMC joint line palpation is asymptomatic.

Selective Tests

Application of the less provocative pressure-shear test produced local joint crepitus, indicating likelihood of first CMC OA changes but not the patient's main pain complaint.

Finkelstein's test reproduced thumb symptoms.

Clinical Diagnosis and Plan

To further explore her beliefs and expectations after the examination.

To explain examination findings that support a primary hypothesis of de Quervain tendinopathy.

To share an understanding of tendon dysfunction based on her existing knowledge and understanding.

Explanation of expected time scales and recovery with the option of referral onward for a corticosteroid injection.

To discuss physiotherapy management options using likely multifactorial contributors for this patient to individualize her care. To include initial advice on pacing activities, e.g. typing, review ergonomics of PC use, minimize and

Continued

Case Study—cont'd

modify lifting, e.g. through biceps with palms supinated rather than in mid position. To further reduce loading and tendon irritation through use of a forearm-based thumb spica splint to support wrist in neutral, limit CMC joint range and thumb abduction with interphalangeal (IP) joint free, for use especially on childcare days. Granddaughter now enrolled in nursery 4 days a week so less loading on a daily basis.

Use of splint at night to reduce symptoms from positioning whilst asleep, to improve sleep duration and quality as essential for recovery.

Discuss the value of building upper limb strength and returning to physical activity – swimming (modified stroke) and Tai Chi for both physical and mental health benefits.

As tendon symptoms settle to build capacity of the tendons to take load through a graded isometric, eccentric and isotonic loading programme.

Outcomes can be measured using NPRS and the Disabilities of the Arm, Shoulder and Hand questionnaire.

REFERENCES

Ahern, M., Skyllas, J., Wajon, A., Hush, J., 2018. The effectiveness of physical therapies for patients with base of thumb osteoarthritis: systematic review and meta-analysis. Musculoskelet. Sci. Pract. 35, 46–54.

Amirfeyz, R., Gozzard, C., Leslie, I.J., 2005. Hand elevation test for assessment of carpal tunnel syndrome. J. Hand Surg. Br. 30, 361–364.

Baker, N., Cham, R., Cidboy, E.H., Cook, J., Redfern, M.S., 2007. Kinematics of the fingers and hands during computer keyboard use. Clin. Biomech. 22, 34–43.

Baldassarre, R., Hughes, T., 2013. Investigating suspected scaphoid fractures. Br. Med. J. 346, 1370–1371.

Barnard, K., Ryder, 2024. Principles of Neuromusculoskeletal Treatment and Management: A Handbook for Therapists, fourth ed. Elsevier, Edinburgh.

Batra, S., Kanvinde, R., 2007. Osteoarthritis of the thumb trapeziometacarpal joint. Curr. Orthop. 21, 135–144.

Batteson, R., Hammond, A., Burke, F., Sinha, S., 2008. The de Quervain's screening tool: validity and reliability of a measure to support clinical diagnosis. Muscoskel. Care 6, 168–180.

Blair, S.J., McCormick, E., Bear-Lehman, J., Fess, E.E., Rader, E., 1987. Evaluation of impairment of the upper extremity. Clin. Orthop. Relat. Res. 221, 42–58.

Brüske, J., Bednarski, M., Grzelec, H., Zyluk, A., 2002. The usefulness of the Phalen test and the Hoffmann-Tinel sign in the diagnosis of carpal tunnel syndrome. Acta Orthop. Belg. 68, 141–145.

Bulstrode, C., Buckwalter, J., Carr, A., Marsh, L., Fairbank, J., Wilson-MacDonald, J., et al., 2002. Oxford Textbook of Orthopaedics and Trauma. Oxford University Press, Oxford.

Butler, D., 2000. The sensitive nervous system. Neuro Orthopaedic Institute, Adelaide.

Butterfield, W.L., Joshi, A.B., Lichtman, D., 2002. Lunotriquetral injuries. J. Am. Soc. Surg. Hand 2 (4), 195–203.

Cakir, M., Samanci, N., Balci, N., Balci, M.K., 2003. Musculoskeletal manifestations in patients with thyroid disease. Clin. Endocrinol. 59, 162–167.

Caldwell, C., Khoo-Summers, L., 2010. Movement system impairment syndromes of the wrist and hand. In: Sahrmann, S.A. (Ed.), Movement System Impairment Syndromes of the Extremities, Cervical and Thoracic Spines. Mosby, St Louis, pp. 165–236.

Calveri Schabrun, S., Te, M., Chipchase, L., 2016. Hand therapy versus corticosteroid injections in the treatment of de Quervain's disease: a systematic review and meta-analysis. J. Hand. Therapy. 29, 3–11.

Cheimonidou, A., Lamnisos, D., Lisacek-Kiosoglous, A., Chimonas, C., Stasinopoulos, D., 2019. Validity and reliability of the Finkelstein test. Trends Med. 19, 1–7.

Christodoulou, L., Bainbridge, L.C., 1999. Clinical diagnosis of triquetrolunate injuries. J. Hand Surg. Br. 24, 598.

Clark, D., Amirfeyz, R., Leslie, I., Bannister, G., 2011. Often atypical? The distribution of sensory disturbance in carpal tunnel syndrome. Ann. R. Coll. Surg. Engl. 93, 470–473.

Court-Brown, C.M., Caesar, B., 2006. Epidemiology of adult fractures: a review injury. Int. J. Care Injured 37, 691–697.

Davis, D.I., Baratz, M., 2010. Soft tissue complications of distal radius fractures. Hand Clin. 26, 229–235.

Dyer, G., Simmons, B., 2011. Rheumatoid thumb. Hand Clin. 27 (11), 73–77.

Eaton, R.G., Glickel, S.Z., 1987. Trapeziometacarpal osteoarthritis. Staging as a rationale for treatment. Hand Clin. 3, 455–471.

Eckhaus, D., 1993. Swan-neck deformity. In: Clark, G.L., Shaw Wilgis, E.F., Aiello, B., Eckhaus, D., Eddington, L.V. (Eds.), Hand rehabilitation, a practical guide. Churchill Livingstone, Edinburgh (Chapter 16).

Eddington, L.V., 1993. Boutonnière deformity. In: Clark, G.L., Shaw Wilgis, E.F., Aiello, B., Eckhaus, D., Eddington, L.V.

(Eds.), Hand rehabilitation, a practical guide. Churchill Livingstone, Edinburgh (Chapter 17).
Elliott, B.G., 1992. Finkelstein's test: a descriptive error that can produce a false positive. J. Hand Surg. Am. 17B, 481–482.
El Miedany, Y., Ashour, S., Youssef, S., Mehanna, A., Meky, F.A., 2008. Clinical diagnosis of carpal tunnel syndrome: old tests, new concepts. Joint Bone Spine 75, 451–457.
Gaston, M.S., Simpson, A.H., 2007. Inhibition of fracture healing. J. Bone Joint Surg. Br. 89-B, 1553–1560.
Gates, D.H., Walters, L.S., Cowley, J., Wilken, J.M., Resnik, L., 2016. Brief report—range of motion requirements for upper-limb activities of daily living. Am. J. Occup. Ther. 70. https://doi.org/10.5014/ajot.2016.015487, 7001350010.
Gelberman, R.H., Boone, S., Osei, D.A., Cherney, S., Calfee, R. P., 2015. Trapeziometacarpal arthritis: a prospective clinical evaluation of the thumb adduction and extension provocative tests. J. Hand Surg. Am. 40 (7), 1285e1291.
Gelberman, R.H., Hergenroeder, P.T., Hargens, A.R., Lundborg, G.N., Akeson, W.H., 1981. The carpal tunnel syndrome. A study of carpal canal pressures. J. Bone Joint Surg. Am. 63, 380–383.
Gollins, C., de Berker, D., 2021. Nails in systemic disease. Clin. Med. 21 (3), 166–169.
González del Pino, J., Delgado-Martínez, A.D., González González, I., Lovic, A., 1997. Value of the carpal compression test in the diagnosis of carpal tunnel syndrome. J. Hand Surg. Br. 22, 38–41.
Goubau, J.F., Goubau, L., Van Tongel, A., Van Hoonacker, P., Kerckhove, D., Berghs, B., 2014. The wrist hyperflexion and abduction of the thumb (WHAT) test: a more specific and sensitive test to diagnose de Quervain's tenosynovitis than the Eichhoff's test. J. Hand Surg. Eur. 39, 286–292.
Gracia-Ibáñez, V., Sancho-Bru, J., Vergaraet, M., 2018. Relevance of grasp types to assess functionality for personal autonomy. J. Hand Ther. 31, 102–110.
Grassi, W., De Angelis, R., Lamanna, G., Cervini, C., 1998. The clinical features of rheumatoid arthritis. Eur. J. Radiol. 27, S18–S24.
Hattam, P., Smeatham, A., 2010. Special Tests in Musculoskeletal Examination. An Evidence-Based Guide for Clinicians. Churchill Livingstone Elsevier, Edinburgh (Chapter 4).
Hengeveld, E., Banks, K., 2014. Maitland's Peripheral Manipulation, fifth ed. Butterworth-Heinemann Elsevier, London.
Heras-Palou, C., Burke, F.D., Dias, J.J., Bindra, R., 2003. Outcome measurement in hand surgery: report of a consensus conference. Br. J. Hand Ther. 8, 70–80.
Hislop, H., Avers, D., Brown, M., 2013. Daniels and Worthingham's Muscle Testing: Techniques of Manual Examination and Performance Testing, ninth ed. W.B. Saunders, Philadelphia.
Kaltenborn F.M. 2002 Manual Mobilization of the joints. vol1 6th Ed The extremities Norli Oslos.
Kalk, W.J., 2005. Endocrinology. In: Shamley, D. (Ed.), Pathophysiology: An Essential Test for the Allied Professions. Elsevier Butterworth Heinemann, Edinburgh.
Kendall, F.P., McCreary, E.K., Provance, P.G., Rodgers, M.M., Romani, W.A., 2010. Muscles Testing and Function, fifth ed. Lippincott Williams and Wilkins, Baltimore.
La Stayo, P., Howell, J., 1995. Clinical provocative tests used in evaluating wrist pain: a descriptive study. J. Hand Ther. 8, 10–17.
Lichtman, D., Wroten, E., 2006. Understanding midcarpal instability. J. Hand Surg. 31 (3), 491–498.
Lindau, T., 2016. The role of arthroscopy in carpal instability. J. Hand Surg. 41 (1), 35–47.
Lundborg, G., Rosén., B., 2004. The two-point discrimination test – time for a re-appraisal? J. Hand Surg. 29b (5), 418, 22.
Mandhkani, M., Rhemrev, S., 2013. Rupture of the ulnar collateral ligament of the thumb – a review. Int. J. Emerg. Med. 6, 31.
Magee, D., Manske, R., 2021. Orthopedic Physical Assessment, seventh ed. Saunders Elsevier, St Louis.
Mathiowetz, V., Kashman, N., Volland, G., Weber, K., Dowe, M., Rogers, S., 1985. Grip and pinch strength: normative data for adults. Arch. Phys. Med. Rehab 66 (2), 69–74.
Montechiarello, S., Miozzi, F., D'Ambrosio, I., Giovagnorio, F., 2010. The intersection syndrome: ultrasound findings and their diagnostic value. J. Ultrasound 13, 70–73.
Morco, S., Bowden, A., 2015. Ulnar drift in rheumatoid arthritis: a review of biomechanical etiology. J. Biomech. 48, 725–728.
Neumann, D.A., 2010. Kinesiology of the musculoskeletal system. In: Foundations for Rehabilitation, second ed. Mosby Elsevier, St Louis (Chapter 8).
Nolte, M., Shauver, M., Chung, K., 2017. Normative values of the Michigan Hand Outcomes Questionnaire for patients with and without hand conditions. Plast. Reconstr. Surg. 140 (3), 425e–433e.
Pellecchia, G.L., 2003. Figure-of-eight method of measuring hand size: reliability and concurrent validity. J. Hand Ther. 16, 300–304.
Prosser, R., Harvey, L., Lastayo, P., Hargreaves, I., Scougall, P., Herbert, R.D., 2011. Provocative wrist tests and MRI are of limited diagnostic value for suspected wrist ligament injuries: a cross-sectional study. J. Physiother. 57, 247–253.
Rainbow, M.J., Wolff, A.L., Crisco, J.J., Wolfe, S., 2016. Functional kinematics of the wrist. J. Hand Surg. 41 (1), 7–21.
Rumsey, N., Clarke, A., White, P., Hooper, E., 2003. Investigating the appearance-related concerns of people with hand injuries. J. Hand Ther. 8, 57–61.
Sela, Y., Seftchick, J., Wang, W., Baratz, M., 2019. Diagnostic clinical value of thumb metacarpal grind, pressure shear, flexion, and extension tests for carpometacarpal osteoarthritis. J. Hand Ther. 32, 35–40.

Staes, F., Banks, K.J., De Smet, L., Daniels, K.J., Carels, P., 2009. Reliability of accessory motion testing at the carpal joints. Man. Ther. 14, 292–298.

Taleisnik, J., 1988. Carpal instability. J. Bone Joint Surg. 70A, 1262–1268.

Tang, P., 2011. Collateral ligament injuries of the thumb metacarpophalangeal joint. J. Am. Acad. Orthop. Surg. 19, 287–296.

Tekeoglu, I., Dogan, A., Demir, G., Dolarm, E., 2007. The pneumatic compression test and modified pneumatic compression test in the diagnosis of carpal tunnel syndrome. J. Hand Surg. Eur. 32, 697–699.

Toemen, A., Dalton, S., Sandford, F., 2011. The intra- and inter-rater reliability of manual muscle testing and a hand-held dynamometer for measuring wrist strength in symptomatic and asymptomatic subjects. Hand Ther. 16, 67–74.

Totten, P., Flinn-Wagner, S., 1992. Functional evaluation of the hand. In: Stanley, B., Tribuzi, S. (Eds.), Concepts in Hand Rehabilitation. FA Davis, New York, p. 128.

Townley, W.A., Swan, M.C., Dunn, R.L., 2010. Congenital absence of flexor digitorum superficialis: implications for assessment of little finger lacerations. J. Hand Surg. Eur. 35, 417–418.

Valdes, K., LaStayo, P., 2013. The value of provocative tests for the wrist and elbow: a literature review. J. Hand Ther. 26, 33–43.

Watson, H.K., Ashmead, D., 4th, Makhlouf, M.V. , 1988. Examination of the scaphoid. J. Hand Surg. Am. 13A, 657–660.

Wolfe, S., Gupta, A., Crisco, J., 1997. Kinematics of the scaphoid shift test. J. Hand Surg. Am. 22 (5), 801–806.

Wollstein, R., Wollstein, A., Rodgers, J., Ogden, T.J., 2013. A hand therapy protocol for the treatment of lunate overload or early Kienbock's disease. J. Hand Ther. 26, 255–260.

13

Examination of the Lumbar Region

Chris Mercer and Amy Kemp

LEARNING OUTCOMES

After studying this chapter, you should be able to:

- Discuss pathological presentations for this region within the context of the multifactorial drivers for the development/persistence of low back pain.
- Explain how clinical reasoning guides history taking in the subjective examination of patients with low back pain.
- Understand the relevance and importance of specific screening questions asked during the subjective examination of a patient with low back pain.
- List the key constituents of a comprehensive physical examination of the lumbar spine and identify how subjective data will guide the physical examination of the lumbar spine.
- Using clinical reasoning to justify selection of tests and interpretation of findings related to common low back pain presentations.
- Consider the sensitivity and specificity of key physical tests for the lumbar spine.
- Discuss the value of functional testing and symptom modification when considering the aggravating factors, whilst understanding that such tests lack the validity and reliability of some physical tests.
- Explain how physical examination findings contribute to reasoning of lumbar spine pain in common clinical presentations.

CHAPTER CONTENTS

Introduction to the Lumbar Spine, 364
Subjective Examination/Taking the Patient's History, 364
Patient's Perspectives on Their Experience, 364
Body Chart, 365
Behaviour of Symptoms, 365
Special/Screening Questions, 367
History of the Present Condition, 367
Past Medical History, 367
Family History, 367
Plan of the Physical Examination, 369
Physical Examination, 370
Observation, 370
Active Physiological Movements, 370
Differentiation or Symptom Modification, 372
Passive Physiological Movements, 373
Muscle Tests, 374
Neurological Tests, 376
Miscellaneous Tests, 377
Palpation, 378
Passive Accessory Intervertebral Movements, 378
Completion of the Examination, 380
Case Study, 381
References, 384

INTRODUCTION TO THE LUMBAR SPINE

The lumbar region consists of the five largest vertebrae in the spine, connecting the ribcage to the pelvis and supporting the body weight, whilst also permitting movement. The lumbar spine is defined here as the region between T12 and the sacrum and includes the joints, discs and their surrounding tissues.

Low back pain (LBP) is the leading cause of years lived with disability globally, having a significant impact on health and social care systems across the world (Wu et al., 2020). It is the main cause of work absenteeism producing economic consequences to society as a result (Lee et al., 2015; Hartvigsen et al., 2018). Although it is very common, only a small number of people with LBP have a clear, identifiable structural/patho-anatomical cause for their pain which can be defined as 'specific' LBP, e.g. nerve root compression (Buchbinder et al., 2018).

Serious pathology can occur in 1% to 2% of LBP presentations and must be screened for, the most common of these being fracture, metastatic disease, infection and cauda equina syndrome (Henschke et al., 2009; Finucane et al., 2020). For a detailed assessment of serious pathologies, the reader is referred to Chapter 9 in Barnard and Ryder (2024).

Whilst there are many pain-sensitive structures in the lumbar spine, such as the nerve roots, intervertebral discs, joints and muscles, it has been shown in multiple studies that abnormalities in these structures are not strongly associated with pain and disability. Conversely, people with no symptoms can have significant abnormalities on imaging (Brinjikji et al., 2015; Romeo et al., 2019). The majority of LBP disorders have no diagnosis, and therefore the term 'nonspecific LBP' (NSLBP) is used. For this reason, people with LBP require a thorough examination that addresses possible biological, psychological and social aspects that may be contributing to the development and persistence of LBP symptoms.

This chapter focuses on the examination of the lumbar spine, exploring features of the subjective and physical examination that will help build a detailed and thorough examination tailored to the individual patient.

SUBJECTIVE EXAMINATION/TAKING THE PATIENT'S HISTORY

Patient's Perspectives on Their Experience

In order to treat the patient appropriately and holistically, it is important that the condition is managed within the context of the patient's social and work environment. This includes the patient's perspectives, experiences and expectations, age, employment, home situation and details of any leisure activities. Research indicates that LBP is influenced by a range of factors, including cognitive factors such as catastrophic thoughts and beliefs, unhelpful expectations, poor motivation, psychological, e.g. depression, anxiety and social, e.g. low job satisfaction, interpersonal relationship stress, cultural factors, as well as physical and lifestyle factors (Synnott et al., 2015). Back pain patients' beliefs, expectations and preferences should be explored and used to inform the clinical reasoning process and determine the most appropriate treatment to support the patient's return to function. Patients' beliefs about pain, their fears of hurting, harming, causing further injury and self-efficacy are important to consider (Main et al., 2010a). Expectations and preferences about treatments for back pain are known to influence the patients' engagement in and adherence to treatment plans.

Features of the 'good back-consultation' Main et al. (2010b)

- To be taken seriously (seen and believed)
- To be given an understandable explanation of what is wrong
- To have patient-centred communication (seeking patients perspectives/preferences)
- To receive reassurance and if possible to be given a favourable outcome
- To be told about what can be done (by the patient him/herself and by the care provider).

Psychosocial factors are important predictors of prognosis, influencing the transition from acute to persistent back pain and disability (Van Tulder et al., 2005). Screening for psychosocial risk can be divided into the following five factors (O'Sullivan et al., 2015):

1. Cognitive: negative beliefs (e.g. 'slipped discs' and 'trapped nerves'), catastrophizing (e.g. thinking the worst) and fear of movement (e.g. believing that 'pain indicates damage').
2. Social and cultural: may influence pain beliefs and stress load.
3. Work-related: compensation and work absenteeism.
4. Lifestyle: sleep, rest, workload, stress and exercise levels; deconditioning secondary to activity avoidance.
5. Individual: patient goals, preferences, expectations and readiness for change.

Both the Örebro Musculoskeletal Pain Questionnaire (ÖMPQ) and STarT Back screening tools have been recommended as validated tools for assessing psychosocial factors and patients at risk of developing more persistent/disabling symptoms, enabling health resources to be targeted (Synnott et al., 2015).

Body Chart

The following information concerning the type and area of the current symptoms can be recorded on a body chart.

Area of Current Symptoms

It is important to be accurate when mapping the area of the symptoms the patient describes, as this provides a baseline for reference, as well as information about potential source of symptoms, or spinal levels that may be involved. Lumbar symptoms can include pain, stiffness, altered sensations (burning, numbness, paraesthesia) or other descriptions such as heaviness or twitching. Symptoms may be local to the spine or may be referred to the trunk, abdomen, groin and lower limbs and need to be clearly mapped as it may indicate the spinal level affected (Albert et al., 2019).

Viscera can refer to the lumbar spine, e.g. bowel, uterus, kidneys, so an understanding of where they can refer to is important in differentiating a potential source of symptoms that may be nonmusculoskeletal in nature (Fig. 3.6) (Boissonault & Bass, 1990).

Areas Relevant to the Region Being Examined

All other relevant areas are checked for symptoms. Widespread symptoms may be an indication of conditions that are not limited to the lumbar spine, such as persistent widespread pain (fibromyalgia), inflammatory arthritis, autoimmune disease, vitamin D deficiency (Pal, 2002).

If areas are symptom free, it is helpful to mark them with ticks (✓) on the body chart as a reference point later on in the course of treatment.

Type and Intensity of Pain

Whilst the nature of the pain the patient describes does not indicate specific structures/mechanisms involved, it is useful to ask the patient to describe their symptoms in their own words, so the clinician can use the same description when talking with the patient to facilitate communication to foster the therapeutic relationship. The intensity of pain can be measured using, for example, a visual analogue scale, a numeric pain scale or simple descriptors such as mild, moderate or severe may be useful for some patients. Other screening tools such as the Pain Detect or Leeds Assessment of Neuropathic Symptoms Scale (LANNS) score may also be helpful for assessing neuropathic pain (Eckeli et al., 2016).

A pain diary may be useful for patients with persistent low back pain to determine the pain patterns and triggering factors over a period of time.

Relationship of Symptoms

If there is more than one area of symptoms, determine the relationship between symptomatic areas—do they come together or separately? For example, the patient could have thigh pain with or without lumbar spine pain. It is possible that there may be related symptoms or two separate sources of symptoms and careful questioning can help to establish this relationship.

Behaviour of Symptoms

Aggravating Factors

For each symptomatic area a series of questions can be asked:

- What movements, activities or positions bring on or make the patient's symptoms worse?

Constant lumbar spine symptoms that do not vary with movement, activity or positions should cause the clinician to consider alternative serious pathologies, such as inflammatory back pain, infection, cancer or a visceral source (see Barnard & Ryder, 2024, Chapter 9). Pain in the lumbar spine that worsens with lying is an unusual presentation and may raise concerns about possible spinal cancer (NASS, 2021).

Constant pain that is worse with rest and eased with movement may indicate inflammatory back pain such as axial spondyloarthropathy (axSpA) (Poddubnyy, 2020).

Details about the aggravating activities will inform reasoning. For example, the patient may complain that driving aggravates symptoms; this position implicates both the lumbar spine (flexion) and neural tissue (slumped position combined with knee extension) and signposts to the clinician those tests that need to be included in the physical examination.

- How long does it take before symptoms are aggravated?
- Is the patient able to maintain this position or movement?
- What happens to other symptoms when this symptom is produced or made worse?

Easing Factors

For each symptomatic area a series of questions can be asked to help determine what eases the symptoms:

What movements and/or positions ease the patient's symptoms? Improvement in symptoms with movement and exercise could be suggestive of inflammatory back pain (Grinnell-Merrick et al., 2020; NASS, 2021).

- How long does it take before symptoms are eased? If symptoms are constant but variable, it is important to know what the baseline is and how long it takes for the symptoms to reduce to that level.
- What happens to other symptoms when this symptom is eased?

Aggravating and easing factors will help to determine the irritability of the patient's symptoms and help in planning the extent and vigour of the physical examination.

The severity can be determined by the intensity of the symptoms and whether the symptoms are interfering with normal activities of daily living, such as work and sleep. This information can be used to determine the direction of the physical examination as well as the aim of treatment and any advice that may be required.

The most relevant subjective information should be highlighted with an asterisk (*), explored in the physical examination and reassessed at subsequent treatment sessions to evaluate treatment intervention.

Twenty-Four-Hour Behaviour of Symptoms

The clinician determines the 24-hour behaviour of symptoms by asking questions about night, morning and evening symptoms. This will help to determine if the pain is mechanical in nature and suitable for physiotherapy management or inflammatory/systemic which may not be appropriate for treatment and may require onward referral.

Night symptoms. Although severe night pain is a recognized red flag for serious pathology, it should be noted that night symptoms are common in people with back pain so other factors need to be considered before onward referral or investigation is considered (Harding et al., 2005; Gerhart et al., 2017). Night pain or pain when turning over in bed is not an indicator of serious pathology; however, back pain that wakes a person from sleep, i.e. is not movement related, and keeps the person awake or forces them to get out of bed is more concerning and may warrant further investigation. People with inflammatory back pain, e.g. axial spondyloarthropathy often describe worsening symptoms when resting at night, with reported waking during the second half of the night due to pain (Grinnell-Merrick et al., 2020).

The following questions may be asked:

- Do you have any difficulty getting to sleep?
- Do your symptoms wake you at night? If so:
  - Which symptoms?
  - How many times in a night?
  - How many times in the past week?
  - What do you have to do to get back to sleep?
- If sleep is an issue, further questioning may be useful to determine management.

Morning and evening symptoms. Morning stiffness lasting less than 30 minutes is more likely to be mechanical and/or degenerative in nature; however, stiffness that lasts more than half an hour may indicate an inflammatory condition such as axial spondyloarthropathy (Jois et al., 2008). Morning stiffness should be taken in context with other potential symptoms associated with inflammatory back pain, such as colitis, iritis, uveitis, dactylitis, enthesitis and psoriasis (NASS, 2021; Table 13.1).

TABLE 13.1 NICE Guidelines 2017 Suggested Guidelines on When to Refer on for Specialist Assessment

If a person has low back pain that started before the age of 45 years and has lasted for longer than 3 months, refer the person to a rheumatologist for a spondyloarthritis assessment if four or more of the following additional criteria are also present:
• low back pain that started before the age of 35 years (this further increases the likelihood that back pain is due to spondyloarthritis compared with low back pain that started between 35 and 44 years) • waking during the second half of the night because of symptoms • buttock pain • improvement with movement • improvement within 48 h of taking nonsteroidal antiinflammatory drugs (NSAIDs) • a first-degree relative with spondyloarthritis • current or past arthritis • current or past enthesitis; current or past psoriasis
If exactly three of the additional criteria are present, perform an HLA-B27 test. If the test is positive, refer the person to a rheumatologist for a spondyloarthritis assessment.

Early diagnosis of axial spondyloarthropathy is crucial to achieve an optimal treatment response (Redeker, 2019). Research suggests that there is often a substantial delay between symptom onset and diagnosis, suggesting an average diagnostic delay of 5–14 years (Yi et al., 2020). Physiotherapists can play a key role in identifying these patients earlier.

Special/Screening Questions

Special questions must always be asked, as they may identify certain precautions or contraindications to the physical examination and/or treatment. The clinician must differentiate between conditions that are suitable for conservative management and those such as systemic disease, neoplastic and other non-neuromusculoskeletal conditions (such as abdominal aortic aneurysm) that require onward referral for specialist assessment and further investigation (Grieve, 1994).

Neurological Symptoms

Neurological symptoms mapped on the body chart may include areas of pins and needles, numbness and weakness.

Careful explanation and questioning is required to rule out possible cauda equina compression (i.e. compression below L1). Has the patient experienced symptoms indicating cauda equina syndrome, i.e. saddle anaesthesia/paraesthesia, sexual or erectile dysfunction, loss of vaginal sensation, bladder and/or bowel sphincter disturbance (loss of control, retention, hesitancy, urgency or a sense of incomplete evacuation) (Lavy et al., 2009; Greenhalgh et al., 2018). Urgent imaging and surgical decompression are required to prevent permanent sphincter paralysis (Greenhalgh et al., 2018; Finucane et al., 2020).

Has the patient experienced symptoms of spinal cord compression (i.e. compression above the L1 level, which may include the cervical and thoracic cord as well as the brain), such as bilateral tingling in hands or feet and/or disturbance of gait? Are there motor, sensory or tonal changes in all four limbs? Does the patient report coordination changes, including gait disturbance?

Responses to these questions on neurological function should inform the physical neurological examination.

History of the Present Condition

For each symptomatic area, the clinician needs to know how long the symptom has been present, whether there was a sudden or slow onset and whether there was a known cause that provoked the onset of symptoms. If the onset was slow, has there been any change in the patient's lifestyle, e.g. work, sport/hobbies, personal circumstances or mental health?

If the onset was sudden, was this related to a specific trauma? It is important to be very clear about the mechanism of the injury, as this may help with diagnosis and decision-making whether the patient needs onward referral.

Are the patient's symptoms getting better, worsening or staying the same, as this can give a good overall picture of any progression of the problem.

- If the patient has more than one area of symptoms, the relationship between the symptoms can be established by asking what happened to other symptoms when each symptom began.

It is helpful to know if the patient has had previous episodes of LBP and if they have, if this episode is similar. Patients should be asked about the frequency and duration of episodes. When were they? Was there a cause? Did they seek treatment? If so, what was the outcome? Did the patient fully recover between episodes? Does the patient perceive the current condition to be better, the same or worse in relation to other previous episodes? If there has been no previous back pain, has the patient had any episodes of stiffness in the lumbar spine, thoracic spine or any other relevant region? Check for a history of trauma or recurrent minor trauma.

Past Medical History

The following information is obtained from the patient and/or the medical notes:

- The details of any relevant medical history related to visceral structures; for example, the pelvic organs, bowel and kidneys can refer to lumbar spine and sacral regions masquerading as musculoskeletal conditions, so it is important to explore to help differentiate the cause of symptoms (Pacheco-Carroza, 2021).

Family History

Has the patient (or any family members) been diagnosed as having rheumatoid arthritis or inflammatory conditions, or psoriasis which may increase the risk to the patient of inherited inflammatory disease. Patients with a family history of ankylosing spondylitis, psoriasis or inflammatory bowel disease (Crohn or ulcerative colitis) in a first or second degree relative have a greater likelihood of developing inflammatory back pain (Ez-Zaitouni et al., 2017).

General Health

Does the patient suffer from any systemic symptoms such as night sweats, malaise, fatigue, fever, nausea or vomiting, stress, anxiety or depression?

It is important to identify the patient's lifestyle choices in detail and explain their relevance. Tobacco smoking and alcohol consumption are among the four most important lifestyle exposures, combined with dietary factors and bodyweight that contribute to risk of developing cancer (Parkin et al., 2011). A history of smoking may also increase the likelihood of a possible vascular cause to a patient's leg symptoms. Both are also significant risk factors for back pain and potentially serious spinal pathology such as pathological fractures and cancer (Finucane et al., 2020). Smoking more than 20 cigarettes a day and drinking more than three units of alcohol a day are risk factors for developing osteoporosis (NICE, 2017).

Weight Loss

Has the patient noticed any recent unexplained weight loss? Unintentional weight loss of greater than 5% total body weight in 3–6 months is concerning and should prompt referral for further medical investigation.

Serious Pathology

The most common serious pathologies to affect the lumbar spine are fractures, metastatic disease, cauda equina syndrome and infection (Finucane et al., 2020). The clinician needs to be aware of risk factors and signs and symptoms to look out for. These are covered in detail in the International Framework for Red Flags, with guidance for clinicians on clinical decision-making related to patients presenting with concerning features (Finucane et al., 2020).

Cardiovascular Disease

Is there a history of cardiac disease or cardiovascular risk factors, e.g. hypertension, angina, diabetes? A history of cardiovascular disease in a patient with leg symptoms may raise suspicion of peripheral vascular disease which can mimic symptoms of spinal stenosis (Jansen et al., 2019). Patients presenting with back and leg symptoms aggravated by walking may have spinal claudication or vascular claudication, so a detailed vascular history will help differentiate the underlying cause (Comer et al., 2020).

Diabetes

Does the patient suffer from diabetes mellitus? Patients with diabetes may develop peripheral neuropathy and vasculopathy, are at an increased risk of infection and may take longer to heal than those without diabetes. It is important to consider the location of any sensory abnormality. Peripheral neuropathy/sensory disturbance tends to present with a stocking distribution of paraesthesia (Lehmann et al., 2020), whereas lumbar radiculopathy will likely fit within a dermatomal distribution.

Osteoporosis

Does the patient have a known history of osteoporosis? Has the patient had appropriate imaging, e.g. an x-ray if fracture suspected and dual-energy x-ray absorptiometry scan for diagnosis of osteoporosis and measurement of bone density? It is essential to know if the patient has had previous fractures in the spine—the most common area to suffer pathological fractures—or if they have had other low-impact fractures in other areas such as the wrist or hip (National Osteoporosis Guidance Group (NOGG), 2021; Finucane et al., 2020). The risk of further fracture increases if the patient is not treated for their osteoporosis (NOGG, 2021). This information would be a caution to physical testing in the physical examination.

Previous Surgery

Has the patient had previous surgery which may be of relevance to the presenting complaint? Patients who have had previous spinal surgery are at significantly higher risk of developing spinal infections occurring in up to 40% of cases (Jeong et al., 2014).

Drug Therapy

What medication is being taken by the patient? Is the patient self-medicating or been prescribed medication for their LBP, for example, strong analgesics, combinations of analgesics, antiinflammatories and/or neuropathic pain medication?

This information is relevant for several reasons:

1. Indicates the severity of the patient's pain experience. Is what they are taking effective and recommended by NICE guidelines for appropriate prescription for LBP and lower limb symptoms? (NICE, 2020.) Alternatively, if the patient has not taken pain medication why might this be, and would a short course be useful? Would the patient benefit from a pharmacological review?
2. Identifies possible risk factors for other causes of spinal pain, for example steroid use of $\geq$ 5 mg for more than 3 months increases the risk of vertebral fracture (NOGG, 2021).
3. Informs the clinician about the patient's general health and highlights medical conditions that may cause back pain, such as abdominal aortic aneurysm, constipation, endometriosis (Goel, 2019).

Investigations and Imaging

Has the patient had any investigations (e.g. blood tests for systemic inflammatory conditions, been radiographed or had any other investigations for this or any similar complaint (magnetic resonance imaging [MRI] and computed tomography [CT] scan). Unless a bony injury, e.g. a fracture is suspected, x-rays should not routinely be done for diagnosis in LBP as they expose the patient to unnecessary radiation for limited clinical information (NICE, 2020). MRI scans are more sensitive and specific for spinal pathology but should only be requested to help plan further interventions or to exclude serious pathology when clinical history and examination have raised significant concerns.

KNOWLEDGE CHECK

1. What features are recognized features of inflammatory back pain?
2. When should x-rays be used for low back pain?
3. Explain the value of asking about a patient's use of medication?
4. What questions would you ask in assessing for symptoms of cauda equina syndrome?

Plan of the Physical Examination

When all this information has been collected, the subjective examination is complete. It is useful at this stage to highlight with asterisks (*), for ease of reference, important findings and particularly one or more functional restrictions. These can then be re-examined at subsequent treatment sessions to evaluate the treatment intervention.

In order to plan the physical examination, the following hypotheses need to be developed from the subjective examination:

- Are there any precautions and/or contraindications to elements of the physical examination that need to be explored further, such as significant neurological involvement, recent fracture, trauma, steroid therapy or rheumatoid arthritis? There may also be certain contraindications to further examination and treatment, e.g. symptoms of cord compression.
- The regions and structures that need to be examined as a possible cause of the symptoms, e.g. lumbar spine, thoracic spine, sacroiliac joint, pubic symphysis, hip, knee, ankle and foot, muscles and nerves. Often it is not possible to examine all of these areas fully at the first attendance and so examination of the structures must be prioritized over subsequent treatment sessions.
- In what way should the physical tests be carried out? Are symptoms severe and/or irritable? Will it be easy or hard to reproduce each symptom? Will it be necessary to use combined movements, repetitive movements, sustained movements or functional activities to reproduce the patient's symptoms?
- If symptoms are severe, physical tests may be carried out just before the onset of symptom production or just at the onset of symptom production; no overpressures will be carried out, as the patient would be unable to tolerate this. If symptoms are nonsevere, physical tests will be carried out to reproduce symptoms fully and may include overpressures and combined movements.
- If symptoms are irritable, physical tests may be examined just before symptom production or just at the onset of provocation, with fewer physical tests being examined to allow for a rest period between tests. If symptoms are nonirritable, physical tests will be carried out to reproduce symptoms fully and may include overpressures and combined movements.
- A physical examination planning form can be useful for clinicians to help guide them through the clinical reasoning process (see Appendix 3.1 and 3.2).

PHYSICAL EXAMINATION

The information from the subjective examination helps the clinician to plan an appropriate physical examination (Jones & Rivett, 2004). The severity, irritability and nature of the condition are the major factors that will influence the choice and priority of physical testing procedures. The first and overarching question the clinician might ask is: 'Is this patient's condition suitable for me to manage?' For example, a patient presenting with cauda equina compression symptoms may only need neurological integrity testing, prior to an urgent medical referral. The second question the clinician might ask is: 'Does this patient have a neuromusculoskeletal dysfunction that I may be able to help?' To answer that, the clinician needs to carry out a full physical examination; however, this may not be possible if the symptoms are severe and/or irritable. If the patient's symptoms are severe and/or irritable, the clinician aims to explore movements as much as possible, within a symptom-free range. If the patient has constant and severe and/or irritable symptoms, then the clinician aims to find physical tests that ease the symptoms. If the patient's symptoms are nonsevere and nonirritable, then the clinician aims to find physical tests that reproduce each of the patient's symptoms.

Each significant physical test that either provokes or eases the patient's symptoms is highlighted in the patient's notes by an asterisk (*) for easy reference. The highlighted tests are often referred to as 'asterisks' or 'markers'.

The order and detail of the physical tests described below need to be appropriate to the patient being examined; some tests will be irrelevant, some tests will be carried out briefly, while it will be necessary to investigate others fully.

Observation

Informal Observation

This should begin as soon as the clinician sees the patient for the first time. This may be in the reception or waiting area, or as the patient enters the treatment room, and should continue throughout the subjective examination. The clinician should be aware of the patient's posture, demeanour, facial expressions, gait and interaction with the clinician, as these may all give valuable information regarding any anxieties the patient may have, possible pain mechanisms and the severity and irritability of the problem.

Formal Observation

The clinician observes the patient's spinal, pelvic and lower-limb posture in standing, from anterior, lateral and posterior views. Any asymmetry in levels at the pelvis and shoulders and in muscle bulk, tone and symmetry should be noted. Skin colour, areas of redness, swelling or sweating should be noted, as these may indicate areas of local pathology, or possibly a systemic or dermatological condition. The clinician should watch the patient performing simple functional tasks or tasks that the patient has identified as being problematic. Observation of gait, of sit-to-stand and dressing/undressing will help to give the clinician a good idea of how the patient is likely to move in the physical examination, and may help to highlight any problems such as hypervigilance and fear avoidance.

Despite widespread beliefs about correct posture, there is no strong evidence that avoiding incorrect posture prevents LBP or that any single spinal curvature is strongly associated with pain (Kwon et al., 2011). Slater et al. (2019) propose changing the narrative around posture and LBP, avoiding a one-size-fits-all approach. The authors suggest considering how to expose people to postures and ways of moving that they have avoided and encourage change in habits that may be provocative. Alterations in posture or movements that relieve symptoms in the acute stage may not be needed long-term.

Active Physiological Movements

For active physiological movements, the clinician notes the:

- quality of movement
- range of movement
- behaviour of pain through the range of movement
- resistance through the range of movement and at the end of the range of movement
- provocation of any muscle spasm.

The active movements with overpressure listed are tested with the patient in standing and are shown in Fig. 13.1. The clinician usually stands behind the patient to be able to see the quality and range of movement. Before starting the active movements, the clinician notes any deformity or deviation in the patient's spinal posture or any muscle spasm. This may include

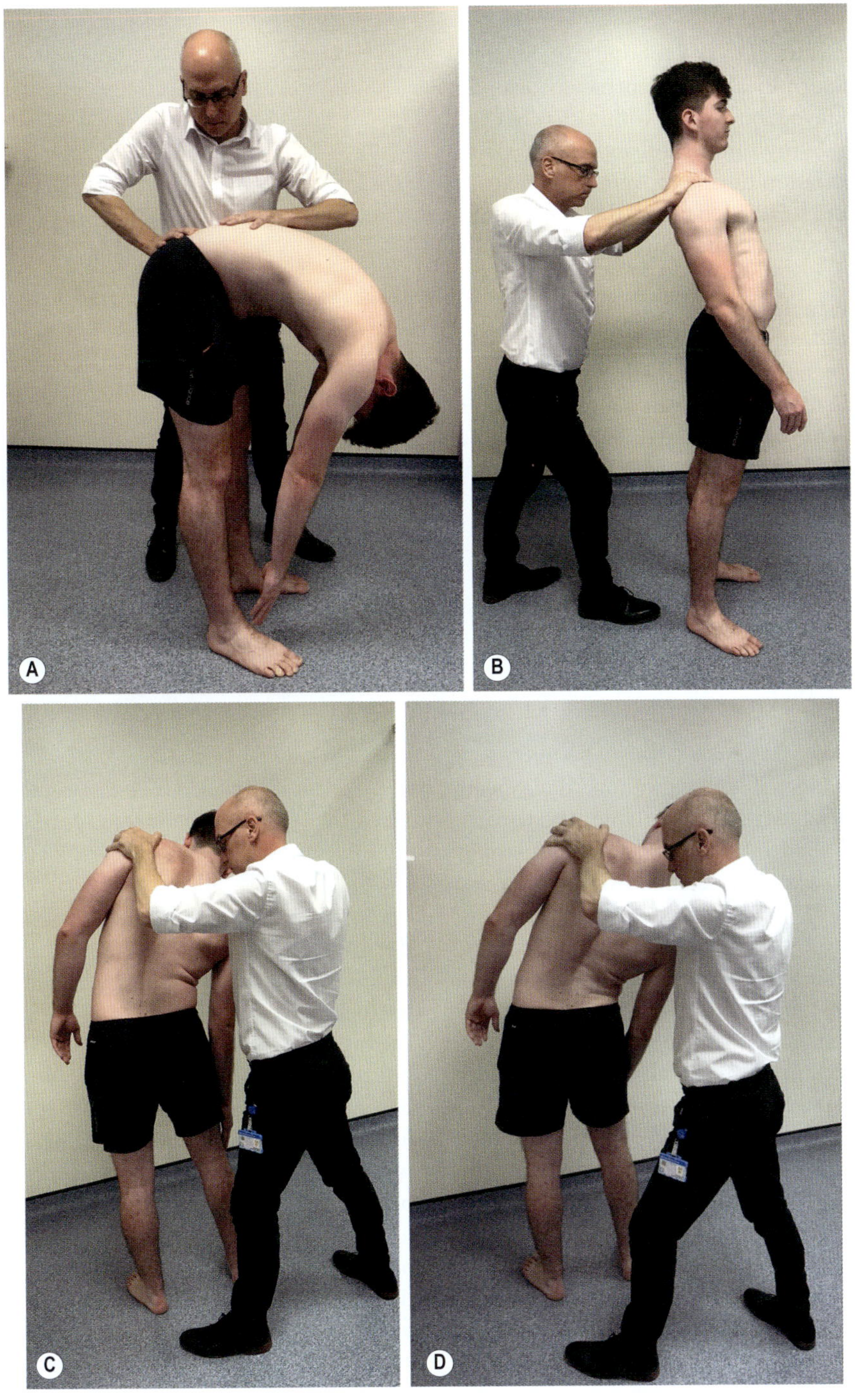

Fig. 13.1 Overpressures to the lumbar spine. (A) Flexion. The hands are placed proximally over the lower thoracic spine and distally over the sacrum. Pressure is then applied through both hands to increase lumbar spine flexion. (B) Extension. Both hands are placed over the shoulders, which are then pulled down in order to increase lumbar spine extension. The clinician observes the spinal movement. (C) Lateral flexion. Both hands are placed over the shoulders, and a force is applied that increases lumbar lateral flexion. (D) Right extension quadrant. This movement is a combination of extension, right rotation and right lateral flexion. The handhold is the same as for extension. The patient actively extends, and the clinician maintains this position, passively rotates the spine, and then adds lateral flexion overpressure.

scoliosis, a lateral shift, or a kyphotic or lordotic posture. Postural deformities can be corrected prior to starting the active movements to see if this changes the patient's symptoms. Symptom response through range is noted, and any deviation during movement can again be corrected to see if this changes the symptoms. Changes in pain response may help to guide the treatment.

Patients may exhibit a range of compensatory movement strategies, some of which may be a way to avoid pain (adaptive), but some of which are likely to be provocative (maladaptive). O'Sullivan (2015) describes typical movement patterns and related tests as part of a subclassification system for patients with low back pain.

Simple movements tested are:

- flexion
- extension
- lateral flexion to the right
- lateral flexion to the left
- lateral glide to the left
- lateral glide to the right
- left rotation
- right rotation.

At the end of range, if no symptoms have been produced and the problem is nonirritable, then overpressure may be applied in order to clear that single movement and to explore further for symptoms (Maitland et al., 2005). If this produces no symptoms and the clinician is still searching for the patient's pain, or is looking to screen the lumbar spine as a source of the pain, then these movements may be combined Fig. 13.2. The order in which the movements are combined will depend on the aggravating activities, and the patient's response to plane movements.

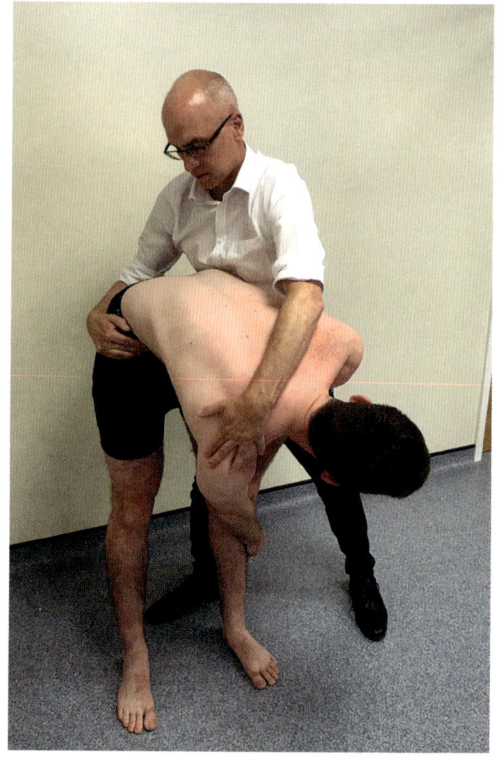

Fig. 13.2 Combined movement of the lumbar spine. The patient moves into lumbar spine flexion, and the clinician then maintains this position and passively adds right lateral flexion.

Hicks et al. (2003) examined the reliability of active movement testing and found good kappa values (mean 0.60 and 95% confidence intervals 0.43–0.73).

Movements may also be repeated to see the effect this has on the patient's symptoms.

Differentiation or Symptom Modification

Additional tests may also be useful to help to differentiate the lumbar spine from the hip and sacroiliac joint in standing. For example, when trunk rotation in standing on one leg (causing rotation in the lumbar spine and hip joint) reproduces the patient's buttock pain, differentiation between the lumbar spine and hip joint may be required. The clinician can increase and decrease the lumbar spine rotation and the pelvic rotation in turn, to find out what effect each has on the buttock pain (Fig. 13.3). If the pain is emanating from the hip then the lumbar movements may have no effect, but pelvic movements may alter the pain; conversely, if the pain is emanating from the lumbar spine, then lumbar spine movements may alter the pain, but pelvic movement may have no effect. The hip can also be placed in a different position, in order to see how much it is contributing to the pain. It can be placed in a more or less provocative position, depending on the subjective aggravating factors and the irritability of the problem, and the pain response noted. Changes to symptom response may guide the clinician towards a more in-depth hip assessment or may equally focus the clinician on the lumbar spine. Compression or distraction of the sacroiliac joints can be added at the same time to see if this helps to change symptoms. Changes in pain may help guide the clinician towards a more in-depth assessment of the sacroiliac joints.

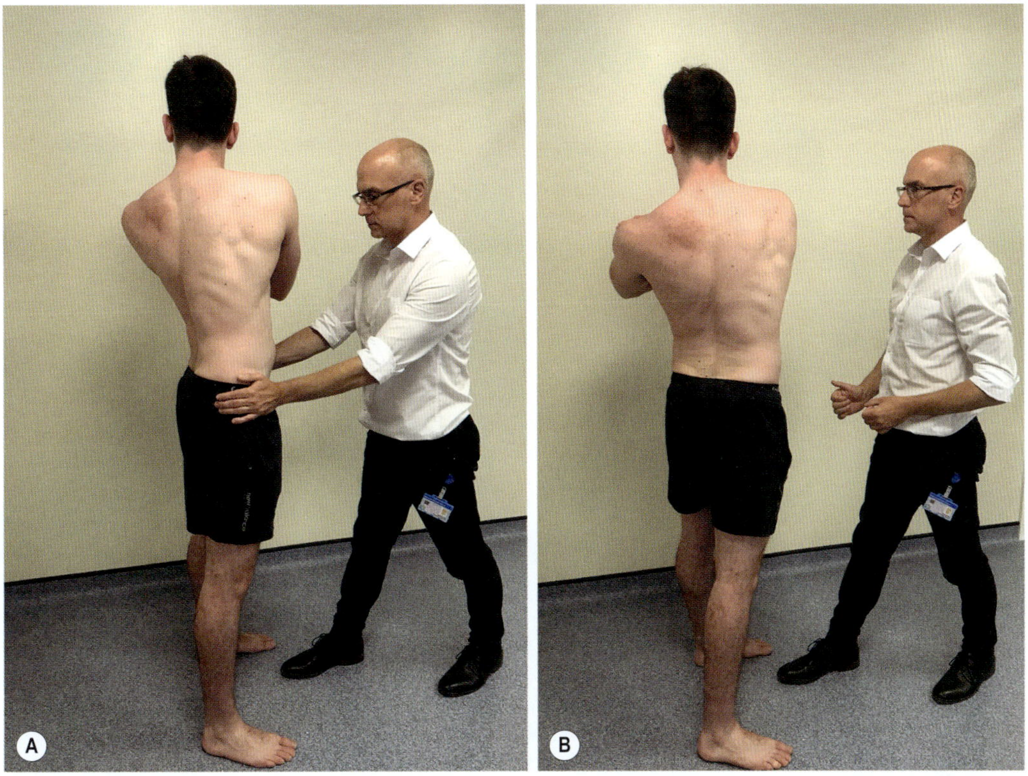

Fig. 13.3 Differentiation between lumbar spine and hip. (A) Lumbar and hip rotation. (B) Lumbar rotation with hips released. The clinician rotates the lumbar spine and the pelvis/hip – identifies symptom response before releasing hips if pain remains unchanged this implicates the lumbar spine.

Some functional ability has already been tested by the general observation of the patient during the subjective and physical examinations, e.g. the posture adopted during the subjective examination and the ease or difficulty of undressing and changing position prior to the examination. Any further functional testing can be carried out at this point in the examination and may include lifting, sitting postures and dressing. Clues for appropriate tests can be obtained from the subjective examination findings, particularly aggravating factors. These may be particularly helpful if the pain is proving difficult to reproduce with the other tests described.

Passive Physiological Movements

Passive physiological intervertebral movements (PPIVMs), which examine the movement at each segmental level, may be used to identify segmental hypomobility and hypermobility (Hengeveld & Banks, 2014). They can be performed with the patient in side-lying position with the hips and knees flexed (Fig. 13.4). The clinician palpates the gap between adjacent spinous processes to feel the range of intervertebral movement during flexion, extension, lateral flexion and rotation. It is usually not necessary to examine all directions of movement, only the movement that has been most provocative or most positive during active movement tests, or the movement that most closely fits the patient's aggravating activities, e.g. if a patient says he has most pain when bending to tie shoelaces, then flexion would be the logical PPIVM choice.

Abbott et al. (2005) evaluated the validity of PPIVMs. Specificity was found to be generally high (0.99–1.00), whereas sensitivity was extremely poor (0.03–0.07). It has been suggested that there is low value in using PPIVMs (flexion and extension) for detecting lumbar instability and their use in ruling out lumbar instability, is not recommended (Stolz et al., 2020). Phillips and Twomey (1996) evaluated the

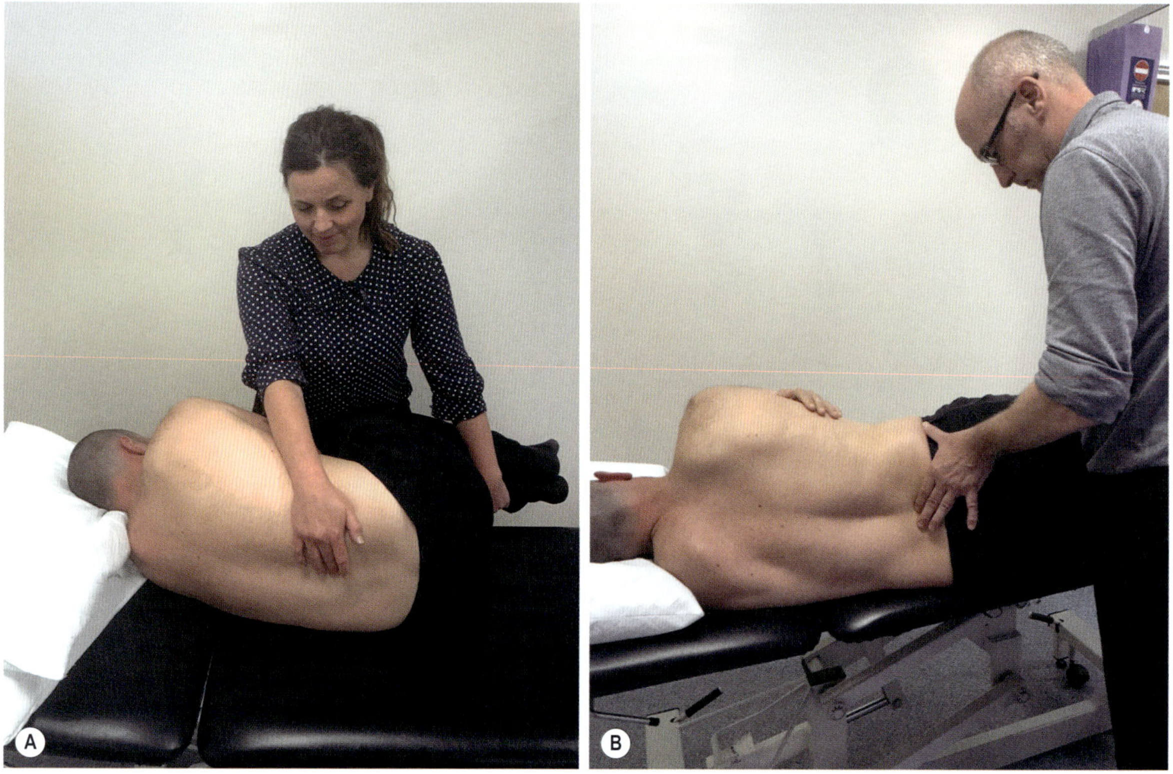

Fig. 13.4 Flexion/extension passive physiological intervertebral movements (PPIVMs) of the lumbar spine. (A) Flexion PPIVM: palpate the interspinous space of the spinal level being assessed. Flex the patient's hips and feel for gapping at the interspinous space. Assess the same movement at other lumbar levels to give an indication of the relative segmental motion. (B) Extension PPIVM: palpate the interspinous space of the spinal level being assessed. Extend the patient's hips and feel for the closing down or coming together of the spinous processes at the interspinous space. Assess the same movement at other lumbar levels to give an indication of the relative segmental motion. One leg may be used for this technique, depending on the relative size of the clinician and the patient.

validity of PPIVMs and passive accessory intervertebral movements (PAIVMs) in combination. Sensitivity and specificity for mobility judgement were not as good as for pain provocation, resulting in an excellent positive and negative likelihood ratio for pain and a fair positive likelihood ratio for mobility assessment.

Muscle Tests

Muscle tests may include examining muscle strength, control, length and isometric muscle testing. Depending on the patient presentation, these tests may not be a priority on day 1 of the examination, but they may well be part of the ongoing patient management and rehabilitation. Assessment should be based on the subjective asterisks (movements or tests that have been found to reproduce the patient's symptoms). If the clinician thinks that the muscle is the main source of symptoms, or a strong contributing factor to the patient's problem, then the muscle control component should be examined on day 1. Patients may complain of a feeling of weakness, of a lack of control of movement, or catches of pain through movement, and these types of descriptions should alert the clinician to the importance of the muscle component of the patient presentation. Muscle may be both a source of symptoms and a contributing factor.

Muscle Strength

The clinician may test the trunk flexors, extensors, lateral flexors and rotators and any other relevant muscle groups, if these are indicated from the subjective examination. For details of these general tests, readers are directed to Hislop and Montgomery (2007) or Kendall et al. (2010). Magee and Manske (2021) describe testing isometric spinal flexion, extension, side flexion and rotation with the patient sitting in a neutral position. More advanced tests are also described, including the dynamic abdominal endurance test, dynamic extensor endurance test, double straight leg lowering test, internal/external abdominal oblique, dynamic horizontal side support (bridge) and back rotators/multifidus tests. There is good evidence to suggest that general exercise and strengthening exercises are likely to be of benefit for people with low back pain (Van Tulder et al., 2005; Clinical Guidelines, 2021; NICE, 2020).

Muscle Control

Many approaches for LBP management focus on modifying motor control which refers to motor, sensory and central processes for control of posture and movement (Hides et al., 2019). There is evidence that patients with LBP can present with both increased activation of trunk muscles as well as inhibition and weakness (Hodges & Moseley, 2003). It is not clear whether these changes in muscle activity are the cause or effect of pain. Changes in muscle activity are thought to be context specific, for example relating to the patient's fear of a specific movement such as bending which may lead to anticipatory guarding and stiffening of the trunk. It is considered that these changes in motor control may be either an adaptive/helpful strategy to avoid further injury or maladaptive, for example, bracing of trunk muscles creating more continuous forces through the spine.

Several systems for subgrouping or profiling motor control aspects in the assessment of patients with LBP have been developed which will be summarized below.

Motor Control Training

In the late 1990s several studies identified a consistent delay in activation of the transversus abdominus (TrA) muscle in patients with a history of LBP with rapid limb movements (Hodges & Richardson, 1999; Hodges et al., 1999). Transverse abdominus is thought to activate in a preparatory or feed forward pattern with EMG analysis showing that in healthy subjects it activates prior to anterior deltoid with rapid arm movements (Hodges & Richardson, 1997a, 1997b). Research also found evidence of atrophy in the multifidus muscles in patients with LBP (Hides et al., 2008). This research led to a focus on teaching patients to isolate the deep anterior and posterior muscles.

The aim of the approach is for an appropriate balance between movement and stiffness as required by the task and the individual (Hides et al., 2019). Assessment can include palpation, observation and ultrasound to assess the timing and quality of activation of these muscles. The assessment process incorporates consideration of pain mechanisms and psychosocial factors and their influence on the patient's presentation. Training can include voluntary contraction of deeper trunk muscles to teach the skill of activating these muscles with the emphasis on integrating these into function and reducing overactivity of more superficial muscles.

The importance of TrA in spinal stability in isolation has been questioned (Cholewicki & VanVliet, 2002; Allison & Morris, 2008; Lederman, 2009). It has also been suggested that asking patients to focus on 'stabilizing' their back with these types of exercises can reinforce a patient's beliefs that there is something wrong with their back. This highlights the importance of exploring the patient's beliefs and concerns about their back pain. O'Sullivan (2018) discusses the importance of the language that we use with patients, giving a clear message that their spine is a strong structure.

Movement system impairment classification system. In this classification system developed and described by Sahrmann (2013), the main inducers of movement impairments are considered to be the repeated movements and sustained alignments of everyday activities. These are thought to result in tissue adaptations leading to a joint moving more readily in a specific direction causing pain. Clinical examination identifies the movement directions that elicit symptoms and the contributing factors, e.g. excessive lumbar flexion and limited hip flexion during forward bending. The effect of the patient correcting the movement impairment on the symptoms is noted. The systematic movement examination consists of tests performed in different positions, such as standing, supine, side-lying, prone, quadruped and sitting. Movements are corrected primarily by limiting any associated lumbar motion and effects on symptoms are noted. Patients are taught the correct way to perform basic mobility activities as well as those relevant to their work or fitness.

O'Sullivan et al. (2006) developed an assessment classification for patients with persistent nonspecific LBP which was found to have good interrater reliability when applied by trained therapists (Dankaerts et al., 2006). They describe maladaptive movement patterns that patients with NSLBP may present with.

These classifications include

- flexion dysfunction,
- flexion/lateral shift pattern,
- passive extension,
- active extension pattern,
- multidirectional instability (Dankaerts et al., 2006).

This assessment system has been further defined as a flexible multidimensional clinical reasoning framework which helps therapists to identify both modifiable and nonmodifiable factors contributing to a patient's pain (O'Sullivan et al., 2018). This framework has been designed for patients with persistent disabling LBP but is felt to be applicable to all patients with nonspecific LBP. This treatment approach consists of:

1. helping patients make sense of pain
2. gradual exposure to challenging/valued tasks through exploring changes in movement to reduce pain
3. lifestyle change—highlighting the importance of factors such as good quality sleep and general activity/health.

The authors describe 'behavioural experiments' in specific case studies. An example of this is a patient presenting with active extension pattern taught to relax back posture with reduced lordosis.

When examining the way a patient moves it is important to consider the dominating pain mechanisms, for example, a patient with mechanical nociceptive pain is more likely to have a direction-specific limitation to movements, whereas those with high levels of fear and anxiety are more likely to display bracing and general overactivity of the trunk muscles limiting movements more globally.

A common theme with the motor control approaches discussed is the importance of using functional assessment looking at specific tasks relevant to the individual patient identified in the subjective examination (Hides et al., 2019).

A systematic review by Saragiotto et al. (2016) found there was no clinically important difference between motor control exercise and other forms of exercises or manual therapy for acute and chronic LBP. The authors of this study suggest that effectiveness of motor control exercises should also be tested on subgroups of patients more likely to respond to this approach. Assessment of patients' general fitness as well as relevant strength in other areas of the body to help achieve functional goals are also important, e.g. strengthening lower limb with squats when retraining a patient with flexion dysfunction (O'Sullivan et al., 2018).

Neurological Tests

Neurological examination includes neurological integrity testing, tests for neural sensitization and other specific nerve tests.

Integrity of the Nervous System

As a general guide, a neurological examination is indicated if the patient has symptoms below the level of the buttock crease, or if reporting altered sensation, weakness or any neurological symptoms.

Dermatomes/peripheral nerves. Light touch and pain sensation of the lower limb are tested using cotton wool and pinprick, respectively. It is always useful to quantify any variations from the normal, as this can then be used as an asterisk and retested at a later date. For example, if sensation to light touch is 4/10 at initial assessment, but then 7/10 following treatment, this identifies an important marker of change for the clinician and the patient. Knowledge of the cutaneous distribution of nerve roots (dermatomes) and peripheral nerves enables the clinician to distinguish the sensory loss due to a root lesion from that due to a peripheral nerve lesion.

It should be noted that sensation may be increased in certain conditions. The clinician should be aware of the possible different descriptions of these sensory variations, e.g. allodynia, hyperalgesia, analgesia and hyperpathia.

Myotomes/peripheral nerves. The following myotomes are tested in sitting or lying or in a position of comfort for the patient. The clinician should take account of the patient's pain when testing muscle power, as pain will often inhibit full cooperation from the patient, and may lead to a false-positive test.

- L2—3—4: hip flexion
- L2—3—4: knee extension
- L4—5—S1: foot dorsiflexion and inversion
- L4—5—S1: extension of the big toe
- L5—S1: eversion foot, contract buttock, knee flexion
- L5—S1: toe flexion

- S1–S2: knee flexion, plantarflexion
- S3–S4: muscles of the pelvic floor, bladder and genital function.

A working knowledge of the muscular distribution of nerve roots (myotomes) and peripheral nerves enables the clinician to distinguish motor loss due to a root lesion from that due to a peripheral nerve lesion. Patients with myotomal weakness of grade 3/5 MRC or less and with more than two spinal root levels of weakness in the lumbar spine should be discussed with an experienced clinician in a timely manner as they will likely need onward referral for investigation.

Reflex testing. The following deep tendon reflexes are tested with the patient relaxed, usually in sitting or lying:

- L3–L4: knee jerk
- S1–S2: ankle jerk.

Any abnormalities in the reflexes might lead to a more extensive examination of the nervous system to exclude CNS involvement (see Chapter 4.) This might include Hoffman's, Clonus, Rhomberg's and cranial nerve testing.

Neural Sensitization Tests

Neural sensitization tests may be carried out in order to ascertain the degree to which neural tissue is responsible for the production of the patient's symptoms.

- passive neck flexion
- straight-leg raise (SLR)
- femoral nerve tension test in side-lying
- slump test.

The choice of test should be guided by the aggravating activities, e.g. a slump test if the patients symptoms are worse with sitting/driving and straight leg raise test (SLR) if symptoms are worse with walking.

Majlesi et al. (2008) found that the slump test was more sensitive (0.84) than the SLR (0.52) in patients with lumbar disc herniations confirmed on MRI. However, the SLR was found to be a slightly more specific test (0.89) than the slump test (0.83).

Further tests may be added in order to bias specific peripheral nerves, such as the sural nerve or common peroneal nerve, depending on the area of symptoms.

Nerves in the lower limb can be palpated at the following points:

- the sciatic nerve two-thirds of the way along an imaginary line between the greater trochanter and the ischial tuberosity
- the common peroneal nerve medial to the tendon of biceps femoris and also around the head of the fibula
- the tibial nerve centrally over the posterior knee crease medial to the popliteal artery; it can also be felt behind the medial malleolus, which is more noticeable with the foot in dorsiflexion and eversion
- the superficial peroneal nerve on the dorsum of the foot along an imaginary line over the fourth metatarsal; it is more noticeable with the foot in plantarflexion and inversion
- the deep peroneal nerve between the first and second metatarsals, lateral to the extensor hallucis tendon
- the sural nerve on the lateral aspect of the foot behind the lateral malleolus, lateral to the tendocalcaneus.

Other Neurological Tests

Plantar Response to Test for an Upper Motor Neuron Lesion (Walker et al., 1990).

Pressure applied from the heel along the lateral border of the plantar aspect of the foot produces flexion of the toes in the normal individual. Extension of the big toe with outward fanning of the other toes is known as a positive Babinski sign or upward going plantar response and indicates an upper motor neuron lesion such as a brain haemorrhage or spinal tumour.

Clonus. The patient's ankle is rapidly dorsiflexed by the clinician in order to elicit a stretch response in the calf. A normal response would be up to 2–4 beats of plantarflexion from the patient. More than this is suggestive of an upper motor neuron problem such as multiple sclerosis (MS).

Coordination. Simple coordination tests can be used if the clinician suspects that there is an issue with control of movement. Upper and lower limbs should be tested. Finger–nose tests and heel–shin sliding tests done bilaterally may help to identify problems with coordination.

Miscellaneous Tests

Examination of Other Areas

It may be appropriate to examine adjacent areas, such as the thoracic spine, the hip or sacroiliac joints, as these may directly refer to the lumbar spine, or they may be contributing factors to the pain in the lumbar spine. Examination of these areas is covered in the respective regional chapters.

Vascular Tests

If the patient's circulation is suspected of being compromised, the pulses of the femoral, popliteal and dorsalis pedis and posterior tibial arteries are palpated in both legs. Capillary refill is also tested in the toes to test the small blood vessel. The toenail beds are squeezed until they blanch and normally revascularize within 3 seconds—a delay indicates small vessel vascular disease. The state of the vascular system can also be determined by the response of symptoms to dependence and elevation of the lower limbs.

The clinician should be vigilant for male patients over the age of 65 who complain of diffuse low back pain which is not mechanical in nature. Abdominal aortic aneurysms may present as low back pain. The clinician should clearly ask about any vascular history when exploring the patient's past medical history.

Leg Length

A difference in leg length of up to 1–1.3 cm is considered normal. Although leg-length discrepancy (LLD) has been listed as risk factor of LBP, there is conflicting evidence on the relationship between LLD and LBP, and hence there is disagreement on the benefits of correcting LLD in people with back pain. Haryoni et al. (2019) found no association between LBP and LLD in a cross-sectional study of college students.

Rannisto et al. (2019) investigating a small sample size of workers with an LLD of 5 mm or more who stood during their workday, identified benefits from correction with insoles with less back pain and greater work presenteeism. A systematic review by Campbell et al. (2018) concluded that there was low-quality evidence that shoe raises reduce pain and improve function in patients with LLD with common painful musculoskeletal conditions including back pain.

Palpation

The clinician palpates the lumbar spine and any other relevant areas. It is useful to record palpation findings on a body chart and/or palpation chart.

The clinician notes the following:

- the temperature of the area
- localized increased skin moisture
- the presence of any swelling
- mobility and feel of superficial tissues, e.g. ganglions, nodules and the lymph nodes in the femoral triangle
- the presence of any muscle spasm
- increased or decreased prominence of bones
- pain provoked or reduced on palpation.

Passive Accessory Intervertebral Movements

The clinician palpates the spine and notes the:

- quality of movement
- range of movement
- resistance through the range and at the end of the range of movement
- behaviour of pain and any other symptoms through the range
- provocation of any muscle spasm.

Lumbar spine (L1–L5) accessory movements can be performed on different parts of the vertebra—central posteroanterior, unilateral posteroanterior and transverse glides, shown in Fig. 13.5. Each can be angled to explore the movement more fully. Lumbar spine accessory movements may need to be examined with the patient in flexion, extension, lateral flexion, rotation or a combination of these positions (Fig. 13.6) or in functional positions that the patient finds uncomfortable or restricted.

Accessory movements can also be tested for other regions suspected to be a source of, or contributing to, the patient's symptoms—these may include the thoracic spine, the hips and the sacroiliac joints.

If the clinician feels that the symptoms may be difficult to reproduce, then s/he may choose to do the accessory movements in a more provocative position, which will be dependent on the aggravating active movements or provocative functional activities. Conversely, if the patient's condition is severe and irritable, the clinician may choose a nonprovocative position for the accessory movements, or may choose to omit them completely from the initial examination.

Hicks et al. (2003) examined the reliability of passive movement testing, palpation and provocation tests for the identification of lumbar segmental instability and found poor kappa values for segmental passive tests (κ range 0.02–0.26) but better reliability (κ range 0.25–0.55) for passive pain provocation tests. Hidalgo et al. (2014) also found that a combination of pain provocative tests demonstrated acceptable inter-examiner reliability in identifying the main pain provocative movement pattern and the level of lumbar segment involvement. A systematic review by Stolz et al. (2020) also concluded that the reliability and validity of segmental motion tests were greater when used in combination rather than in isolation.

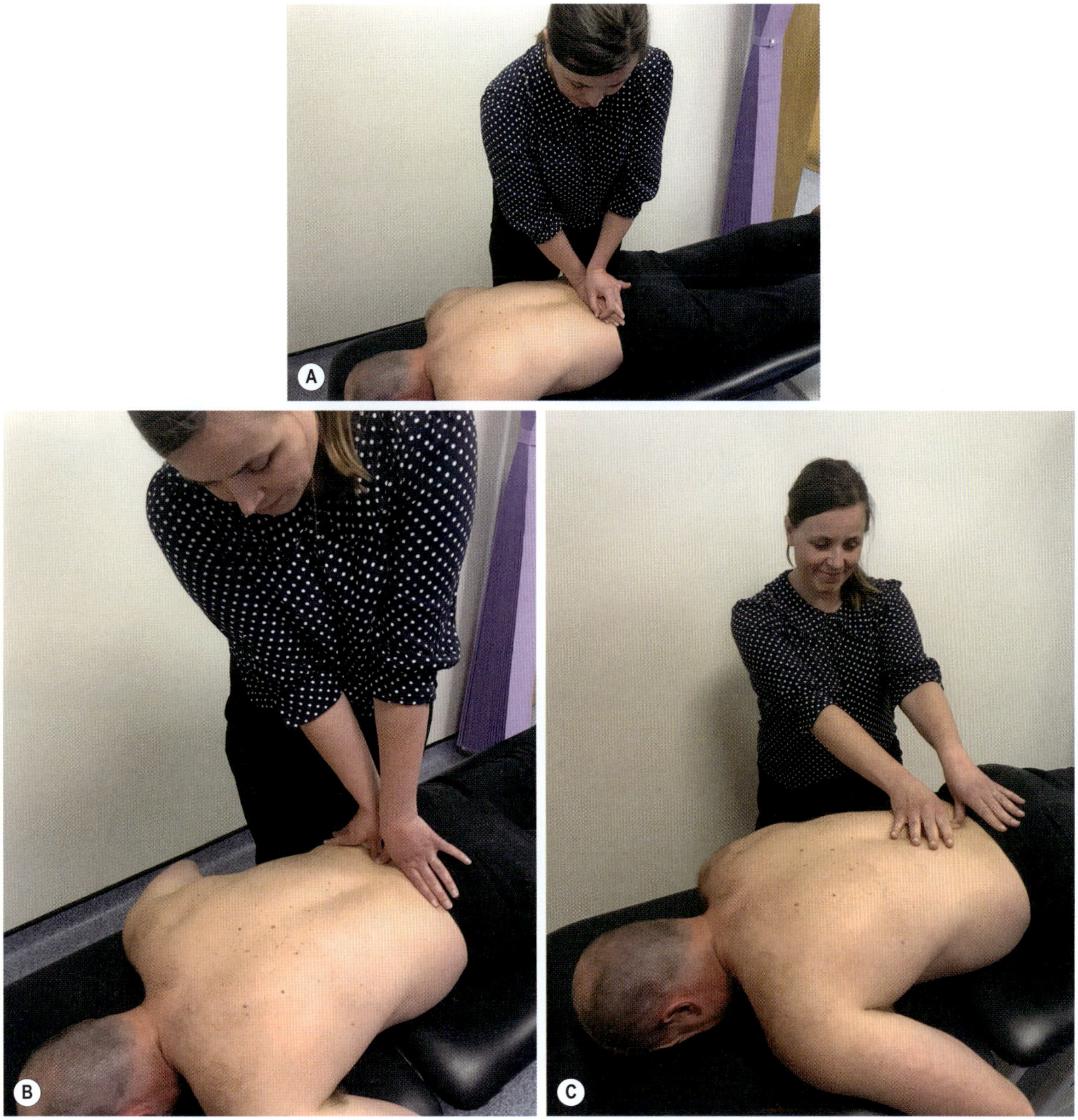

Fig. 13.5 Lumbar spine accessory movements. (A) Central posteroanterior. The pisiform grip is used to apply a posteroanterior pressure on the spinous process. (B) Unilateral posteroanterior. Thumb pressure is applied to the transverse process. (C) Transverse. Thumb pressure is applied to the lateral aspect of the spinous process.

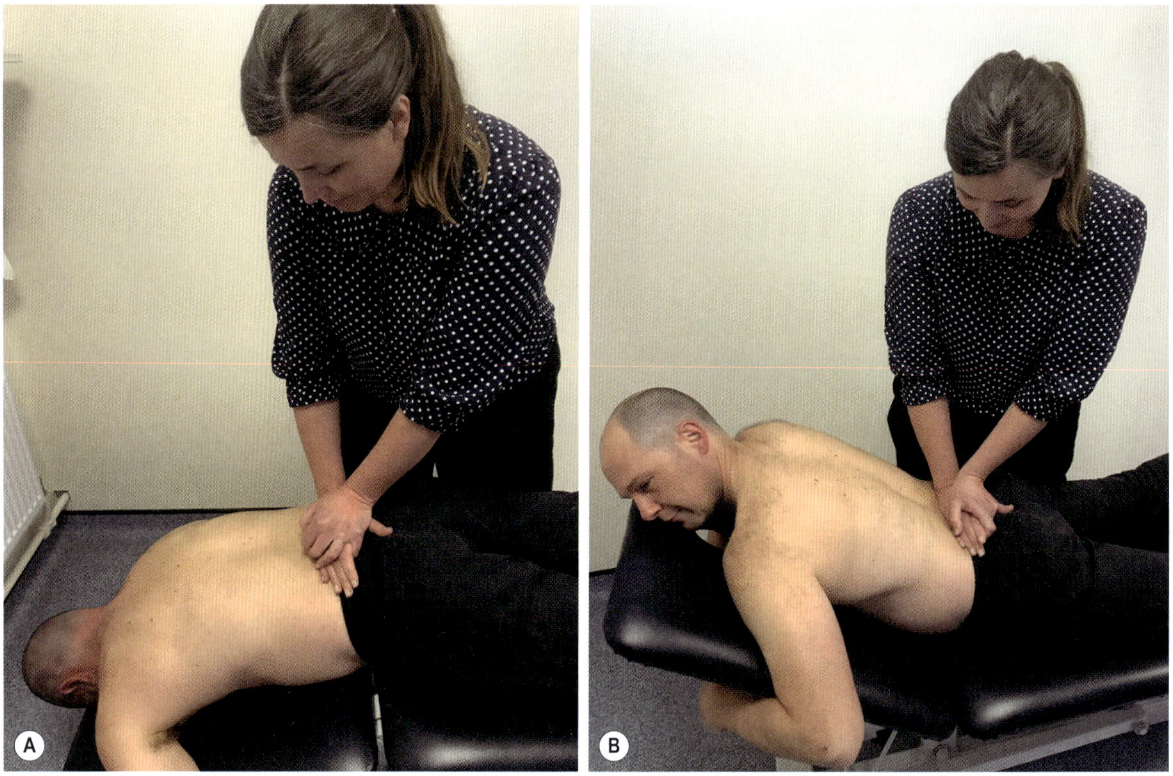

Fig.13.6 Posteroanterior pressure in (A) flexion, (B) extension.

> **KNOWLEDGE CHECK**
> 1. What level of motor weakness would prompt you to seek further investigation for your patient?
> 2. What tests might you include in your physical examination for a patient with a cardiovascular history to differentiate a possible vascular cause of leg pain?
> 3. What do the abbreviations PAIVM and PPIVM mean, and why are they useful in examining a patient with low back pain?
> 4. Explain using examples the differences between adaptive and maladaptive movement strategies.

COMPLETION OF THE EXAMINATION

The subjective and physical examinations produce a large amount of information which needs to be fully and accurately recorded. It is important, however, that the clinician does not examine in a rigid and formulaic manner. Each patient presents differently, and this needs to be reflected in the examination process and adapted to the individual.

A tailored and personalized examination that fully involves the patient will help build a strong therapeutic relationship and give the best chance of a positive outcome from treatment.

Following the examination, the clinician should fully explain what they have found and what that means, and working with the patient through a shared decision-making process, should formulate an agreed plan of the next steps (Hoffman et al., 2020).

For guidance on treatment and management principles, the reader is directed to the companion textbook (Barnard and Ryder, 2024).

REVIEW AND REVISE QUESTIONS

1. What percentage of people with LBP will have serious spinal pathology?
2. What are the limitations of imaging in diagnosis of LBP?
3. What are the five psychosocial factors identified by O'Sullivan as predictors for persistent pain and disability?
4. Identify the visceral organs that refer into the lumbar spinal region.
5. What can cause a person to have widespread symptoms?
6. What are the subjective examination findings and physical tests to identify possible cord compression?
7. Identify four lifestyle choices that increase the risk of developing cancer.
8. Patients with LBP have reduced motor activity. TRUE/FALSE?
9. When applying PAIVMs what should the clinician note?
10. When examining a patient presenting with non-irritable symptoms; what active movement testing can the clinician apply to screen the lumbar spine as a source of the pain?

Case Study Mr M

Male, aged 38 years old

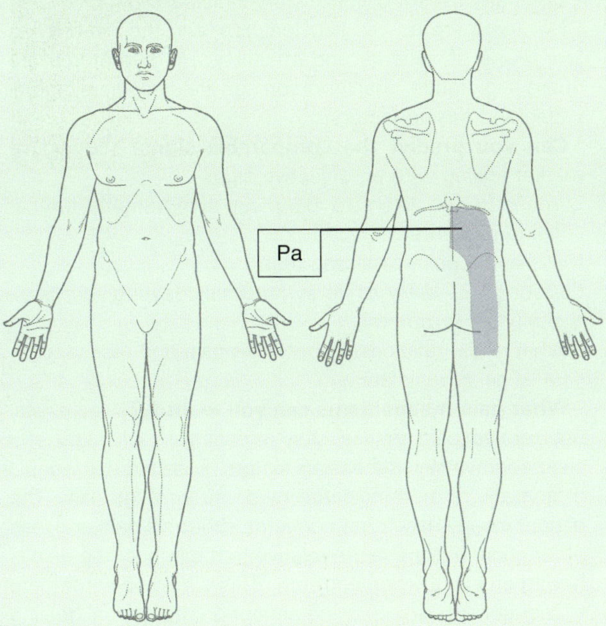

Pa—
Aggravating factors—
Sitting > 30 min
Bending
Twisting
Easing factors—
Stand and move
Lean backwards

24-h pattern—
Wakes up on turning in bed but able to get back to sleep. Pain generally better in the mornings although some stiffness for 5–10 min. During the day pain activity dependent. Evening symptoms depend on level of activity during the day.

No symptoms anywhere else

HPC
Back pain came on after long drive (4 h) 3 weeks ago. Pain in lumbar spine and posterior thigh started at the same time. Pain constant low level but can be severe and restricting.

Overall Pain Improving

Lifestyle/Occupation/Home Life
Self-employed plasterer. Married with two children aged 3 and 1. Surfs at weekends and runs 3/7 a week 5–10 km.

Impact on Function/Beliefs and Expectations
Unable to work at present due to the level of pain and doesn't feel will cope with the amount of driving. Finding it difficult to play with children. Unable to run or surf which is making him feel low, keen to return to previous level of fitness. Concerned about loss of income.

PMH
Otherwise in good general health.
Previous history of knee surgery on the left, no residual issues.
History of psoriasis.

Case Study Mr M—cont'd

DH/Investigations

Prescribed naproxen from GP which does relieve pain to a certain extent.
Tried ibuprofen and paracetamol which were not helpful.
No other medication currently.
No relevant investigations.

FH nil of note. No history of any inflammatory joint conditions, inflammatory bowel disease, uveitis or enthesopathy.

Clinical Reasoning

There are very few concerning features with this presentation. This patient is young and has clear mechanical aggravating and easing factors for his pain. His pain has started to improve within the normal healing times expected for this type of presentation. There are no inflammatory features to the nature of his pain in terms of any diurnal pattern. He is not woken with the pain, and he has no prolonged morning stiffness. He does however have constant low-level pain as well as psoriasis, both of which can be features of inflammatory back pain. At this stage on balance, his symptoms are less likely to be inflammatory in nature and more likely to be mechanical. He therefore does not require onward referral for further investigation.

He does have some psychosocial factors that need to be addressed with him to help his recovery. He has understandable worries about money and his ability to work as well as his ability to play with his children. These are legitimate concerns, and he needs to be reassured that his symptoms are likely to improve significantly over the next 3 weeks or so. He should be able to return to normal work, social and sporting activities, given the mechanical nature of his problem and the fact that he has had no previous episodes and he is otherwise fit and well.

- **Yellow flags**—patient starting to feel quite low about being unable to exercise however patient optimistic about his recovery and keen to get back to normal activities (**pink flag**).
- **Black flags**—financial concerns related to loss of income. Patient's work is quite heavy, and it is difficult to modify his work load as he works alone. However, he is expected to make a full recovery and be able to return to full duties.
- **Red flag** symptom—no concerning features. Patient's symptoms are constant; however, his symptoms are acute in nature and improving over time.
- **Evaluation of severity, irritability and nature**
- **Severity (Pa)**—moderate, taking regular naproxen, unable to work (NPRS of 5/10).
- **Irritability (Pa)—low** (symptoms with sitting >30 min, eases quickly with stretching backwards/standing.
- **Nature**—Acute mechanical back pain. Possible neurogenic component with radiation to the posterior thigh fitting with S1 dermatome.
- **What are you treating?** Likely mechanical back pain. Although the patient has a history of psoriasis and a constant background ache, his pain is recent onset, and there are no other features of inflammatory back pain.
- **Main functional limitation**—sitting

Subjective Markers (Link to Genics)

1. Sitting for greater than 30 min without back/posterior thigh pain.
2. Be able to return to work full time with manageable levels of pain.
3. Be able to play with his children.
4. Return to previous level of fitness, running 5–10 km and surfing.

Does any aspect of the history indicate caution?

No, there are no red flag features, and the patient has low levels of severity and irritability. His symptoms are improving, rather than worsening. He has clear aggravating and easing factors.

Can you predict the comparable signs? (Subjective marker linking with an objective sign)

Lumbar flexion likely to be most symptomatic lumbar spine movement.
May have a positive slump test.
L4/5 or L5/S1 likely to be symptomatic level given distribution of symptoms.

What is the relationship between pain and resistance?

Pa—Pain > resistance

What pain mechanisms can you identify? Mechanical nociceptive pain with a clear mechanism of injury and clear aggravating and easing factors. Possible neurogenic or somatic referral indicated by posterior thigh pain. The patient clearly has some concerns about his pain and loss of function, but these are relative to the impact the pain is having on his function currently. This would be something to monitor and reassure the patient on the normal healing times of these types of presentations, encouraging him to gradually return to exercise and work.

Analysis of percentage weighting (Pain source)—Myogenic 20%, atherogenic 50%, neurogenic 30%.

Analysis of percentage weighting (driver of pain/contributing factors) The patient's symptoms are acute in nature and are improving within expected time frames. The patient's work as a plasterer involves sustained, sometimes awkward postures and heavy lifting as well as

Case Study Mr M—cont'd

long drives which has made it difficult for him to return to work. The patient was previously fit and active, and he is keen to return to this which is potentially a positive prognostic indicator.

Hypotheses to test/working diagnosis? (Differentiate between genics)

1. Reduced work capacity possibly some loss of endurance trunk muscles.
2. Lumbar spine active/passive movement (muscle vs joint).
3. Possible dysfunctional movement pattern particularly flexion.
4. Neural mechanosensitivity sciatic nerve.

Planning the Physical Examination

Observation position of lumbar spine in sitting, particularly when driving. Does the patient sit with excessive lumbar flexion or in a position of active extension?

Observe movements of lumbar spine, particularly flexion which is most likely to be the most provocative movement. Observe where movement is originating from (quality, range and reproduction of any symptoms). Are there any maladaptive movement patterns?

Muscles

This could be tested in a functional way, related to the patient's goal of returning to running. For instance, the therapist could look at the patient's ability to do a controlled single leg squat or lunge. This may not be a priority for day 1 but would be part of the therapist's plan.

Neurological integrity testing of the lower limb.

Neurodynamic testing—slump would be the most appropriate test to use given patient's symptoms are worse in sitting.

Main clinical findings for Mr M included

The patient adopted a sitting posture of end range lumbar flexion, when this was corrected, there was a subjective improvement in his pain. Lumbar flexion was limited to around ½ expected range reproducing the patient's back and posture thigh pain. There was relatively excessive movement in the lower lumbar spine into flexion with some stiffness into extension. Lower limb neurology was normal including sensation testing, muscle strength and reflexes.

Slump was positive at −45 degrees knee extension, reproducing all the patient's back and leg pain. He was locally tender and stiff on palpation of L5 unilaterally on the right which reproduced all his leg pain when palpated in a degree of flexion.

At subsequent sessions, the patient was found to have more difficulty with balance and control on the right leg with functional tests such as a single leg squat and lunge.

Management included

Education and advice

Advice and education on the nature of his pain presentation and the normal healing times. Advice to remain active and to gradually return to activity as his symptoms started to improve.

Manual therapy L5 which improved the patient's pain-free lumbar spine movement and increased pain-free range with slump testing. This helped to then engage the patient with a home exercise programme.

Home exercise programme

1. Self-mobilisation L5.
2. Lumbar extension range of motion exercise to improve relative flexibility in this movement.
3. Advice on posture/retraining movement patterns to focus on more hip flexion and anterior pelvic tilt. Use mirror/video to help patient's awareness. Integrate into functional tasks such as bending and lifting without and then with load.
4. Functional exercise to work towards patient's goal of returning to surfing and running—balance, proprioception, lower limb strengthening.

Outcome

Over the course of three treatment sessions, the patient had regained pain-free movement in his lumbar spine. He was able to return to work with only a slight ache in his lower back at the end of a working day. He was encouraged to start a gradual return to running.

REFERENCES

Abbott, J.H., McCane, B., Herbison, P., Moginie, G., Chapple, C., Hogarty, T., 2005. Lumbar segmental instability: a criterion-related validity study of manual therapy assessment. BMC Musculoskelet. Disord. 6 (56), 1–10.

Albert, H.B., Hansen, J.K., Sogaard, H., Kent, P., 2019. Where do patients with MRI confirmed single level radiculopathy experience pain, and what is the clinical interpretability of these pain patterns? A cross-sectional diagnostic accuracy study. Chiropr. Man. Ther. 27, 50.

Allison, G.T., Morris, S.L., 2008. Transversus abdominus and core stability: has the pendulum swung? Br. J. Sports Med. 42, 930–931.

Barnard, K., Ryder, D., 2024. Principles of Musculoskeletal Treatment and Management: A Handbook for Therapists, fourth ed. Elsevier, Edinburgh.

Boissonault, W.G., Bass, C., 1990. Pathological origins of trunk and neck pain: part 1- pelvic and abdominal visceral disorders. J. Orthop. Sports Phys. Ther. 12 (5), 192–207.

Brinjikji, W., Luetmer, P.H., Comstock, B., Bresnahan, B.W., Chen, L.E., Deyo, R.A., et al., 2015. Systematic literature review of imaging features of spinal degeneration in asymptomatic populations. AJNR Am. J. Neuroradiol. 36, 811–816.

Buchbinder, R., van Tulder, M., Öberg, B., Costa, L.M., Woolf, A., Schoene, M., et al., 2018. Low back pain: a call for action. Lancet 391 (10137), 2384–2388.

Campbell, T., Ghaedi, B., Ghogomu, E.T., Welch, V., 2018. Shoe lifts for leg length discrepancy in adults with common painful musculoskeletal conditions: a systematic review of the literature. Arch. Phys. Med. Rehabil. 99, 981–993.

Cholewicki, J., VanVliet, J., 2002. Relative contribution of trunk muscles to the stability of the lumbar spine during isometric exertions. Clin. Biomech. 17 (2), 99–105.

Clinical guidelines to address low back pain: using the evidence to guide physical therapist practice. J. Orthop. Sports Phys. Ther. 51 (11), 2021, 533–534. https://www.jospt.org/doi/10.2519/jospt.2021.0507.

Comer, C., Finucane, L., Mercer, C., Greenhalgh, S., 2020. Shades of grey- the challenge of 'grumbling' cauda equina symptoms in older adults with lumbar spinal stenosis. Musculoskelet. Sci. Pract. 45, 102049.

Dankaerts, W., O'Sullivan, P., Burnett, A., Straker, L., 2006. Altered patterns of superficial trunk muscle activation during sitting in non-specific chronic low back pain patients: importance of subclassification. Spine 31, 2017–2023.

Eckeli, F.D., Teixeira, R.A., Gouvea, A.L., 2016. Neuropathic pain evaluation tools. Rev. Dor. Sao. Paulo. 17 (Suppl. 1), S20–S22.

Ez-Zaitouni, Z., Hilkens, A., Gossec, L., Berg, I.J., Landewe, R., Ramonda, R., et al., 2017. Is the current ASAS expert definition of a positive family history useful in identifying axial spondyloarthritis? Results from the SACE and DESIR cohorts. Arthritis Res. Ther. 19 (118), 1335–1338.

Finucane, L., Downie, A., Mercer, C., Greenhalgh, S.M., Boissonault, W.G., Pool-Goudzwaard, A.L., et al., 2020. International framework for red flags for potential serious spinal pathology. J. Orthop. Sports Phys. Ther. 50 (7), 350–372.

Gerhart, J.I., Burns, J.W., Post, K.M., Smith, D.A., Porter, L.S., Burgess, H.J., et al., 2017. Relationships between sleep quality and pain-related factors for people with chronic low back pain: tests of reciprocal and time of day effects. Ann. Behav. Med. 51 (3), 365–375.

Goel, S., 2019. Non-spinal causes of back pain: an 'undiagnosed' diagnosis. J. Med. Res. Innov. 3 (2), e000172–e000172. https://doi.org/10.32892/jmri.172.

Greenhalgh, S., Finucane, L., Mercer, C., Selfe, J., 2018. Assessment and management of cauda equina syndrome. Musculoskelet. Sci. Pract. 37, 69–74.

Grieve, G.P., 1994. The masqueraders. In: Boyling, J.D., Palastanga, N. (Eds.), Grieve's Modern Manual Therapy, second ed. Churchill Livingstone, Edinburgh, p. 745.

Grinnell-Merrick, L.L., Lydon, E.J., Mixon, A.M., Saalfeld, W., 2020. Evaluating Inflammatory Versus Mechanical Back Pain in Individuals with Psoriatic Arthritis: A Review of the Literature. Rheumatol Ther. 7 (4), 667–684. https://doi.org/10.1007/s40744-020-00234-3. Epub 2020 Sep 15. PMID: 32935330, PMCID: PMC7695767.

Harding, I., Davies, E., Buchanan, E., Fairbank, J.T., 2005. The symptom of night pain in a back pain triage clinic? Spine 30 (17), 1985–1988.

Hartvigsen, J., Hancock, M., Kongsted, A., Louw, Q., Ferreira, M.L., et al., 2018. What low back pain is and why we need to pay attention. Lancet 391, 2356–2367.

Haryoni, I., Karawilarang, M., Prastowo, N., 2019. Leg length discrepancy in college students and its association with low back pain: a preliminary study. J. Anthr. Sport Phys. Educ. 3 (20), 15–18.

Hengeveld, E., Banks, K., 2014. Maitlands's vertebral manipulation. Churchill Livingston, Edinburgh.

Henschke, N., Maher, C.G., Refshauge, K.M., Herbert, R.D., Cumming, R.G., Beasel, J., et al., 2009. Prevalence of and screening for serious spinal pathology in patients presenting to primary care settings with acute low back pain. Arthritis Rheumatol. 60, 3072–3080.

Hicks, G.E., Fritz, J.M., Delitto, A., Mishock, J., 2003. Interrater reliability of clinical examination measures for identification of lumbar segmental instability. Arch. Phys. Med. Rehabil. 8412, 1858–1864.

Hidalgo, B., Hall, T., Nielens, H., Detrembleur, C., 2014. Intertester agreement and validity of identifying lumbar pain provocative movement patterns using active and passive accessory movement tests. J. Manip. Physiol. Ther. 37, 105–115.

Hides, J., Donelson, R., Lee, D., Prather, H., Sahrmann, S.A., Hodges, P.W., 2019. Convergence and divergence of exercise-based approaches that incorporate motor control for the management of low back pain. J. Orthop. Sports Phys. Ther. 49 (6), 363–483.

Hides, J., Glimore, C., Stanton, W., Bohlscheid, E., 2008. Multifidus size and symmetry among chronic LBP and healthy asymptomatic subjects. Man. Ther. 13, 43–49.

Hislop, H., Montgomery, J., 2007. Daniels and Worthingham's Muscle Testing: Techniques of Manual Examination, eight ed. WB Saunders, Birmingham, AL, p. 210.

Hodges, P., Cresswell, A., Thorstensson, A., 1999. Preparatory trunk motion accompanies limb movement. Exp. Brain Res. 124, 69–79.

Hodges, P.W., Moseley, L., 2003. Pain and motor control of the lumbopelvic region: effect and possible mechanisms. J. Electromyogr. Kinesiol. 13, 361–370.

Hodges, P.W., Richardson, C.A., 1997a. Contraction of the abdominal muscles associated with movement of the lower limb. Phys. Ther. 77 (2), 132–142.

Hodges, P.W., Richardson, C.A., 1997b. Feedforward contraction of transversus abdominus is not influenced by the direction of arm movement. Exp. Brain Res. 114, 362–370.

Hodges, P.W., Richardson, C.A., 1999. Altered trunk muscle recruitment in people with low back pain with upper limb movement at different speeds. Arch. Phys. Med. Rehabil. 80, 1005–1012.

Hoffman, T.C., Lewis, J., Maher, C.G., 2020. Shared decision making should be an integral part of physiotherapy practice. Physiotherapy 107, 43–49.

Jansen, S.C.P., Hoorweg, B.B., Hoeks, S.E., Van den Houten, M.M.L., Scheltinga, M.R.M., Teijink, J.A.W., et al., 2019. A systematic review and meta-analysis of the effects of supervised exercise therapy on modifiable cardiovascular risk factors in intermittent claudication. J. Vasc. Surg. 69, 1293–1308.

Jeong, S.J., Choi, S.W., Youm, J.Y., Kim, H.W., Ha, H.G., Yi, J.S., 2014. Microbiology and epidemiology of infectious spinal disease. J. Korean Neurosurg. Soc. 56, 21e7.

Jois, R.N., Macgregor, A.J., Gaffney, K., 2008. Recognition of inflammatory back pain and ankylosing spondylitis in primary care. Rheumatology 47 (9), 1364–1366.

Jones, M.A., Rivett, D.A., 2004. Clinical reasoning for manual therapists. Butterworth-Heinemann, Edinburgh.

Kendall, F.P., McCreary, E.K., Provance, P.G., Rodgers, M., 2010. Muscles Testing and Function, fifth ed. Lippincott Williams and Wilkins, Baltimore.

Kwon, B.K., Roffey, D.M., Bishop, P.B., Dagenais, S., Wai, E., 2011. Systematic review: occupational physical activity and low back pain. Occup. Med. 61, 541–548.

Lavy, C., James, A., Wilson-McDonald, J., Fairbank, J., 2009. Cauda equina syndrome. Br. Med. J. 338, 881–884.

Lederman, E., 2009. The myth of core stability. J. Bodyw. Mov. Ther. 14 (1), 84–98.

Lee, H., Hubscher, M., Moseley, G.L., 2015. How does pain lead to disability? A systematic review and meta-analysis of mediation studies in people with low back and neck pain. Pain 156, 988–997.

Lehmann, H.C., Wunderlich, G., Fink, G.R., Sommer, C., 2020. Diagnosis of peripheral neuropathy. Neurol. Res. Pract. 2, 20.

Magee, D., Manske, R., 2021. Orthopedic Physical Assessment, seventh ed. Saunders Elsevier, St Louis.

Main, C.J., Buchbinder, R., Porcheret, M., Foster, N., 2010a. Addressing patient beliefs and expectations in the consultation. Best Pract. Res. Clin. Rheumatol. 24, 219–225.

Main, C.J., Foster, N., Buchbinder, R., 2010b. How important are back pain beliefs and expectations for satisfactory recovery from back pain? Best Pract. Res. Clin. Rheumatol. 24, 205–217.

Maitland, G.D., Hengeveld, E., Banks, K., English, K., 2005. Maitland's Vertebral Manipulation, seventh ed. Butterworth-Heinemann, Edinburgh.

Majlesi, J., Togay, H., Unalan, H., Toprak, S., 2008. The sensitivity and specificity of the Slump and the straight leg raising tests in patients with lumbar disc herniation. J. Clin. Rheumatol. 14, 87–91.

NASS. What Is Axial SpA (AS)? 2021. NASS website. https://nass.co.uk/about-as/what-is-as/.

National Osteoporosis Guidance Group (NOGG), 2021. Clinical Guidance for the Effective Identification of Vertebral Fractures. National Osteoporosis Guidance Group, London.

NICE, 2017. Osteoporosis quality standard (QS149). National Institute for health and Care Excellence. Available online at: www.nice.org.uk/guidance/qs149.

NICE, 2020. Low back pain and sciatica in over 16s: assessment and management NICE guideline (NG59). Published Nov 2016. Updated December 2020. Available online at: https://www.nice.org.uk/guidance/ng59.

O'Sullivan, P., 2006. Classification of lumbopelvic disorders — why is it essential for management? Man. Ther. 11, 169–170.

O'Sullivan, P., Dankaerts, W., O'Sullivan, K., Fersum, K., 2015. Multidimensional approach for the targeted management of low back pain. In: Jull, G., et al. (Eds.), 2015 Grieve's Modern Musculoskeletal Physiotherapy, fourth ed. Elsevier, Edinburgh.

O'Sullivan, P.B., Caneiro, J.P., O'Keeffe, M., Smith, A., Dankaerts, W., Fersum, K., et al., 2018. Cognitive functional

therapy: an integrated behavioural approach for the targeted management of disabling low back pain. Phys. Ther. 98 (5), 408–423.
Pacheco-Carroza, E.A., 2021. Visceral pain, mechanisms and implications in musculoskeletal practice. Med. Hypotheses 153, 110624. https://doi.org/10.1016/j.mehy.2021.110624.
Pal, B., 2002. Paraesthesia. Br. Med. J. 324, 1501.
Parkin, D.M., Boyd, L., Walker, L.C., 2011. The fraction of cancer attributable to lifestyle and environmental factors in the UK in 2010. Br. J. Cancer 105, S77–S81.
Phillips, D.R., Twomey, L.T., 1996. A comparison of manual diagnosis with a diagnosis established by a uni-level lumbar spinal block procedure. Man. Ther. 1 (2), 82–87.
Poddubnyy, D., 2020. Classification vs diagnostic criteria: the challenge of diagnosing axial spondyloarthritis. Rheumatology 59, iv6–iv17. https://doi.org/10.1093/rheumatology/keaa250.
Rannisto, S., Okuloff, A., Uitti, J., Paananen, M., Eannisto, P., Malmivaara, A., et al., 2019. Correction of leg-length discrepancy among meat cutters with low back pain: a randomized controlled trial. BMC Musculoskelet. Disord. 20, 105.
Redeker, I., Callhoff, J., Hoffman, F., Haibel, H., Sieper, J., Zink, A., et al., 2019. Determinants of diagnostic delay in axial spondyloarthritis: an analysis based on linked claims and patient-reported data. Rheumatology 58 (9), 1634–1638.
Romeo, V., Covello, M., Salvatore, E., Parente, C.A., Abbenante, D., Biselli, R., et al., 2019. High prevelance of spinal magnetic resonance imaging findings in asymptomatic young adults (18–22 yrs) candidate to air force flight. Spine 44 (12), 872–878.
Sahrmann, S.A., 2013. Diagnosis and Treatment of Movement Impairment Syndromes. Elsevier, St Louis.
Saragiotto, B.T., Maher, C.G., Yamato, T.P., Costa, L.O., Menezes Costa, L.C., Ostelo, R.W., Macedo, L.G., 2016. Motor control exercise for chronic non-specific low-back pain. Cochrane Database Syst. Rev. 2016 (1), CD012004. https://doi.org/10.1002/14651858.CD012004.
Slater, D., Korakakis, V., O'Sullivan, P., Nolan, D., O'Sullivan, K., 2019. 'Sit up straight': time to re-evaluate. J. Orthop. Sports Phys. Ther. 49 (8), 562–564.
Stolz, M., Piekartz, H., Hall, T., Schindler, A., Ballenberger, N., 2020. Evidence and recommendations for the use of segmental motion testing for patients with LBP – a systematic review. Musculoskelet. Sci. Pract. 45, 102076.
Synnott, A., O'Keeffe, M., Bunzli, S., Dankaerts, W., O'Sullivan, P., O'Sullivan, K., 2015. Physiotherapists may stigmatise or feel unprepared to treat people with low back pain and psychosocial factors that influence recovery: a systematic review. J. Physiother. 61 (2), 68–76.
Van Tulder, M., Kovacs, F., Muller, G., Airaksinen, O., Balague, F., Broos, L., et al., 2005. Back pain Europe: European guidelines on the management of persistent low back pain. Available online at: http://www.backpaineurope.org.
Walker, H.K., Hall, W.D., Hurst, J.W., 1990. Clinical Methods: The History, Physical, and Laboratory Examinations, third ed. Boston, Butterworths.
Wu, A., March, L., Zheng, X., Huang, J., Wang, X., Zhao, J., et al., 2020. Global low back pain prevalence and years lived with disability 199–2017: estimates from the Global Burden of Disease Study 2017. Ann. Transl. Med. 8 (6), 229. https://doi.org/10.21037/atm.2020.02.175.
Yi, E., Ahuja, A., Rajput, T., George, A., Park, Y., 2020. Clinical, economic and humanistic burden associated with delayed diagnosis of axial spondyloarthritis: a systematic review. Rheumatol. Ther. 7, 65–87.

14

Examination of the Pelvis

Claire Small

LEARNING OUTCOMES

After studying this chapter, you should be able to:

- Outline the key anatomical structures and biomechanical functions of the pelvic girdle to inform an understanding of common pathological presentations in this region.
- Understand the multifactorial nature of pelvic girdle pain and the important role psychosocial factors may play in persistent pelvic pain.
- Identify how clinical reasoning guides history taking in the subjective examination of people with pelvic girdle pain, informed by the location, behaviour and nature of symptoms, and the value of screening questions.
- Use the information gained from the subjective examination to establish a working hypothesis on which to base the physical examination.
- List the key components of a comprehensive physical examination of the pelvic girdle region with consideration of the sensitivity and specificity of key physical tests for the pelvic girdle region.
- Understand how observation of a patient's posture and functional activities including the assessment of form and force closure contributes to the reasoning process in confirming a working hypothesis.
- Discuss the reliability and clinical utility of the physical tests for the pelvic girdle.
- Use the information gained from the subjective and physical examination to establish/confirm a working hypothesis and treatment plan.

CHAPTER CONTENTS

Introduction to the Pelvic Region, 388
Subjective Examination/Taking the Patient's History, 390
Patients's Perspective on Their Experience, 390
Body Chart, 390
Behaviour of Symptoms, 391
Special/Screening Questions/General Health, 392
History of the Present Condition, 392
Past Medical History, 392
Plan of the Physical Examination, 393
Physical Examination, 393
Observation, 393
Functional Testing, 393
Active Physiological Movements, 393
Pain Provocation Tests, 395
Passive Accessory Movements, 397
Muscle Tests, 398
The Pelvic Floor, 399
Palpation, 399
Completion of the Examination, 400
Case Study, 401
References, 404

INTRODUCTION TO THE PELVIC REGION

The primary function of the lumbo-pelvic hip region is to transfer and attenuate the forces generated by the trunk and lower limbs due to body weight, gravity and activity (Snijders et al., 1993). The region must be both solid/stable to achieve force transmission and mobile to achieve force attenuation or shock absorption as well as permit effective function. A solid bony ring or interlocking joints would not allow an effective gait pattern or other movements while an excessively mobile joint would be unable to cope with the large forces transmitted through the joints with weightbearing and plyometric activities. A lack of motion limits the ability to attenuate force through the region during movements and risks overloading joints causing inflammation and degeneration.

It is important to differentiate pelvic girdle pain and dysfunction from low-back pain and dysfunction in order to be as accurate and effective with treatment as possible. Isolated sacroiliac joints (SIJ) pain is reported to be as high as 15% in people with chronic low back and pelvic pain below L5/S1 (Dreyfuss et al., 2004), and so it is important to develop skills in the assessment and differential diagnosis of this region.

Due to its role in load transfer between the trunk and lower limbs, consideration should also be given to the role the pelvis may play in relation to symptoms elsewhere.

The pelvic girdle consists of two innominate bones and one sacrum. There are three joints, two joints posteriorly between the ilial portion of the innominate and the sacrum forming the SIJ and the one anteriorly between the pubic bone portions of the innominates forming the symphysis pubis (Fig. 14.1).

The sacroiliac joints are auricular-shaped diarthrodial joints. The anterior third is a synovial joint, while the posterior two-thirds is composed of ligamentous structures with no specific joint capsule. The SIJ is covered by two different cartilages. The concave sacral surface is covered by thick hyaline articular cartilage while the convex ilial surfaces are lined with thin fibrocartilage. The joint surfaces have interlocking ridges and grooves which enhance the stability of the joint. Several ligaments are important in maintaining the integrity of the SIJ: the ventral SIJ ligaments, interosseous ligaments, long dorsal SIJ ligament, sacrotuberous, sacrospinous and iliolumbar ligaments, as shown in Fig. 14.1.

The SIJ has a widespread pattern of innervation from the ventral rami of L5–S4. This may be the reason for such wide variations in the clinical pain patterns reported by patients with SIJ pain (Lee, 2010).

The pubic symphysis has two osseous surfaces covered by hyaline cartilage separated by a fibrocartilaginous disc. The supporting ligaments include the

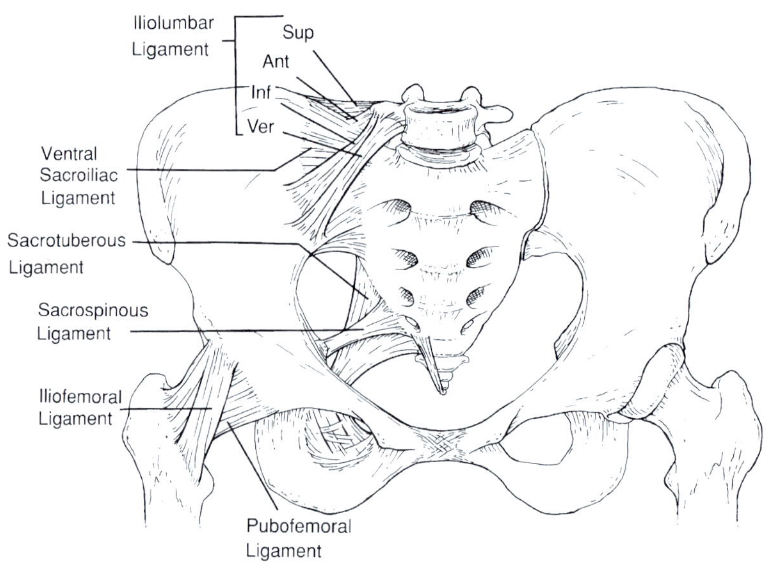

Fig. 14.1 The ligaments of the pelvic girdle viewed from the anterior aspect. *Ant*, Anterior; *Inf*, inferior; *Sup*, superior; *Ver*, vertical. (From Lee 2010, with permission.)

superior, anterior and posterior ligaments and the inferior arcuate ligament. The pubic symphysis is supplied by the pudendal (S2–S3–S4) and/or genitofemoral nerve (L1–L2) and/or ilioinguinal/iliohypogastric nerves (L1–L2).

While small, movement occurs in all three planes of the joint (Sturesson, 1989; Sturesson et al., 1997, 2000; Hungerford et al., 2001), and movement is maintained throughout life (Vleeming et al., 1992, 1997). The movement at the SIJ is 1–3 degrees of rotation and 2–4 mm of translation.

There are three primary movements (Fig. 14.2):

Nutation—the sacral base moves inferiorly and anteriorly and rotates. The movement is resisted by the ridges and depressions of the articular surfaces and the posterior, interosseous and sacrotuberous ligaments.

Counternutation—the sacral base moves superiorly and posteriorly and rotates. Motion in this direction is opposed by the posterior sacroiliac ligament, supported by the multifidus muscle.

Torsion—the sacrum rotates within the innominate bones. Any motion of the SIJ is accompanied by pubic symphysis motion.

Form Closure (Vleeming et al., 1997) refers to the shape, structure and orientation of the SIJs that work to provide stability. The wedge shape of the sacrum also contributes to form closure with the effect of body weight lodging it firmly between the ilia.

A balance of form and *Force Closure* permit load to be transferred effectively across the trunk, pelvis and lower extremities (Vleeming et al., 1990, 1997). Because the amount and orientation of these joint forces vary at any one time depending on the nature and speed of the activity being undertaken, the amount of load transfer and shock absorption are also variable. The joint position will vary depending on the activity, and so the level of Form Closure will also change. Force Closure assists in load transfer through joint compression generated by tension in the ligaments, muscles and fascia of the SIJ, pelvis and trunk. It is dependent upon effective neuromotor control. Any alteration to an individual's bony or ligamentous structural integrity or neuromotor control may result in alterations to form and force closure mechanisms, resulting in pain and dysfunction (Richardson et al., 2002).

The muscles that attach to the pelvis and its associated ligaments and fascia are extensive. Muscle contraction supports stability by either directly or indirectly producing joint compression. Muscles that cross the joint, for example, gluteus maximus, piriformis and the transverse and oblique abdominals are able to compress the joint directly. Other key muscles involved in lumbo-pelvic hip function include the

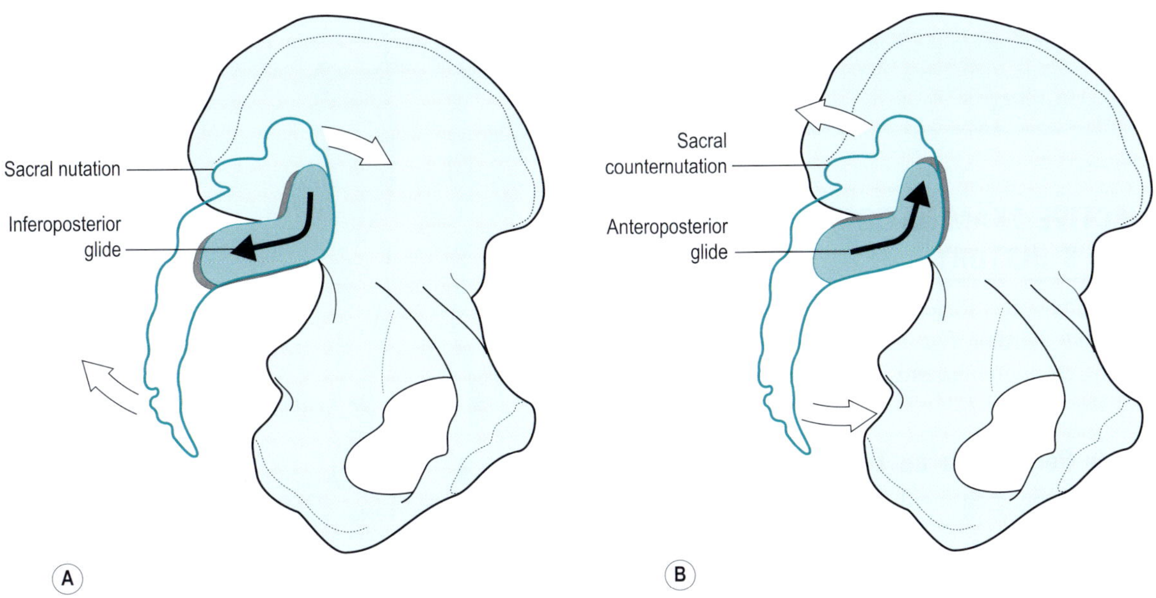

Fig. 14.2 Movements of the sacroiliac joint. (From Lee 2010, with permission.)

multifidus and the erector spine, the rectus abdominis, the pelvic floor and pelvic wall and the thoracolumbar fascia.

O'Sullivan and Beales developed a classification system for pelvic girdle pain (O'Sullivan & Beales, 2007a). It acknowledges the often complex and multifactorial nature of pelvic dysfunction which can be associated with reduced or increased force closure of the pelvic girdle, the effect this may have on pain-sensitive pelvic structures and the interaction of passive coping strategies, faulty belief systems and anxiety and depression. They hypothesize that a motor control system can become dysfunctional in response to pain or may itself produce pain due to abnormal tissue strain. This can result in ongoing peripheral pain sensitization (Beales et al., 2020).

Examination of the pelvic region is not performed in isolation and will always include some aspects of assessment of the lumbar spine (see Chapter 13) and hip (see Chapter 15). It is not unusual for there to be concomitant symptoms and dysfunction in the lumbar spine, pelvis and hip, all of which will need to be assessed and managed.

KNOWLEDGE CHECK

1. What is the primary function of the pelvis and associated joints?
2. What do Form and Force Closure refer to?
3. Which ligaments provide stability to the sacroiliac joints?
4. What type of joint is the pubic symphysis?
5. The sacroiliac joint does not refer pain below the ankle. TRUE/FALSE

SUBJECTIVE EXAMINATION/TAKING THE PATIENT'S HISTORY

Within this chapter, focus is given to elements specific to the pelvic girdle. For details regarding common assessment components and clinical reasoning considerations see Chapter 5.

Patients's Perspective on Their Experience

Patients seeking treatment tend to fall into four different groups:

1. Pregnant women with symptoms they have been experiencing for a short period of time
2. Postpartum women. This group may have had symptoms for a short time only or may have persistent pain symptoms which have not been managed or not managed effectively
3. Patients with underlying inflammatory conditions who may or may not have received a diagnosis
4. People with long-term symptoms who have often seen a number of clinicians

In all cases, there is often a great deal of misinformation about the causes of pelvic girdle pain. Pregnant and postpartum women often think their problems are due to ligamentous laxity, and people with persistent symptoms have often been told that their pelvis is "out" or unstable. This is often information that has been provided by a clinician based on our previous understanding of pelvic function. There is no evidence to support any of these scenarios (Beales et al., 2020).

Body Chart

Area and Nature of Symptoms

Area of Current Symptoms. Guided SIJ anaesthetic injection studies show that pain from the SIJ presents very similarly to pain referred into the lower limb from the lumbar spine—it can refer to the buttock, the groin, the anterior and posterior thigh and into the calf and foot (Schwarzer et al., 1995; Dreyfuss et al., 1996; van der

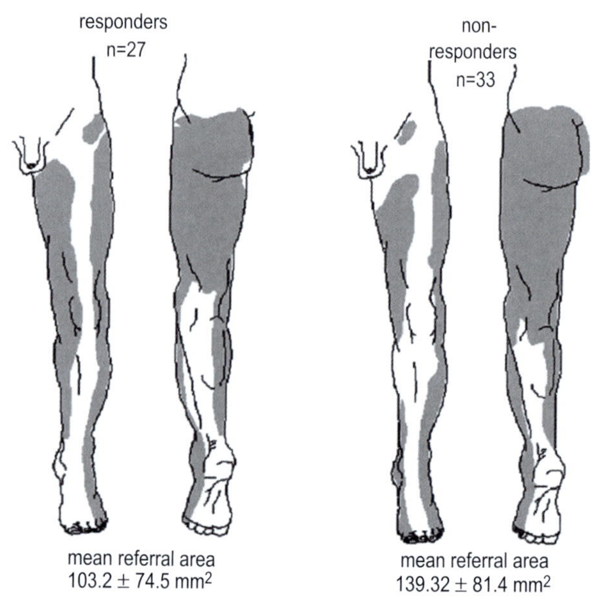

Fig. 14.3 Distribution of pain referral in patients with sacroiliac joint mediated symptoms. (van der Wurff et al., 2006.)

Wurff et al., 2006; Visser et al., 2013) (Fig. 14.3). Pain over the posterior superior iliac spine (PSIS) and sacral sulcus is the most common area of symptoms—80%–100% of patients who respond to SIJ injection had pain over their PSIS—but pain in that location is not diagnostic of SIJ-mediated pain (Dreyfuss et al., 1996; van der Wurff et al., 2006).The area is referred to as Fortin's area, as this was the location of pain identified by Fortin et al. (1994, 1997) when they injected healthy SIJs with an irritant solution.

Extraarticular sources of pain, e.g. the dorsal sacroiliac, or long dorsal ligament are relatively common sources of postpartum pelvic pain (Vleeming et al., 2002) and chronic pelvic pain (Dreyfuss et al., 1996; Fortin et al., 1999).

Ischial pain can be referred from the pelvic floor (Pastore & Katzman, 2012). Recently ischiofemoral impingement resulting in inflammation and oedema in the ischiofemoral space and quadratus femoris has been identified as a cause of atypical groin and/or posterior buttock pain. It is thought that this is caused by abnormal contact between the lesser trochanter of the femur and the ischium (Stafford & Villar, 2011).

Quality and Intensity of Symptoms. Studies have shown that the quality and intensity of symptoms are not diagnostic of any specific tissue pathology, but it is important to ask about these elements to gain a full understanding of the patient's presentation, including symptoms other than pain, such as stiffness, weakness, paraesthesia or numbness.

Other Symptoms. Patients with pelvic girdle pain commonly have other symptoms and problems. These can include bladder and bowel disorders, gut issues, sexual dysfunction, hormonal issues, problems with menstruation and other systemic conditions. Specific questions regarding signs and symptoms of inflammatory arthropathies should also be included in the subjective examination.

Relationship of Symptoms. As pelvic girdle pain is often widespread with more than one tissue source of symptoms, establishing when and how each symptom area is brought on, will help determine if it is likely that there are multiple sources of pain. This will help in planning the physical examination and what regions need to be examined.

Behaviour of Symptoms

Aggravating/Easing Factors

Identifying aggravating and easing factors is important but there are no specific activities that are diagnostic of the SIJ or pubic symphysis as the source of symptoms. The pelvic girdle questionnaire developed by Stuge et al. (2011) is useful in establishing problematic activities and the extent to which these limit the patient's function.

Commonly cited aggravating factors for the SIJ are standing on one leg, turning over in bed, getting in or out of bed, sloppy standing with uneven weight distribution through the legs, habitual work stance, stepping up on the affected side and walking (Huijbregts, 2004) however studies using pain provocation test procedures show that these aggravating activities are just as commonly associated with the lumbar spine (Young et al., 2003; Dreyfuss et al., 2004; Visser et al., 2013).

Although no particular easing factors have been found to be associated with the proven presence of SIJ pain, understanding what the patient reports helps their symptoms may guide treatment. For example, symptoms from the SIJ may be eased by crook-lying, sitting with the pelvis posteriorly tilted and stooping forwards in standing. The effect of pelvic compression and/or applying a sacroiliac stabilization belt may also be helpful, e.g. in pregnant women (Ostgaard et al., 1994) or patients with groin pain (Mens et al., 2006).

Twenty-Four-Hour Behaviour of Symptoms

Night symptoms. Although severe night pain is a recognized red flag, it should be noted that night symptoms are common in back pain (Harding et al., 2004). SIJ patients often report turning in bed as being painful and difficult to perform, but this is not diagnostic (Van der Wurff et al., 2000a, 2000b).

Pregnant women often report difficulty finding a comfortable position to sleep in. Questions should be asked about pillow support between their knees and under then stomachs as this often makes it more comfortable for them.

Morning and evening symptoms. It is important to question the patient closely about morning stiffness. Many patients with lumbo-pelvic hip pain report some element of morning stiffness, especially if they are older, but stiffness of a mechanical nature generally eases within about 30 minutes (Suresh, 2004). Stiffness lasting longer than an hour is more likely to be associated with inflammatory arthropathies (Yazici et al., 2004; Solomon et al., 2010).

Special/Screening Questions/General Health

The importance of asking questions relating to the visceral system, possible systemic conditions and the general health of the patient has been discussed previously and is covered in detail in Chapter 3 (Goodman et al., 2018).

Obstetric History

Due to an increased incidence of pelvic pain in women postpartum, a full obstetric history should be taken. Is the patient pregnant? How many children has she given birth to? When was she last pregnant? Has she had caesarean sections? Did she suffer trauma to her pelvic floor during delivery through instrumental deliveries with forceps and ventouse? Did she have episiotomies and/or tears?

It is common for low-back and pelvic pain to be associated with pregnancy, although the underlying mechanism remains unclear. A number of factors have been proposed and have included an increase in the load on the lumbar spine because of weight gain, hormonal changes causing hypermobility of the SIJ and pubic symphysis (Hagen, 1974) and an increase in the abdominal sagittal diameter (Ostgaard et al., 1993). Little evidence supports the hypothesis that the pain is related to alteration in posture (Bullock et al., 1987; Ostgaard et al., 1993).

There are no studies showing a causal relationship between relaxin and reduced stability in the pelvic girdle or a relationship between relaxin and pelvic girdle pain (Petersen et al., 1994; Hansen et al., 1996). Relaxin is not detectable after 3 months postpregnancy and is unlikely to be the cause of symptoms (Sapsford et al., 1999).

History of the Present Condition

The main information to be gathered during this part of the exam is the mode of onset. Was it sudden or did it come on gradually? Was there a history of trauma? It is commonly assumed that there is often a traumatic event causing SIJ pain; however, only 40% of patients have been found to relate a traumatic incident to the onset of symptoms (Dreyfuss et al., 1996; Visser et al., 2013).

Questions should also be asked about the patient's working habits, hobbies and sporting activities to understand repeated misuse or overuse, as well as any change in the patient's lifestyle, e.g. a new job or hobby or a change in sporting activity.

Past Medical History

The following information is important in pelvic girdle pain.

- Relevant medical history: pelvic inflammatory or other visceral disease, systemic illnesses or injuries to the limbs.
- The history of any previous episodes: How many? When were they? What was the cause? What was the duration of each episode? Did the patient fully recover between episodes? Does the patient perceive the current condition to be better, the same or worse in relation to the previous episode?
- Ascertain the effects of any previous treatment for the same or a similar problem.

Imaging and Investigations

Routine spinal radiographs are not considered necessary prior to conservative treatment as they are only likely to identify the normal age-related degenerative changes, which do not necessarily correlate with the symptoms experienced by the patient (NICE Guidelines 2020 (NG59)). If the history suggests serious spinal pathology, fractures, inflammatory arthropathy or other nonmechanical conditions, imaging may be deemed appropriate, especially in young patients under 20 years or the elderly. Patients who have failed to respond to conservative management or who do not have a definitive diagnosis may also be considered appropriate to refer for imaging (Royal College of Radiologists, 2007). X-ray and magnetic resonance imaging (MRI) are usually the first choice of imaging, but bone scans and computed tomography (CT) may be used for investigating specific suspected conditions. Blood tests are useful for inflammatory conditions, infections and other systemic.

In complex cases where determining the tissue source of pain is difficult, local anaesthetic joint injections may be useful in aiding diagnosis.

KNOWLEDGE CHECK

1. Where do patients with pain from the sacroiliac joint commonly report symptoms?
2. What aggravating factors are common in patients with pelvic girdle pain?
3. Name four other nonmusculoskeletal structures that should be discussed as part of an effective history-taking process.
4. Name four groups that commonly present with pelvic girdle pain and dysfunction.
5. List five questions you should ask a patient about their obstetric history if relevant.

Plan of the Physical Examination

The complex nature of people presenting with lumbo-pelvic hip pain means that an extensive examination is usually required to establish the sources of the symptoms and the causes of tissue strain. This includes the joints, muscles and neural structures associated with the SIJ, pubic symphysis, thoracic and lumbar spine and hip. Other regions need consideration depending on the aggravating activities, e.g. the shoulder if tennis is a functional problem, and the knee, ankle and foot if bending and lifting causes problems. It is usually not possible to examine all regions fully at the first attendance, and so examination of the structures must be prioritized and assessed over several treatment sessions.

In considering isolated examination of the pelvis, the tests can be divided into:

- Tests of function
- Pain provocation tests
- Tests of form closure
- Tests of force closure and motor control

PHYSICAL EXAMINATION

Observation

Pelvic asymmetries are not diagnostic of dysfunction, but, as for other regions of the body, postural asymmetries may be reflective of dysfunction; therefore a postural assessment in both standing and supine should be undertaken to determine in any deviations are observable. Changes are often reflective of muscle tightness and changes in motor control.

Key areas to examine include:

- any deformity of the spine, e.g. scoliosis, lateral shift
- any asymmetry in levels at the pelvis—the iliac crests, the anterior or PSISs
- the level of the greater trochanters compared with the level of the iliac crests
- muscle bulk, tone and symmetry
- skin colour, areas of redness, swelling or sweating

Functional Testing

Examination of functional movements that the patients report as problematic is important to give the clinician a good understanding of how the patient moves, what muscle groups they use, their willingness to move and any fear avoidance or hypervigilant behaviour.

There are no isolated active physiological movements at the SIJ since the pelvic girdle moves with the lumbar spine. SIJ movements are therefore tested with the active physiological movements of the lumbar spine and hip joints (Kapandji, 2008).

Active Physiological Movements

It has been well established that the SIJ has 1–3 degrees of rotation and 2–4 mm of translatory movement. This small amount of movement is impossible to detect with the human eye or with palpation, and therefore assessment of active movement is a *qualitative* assessment of load transfer and load tolerance rather than a quantitative assessment of range of movement.

Palpation of the innominate bones with movement may assist the clinician in this qualitative assessment, but it is no longer considered a mechanism to quantify movement at the SIJ (Palsson et al., 2019).

Three elements should be examined with all active movements:

- Range—the amount of overall movement of the body
- Quality—the relative movement in various body regions, the symmetry of the movement, the segmental spinal motion and how the patient uses their neuromotor system to produce the movement
- Response—the presence of pain, tightness or other symptoms in response to movement

Forward Flexion

The patient is instructed to bend forwards towards their toes, and the clinician notes the natural movement pattern of the patient. Specifically, the clinician should note:

- the relative movement of the pelvic girdle as it rotates over the femoral heads to see if it occurs symmetrically
- the intersegmental spinal movement
- any spinal rotation and the symmetry of the paravertebral muscles.

Return From Flexion

As the patient returns from the forward flexion position, the sequence of the lumbo-pelvic hip movement should be noted. This movement should be initiated with the gluteal muscles rotating the innominates posteriorly followed by extension of the flexed spine by the erector spinae once a neutral pelvic position has been achieved. Clinically, patients with lumbo-pelvic hip dysfunction commonly demonstrate early and excessive activation of the erector spinae with poor gluteal activity resulting in spinal hyperextension and a tendency to 'collapse' into passive hip extension at end of range.

Standing Hip Flexion Test (Gillet Test) (Fig. 14.4)

This test is also known as the Gillet test. It is no longer used as a test of SIJ movement but as a test of the ability of the lower limb, pelvis and trunk to transfer load. In single-leg stance, both the weight-bearing and non-weight-bearing innominates rotate posteriorly relative to the sacrum which is relatively nutated. This is the close-packed position of the SIJ and requires both effective form closure and force closure (Hungerford & Gilleard, 2007).

As the patient transfers their weight from two legs to a single-leg stance position, the clinician observes the patient's ability to maintain a stable position of the pelvis and acetabulum over the femur. No lateral shift, pelvic hitching or spinal or trunk movement should be observed, and the patient should also be able to maintain a stable lower limb position with no rotation or abduction/adduction of the thigh (Hungerford & Gilleard, 2007; Lee, 2015).

The clinician may like to challenge the patient's ability to load transfer during function further by progressing from a position of one leg standing to asking them to perform a small knee bend. As a more dynamic movement, this action requires greater motor control.

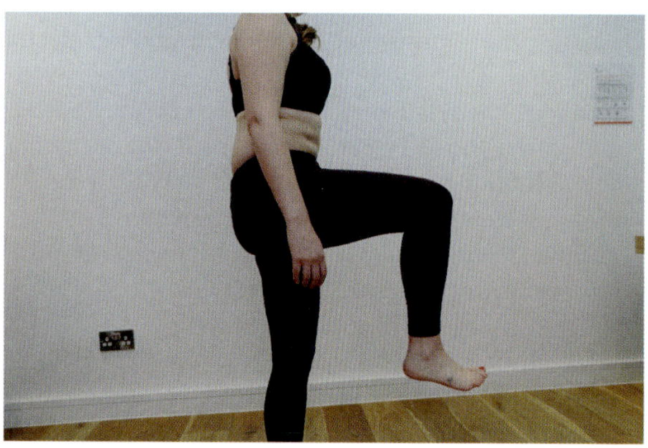

Fig. 14.4 Standing hip flexion (Gillet) test.

Hip Flexion Test

The second component of the Gillet test is active hip flexion in standing to assess the ability of the patient to flex the hip of the non-weight-bearing/stance leg. In this component, the patient should be able to actively flex their non-weight-bearing hip to 90 degrees with minimal movement of the innominate and pelvis. There should be no hitching or excessive posterior rotation of the innominate. The patient should have adequate hip strength and range of motion to flex the hip joint against gravity. Additionally, no or minimal extension of the knee joint should be observed; the knee joint and shin should stay relaxed with minimal activity of the rectus femoris being required. Patients with hip pathology commonly 'fail' the Gillet test, demonstrating poor movement patterns due to weakness or restricted joint mobility.

Active Straight-Leg Raise Test (Fig. 14.5A and B)

The active straight-leg raise test (ASLR) (Mens et al., 1999, 2001, 2002) is a validated test of load transfer between the lower limb and the trunk. When the lumbo-pelvic/hip region is functioning optimally, the individual is able to lift the leg about 20 cm from the plinth with no/minimal effort (Graded 0–5 on an 'effort scale') while maintaining a stable position of the pelvis and thorax. When the patient has ineffective load transfer, increased effort levels are reported (with or without pain) and several different compensation mechanisms may be seen (O'Sullivan et al., 2002).

The ASLR test can be used to identify possible strategies to optimise load transfer. A study by Mens et al. (1999) demonstrated that the application of a compressive force across the pelvis reduces the effort of lifting the leg, suggesting improved load transfer.

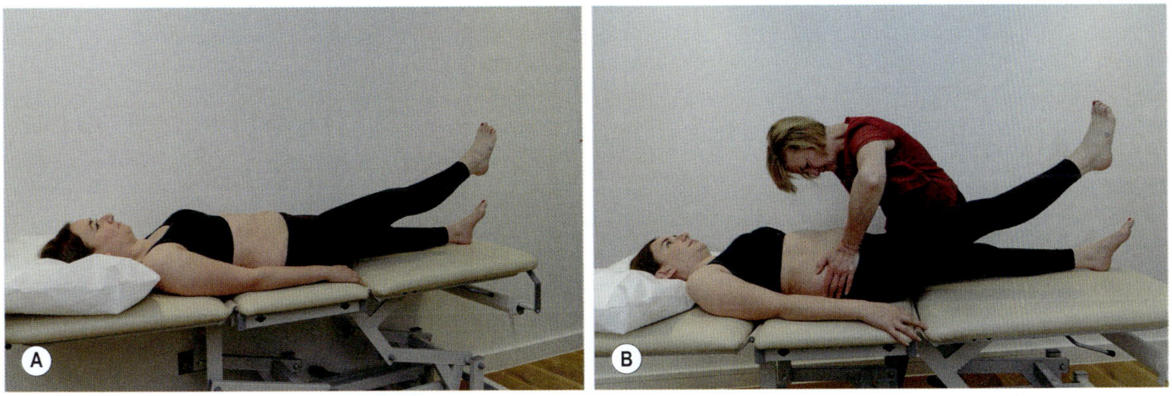

Fig. 14.5 (A) Active straight-leg raise test. (B) Active straight-leg raise test with posterior compression.

Rehabilitation may include motor control activation or muscle strength work. Lee (2010) proposed varying the location and direction of the compression applied during the ASLR test may result in greater effort reduction, indicative of improved load transfer. They suggest that this may help clinicians prescribe appropriate exercises to improve neuromuscular function and load transfer. To date, there is no evidence to support any correlation between the direction and position of the compression and changes in motor control.

If compression makes the leg harder to lift, it is considered a sign of excessive force closure. Interventions may include manual therapy, soft tissue work, muscle stretching or muscle relaxation techniques. The ASLR can be used to reassess the effectiveness of any rehabilitation strategy.

The test:

The patient lies supine on the plinth with both legs extended.

The clinician asks the patient to lift one leg about 20 cm off the bed and grades the effort required to do this on a scale of 0–5. This leg is then lowered to the plinth and the test is repeated with the other leg. The patient is then asked about any difference in the 'effort scale' for the two sides.

The clinician also notes the movement strategy used to perform the task. The pelvis, thorax and ribs should stay relatively stable while the hip flexors and knee extensors lift the leg. No overactivity of the musculature of the truck or pelvis should be evident. Things to look for include bracing and rigidity of the ribs and truck, bulging of the abdominals as a Valsalva manoeuvre and extension of the spine.

Pain Provocation Tests

One of the most important elements of assessing individuals with lumbo-pelvic/hip pain is the need to establish the source of the pain in terms of the joint region. While this does not necessarily tell you *WHY* the individual has their symptoms, it does help establish objective markers for symptom improvement and can assist in determining management strategies. A number of studies have demonstrated that a battery of tests that stress the sacroiliac structures can be used to identify if the SIJ is a source of pain in a patient's presentation. None of them are considered to stress specific structures and are not, therefore, tissue-specific. These tests have been shown to possess acceptable levels of reliability provided they are highly standardized. A number of studies have confirmed that three or more SIJ pain provocation tests have the greatest predictive power in relation to controlled, comparative SIJ blocks. Using 3/6 positive tests as the diagnostic criteria, sensitivity has been shown to be 78%–79% and specificity 85%–94%. A positive test occurs when the familiar pain of which a patient complains is provoked. In all cases, the provocation of pain and its location is noted.

Distraction/Anterior Gapping Test (Fig. 14.6) (Laslett et al., 2005)

In this test, the pelvic girdle is distracted anteriorly and compressed posteriorly.

The patient lies supine on the plinth with the legs extended. The clinician places the heels of their crossed hands against the inside aspects of each ASIS and applies a slow, steady posterolateral force, distracting the anterior portion of the SIJ and the pubic symphysis.

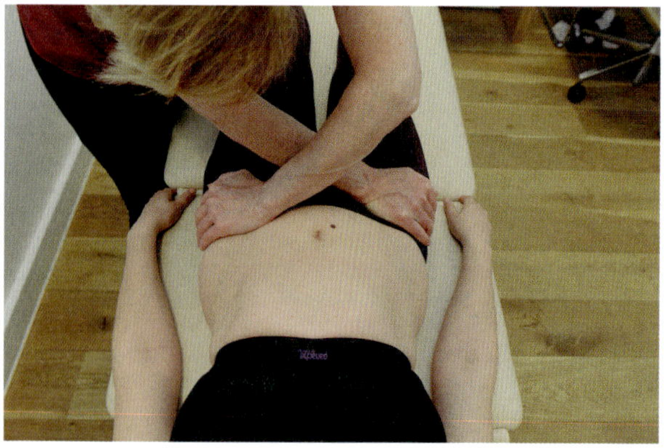

Fig. 14.6 Distraction/anterior gapping.

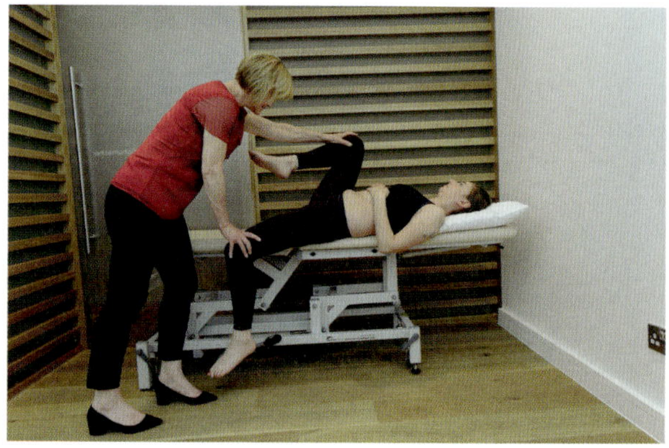

Fig. 14.8 Pelvic torsion/Gaenslen's test.

Thigh Thrust Test/Posterior Shear Test (Fig. 14.7) (Laslett et al., 2005)

The patient lies in supine, close to the edge of the plinth. The clinician flexes the hip and knee closest to the side of the plinth to 90 degrees of hip flexion. They then place both hands cupped together over the knee and drop their forearms along the length of the femur to ensure the force can be directed at the correct angle. Using their body weight, a slow, downward force is applied through the knee and along the length of the femur. Both sides should be tested to check for pain provocation.

Gaenslen's/Pelvic Torsion Test (Fig. 14.8) (Laslett et al., 2005; van der Wurff et al., 2000a, 2000b)

The patient lies in supine, close to the edge of the plinth. The clinician flexes the hip and knee away from the edge of the plinth and asks the patient to hold this position. The clinician then takes the leg closest to the edge of the plinth into an extension over the side of the plinth and applies a downward force, while at the same time applying a force to the other leg to flex it further. The test should be performed bilaterally to stress the pelvic girdle with different forces.

Compression Test/Posterior Gapping (Fig. 14.9) (Laslett et al., 2005)

The patient lies on their side with the hips and knees flexed comfortably to ensure a stable position of the patient. The clinician palpates the upper region of the iliac crest using the palms of both hands and applies a downward force, creating compression across the pelvic girdle.

Sacral Thrust Test (Fig. 14.10) (Laslett et al., 2005)

The patient lies in prone with the legs extended. The clinician places the heel of one hand over the sacrum

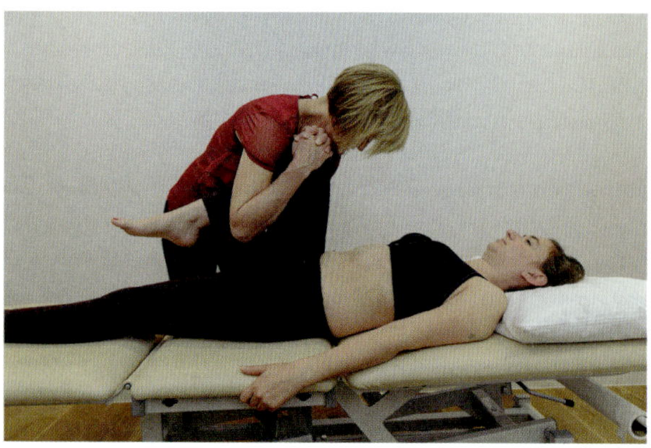

Fig. 14.7 Thigh thrust test/posterior shear.

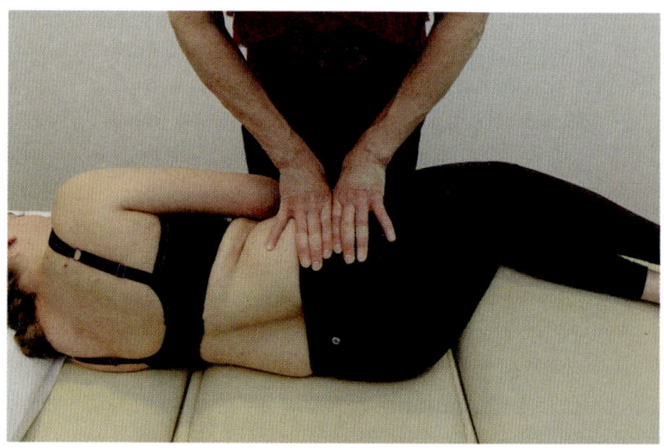

Fig. 14.9 Compression test/posterior gapping.

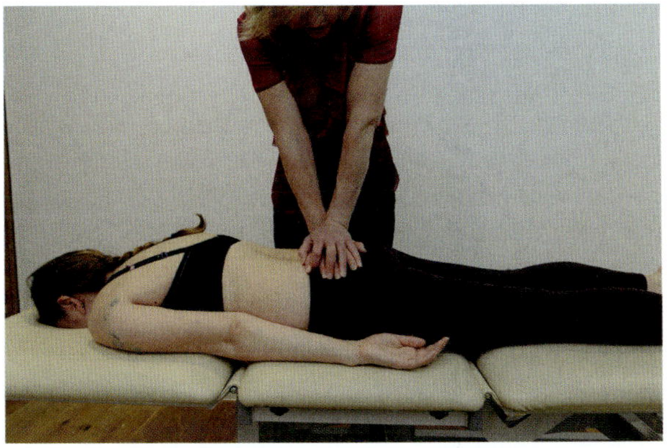

Fig. 14.10 Sacral thrust technique.

and reinforces it with their other hand. They then apply a downward force to the sacrum stressing both sides of the SIJ.

Centralization

There is evidence that a positive result to a cluster of SIJ pain provocation tests is sometimes seen as a false positive in cases of discogenic low back pain (i.e. pain that is not of SIJ origin). These cases can be identified by asking the patient to undertake a series of repeated lumbar extension movements and observing the symptoms centralize (Laslett et al., 2005).

The centralization phenomenon was first described by McKenzie (McKenzie & May, 2003). It has been found to be highly specific for diagnosing discogenic pain and is not observed in patients with confirmed SIJ pain or zygapophyseal joint pain.

While these pain provocation tests are extremely useful in establishing whether the SIJ is a source of pain, they do not help the clinician determine *WHY* the SIJ is painful and therefore are not helpful in determining *HOW* to treat the patient's problem effectively (Palsson et al., 2019).

Passive Accessory Movements

Sacroiliac Joint

The SIJ has accessory motion in both the vertical (superior/inferior) and transverse (AP/PA) planes. Tests for these movements are described by Diane Lee (Lee, 2010) and are considered tests of effective form closure (Lee & Vleeming, 1998). Buyruk et al. (1997) and Damen et al. (2002) demonstrated that it is asymmetrical stiffness and range between the SIJs on either side of the body that correlate with and are prognostic for pelvic girdle pain and dysfunction. The test, therefore, assesses for symmetry of movement between sides.

Vertical Translation (Fig. 14.11)

The patient is positioned in crook lying with the knees comfortably supported over a pillow or the clinician's knee and the arms by the sides to ensure the patient is as relaxed as possible.

The clinician places one hand underneath the iliac crest and onto the sacrum at the level of the PSIS. The other hand is placed over the knee. It is important to determine the plane of the joint by applying a gentle force through the femur in a cranio-caudad direction, varying the inclination from a more medial direction to a more lateral one. One of these planes will meet with the least amount of resistance, and this can be considered the plane of the joint.

The clinician then applies a cranial/caudal oscillatory force through the femur to assess the joint movement and compares this movement with that of the other SIJ to determine if there is a symmetrical or asymmetrical motion.

AP/PA Translation (Fig. 14.12)

The position of the patient is identical to testing for vertical translation, as is the position of the clinician's hands on the sacrum at the level of the joint line. The heel of the other hand is placed over the ASIS and the fingers over the rest of the iliac crest. Again, the plane of the joint is determined by applying a gentle AP force varying the angle from slightly medially to slightly laterally until the plane with the least amount of

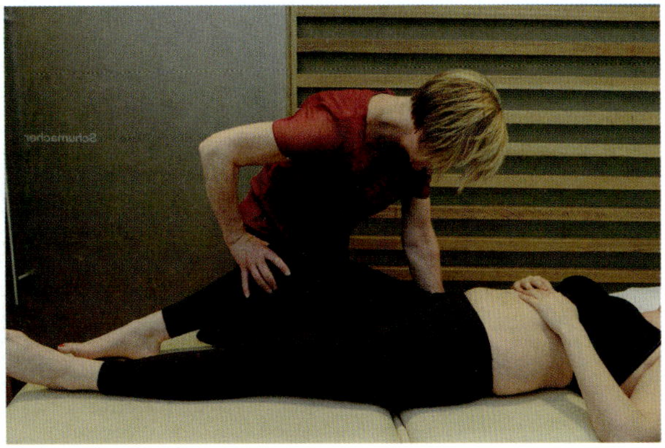

Fig. 14.11 Vertical translation of the sacroiliac joint.

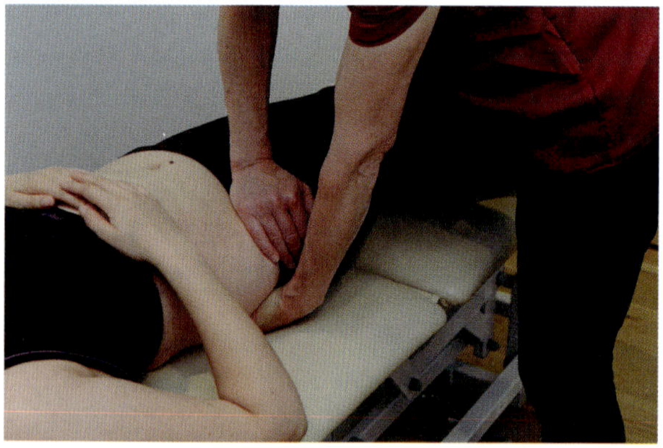

Fig. 14.12 AP translation of the sacroiliac joint.

resistance is identified. The amount and quality of the joint motion is determined and compared with the other side for symmetry.

Pubic symphysis. The historical medical approach to the pelvis has resulted in many misunderstandings about the causes of pelvic girdle pain. One of the most common myths is that pain arising in the region of the pubic symphysis occurs due to ligamentous laxity in the region and resulting 'instability' of the joint.

While instability of the pubic symphysis is a feasible pathology, it usually required significant trauma such as a fall or other accident to disrupt the strong ligamentous structures of the pubis. In cases of hypermobility, a firm end feel should still be present.

To date, no studies have clearly demonstrated the presence of ligamentous laxity/hypermobility in pregnant or postpartum women; nor have any studies demonstrated evidence of instability in this group. Commonly studies have cited increases in the interpubic distance as measured on x-ray or CT, as evidence for pubic symphysis separation, but this technique has not been validated as a measurement tool for instability.

To test for the quality and quantity of the vertical translatory movement of the pubic symphysis, the clinician places the heel of one hand on the superior pubic rami of one innominate and the other hand on the inferior pubic rami of the other. With one hand stable, a vertical translation force is applied with the other hand directly to the pubic rami. A firm end feel denotes a stable joint.

Muscle Tests

Muscle testing may include examining strength, control and length testing of the muscles of the trunk and hip. Assessment of the abdominals, spinal extensors and pelvic floor muscles is essential as they work together to produce effective force closure of the pelvic girdle. Assessment of transversus abdominis (TrA) and multifidus is covered in Chapter 12 on the Lumbar Spine.

Rectus Abdominis

The rectus abdominis is examined for any diastasis recti. This is a stretching of the linea alba between the two rectus abdominis muscles resulting in an abnormal widening of the gap between the muscles. While diastasis recti is most commonly seen in pregnant and postpartum women, it can also occur in men and other female patients. It occurs as a result of excessive intra-abdominal pressure or altered abdominal wall function and load distribution resulting in a stretching of the ligamentous linea alba.

During the third trimester, 100% of pregnant women will have some element of diastasis (da Mota et al., 2015). Postpartum, it takes 2–3 months for the linea alba to regain its normal tension and the gap between the abdominal muscles to reduce. There is evidence to suggest that little change in the inter-rectus distance (IRD) occurs spontaneously after 8–12 weeks postpartum (Coldron et al., 2008).

Recent studies have identified that problems with rectus diastasis are less related to the size of the gap and more related to an individual's ability to generate tension across the linea alba to effectively control the intra-abdominal pressure distribution and load transfer (Lee & Hodges, 2016). It is probably for this reason that there is little agreement in the literature as to what constitutes a normal diastasis and what can be considered abnormal or dysfunctional.

The following is what is being advocated regarding assessment:

1. A measure of the IRD. Beer et al. (2009) used ultrasound imaging to measure the width of the linea alba in healthy, nulliparous women. They found high variability in the IRD at all three levels they measured.
   At the xiphoid process—7 ± 5 mm
   3 cm above the umbilicus—13 ± 7 mm
   2 cm below the umbilicus—8 ± 6 mm

IRDs wider than these were considered abnormal, but the large variability makes the clinical validity of measurement alone questionable.

2. Lee and Hodges (2016) investigated the function of the abdominal wall during a short head/neck curl-up task. In healthy subjects, there was no change in the IRD measured with US during the curl-up task but additionally, the authors stated there was no distortion observed during the task. In defining distortion, the authors refer to doming, sagging or undulations in the linea alba observed during the head-lifting task. Women with diastasis recti demonstrated increased distortion of their abdominal wall as well as an altered ability to transfer load through the trunk during the OLS and ASLR tasks, again suggesting that it is not only the size of the IRD that is clinically relevant but also the function of the abdominal muscles.

The Pelvic Floor

Sixty-six percent of women with diastasis recti have at least one form of pelvic floor dysfunction such as urinary or faecal incontinence or pelvic organ prolapse (Smith et al., 2008).

In considering load and pressure distribution throughout the abdominal region, assessment of pelvic floor function becomes an essential requirement as part of a comprehensive examination of the pelvis. This is usually the domain of a specialist pelvic floor or women's health therapist and involves the internal digital examination of the vagina and/or rectum to assess various components of pelvic floor structure and function including—the position of the pelvic organs, integrity of the pelvic ligaments and sphincters, muscle tone, muscle strength and endurance, the symmetry of muscular contraction, anatomical changes in the muscles including trigger points, tightness and the presence of scar tissue and areas of pain and discomfort.

It is now recognized that overactivity of the pelvic floor muscles can be a source of pelvic girdle pain and can contribute to low back pain, pelvic girdle pain and hip pain and dysfunction (Arab et al., 2010). In long-standing low back, pelvic and hip pain, the contribution and role of pelvic floor dysfunction has often not been considered or addressed and can be a key factor in ensuring effective management of this patient group.

Muscle Length

Altered muscle function can adversely influence the movement and function of the pelvis. Sahrmann (2002) and Lee (2010) proposed that the muscles most commonly seen to tighten in patients with pelvic pain include the latissimus dorsi, erector spinae, the oblique abdominals, hamstrings, psoas major, rectus femoris, TFL, the hip adductors, piriformis and the deep external rotators of the hip. As well as muscle length tests, clinical palpation of these muscles is useful. While no validated clinical tests exist for palpation, it is hypothesized that the presence of tightness, tenderness, rigidity or spasm on palpation may be evidence of overactivity and excessive recruitment of these muscles. Altered recruitment may in turn contribute to altered load transfer across the lumbo-pelvic hip region. Increased levels of activity and shortening may be a source of pain as well as contributing to altered function. There is no specific evidence in the pelvic region that pain and dysfunction are associated with both increases and decreases in the activity of specific muscle groups, but there is evidence for these changes in both lumbar and cervical pain conditions (Hodges et al., 2013; Gizzi et al., 2015).

Palpation

While palpation may help identify the general area of tissue tenderness, it has poor specificity. The clinician palpates over the pelvis, including the sacrum, SIJs, pubic symphysis, long dorsal ligament (Vleeming et al., 2008) and any other relevant areas. Tenderness of bony sites may be indicative of osteoporotic, stress or avulsion fractures

KNOWLEDGE CHECK

1. The Gillet Test is a test that assesses movement of the sacroiliac joints (SIJ). (TRUE/FALSE)
2. How do you use the tests of SIJ accessory motion as part of the clinical reasoning process?
3. Which muscles are commonly tight or overactive in patients with pelvic girdle pain?
4. Why would you refer someone with pelvic girdle pain for a pelvic floor assessment?
5. What causes diastasis recti? How do you measure it? How large does it need to be before it is considered a problem?

COMPLETION OF THE EXAMINATION

On completion of the subjective and physical examination of the lumbo-pelvic hip region, the clinician should consider the following in establishing a working diagnosis:

- Can a mechanical musculoskeletal diagnosis be established or should further investigations be undertaken for other pathology or systemic disease?
- Which structures are a source of symptoms based on various pain provocation tests?
- Which structures are likely to be contributing to the development and maintenance of the patient's signs and symptoms based on examination of function, and active and passive movement?
- Which structures can be ruled out?
- Is this a problem of form closure and/or force closure?
- Is force closure insufficient due to poor motor control/strength or excessive due to muscle overactivity?
- What are the relative contributions of the biological, social and psychological systems in the patient's presentation?

For guidance on treatment and management principles, the reader is directed to the companion textbook (Barnard & Ryder, 2024).

REVIEW AND REVISE QUESTIONS

1. Identify three common pathologies/conditions that may be associated with pelvic girdle pain.
2. What does the term **load transfer** mean?
3. Name five muscle groups that are important in optimal load transfer across the pelvis.
4. Why is pelvic floor function an important consideration in pelvic girdle pain?
5. What is Fortin's finger test?
6. What is the close-packed position of the SIJ? Which ligamentous structures does it tension?
7. Where can the SIJ refer pain to in the lower limb?
8. What role does imaging play in the diagnosis of pelvic girdle pain?
9. Which tests would you use to determine if the SIJ is a source of pain symptoms in a patient's presentation?
10. What does the active straight leg raise assess?

Case Study

Case Study—PostPartum Pelvic Girdle Pain

Patient Information:

A 28-year-old female—Mrs. N

Social History:

Six months postpartum with first child. Lives at home with husband and daughter. Currently on maternity leave from role in banking. Sedentary job—computer-based work.

Body Chart:

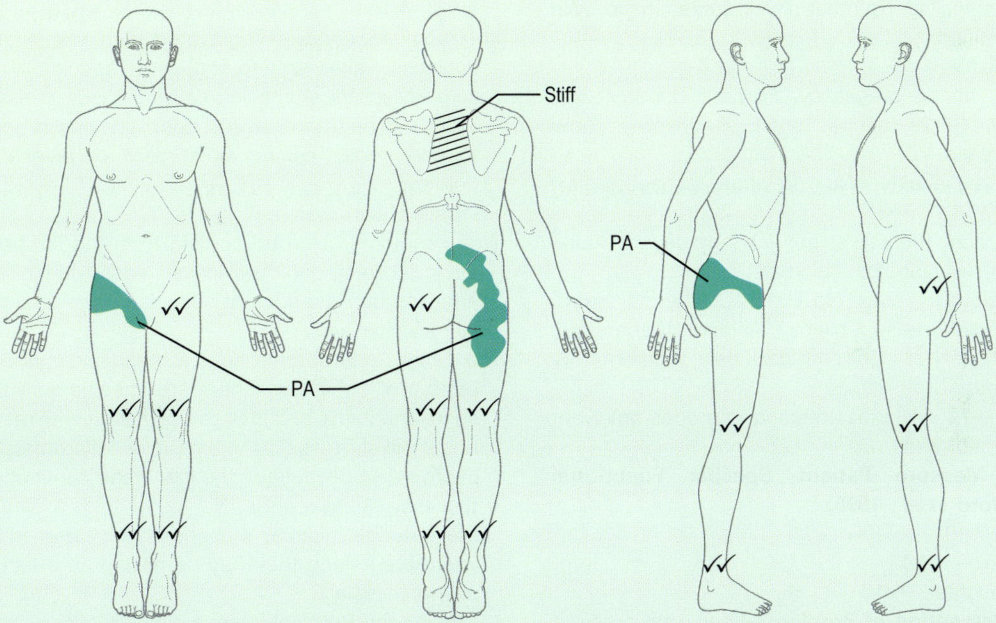

Pa—Constant low-level ache that increases in intensity and area with activity and spreads into buttock, down leg and around into the front of the pelvis and hip area and pubic symphysis. Leg feels weak with walking

- Constantly 4/10—increasing to 7/10 with activity

Aggravating factors—sit to stand

- walking—especially to begin with and after about 10 min. Has to stop after about 20 min. Unable to go for long walks with baby in pram
- bending over to pick up daughter from cot or bath
- climbing stairs

Easing factors—rest/avoiding activities

- Sitting and lying on back for short periods—but pain returns with movement
- Has to sit down after walking for 20 min and rest for a few minutes and can then get up and walk again. Pain gets worse as walks more.

24-h pattern—AM—Feels better in AM after a night's sleep.

AM–PM—activity-dependent. Feels very tired and quite sore by the end of the day.

PM—difficult to find a comfortable position. Problems rolling over in bed. Sleep—no issues although is still getting up to feed.

Other symptom areas

No left buttock/leg pain. No pain in lower legs

No P&N/numbness

No CES

No urinary incontinence—but some sense of urgency since delivery. No anal incontinence. No problems with sexual function.

HPC:

Some low back and pelvic pain during the last trimester. Worked to 36 weeks. Low back pain was better once finished work and was able to move around more regularly. Pain went initially once the baby was delivered—no treatment.

About 3 months ago—started to notice pain in right low back that gradually spread around the pelvis and into

Continued

Case Study—cont'd

the hip and pubic symphysis region. Radiated into the right buttock and down the back of the right thigh.

Tried running at about 3 months postpartum but felt very weak and low back/buttock was sore, so has not run since. Has not been back to Pilates classes.

Had been doing regular 'pregnancy Pilates' during pregnancy. Previously ran about 5 km—three times a week but stopped at 12 weeks and started Pilates as was concerned about doing impact exercise while pregnant.

S/B GP for 6-week postpartum check—episiotomy scar checked for healing. No other physical examination. No issues identified.

Obstetric History:

No problems during pregnancy. Forceps delivery with episiotomy—Gr 2—required stitches—unknown how many. Baby 9lb 4oz.

No other pregnancies. No previous gynaecological problems.

PHx—stiff, achy thoracic spine with long days at work. No other relevant PHx. No investigations.

GH—No relevant issues. No THREAD (Thyroid, Heart, Rheumatoid disease, Epilepsy, Asthma, Diabetes)

No family history of significant back pain, inflammatory conditions.

Medication—nil. Still breastfeeding—so does not want to take medication.

Outcome Measure—Patient Specific Functional Scale (Stratford et al., 1995)

Sit to stand—7/10

Walking 30 min—4/10

Picking up daughter—5/10

Patient's Perception of Problem—Feels that problem is most likely related to muscle weakness as a result of pregnancy. Worried that pelvis is unstable because of ligamentous laxity. Has tried to do pelvic floor and abdominal exercises as per exercise sheet given at the time of delivery, but gave up—unsure if she is doing them correctly and don't seem to be of any help.

Clinical Reasoning

Mrs. N has historically been fit and active with no significant past history. Changes to her posture, abdominal strength and control with pregnancy did not resolve completely after delivery, and it is likely that she has ineffective force closure across the pelvic girdle. There are no observable red flags or anything that is suggestive of systemic disease.

There are no symptoms suggestive of any neurological involvement (paraesthesia, numbness) although patient reports that leg feels weak with walking so a neurological examination is required.

Working hypothesis:

1. Poor force closure at the SIJ due to poor motor control/ muscles weakness of the abdominals, gluteals and pelvic floor
2. Secondary tissue strain on the lumbar spine, pubic symphysis and possibly the hip joint
3. Poor movement patterns due to altered posture and changes in centre of gravity during pregnancy

Evaluation of Severity, Irritability and Nature:

Severity—Moderate—Affecting function but not sleep. NPRS 4/10

Irritability—Moderate—Aggravated with many functional activities. Takes time to settle with specific rest.

Nature—Mechanical irritation causing tissue stress of the lumbar spine, sacroiliac and pubic symphysis secondary to poor motor control as a result of pregnancy and delivery.

Source of symptoms:

The symptoms could be coming from the lumbar spine, sacroiliac joint, pubic symphysis and/or hip joint as the area and behaviour is not specific to one structure.

Pain Mechanisms:

The patient's symptoms have a mechanical, nociceptive pattern of behaviour. There are specific activities that aggravate them, and they can be eased with rest. There is also likely to be an element of inflammatory nociceptive pain because of the low-grade continuous ache that the patient reports. No yellow flags are evident in the patient's history, but she is a new mother with interrupted sleep that may be having an effect on her pain processing.

Planning the Physical Examination

The SIN is moderate so structures can be examined fully, but high-level functional movements/impact activities will not need to be assessed to establish objective markers. Objective markers/comparable signs should be straightforward

- Forward flexion test
- One leg standing test

Because it is not possible to narrow the source of symptoms down, it is important to examine all relevant structures in an attempt to rule some of them out as a source of symptoms. Tests should include manual segmental examination of the lumbar spine and the hip quadrant/FADIR test.

A neurological examination is required.

Physical Examination

Observation

- Wider base of support in standing
- Some anterior tilt of pelvis

Case Study—cont'd

- Poor abdominal muscle tone
- Flat thoracic spine

In standing—low back and sacral pain. Pain over the pubic symphysis radiating to the adductors

Active Movements:

- Forward bending—initiated with hip movement. Limited lumbar flexion—to knee. Pain limited. Pain in low back with cervical flexion. No obvious deviation in pelvic movement
- Return to standing—bends knees and uses hands to push back to standing. Poor gluteal function and overuse of erector spinae
- Extension—10 degrees. Pain increased in low back and pubic symphysis. Poor abdominal activation in return to neutral standing
- Lateral flexion—stiff bilaterally. Fingers to half thigh. Limited lumbar spinal movement
- One leg standing—difficult to stand on either leg. Painful in low back and pubic region. Difficult to weight bear and to flex hip bilaterally.
- Sit to stand—poor movement pattern. Uses hands to push up from seat, extension of lumbar spine, poor gluteal activation/hip extension

Neurological Examination NAD

Supine lying—right pelvis 'appears' elevated relative to left

Hip joint

- Hip Flexion—pubic pain EOR bilaterally
- Hip Abduction—pull in pubic symphysis at EOR bilaterally (40 degrees)
- Hip Quadrant/FADIR—NAD

Pain provocation tests:

- Positive compression test
- Positive thigh thrust test right
- Positive Gaenslen's test bilaterally

ASLR—pain in low back and pubic symphysis with right SLR. Effort R—3/5. L 1/5.

Passive Accessory Movements—SIJ—AP/vertical translation—normal

- Pubic symphysis—normal

Lumbar spine—manual segmental examination—tender erector spinae—increased tone/tenderness. Hypermobility and pain—L4/5/S1

Muscle control and strength:

- Inter-rectus distance—3 fingers at level below umbilicus
- Poor tone in transversus abdominis (TrA) with cueing
- Doming of linea alba with curl up. No change with cueing of TrA

Muscle tone—tenderness and tightness in adductors/piriformis

Palpation—tender over the pubic symphysis

- Tender over the right SIJ (Fortin's area)

Analysis of patient's problem:

Pain provocation tests identify the sacroiliac joint as a likely source of symptoms. Tenderness on palpation of the pubic symphysis and lumbar spine also suggest tissue stress on these areas. The patient demonstrates several elements of poor muscle strength as well as muscle tightness/overactivity indicating poor movement patterns and motor control. This confirms the suspected hypothesis of ineffective force closure. Testing for changes in force closure identify no problems, and the hip joint FADIR test is clear indicating that the hip joint is unlikely to be a source of symptoms.

Management (Day One):

1. Education and advice—explained to the patient that her pelvis was not unstable but that she was lacking the required muscle support and control to support her spine and pelvic effectively, and this was putting stress on various structures, causing pain. At the same time, some of her muscles were working too hard to try and support her body, and these were also a source of pain.
2. Re-education of sit to stand pattern using gluteals and encouraging hip flexion
3. Manual therapy—LxSp Flex PPIVMs to improve lumbar spine mobility
4. Soft tissue work to adductors and piriformis—to reduce tissue tension and pain
5. Home exercise programme—transversus abdominis activation to improve load transfer across the abdominals and pelvis
   - Gluteal strength work
   - Sit-to-stand exercises
   - Roll down—to improve spinal flexion and facilitate gluteal function with return from flexion

Ongoing Management:

1. Education on pelvic floor function using diagrams and analogies. Development of co-activation pattern with transversus abdominis
2. Education on other functional movements—bending and lifting—encourage more effective gluteal function
3. Progressive strength programme for abdominals and gluteals—squats, split squats, step-ups, Romanian

Continued

Case Study—cont'd

deadlifts, lower abdominal leg lowering. Progression to plyometric exercises—jumping, hopping.

4. Graduated return to running programme
5. Mobility exercises to improve and maintain spinal range—including area of thoracic stiffness

Outcome

Mrs. N had six sessions of physiotherapy over 10 weeks. She was discharged pain-free and referred to see a strength and conditioning coach to improve her strength and endurance so that she could increase her running and ensure she had the necessary functional capacity to care for her daughter—bending and lifting, moving pram in and out of car, up and down stairs. Mrs. N was aware that she needed to improve her physical fitness to ensure she remained pain-free with increased levels of activity and demands. She was also aware that she needed to be physically and mentally well as she was planning on getting pregnant again in the next 6 months and wanted to ensure she did not have problems. She was enjoying being more active, although it was challenging to find the time to care for herself with a young baby.

REFERENCES

Arab, A.M., Behbahani, R.B., Lorestani, L., Azari, A., 2010. Assessment of pelvic floor muscle function in women with and without low back pain using transabdominal ultrasound. Man. Ther. 15, 235–239.

Beales, D., Slater, H., Palsson, T., O'Sullivan, P., 2020. Understanding and managing pelvic girdle pain from a person-centred biopsychosocial perspective. Musculoskelet. Sci. Pract. 48, 102152.

Beer, G.M., Schuster, A., Seifert, B., Manestar, M., Mihic-Probst, D., Weber, S.A., 2009. The normal width of the linea alba in nulliparous women. Clin. Anat. 22, 706.

Bullock, J.E., Jull, G.A., Bullock, M.I., 1987. The relationship of low back pain to postural changes during pregnancy. Aust. J. Physiother. 33, 10–17.

Buyruk, H.M., Stam, H.J., Snijders, C.J., Vleeming, A., Lameris, J.S., Holland, W.P.J., 1997. Measurement of sacroiliac joint stiffness with colour Doppler imaging and the importance of asymmetrical stiffness in sacroiliac pathology. In: Vleeming, A., Mooney, V., Dorman, T., Snijders, C., Stoekart, R. (Eds.), Movement, Stability and Low Back Pain. Churchill Livingstone, Edinburgh, p. 297.

Coldron, Y., Stokes, M.J., Newham, D.J., Cook, K., 2008. Postpartum characteristics of rectus abdominis on ultrasound imaging. Man. Ther. 13, 112–121.

Damen, L., Buyruk, H.M., Güler-Uysal, F., Lotgering, F.K., Snijders, C.J., Stam, H.J., 2002. The prognostic value of asymmetric laxity of the sacroiliac joints in pregnancy-related pelvic pain. Spine 27, 2820.

Dreyfuss, P., Dreyer, S.J., Cole, A., Mayo, K., 2004. Sacroiliac joint pain. J. Am. Acad. Orthop. Surg. 12, 255–265.

Dreyfuss, P., Michaelsen, M., Pauza, K., McLarty, J., Bogduk, N., 1996. The value of medical history and physical examination in diagnosing sacroiliac joint pain. Spine 21, 2594–2602.

Fernandes da Mota, P.G., Pascoal, A.G., Carita, A.I., Bø, K., 2015. Prevalence and risk factors of diastasis recti abdominis from late pregnancy to 6 months postpartum, and relationship with lumbo-pelvic pain. Man. Ther. 20, 200–205.

Fortin, J.D., Aprill, C.N., Ponthieux, B., Pier, J., 1994. Sacroiliac joint pain referral patterns II: clinical evaluation. Spine 19, 1483.

Fortin, J.D., Kissling, R.O., O'Connor, B.L., Vilensky, J.A., 1999. Sacroiliac joint innervation and pain. Am. J. Orthop. 28, 687–690.

Fortin, J.D., Pier, J., Falco, F., 1997. Sacroiliac joint injection: pain referral mapping and arthrographic findings. In: Vleeming, A., Mooney, V., Dorman, T., Snijders, C., Stoekart, R. (Eds.), Movement, Stability and Low Back Pain. Churchill Livingstone, Edinburgh, p. 271.

Gizzi, L., Muceli, S., Petzke, F., Falla, D., 2015. Experimental muscle pain impairs the synergistic modular control of neck muscles. PLoS One 10 (9), e0137844.

Goodman, C., Heick, J., Lazaro, R., 2018. Differential Diagnosis for Physical Therapists: Screening for Referral, sixth ed. Elsevier, St Louis.

Hagen, R., 1974. Pelvic girdle relaxation from an orthopaedic point of view. Acta Orthop. Scand. 45, 550–563.

Hansen, A., Jensen, D.V., Larsen, E., Wilken-Jensen, C., Petersen, L.K., 1996. Relaxin is not related to symptom-giving pelvic girdle relaxation in pregnant women. Acta Obstet. Gynecol. Scand. 75, 245–249.

Harding, I., Davies, E., Buchanan, E., Fairbank, J., 2004. Is the symptom of night pain important in the diagnosis of serious spinal pathology in a back pain triage clinic? Spine J. 4, S30.

Hodges, P.W., Coppieters, D., MacDonald, I., Cholewicki, J., 2013. New insight into motor adaptation to pain revealed by a combination of modelling and empirical approaches. Eur. J. Pain 17, 1138–1146.

Huijbregts, P., 2004. Sacroiliac joint dysfunction: evidence-based diagnosis. Reh. Med. 8, 14–37.

Hungerford, B., Gilleard, W., 2007. The pattern of intrapelvic motion and lumbopelvic muscle recruitment alters in the presence of pelvic girdle pain. In: Vleeming, A., Mooney, V., Stoeckart, R. (Eds.), Movement, Stability, and Lumbopelvic Pain: Integration and Research. Churchill Livingstone, Edinburgh, pp. 361–376.

Hungerford, B., Gilleard, W., Lee, D., 2001. Alterations of sacroiliac joint motion patterns in subjects with pelvic motion asymmetry. In: Proceedings from the Fourth World Interdisciplinary Congress on Low Back and Pelvic Pain. Montreal, Canada.

Kapandji, I.A., 2008. The Physiology of the Joints, sixth ed. Churchill Livingstone, Edinburgh.

Laslett, M., Aprill, C.N., McDonald, B., Young, S.B., 2005. Diagnosis of sacroiliac joint pain: validity of individual provocation tests and composites of tests. Man. Ther. 10, 207–218.

Lee, D., 2010. The Pelvic Girdle: An Integration of Clinical Expertise and Research, fourth ed. Churchill Livingstone, Edinburgh.

Lee, D., 2015. The Pelvic Girdle: An Approach to the Examination and Treatment of the Lumbo-Pelvic-Hip Region, second ed. Churchill Livingstone, Edinburgh.

Lee, D., Hodges, P., 2016. Behavior of the linea alba during a curl-up task in diastasis rectus abdominis: an observational study. J. Orthop. Sports Phys. Ther. 46, 580–589.

Lee, D.G., Vleeming, A., 1998. Impaired load transfer through the pelvic girdle – a new model of altered neutral zone function. In: Proceedings from the 3rd Interdisciplinary World Congress on Low Back and Pelvic Pain. Vienna, Austria.

McKenzie, R., May, S., 2003. The Lumbar Spine: Mechanical Diagnosis and Therapy, second ed. Spinal Publications New Zealand Ltd., Waikanae, New Zealand.

Mens, J.M., Damen, L., Snijders, C.J., Stam, H.J., 2006. The mechanical effect of a pelvic belt in patients with pregnancy-related pelvic pain. Clin. Biomech. (Bristol, Avon) 21, 122–127.

Mens, J.M., Vleeming, A., Snijders, C.J., Koes, B.W., Stam, H.J., 2001. Reliability and validity of the active straight leg raise test in posterior pelvic pain since pregnancy. Spine 26, 1167–1171.

Mens, J.M., Vleeming, A., Snijders, C.J., Koes, B.W., Stam, H.J., 2002. Validity of the active straight leg raise test for measuring disease severity in patients with posterior pelvic pain after pregnancy. Spine 27, 196–200.

Mens, J.M., Vleeming, A., Snijders, C.J., Stam, H.J., Ginai, A.Z., 1999. The active straight leg raising test and mobility of the pelvic joints. Eur. Spine J. 8, 468.

NICE Guidelines, 2020. Low back pain and sciatica in over 16s: assessment and management. Assessment and non-invasive treatments. NICE Guideline (NG 59). Methods, evidence and recommendations. November 2016. Updated December 2020.

O'Sullivan, P.B., Beales, D., Beethan, J.A., Cripps, J., Graf, F., Lin, I.B., et al., 2002. Altered motor control strategies in subjects with sacroiliac joint pain during the active straight-leg-raise test. Spine 27, E1–E8.

Ostgaard, H.C., Andersson, G.B., Schultz, A.B., Miller, J.A., 1993. Influence of some biomechanical factors on low-back pain in pregnancy. Spine 18, 61–65.

Ostgaard, H.C., Zetherström, G., Roos-Hansson, E., Svanberg, B., 1994. Reduction of back and posterior pelvic pain in pregnancy. Spine 19, 894–900.

O'Sullivan, P.B., Beales, D.J., 2007a. Diagnosis and classification of pelvic girdle pain disorders – part 1: a mechanism based approach within a biopsychosocial framework. Man. Ther. 12, 86–97.

Palsson, T.S., Gibson, W., Darlow, B., Bunzli, S., Lehman, G., Rabey, M., et al., 2019. Changing the narrative in diagnosis and management of pain in the sacroiliac joint area. Phys. Ther. 99, 1511–1519.

Pastore, A.E., Katzman, W.B., 2012. Recognizing myofascial pelvic pain in the female patient with chronic pelvic pain. J. Obstet. Gynecol. Neonatal Nurs. 41, 680–691.

Petersen, L.K., Hvidman, L., Uldbjerg, N., 1994. Normal serum relaxin in women with disabling pelvic pain during pregnancy. Gynecol. Obstet. Invest. 38, 21–23.

Richardson, C.A., Snijders, C.J., Hides, J.A., Damen, L., Pas, M.S., Storm, J., 2002. The relationship between the transversely orientated abdominal muscles, sacroiliac joint mechanics, and low back pain. Spine 27, 399–405.

Royal College of Radiologists, 2007. Making the Best Use of a Department of Clinical Radiology. Guidelines for Doctors, sixth ed. Royal College of Radiologists, London.

Sahrmann, S.A., 2002. Diagnosis and Treatment of Movement Impairment Syndromes. Mosby, St Louis.

Sapsford, R., Bullock-Saxton, J., Sue Markwell, S., 1999. Women's Health: A Textbook for Physiotherapists. W.B. Saunders, London.

Schwarzer, A.C., Aprill, C.N., Bogduk, N., 1995. The sacroiliac joint in chronic low back pain. Spine 20, 31–37.

Smith, M.D., Russell, A., Hodges, P.W., 2008. Is there a relationship between parity, pregnancy, back pain and incontinence? Int. Urogynecol. J. Pelvic Floor Dysfunct. 19, 205–211.

Snijders, C.J., Vleeming, A., Stoeckart, R., 1993. Transfer of lumbosacral load to iliac bones and legs part 1:

biomechanics of self-bracing of the sacroiliac joints and its significance for treatment and exercise. Clin. Biomech. 8, 285–294.

Solomon, L., Warwick, D., Nayagam, S., 2010. Apley's System of Orthopaedics and Fractures, ninth ed. Arnold, London.

Stafford, G.H., Villar, R.N., 2011. Ischiofemoral impingement. J. Bone Joint Surg. 93, 1300–1302.

Stratford, P., Gill, C., Westaway, M., Binkley, J., 1995. Assessing Disability and Change on Individual Patients: A Report of a Patient Specific measure. Physiother Can. 47, 258–263.

Stuge, B., Garratt, A., Krogstad Jenssen, H., Grotle, M., 2011. The pelvic girdle questionnaire: a condition-specific instrument for assessing activity limitations and symptoms in people with pelvic girdle pain. Phys. Ther. 91, 1096–1108.

Sturesson, B., 1997. Movement of the sacroiliac joint: a fresh look. In: Vleeming, A., Mooney, V., Stoeckart, R. (Eds.), Movement, Stability, and Lumbopelvic Pain: Integration and Research. Churchill Livingstone, Edinburgh, p. 171.

Sturesson, B., Uden, A., Vleeming, A., 2000. A radiostereometric analysis of movements of the sacroiliac joints during the standing hip flexion test. Spine 25 (3), 364–368.

Sturesson, B.E.N.G.T., Selvik, G.Ö.R.A.N., Uden, A., 1989. Movements of the sacroiliac joints. A roentgen stereophotogrammetric analysis. Spine 14 (2), 162–165.

Suresh, E., 2004. Diagnosis of early rheumatoid arthritis: what the non-specialist needs to know. J. R. Soc. Med. 97, 421–424.

van der Wurff, P., Buijs, E.J., Groen, G.J., 2006. Intensity mapping of pain referral areas in sacroiliac joint pain patients. J. Manip. Physiol. Ther. 29, 190–195.

van der Wurff, P., Hagmeijer, R.H.M., Meyne, W., 2000a. Clinical tests of the sacroiliac joint: a systematic methodological review. Part 1: reliability. Man. Ther. 5, 30–36.

van der Wurff, P., Hagmeijer, R.H.M., Meyne, W., 2000b. Clinical tests of the sacroiliac joint: a systematic methodological review. Part 1: reliability. Man. Ther. 5 (1), 30–36.

Visser, L.H., Nijssen, P.G., Tijssen, C.C., van Middendorp, J.J., Schieving, J., 2013. Sciatica-like symptoms and the sacroiliac joint: clinical features and differential diagnosis. Eur. Spine J. 22, 1657–1664.

Vleeming, A., Albert, H.B., Ostgaard, H.C., Sturesson, B., Stuge, B., 2008. European guidelines for the diagnosis and treatment of pelvic girdle pain. Eur. Spine J. 17, 794–819.

Vleeming, A., de Vries, H.J., Mens, J.M., van Wingerden, J.P., 2002. Possible role of the long dorsal sacroiliac ligament in women with peripartum pelvic pain. Acta Obstet. Gynecol. Scand. 81, 430–436.

Vleeming, A., Mooney, V., Dorman, T., Snijders, C., Stoeckart, R. (Eds.), 1997. Movement, Stability and Low Back Pain: The Essential Role of the Pelvis. Churchill Livingstone, Edinburgh.

Vleeming, A., Van Wingerden, J.P., Dijkstra, P.F., Stoeckart, R., Snijders, C.J., Stijnen, T., 1992. Mobility in the sacroiliac joints in the elderly: a kinematic and radiological study. Clin. Biomechan. 7 (3), 170–176.

Vleeming, A., Volkers, A.C., Snijders, C.J., Stoeckart, R., 1990. Relation between form and function in the sacroiliac joint. Part II: biomechanical aspects. Spine 15 (2), 133.

Yazici, Y., Pincus, T., Kautiainen, H., Sokka, T., 2004. Morning stiffness in patients with early rheumatoid arthritis is associated more strongly with functional disability than with joint swelling and erythrocyte sedimentation rate. J. Rheumatol. 31, 1723–1726.

Young, S., Aprill, C., Laslett, M., 2003. Correlation of clinical examination characteristics with three sources of chronic low back pain. Spine J. 3, 460–465.

15

Examination of the Hip Region

Kieran Barnard and Andrew Kemp

LEARNING OUTCOMES

After studying this chapter, you should be able to:

- List the key constituents of a thorough subjective examination.
- Understand the difference between mechanical and non-mechanical pathology and look out for clues in the subjective examination which might lead you to suspect a non-mechanical cause.
- Understand the value of special questions in relation to hip pathology.
- Be able to hypothesize which structures might be at fault based on the location of symptoms and the aggravating factors.
- List the key constituents of a thorough physical examination.
- Have a basic appreciation of common intraarticular and extraarticular pathologies around the hip joint.
- Have an appreciation of the sensitivity and specificity of key physical tests.

CHAPTER CONTENTS

Introduction, 407
Subjective Examination/Taking the Patient's History, 408
Patient's Perspectives on Their Experiences, 408
Body Chart, 408
Behaviour of Symptoms, 408
Special Questions/Screening, 409
History of the Present Condition, 409
Past Medical History, 410
Plan of the Physical Examination, 410
Physical Examination, 411
Observation, 411
Active Physiological Movements, 412
Passive Physiological Movements, 414
Tests for Intraarticular Structures, 414
Tests for Extraarticular Structures, 417
Muscle Tests, 420
Neurological Tests, 421
Miscellaneous Tests, 421
Palpation, 422
Accessory Movements, 422
Completion of the Examination, 423
Case Study, 425
References, 428

INTRODUCTION

The hip is a large, congruent and stable joint. The hip region may become symptomatic due to intraarticular or extraarticular pathology. Intraarticular pathology may be of traumatic origin, for example, in the case of a fractured neck of femur, or may present more gradually. Hip pain of insidious onset may represent, for example, degenerative pathology such as osteoarthritis (OA) or femoroacetabular impingement (FAI) caused by morphological changes within the hip joint.

Although clinically both hip OA and FAI may lead to groin pain, the presentation is often quite different. OA is often characterized by stiffness in the hip when moving from a static position, particularly first thing in the morning when getting out of bed. FAI, however, often causes pain during flexion and twisting movements. Typically, OA affects the older population, whilst FAI is more likely to affect the young adult.

Extraarticular pathology may also present as an acute or more insidious onset. Acute trauma when accelerating or twisting during sport might represent an adductor muscle strain if felt in the groin or a hamstring injury if felt in the buttock or upper thigh. Overuse or biomechanical stresses may cause extra-articular symptoms of more gradual onset. For example, persistent medial torsion of the femur due to reduced endurance of the hip abductors and lateral rotators may in time cause a gluteal tendinopathy, leading to lateral hip pain during walking or running. The clinician must also be mindful of less common conditions such as inflammatory or infective pathologies, for example rheumatoid or septic arthritis.

This chapter will outline the questions asked and the core physical tests necessary to perform a thorough examination of the hip region. The order of the subjective questioning and the physical tests described below can be altered as appropriate for the patient being examined. The reader is directed to Chapters 3 and 4, respectively, for further details on the principles of the subjective and physical examinations.

SUBJECTIVE EXAMINATION/TAKING THE PATIENT'S HISTORY

Patient's Perspectives on Their Experiences

Patients' perspectives and experiences may be relevant to the onset and progression of their problem and are therefore recorded. The patient's age, employment, home situation and details of any leisure activities are also recorded. Factors from this information may indicate direct and/or indirect mechanical influences on the hip. The reader is directed to Chapter 3 for further information.

Body Chart

The following information concerning the type and area of current symptoms can be recorded on a body chart (see Fig. 3.2).

Area of Current Symptoms

Lesions of the hip joint commonly refer symptoms into the groin, anterior thigh and knee. Ascertain which is the worst symptom and record where the patient feels the symptoms are coming from.

Areas Relevant to the Region Being Examined

Symptoms around the hip may be referred from more proximal anatomy, including arthrogenic, myogenic or neurogenic structures in the region of the lumbar spine or sacroiliac joints. Groin and medial thigh pain, for example, may be referred from the upper lumbar spine or may result from a peripheral neuropathy affecting the obturator nerve. Symptoms may also arise as a result of contributing factors such as weak hip lateral rotators or a pronated foot leading to medial femoral torsion (Lack et al., 2014).

The reader is directed to Chapter 3 to fully appreciate other aspects of the body chart to be considered, including the quality, intensity and depth of the pain; whether the symptoms are constant or intermittent; or indeed whether there are any abnormal sensations which could, for example, be referred from upper lumbar nerve roots.

Relationship of Symptoms

Determine the subjective relationship between symptomatic areas—do they come on together or separately? For example, the patient could have lateral thigh pain without back pain, or the pains may always be present together. Consider clarifying questions as explored in Chapter 3.

Behaviour of Symptoms

Aggravating Factors

For each symptomatic area, establish what movements and/or positions aggravate the patient's symptoms. Specific structures in the region of the hip may be implicated by correlating the area of symptoms with certain aggravating factors. For example, groin pain which is aggravated by putting on shoes (flexion) may be more indicative of an arthrogenic hip joint problem than, for example, a femoral nerve peripheral neuropathy.

It is important for the clinician to be as specific as possible when hunting for aggravating factors. Where possible, break the movement or activity down as this may provide clues for what to expect during the physical examination. 'What is it about ...?' is a useful question to ask. Groin pain aggravated by 'gardening', for example, does not offer as much information as groin pain aggravated by 'weeding a flower bed' (flexion) or 'pruning a high hedge' (extension).

Easing Factors

For each symptomatic area, the clinician asks what movements and/or positions ease the patient's symptoms. This helps to confirm the relationship between the symptoms as well as determine the level of irritability (see Chapter 3).

Occasionally, particularly with symptoms that are irritable or with a patient who is catastrophizing, it is difficult to establish clear and distinct aggravating factors. When this is the case it may be worth starting with the easing factors and working backwards. For example, if sitting down eases symptoms, it may be worth asking: 'Does that mean that standing makes your groin pain worse?'

At this point the clinician synthesizes the information gained from the aggravating and easing factors and has a working hypothesis of the structure(s) which might be at fault. Beware of, and do not dismiss, symptoms which do not conform to a mechanical pattern as this may be a sign of serious pathology.

Twenty-Four-Hour Behaviour of Symptoms

The clinician determines the 24-hour behaviour of symptoms by asking questions about night, morning and evening symptoms. See Chapter 3 for more details.

Night symptoms. It is important to establish whether the patient has pain at night. If so, it is crucial to establish whether the pain is position dependent. The clinician may ask: 'Can you find a comfortable position in which to sleep?' or 'What is the most/least comfortable position for you?' Pain which is position-dependent is mechanical; pain which is not position-dependent and unremitting is non-mechanical and should arouse suspicion of more serious pathology.

Position-dependent pain may give clues as to the structure(s) at fault; for example, patients with trochanteric pain syndrome often have trouble sleeping and lying on the symptomatic side.

Morning and evening symptoms. The clinician determines the pattern of the symptoms first thing in the morning, through the day and at the end of the day. This information may provide clues as to the pain mechanisms driving the condition and the type of pathology present. For example, early-morning pain and stiffness lasting for more than half an hour may indicate inflammatory-driven pain.

Special Questions/Screening

Hip-specific special questions may help in the generation of a clinical hypothesis. Such questions may include:

Squatting	Groin pain on squatting may implicate intraarticular pathology as a source of symptoms.
Locking/catching	Locking, clicking and/or catching in the groin may be associated with FAI (Griffin et al., 2016).
Crepitus	Crepitus with groin pain in the older patient may indicate degenerative change.

History of the Present Condition

For each symptomatic area the clinician needs to know how long the symptom has been present, have they changed over time and whether there was a sudden or slow onset and whether there was a known cause that provoked the onset of the symptom. If the onset was slow, the clinician finds out if there has been any change in the patient's lifestyle, e.g. a new job or hobby or a change in sporting activity or training schedule. The stage of the condition is established: are the symptoms getting better, staying the same or getting worse?

The clinician ascertains whether the patient has had this problem previously. If so, how many episodes has s/he had? When were they? What was the cause? What was the duration of each episode? And did the patient fully recover between episodes? If there is no previous history, has the patient had any episodes of pain and/or stiffness in the lumbar spine, knee, foot, ankle or any other relevant region?

To confirm the relationship between the symptoms, the clinician asks what happened to other symptoms when each symptom began. Symptoms which came on at the same time may indicate that the areas of symptoms are related. This evidence is further strengthened if there is a subjective relationship (symptoms come on at the same time or one is dependent on the other) and if the aggravating factors are the same or similar.

Has there been any treatment to date? The effectiveness of any previous treatment regime may help to guide patient management. Has the patient seen a specialist or had any investigations which may help with clinical diagnosis, such as blood tests, x-ray or magnetic resonance imaging (MRI)?

The mechanism of injury gives the clinician some important clues as to the injured structure around the hip, particularly in the acute stage, when a full physical examination may not be possible. For example, sudden buttock pain on sprinting may implicate the hamstring origin, whilst groin pain during extreme flexion activities such as hurdling or martial arts might implicate FAI pathology.

Past Medical History

A detailed medical history is vitally important to identify certain precautions or contraindications to the physical examination and/or treatment (see Table 3.3). As mentioned in Chapter 3, the clinician must differentiate between conditions that are suitable for conservative treatment and systemic, neoplastic and other non-musculoskeletal conditions, which require referral to a medical practitioner. Previous pelvic surgery or interventions that may be relevant such as a hernia repair or guided hip injection is noted.

Plan of the Physical Examination

In order to plan the physical examination, the following questions need to be considered:

- How extensive will the examination be? Is each area of symptoms severe and/or irritable (see Chapter 3)? Will it be necessary to stop short of symptom reproduction to reproduce symptoms partially or fully? If symptoms are severe, physical tests are carried out to just short of symptom production or to the very first onset of symptoms; no overpressures will be carried out, as the patient would be unable to tolerate this. If symptoms are irritable, physical tests need to be performed to just short of symptom production or just to the onset of symptoms, with fewer physical tests being performed to allow for a rest period between tests. Another way to develop the clinician's reasoning is to consider what to expect from each physical test. Will it be easy or hard to reproduce each symptom? Will it be necessary to use combined movements or repetitive movements? Will a particular test prove positive or negative? Will the pain be direction-specific? Synthesizing evidence from the subjective examination and in particular the aggravating and easing factors will provide substantial evidence as to what to expect in the physical examination.
- What are the predominant pain mechanisms which might be driving the patient's symptoms? What are the active 'input mechanisms' (sensory pathways): are symptoms the product of a mechanical, inflammatory or ischaemic nociceptive process? What are the 'processing mechanisms': how has the patient processed this information? What are his or her thoughts and feelings about the pain? Finally, what are the 'output mechanisms': what is the patient's physiological, psychological and behavioural response to the pain? Clearly establishing which pain mechanisms may be causing and/or maintaining the condition will help the clinician manage both the condition and patient appropriately. The reader is directed to Gifford (1998), Jones et al. (2002) and Thacker (2015) for further reading.
- Are there any precautions and/or contraindications to elements of the physical examination that need to be explored further, such as neurological involvement, recent fracture, trauma, steroid therapy or rheumatoid arthritis? There may also be certain contraindications to further examination and treatment, e.g. symptoms of spinal cord or cauda equina compression.
- What are the possible arthrogenic, myogenic and neurogenic structures which could be causing the patient's symptoms: what structures could refer to the area of pain? And what structures are underneath the area of pain? For example, medial thigh pain could theoretically be referred from the lumbar spine or the sacroiliac joint. The structures directly under the medial thigh could also be implicated, for

example, the hip joint, the adductor muscles or the obturator nerve.

- In addition, are there any contributing factors which could be maintaining the condition? These could be:
  - physical, such as weak hip lateral rotators causing medial femoral torsion
  - environmental, for instance, driving for a living
  - psychosocial, such as fear of serious pathology
  - behavioural, for instance, excessive rest in an attempt to help the area heal.
- The clinician decides, based on the evidence, which structures are most likely to be at fault and prioritizes the physical examination accordingly. It is helpful to organize structures into ones that 'must, should and could' be tested on day 1 and over subsequent sessions. This will develop the clinician's clinical reasoning and avoid a recipe-based hip assessment. Where possible, it is advisable to clear an area fully. For example, if the clinician feels the lumbar spine needs to be excluded on day 1, s/he needs to assess this area fully, leaving no stone unturned, to implicate or negate this area as a source of symptoms. This approach will avoid juggling numerous potential sources of symptoms for several sessions, which may lead to confusion.
- A physical planning form can be useful for clinicians to help guide them through the clinical reasoning process (see Appendix 3.1).

KNOWLEDGE CHECK

1. How might osteoarthritis and femoroacetabular impingement present respectively?
2. What might unremitting night pain indicate?
3. Sudden buttock pain on sprinting might indicate which pathology?
4. Might groin pain on squatting indicate intraarticular or extraarticular pathology?
5. What might groin pain and crepitus indicate?

PHYSICAL EXAMINATION

The information from the subjective examination helps the clinician to plan an appropriate physical examination. The severity, irritability and nature of the condition are the major factors that will influence the choice and priority of physical testing procedures. The first and overarching question the clinician might ask is: 'Is this patient's condition suitable for me to manage as a therapist?' For example, a patient presenting with cauda equina compression symptoms may only need neurological integrity testing, prior to an urgent medical referral. The nature of the patient's condition has had a major impact on the physical examination. The second question the clinician might ask is: 'Does this patient have a musculoskeletal dysfunction that I may be able to help?' To answer that, the clinician needs to carry out a full physical examination; however, this may not be possible if the symptoms are severe and/or irritable. If the patient's symptoms are severe and/or irritable, the clinician aims to explore movements as much as possible, within a symptom-free range. If the patient has constant and severe and/or irritable symptoms, then the clinician aims to find physical tests that ease the symptoms. If the patient's symptoms are non-severe and non-irritable, then the clinician aims to find physical tests that reproduce each of the patient's symptoms.

Each significant physical test that either provokes or eases the patient's symptoms is highlighted in the patient's notes by an asterisk (*) for easy reference. The highlighted tests are often referred to as asterisks or markers.

The order and details of the physical tests described below need to be appropriate to the patient being examined; some tests will be irrelevant and some tests will be carried out briefly, while it will be necessary to investigate others fully. It is important for the reader to understand that not all physical tests are equal and that the reliability, sensitivity and specificity will vary markedly between tests (see Chapter 4). The author has chosen to present the most clinically useful tests according to the literature. None of these physical tests should, however, take the place of a thorough subjective examination. A good subjective history when examining the hip region is crucial in helping to determine the diagnosis in the vast majority of cases (Reiman & Thorborg, 2014). The clinician needs to have a clear clinical hypothesis after the subjective examination, and the purpose of the physical examination is to confirm or refute this hypothesis.

Observation

Informal Observation

The clinician needs to observe the patient in dynamic and static situations; the quality of lower-limb and general movement is noted, as are the postural characteristics and facial expression. Informal observation will have begun from the moment the clinician begins the subjective examination and will continue to the end of the physical examination.

Formal Observation

Observation of posture. The clinician examines the patient's spinal and lower-limb posture from anterior, lateral and posterior views in standing and where necessary in functional positions related to the patient's complaint. Specific observation of the pelvis involves noting its position in the sagittal, coronal and horizontal planes: in the sagittal plane, there may be excessive anterior or posterior pelvic tilt; in the coronal plane, there may be a lateral pelvic tilt; and in the horizontal plane, there may be rotation of the pelvis. These abnormalities will be identified by observing the relative position of the iliac crest, the anterior and posterior iliac spines, skin creases (particularly the gluteal creases) and the position of the pelvis relative to the lumbar spine and lower limbs. In addition, the clinician notes whether there is even weight bearing through the left and right leg. The clinician passively corrects any asymmetry to determine its relevance to the patient's problem.

Observation of muscle form. The clinician observes the muscle bulk and muscle tone of the patient, comparing left and right sides. It must be remembered that the level and frequency of physical activity as well as the dominant side may well produce differences in muscle bulk between sides. Some muscles are thought to shorten under stress, while other muscles weaken, producing muscle imbalance. Patterns of muscle imbalance are thought to produce the postures mentioned above.

Observation of soft tissues. The clinician observes the quality and colour of the patient's skin and any area of swelling or presence of scarring and takes cues for further examination.

Observation of balance. Balance is provided by vestibular, visual and proprioceptive information. This rather crude and non-specific test is conducted by asking the patient to stand on one leg with the eyes open and then closed. If the patient's balance is as poor with the eyes open as with the eyes closed, this suggests a vestibular or proprioceptive dysfunction (rather than a visual dysfunction). The test is carried out on the affected and unaffected sides; if there is greater difficulty maintaining balance on the affected side, this may indicate some proprioceptive dysfunction.

As well as monitoring the ability of the patient to balance on one leg, the clinician also pays close attention to the patient's pelvis. A pelvis that drops on the unsupported side indicates abductor weakness on the standing leg and is known as a positive Trendelenburg sign (Fig. 15.1). A positive Trendelenburg sign is a common finding in patients who have undergone hip joint arthroplasty, and hip abductor function may be particularly compromised when the surgeon has employed a lateral approach to the hip (Berstock et al., 2015). Abductor weakness leads to increased adduction and altered pelvic kinematics during gait and may be associated with gluteal tendinopathy (Grimaldi & Fearon, 2015; Grimaldi et al., 2015; Allison et al., 2016).

Observation of gait. Analyze gait on even/uneven ground, slopes, stairs and running. Note the stride length and weight-bearing ability. Inspect the feet, shoes and any walking aids. The typical gait patterns that might be expected in patients with hip pain are the gluteus maximus gait, the Trendelenburg gait and the short-leg gait (see Chapter 4 for further details).

Observation of function. If possible, meticulously examine a functional task related to the patient's presenting complaint, such as squatting, pivoting or climbing stairs. Does pain occur at any phase of that particular movement, e.g. taking weight through the leg when stepping up? It may be possible at this stage to modify the activity to see if symptoms change by, for example, adjusting pelvic rotation.

Active Physiological Movements

Active physiological movements of the hip include flexion, extension, abduction, adduction, medial rotation and lateral rotation (Table 15.1). All movements may be performed bilaterally in supine, with the exception of extension, which may be more readily appreciated in prone. Movements are overpressed if symptoms allow (Fig. 15.2).

The clinician establishes the patient's symptoms at rest, prior to each movement, and passively corrects any movement deviation to determine its relevance to the patient's symptoms. The following are noted:

- quality of movement
- range of movement

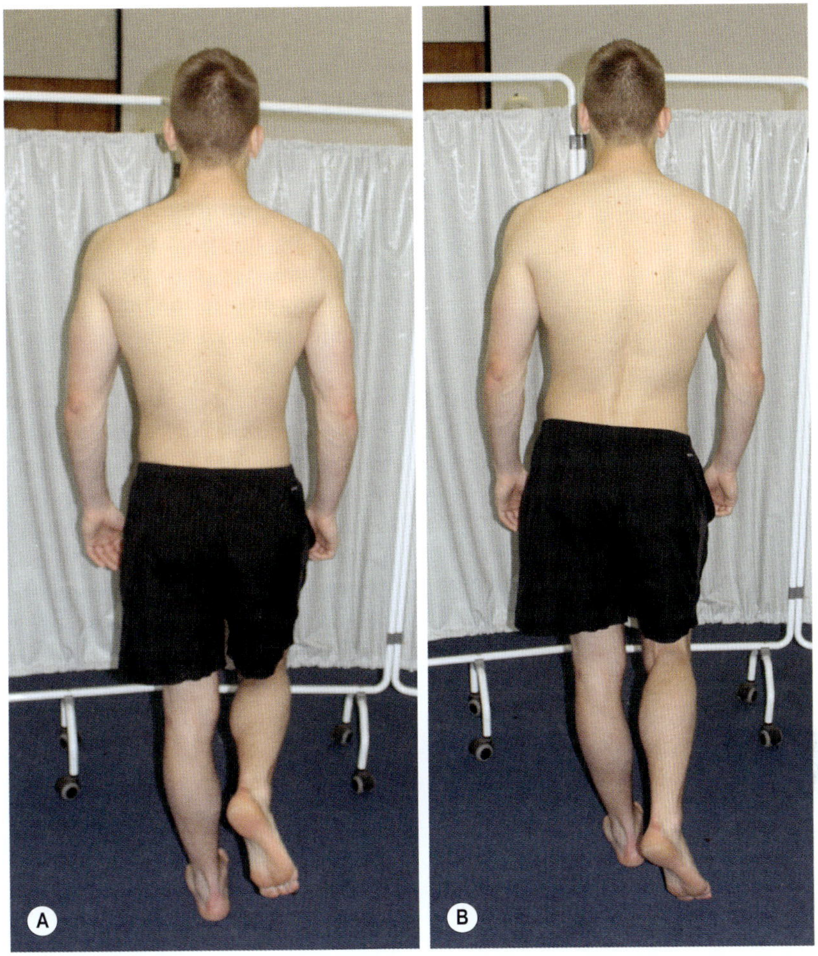

Fig. 15.1 Trendelenburg Test. (A) The patient stands on the affected leg. (B) Positive test indicated by the pelvis dropping on the unsupported side.

- behaviour of pain through the range of movement
- resistance through the range of movement and at the end of the range of movement
- provocation of any muscle spasm.

In a similar way to the manipulation of a symptomatic physical task, the thoughtful clinician may be able to manipulate physiological movements to help differentiation between tissues. For example, when trunk rotation with the patient standing on one leg (causing rotation in the lumbar spine and hip joint) reproduces the patient's buttock pain, differentiation between the lumbar spine and hip joint may be required. The clinician can increase and decrease the lumbar spine rotation and the pelvic rotation in turn, to find out what effect each movement has on the buttock pain. If the pain is coming from the hip then the lumbar spine movements will have no effect on the pain, but pelvic movements will alter the pain; conversely, if the pain is coming from the lumbar spine then lumbar spine movements will affect the pain but pelvic movement will have no effect.

It may be necessary to examine other regions to determine their relevance to the patient's symptoms; they may be the source of the symptoms, or they may be contributing to the symptoms. The most likely regions are the lumbar spine, sacroiliac joint, knee, foot and ankle. These regions can be quickly screened; see Chapter 4 for further details. Contrary to what the

TABLE 15.1 Active Physiological Movements With Possible Modifications

Active Physiological Movements	Modifications
Flexion	Repeated
Extension	Speed altered
Abduction	Combined, e.g.
Adduction	• Flexion with rotation
Medial rotation	• Rotation with flexion
Lateral rotation	Compression or distraction, e.g.
• Lumbar spine	• Through greater tuberosity with flexion
• Sacroiliac joint	Sustained
• Knee	Injuring movement
• Ankle and foot	Differentiation tests
	Functional ability

name might suggest, however, performing a clearing test on the lumbar spine, for example, does not fully negate this region as a source of symptoms, and if there is any doubt, the clinician is advised to assess the suspected area fully (see relevant chapter).

Passive Physiological Movements

All the active movements described above can be examined passively with the patient usually in supine, comparing left and right sides. In the presence of OA, the clinician may expect a limitation to flexion, abduction and internal rotation, slight limitation of extension and no limitation of lateral rotation (Cyriax, 1982).

Comparison of the response of symptoms to the active and passive movements can help to determine whether the structure at fault is non-contractile (articular) or contractile (extraarticular) (Cyriax, 1982). If the lesion is non-contractile, such as a ligament, then active and passive movements will be painful and/or restricted in the same direction. If the lesion is in a contractile tissue (i.e. muscle) then active and passive movements are painful and/or restricted in opposite directions. For example, a hip adductor strain may be painful during active adduction and passive abduction. Such patterns are, however, theoretical, and a muscle strain may be more readily assessed by contracting muscle isometrically, where there will be little or no change in the length of non-contractile tissue.

Tests for Intraarticular Structures

As well as testing the active and passive physiological range, the clinician may employ specific tests to bias different structures around the hip. The reliability, sensitivity and specificity of these tests are variable. The author has chosen to present the most clinically useful tests according to the literature. The intraarticular tests include tests for hip impingement and fracture.

Hip Impingement

FAI is a morphological hip condition leading to groin pain during flexion and twisting movements, typically in young adults. It is still a relatively poorly understood condition (Cannon et al., 2020). The 2016 Warwick International Agreement on femoroacetabular impingement syndrome sought to add clarity to the diagnosis and management of FAI. The consensus document defines FAI as 'a motion-related clinical disorder of the hip with a triad of symptoms, clinical signs, and imaging findings' (Griffin et al., 2016). Pain is thought to arise from 'premature contact between the proximal femur and the acetabulum' (Griffin et al., 2016). This 'premature contact' is thought to be caused by an abnormality in the shape of the femoral head (known as a cam deformity), an abnormal morphology of the acetabulum rim (known as a pincer deformity) or indeed a combination of the two (Cannon et al., 2020). The long-term prognosis of FAI is unclear (Cannon et al., 2020), but the condition may lead to osteoarthritic change if untreated (Griffin et al., 2016).

The triad of features leading to diagnosis according to the Warwick consensus includes

- **Symptoms**—Pain is typically felt in the hip/groin region. There may be clicking, catching, locking, stiffness restricted range and sometimes giving way.
- **Clinical Signs**—There is no one clinical sign which implicates FAI as a pathology but rather a battery of tests may be helpful. Below we describe three of the most widely used clinical tests: internal rotation over pressure (IROP), flexion adduction internal rotation (FADDIR) and flexion abduction external rotation (FABER). These tests appear clinically useful (Reiman et al., 2015a; Pacheco-Carrillo & Medina-Porqueres, 2016); however, in general terms these

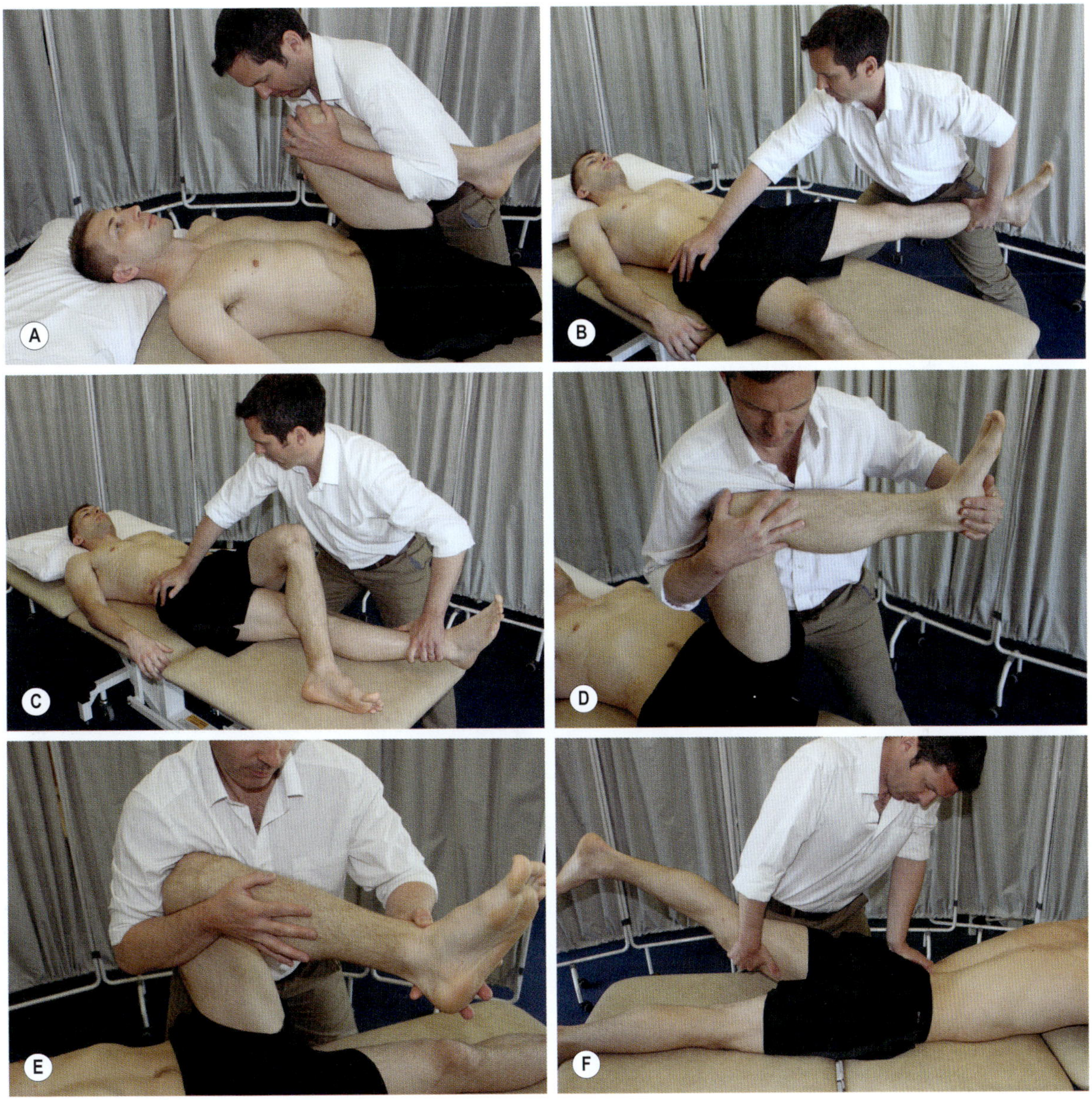

Fig. 15.2 Overpressures to the Hip Joint. (A) Flexion. Both hands rest over the knee and apply overpressure to hip flexion. (B) Abduction. The right hand stabilizes the pelvis while the left hand takes the leg into abduction. (C) Adduction. With the left leg crossed over the right leg, the right hand stabilizes the pelvis, and the left hand takes the leg into adduction. (D) Medial rotation. The clinician's trunk and right hand support the leg. The left hand and trunk then move to rotate the hip medially. (E) Lateral rotation. The clinician's trunk and right hand support the leg. The left hand and trunk then move to rotate the hip laterally. (F) Extension. In prone, the left hand supports the pelvis whilst the right hand takes the leg into extension.

tests are sensitive but not specific, so the clinician should be mindful of false positives.

- **Diagnostic Imaging**—Whilst not all clinicians will have access to imaging, it is helpful to have an appreciation of the imaging which may be useful in the diagnosis of FAI. A plain anteroposterior x-ray of the pelvis and a lateral view of the hip may be helpful in the first instance to check for cam or pincer morphologies followed by MRI if more detailed imaging is desired, for example to identify a labral tear. An MRI arthrogram (involving the injection of gadolinium before imaging) is more invasive but usually more accurate in detecting labral tears and articular cartilage defects (Griffin et al., 2016).

Internal Rotation Over Pressure

With the patient lying in supine position, the affected hip is flexed to 90 degrees. The clinician stabilizes at the pelvis and internally rotates the hip to the end of range with some overpressure (Fig. 15.3). The IROP test is deemed positive if the patient's pain is reproduced. The IROP test has a sensitivity of greater than 80% (Maslowski et al., 2010; Pacheco-Carrillo & Medina-Porqueres, 2016), but a specificity as low as 17%.

Flexion Adduction Internal Rotation

The patient lies supine with one knee flexed. The clinician fully flexes the hip and then adducts and internally rotates the femur (Fig. 15.4). This movement approximates the anterior aspect of the femoral neck with the acetabulum. The test is positive if it reproduces pain, clicking, catching or locking. The sensitivity of the FADDIR has been reported as excellent—94% (with MRI arthrogram as a reference), with a poor specificity of 8% (Reiman et al., 2015b).

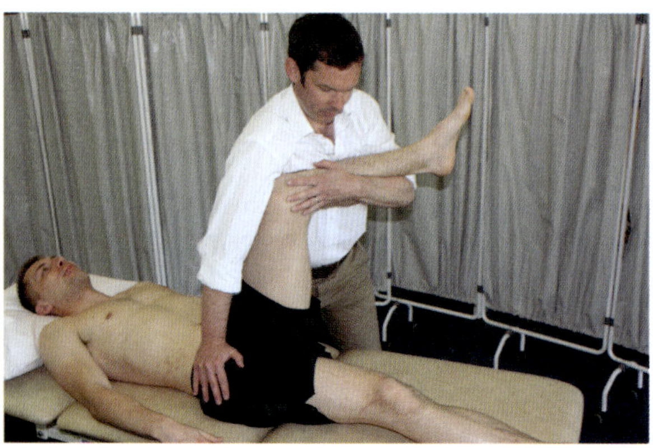

Fig. 15.3 Internal Rotation Over Pressure (IROP). The clinician stabilizes at the pelvis and internally rotates the hip to the end of range with some overpressure.

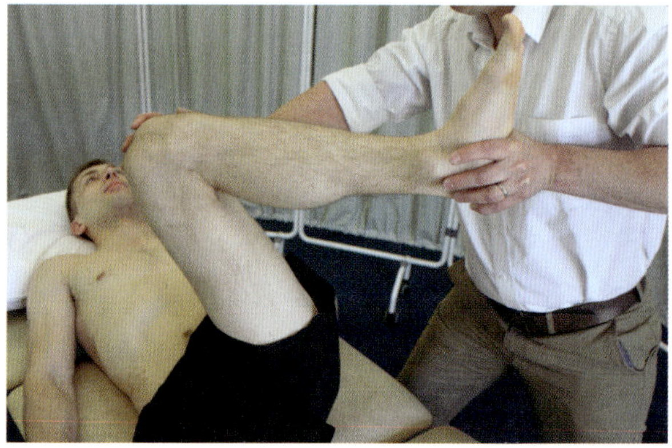

Fig. 15.4 Flexion, Adduction, Internal rotation (FADDIR). The clinician fully flexes the hip and then adducts and internally rotates the femur.

Flexion Abduction External Rotation

The FABER test has also been found to be a sensitive test in detecting FAI, at 82%, but again the test lacks specificity, at 25% (Maslowski et al., 2010). With the patient lying supine, the foot of the symptomatic leg is placed on the knee of the asymptomatic leg. The clinician then stabilizes the pelvis and adds some gentle downward pressure to the knee (Fig. 15.5). A positive

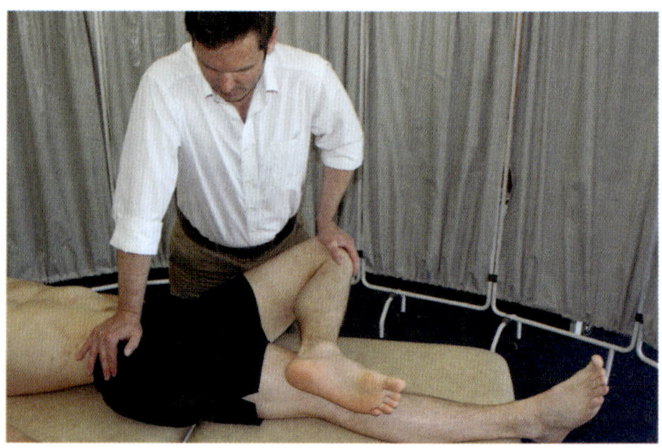

Fig. 15.5 Flexion, Abduction, External Rotation (FABER) Test. The foot of the symptomatic leg is placed on the knee of the asymptomatic leg so the symptomatic leg lies in a flexed, abducted and externally rotated position. The clinician then stabilizes the pelvis and adds some gentle downward pressure to the knee.

test is indicated by reproduction of the patient's ipsilateral hip pain (Pacheco-Carrillo & Medina-Porqueres, 2016). In addition to the presence of FAI, a positive FABER test may also indicate iliopsoas spasm or sacroiliac joint dysfunction (Magee & Manske, 2021).

Fracture

Some tests have been advocated in the diagnosis of fracture and stress fracture to the femur. Indeed, the two tests presented below show good discriminative ability (Reiman et al., 2015b).

Patellar Pubic Percussion Test

In this test, the clinician sits or stands by the symptomatic leg and places a stethoscope over the pubic symphysis. The patella of the leg being tested is then tapped or a tuning fork is used, and the sound is noted (Fig. 15.6). The quality of the sound is then compared to the contralateral side. If the sound is duller ipsilaterally, then the test is considered positive. The sensitivity and specificity may be as high as 95% and 86%, respectively (Reiman et al., 2013, 2015b).

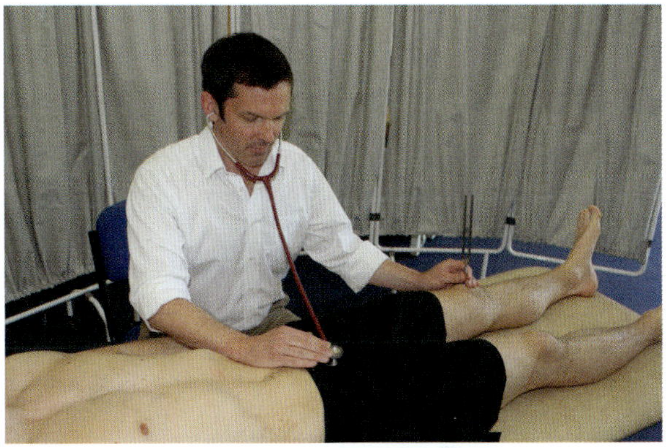

Fig. 15.6 Patellar Pubic Percussion Test. The clinician sits or stands by the symptomatic leg and places a stethoscope over the pubic symphysis. The patella of the leg being tested is then tapped or a tuning fork is used and the sound is noted.

Fulcrum Test

Another test which has shown good sensitivity and specificity in the diagnosis of fracture is the fulcrum test. The patient sits on the treatment couch with the clinician on the symptomatic side. The clinician's hand rests on the asymptomatic thigh with the patient's symptomatic thigh resting on the clinician's forearm. The patient leans back slightly and the clinician places a downward pressure on the symptomatic side at the knee (Fig. 15.7). A positive test is indicated by apprehension and the reproduction of symptoms. Sensitivity and specificity have been reported at 93% and 75%, respectively (Reiman et al., 2013, 2015b).

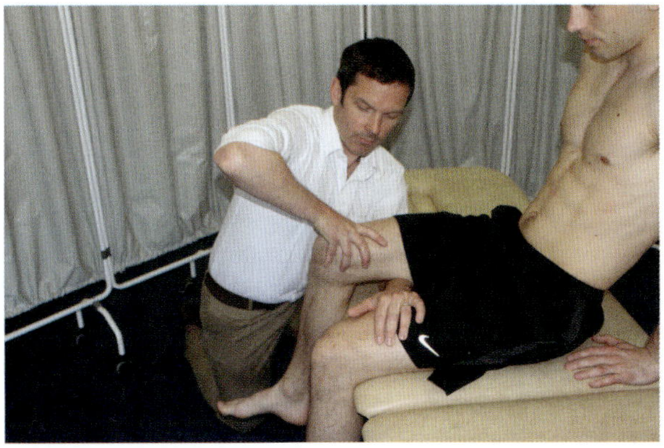

Fig. 15.7 Fulcrum Test. The patient sits on the treatment couch with the clinician on the symptomatic side. The clinician's hand rests on the asymptomatic thigh with the patient's symptomatic thigh resting on the clinician's forearm. The patient leans back slightly, and the clinician places a downward pressure on the symptomatic side at the knee.

Tests for Extraarticular Structures

Tests for symptoms emanating from extraarticular structures will now be presented. These have been categorized as tests for gluteal tendinopathy and sports-related groin pain.

Gluteal Tendinopathy

It is now acknowledged that lateral hip pain is more multi-factorial than once thought. What used to be termed 'trochanteric bursitis' is now described as 'trochanteric pain syndrome' or simply 'lateral hip pain'. It is now widely recognized that the primary source of lateral hip pain is gluteal tendinopathy, particularly tendinopathy of the gluteus medius and minimus tendons (Grimaldi & Fearon, 2015; Grimaldi et al., 2015; Reid, 2016; Ladurner et al., 2021). Gluteal tendinopathy is not thought to be an inflammatory pathology as rubor, erythema and oedema are uncommon features, with only pain being a common feature (Reid, 2016). Furthermore inflammatory cells are not always present in the tendinopathic tendon (Jomaa et al., 2020).

Treatment of gluteal tendinopathy should therefore focus on regaining the loading capacity of the musculotendinous unit. Indeed, a recent large multi-centred randomized controlled trial suggests that education and exercise perform better than steroid injection in the management of gluteal tendinopathy (Mellor et al., 2018). Further level 1 research evidence suggests that extracorporeal shockwave therapy may also be a useful adjunct in the management of chronic gluteal tendinopathy (Ramon, 2020).

MRI is the gold standard imaging in the detection of gluteal tendinopathy (Grimaldi et al., 2015). In the absence of (or as an adjunct to) imaging, it is important to recognize that there is a lack of consensus as to which tests possess the greatest diagnostic accuracy in the detection of gluteal tendinopathy. It is good practice therefore to employ a battery of clinical tests (Grimaldi et al., 2015).

Resisted External Derotation Test

The resisted external derotation test has demonstrated good sensitivity (88%) and excellent specificity (97.3%) in the diagnosis of gluteal tendinopathy (Reiman et al., 2013, 2015b). The patient lies in supine with the symptomatic hip at 90 degrees of flexion. The clinician fully externally rotates the hip, and the patient is asked to return the leg actively to neutral against the clinician's resistance (Fig. 15.8). A positive test is indicated by the reproduction of pain (Reiman et al., 2015b).

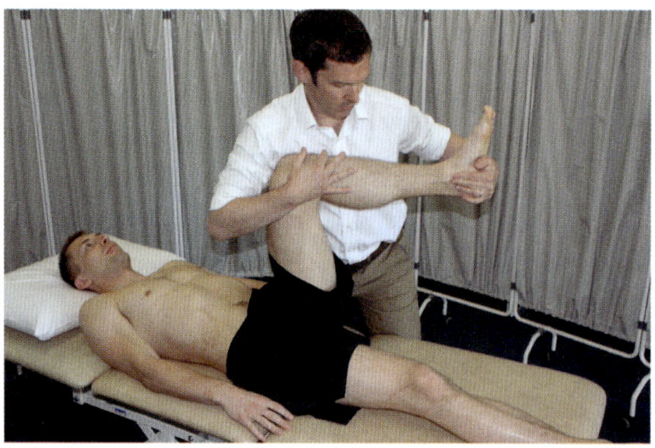

Fig. 15.8 Resisted External Derotation Test. The patient lies in supine with the symptomatic hip at 90 degrees of flexion. The clinician fully externally rotates the hip, and the patient is asked actively to return the leg to neutral against the clinician's resistance.

Sustained Single-Leg Stance

Grimaldi and Fearon (2015) recommend the single-leg stance as a valid and simple test in the diagnosis of gluteal tendinopathy. They point out that several variations of the test are described in the literature. They recommend a simple one-leg stance on the symptomatic side for 30 seconds with the clinician offering balance support at the fingertips, as suggested by Lequesne et al. (2008; Fig. 15.9). Those with poorer hip abductor endurance may develop an adducted hip during this test, increasing the compressive load over the lateral hip and causing pain. The test is positive if pain is reproduced within the 30-second period. Lequesne et al. (2008) found the test to have excellent sensitivity and specificity at 100% and 97.3%, respectively, in the identification of gluteal tendinopathy.

Palpation

Pain on palpation around the greater trochanter is generally considered an important sign in the diagnosis of gluteal tendinopathy (Grimaldi et al., 2015). However, when comparing to MRI findings, despite good

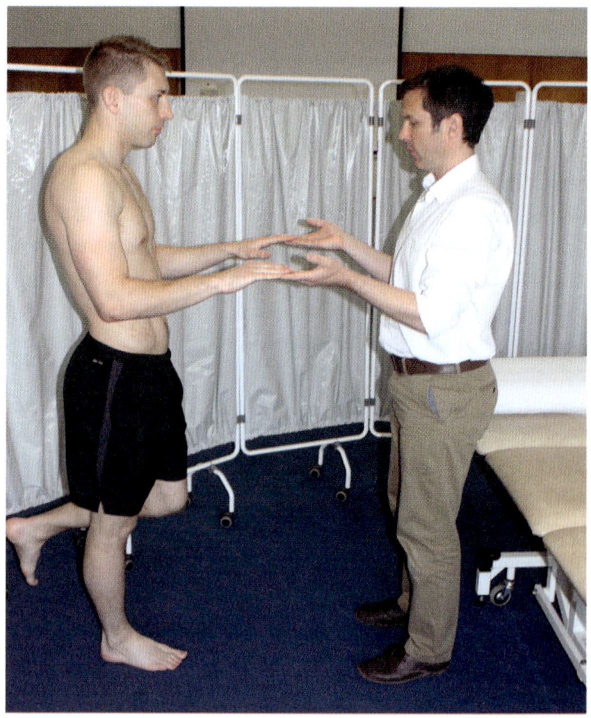

Fig. 15.9 Sustained Single-Leg Stance. The patient stands on the symptomatic leg for 30 seconds with the clinician offering balance support at the fingertips.

sensitivity (80%), Grimaldi et al. (2016) found the sensitivity of palpation to be poor at 47%, so the clinician should be aware of false positives.

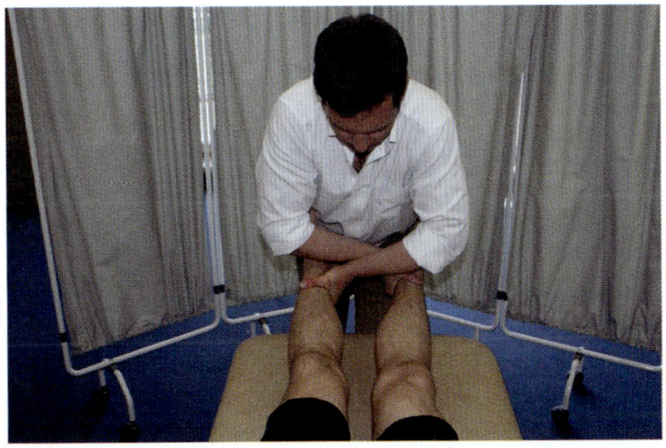

Fig. 15.10 Double Adductor Test. The clinician lifts the legs passively into slight flexion and asks the patient to adduct maximally against manual resistance.

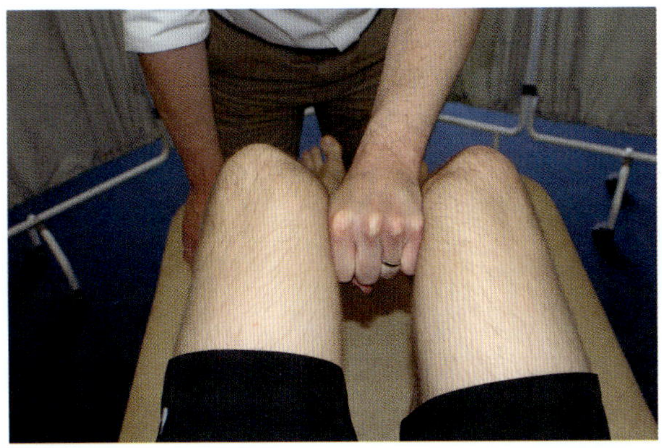

Fig. 15.11 Squeeze Test. With the knees flexed to 45 degrees, the patient is asked to squeeze the clinician's clenched fist which is placed between the patient's knees.

Groin Hernia

Although not a musculoskeletal disorder as such, it is helpful for the clinician to have an appreciation of groin hernia as it may present as discomfort in the groin region. Groin hernias comprise inguinal and femoral hernias. A hernia occurs when tissue such as part of the intestine protrudes through a weakness in the abdominal wall. Seventy-five per cent of all hernias occur in the inguinal region with a 9:1 male predominance (LeBlanc et al., 2013). Often an inguinal hernia presents as a bulge or swelling in the groin region or as an enlarged scrotum in men. During physical examination, the clinician inspects the groin region for swelling or a bulge during Valsava manoeuvres or with a cough. The inguinal bulge if present often disappears with lying. Whilst the sensitivity and specificity in detecting groin hernia has been reported as 75% and 96%, respectively (van den Berg et al., 1999), ultrasonography may be required in women as hernias can be more difficult to detect than in men (Shakil et al., 2020).

Sports-Related Chronic Groin Pain

Often despite hernia being ruled out clinically and with imaging, chronic sports-related groin pain persists and such presentations are often confounding to many practitioners (Zuckerbraun et al., 2020). Whilst sports-related hip injuries are varied (Reiman et al., 2013), the aim of the following tests is to place stress across the common adductor origin and pubic symphysis (Reiman et al., 2015b). In so doing it may be possible to establish if this region may be the source of the patient's symptoms. In general terms these tests are specific with moderate sensitivity.

Double Adductor Test

The patient lies supine with the legs extended. The clinician lifts the legs passively into slight flexion and asks the patient to adduct maximally against manual resistance (Fig. 15.10). A positive test is indicated by the reproduction of the patient's symptoms (Reiman et al., 2013). The sensitivity for this test is 54% and the specificity is 93% (Reiman et al., 2015b).

Squeeze Test

Similarly to the double adductor test, in this test the patient contracts the adductors of both hips simultaneously. This time the knee is flexed to 45 degrees, and the patient is asked to squeeze the clinician's clenched fist, which is placed between the patient's knees (Fig. 15.11). A positive test is indicated by the

TABLE 15.2 Summary of the Sensitivity and Specificity of the Presented Tests for Intraarticular and Extraarticular Pathologies

	Pathology	Test	Sensitivity	Specificity	Reference
Intraarticular Structures	Hip impingement	IROP	High > 80%	Low 17%	Maslowski et al. (2010), Pacheco-Carrillo and Medina-Porqueres (2016)
		FADDIR	Very high 94%	Very low 8%	Reiman et al. (2015b)
		FABER	Moderate to high 82%	Very low 25%	Maslowski et al. (2010)
	Fracture	Patella pubic percussion test	Very high 95%	High 86%	Reiman et al. (2013, 2015b)
		Fulcrum test	Very high 93%	Moderate 75%	Reiman et al. (2013, 2015b)
Extraarticular Structures	Gluteal tendinopathy	Resisted external de-rotation test	High 88%	Very high 97.3	Reiman et al. (2013, 2015b)
		Sustained single leg stance	Very high 100%	Very high 97.3	Lequesne et al. (2008)
		Palpation	Moderate to high 80%	Low 47%	Grimaldi et al. (2016)
	Groin hernia	Physical examination	Moderate to high 75%	Very high 96%	van den Berg et al. (1999)
	Sports-related groin pain	Double adductor test	Low 54%	Very high 93%	Reiman et al. (2015b)
		Squeeze test	Low 43%	Very high 91%	Reiman et al. (2015b)

reproduction of the patient's symptoms (Reiman et al., 2013). The diagnostic accuracy of the squeeze test is similar to the double adductor test, with a sensitivity of 43% and a specificity of 91% (Reiman et al., 2015b).

A summary of the sensitivity and specificity of the presented tests for intraarticular and extraarticular pathologies is presented in Table 15.2.

Muscle Tests

Muscle tests include those examining muscle strength, control and length as well as isometric muscle testing.

Muscle Strength

For a true appreciation of a muscle's strength, the clinician tests the muscle isotonically through the available range. During the physical examination of the hip, it may be appropriate to test the hip flexors, extensors, abductors, adductors, medial and lateral rotators as well as any other relevant muscle group.

Greater detail may be required to test the strength of muscles, in particular those thought prone to become weak, that is, rectus abdominis, gluteus maximus, medius and minimus, vastus lateralis, medialis and intermedius, tibialis anterior and the peronei (Jull & Janda, 1987; Sahrmann, 2002). Testing the strength of these muscles is described in Chapter 4.

Muscle Control

The relative strength of muscles is considered to be more important than the overall strength of a muscle group (Janda, 1994, 2002; White & Sahrmann, 1994; Sahrmann, 2002). Relative strength is assessed indirectly by observing posture, as already mentioned, by the quality of active movement, noting any changes in muscle recruitment patterns and by palpating muscle activity in various positions.

Muscle Length

The clinician may test the length of muscles, in particular those thought prone to shortening (Janda, 1994), that is, erector spinae, quadratus lumborum, piriformis, iliopsoas, rectus femoris, tensor fasciae latae, hamstrings, tibialis posterior, gastrocnemius and soleus (Jull & Janda, 1987; Sahrmann, 2002). Testing the length of these muscles is described in Chapter 4.

Isometric Muscle Testing

Isometric muscle testing may help to differentiate whether symptoms are arising from contractile or non-contractile tissue. Isometric testing is described in detail in Chapter 4.

It may be appropriate to test the hip joint flexors, extensors, abductors, adductors, medial and lateral rotators (and other relevant muscle groups) in a resting position and, if indicated, in different parts of the physiological range. The clinician notes the strength and quality of the contraction, as well as any reproduction of the patient's symptoms.

Neurological Tests

Neurological examination includes neurological integrity testing and neurodynamic tests.

Integrity of the Nervous System

The integrity of the nervous system is tested if the clinician suspects that the symptoms are emanating from the spine or from a peripheral nerve.

Dermatomes/peripheral nerves. Light touch and pain sensation of the lower limb are tested using cotton wool and pinprick, respectively, as described in Chapter 4. Knowledge of the cutaneous distribution of nerve roots (dermatomes) and peripheral nerves enables the clinician to distinguish the sensory loss due to a root lesion from that due to a peripheral nerve lesion. The cutaneous nerve distribution and dermatome areas are shown in Chapter 4.

Myotomes/peripheral nerves. The following myotomes are tested (see Chapter 4 for further details):

- L2: hip flexion
- L3: knee extension
- L4: foot dorsiflexion and inversion
- L5: extension of the big toe
- S1: eversion of the foot, contract buttock, knee flexion
- S2: knee flexion, toe standing
- S3—S4: muscles of pelvic floor, bladder and genital function.

A working knowledge of the muscular distribution of nerve roots (myotomes) and peripheral nerves enables the clinician to distinguish the motor loss due to a root lesion from that due to a peripheral nerve lesion. The peripheral nerve distributions are shown in Chapter 4.

Reflex testing. The following deep tendon reflexes are tested (see Chapter 4):

- L3—L4: knee jerk
- S1: ankle jerk.

Neurodynamic Tests

The following neurodynamic tests may be carried out in order to ascertain the degree to which neural tissue is responsible for the production of the patient's symptom(s):

- passive neck flexion
- straight-leg raise
- passive knee bend
- slump.

These tests are described in detail in Chapter 4.

Miscellaneous Tests

Vascular Tests

If the circulation is suspected of being compromised, the clinician palpates the pulses of the femoral, tibial, popliteal and dorsalis pedis arteries. The clinician then checks for skin and temperature changes as well as capillary refill of the nail beds. The state of the vascular system can also be determined by the response of symptoms to positions of dependence and elevation of the lower limbs. Refer to Chapter 8 in the companion text (Barnard & Ryder, 2024) for further information.

Leg Length

True leg length, which tends to be congenital, is measured from the anterior superior iliac spine to the medial or lateral malleolus. Apparent leg length, which results from compensatory change such as a pronated foot or spinal scoliosis, is measured from the umbilicus to the medial or lateral malleolus. A difference in leg length of up to 1–1.5 cm is considered normal (Magee, 2014).

Palpation

The clinician palpates the hip region and any other relevant area. It is useful to record palpation findings on a body chart (see Fig. 3.2) and/or palpation chart (see Fig. 4.34).

The clinician notes the following:

- the temperature of the area
- localized increased skin moisture
- the presence of oedema. This can be measured using a tape measure and left and right sides compared.
- mobility and feel of superficial tissues, e.g. ganglions, nodules, lymph nodes in the femoral triangle
- the presence or elicitation of any muscle spasm
- tenderness of bone (the greater trochanter may be tender because of trochanteric bursitis and the ischial tuberosity because of ischiogluteal bursitis); inguinal area tenderness may be due to iliopsoas bursitis, ligaments, muscle (Baer's point, for tenderness/spasm of iliacus, lies a third of the way down a line from the umbilicus to the anterior superior iliac spine), tendon, tendon sheath, trigger points and nerve.

Palpable nerves which may be relevant to assessment of the hip region are as follows:

- The sciatic nerve can be palpated two-thirds of the way along an imaginary line between the greater trochanter and the ischial tuberosity with the patient in prone.
- The common peroneal nerve can be palpated medial to the tendon of biceps femoris and also around the head of the fibula.
- The tibial nerve can be palpated centrally over the posterior knee crease medial to the popliteal artery; it can also be felt behind the medial malleolus, which is more noticeable with the foot in dorsiflexion and eversion.
- Increased or decreased prominence of bones.
- Pain provoked or reduced on palpation.

Accessory Movements

It may be useful to use the palpation chart and movement diagrams (or joint pictures) to record findings. These are explained in detail in Chapter 4.

The clinician notes the following:

- quality of movement
- range of movement
- resistance through the range and at the end of the range of movement
- behaviour of pain through the range
- provocation of any muscle spasm.

Hip joint accessory movements are shown in Fig. 15.12 and are listed in Table 15.3. Following accessory movements to the hip region, the clinician reassesses all the physical asterisks (movements or tests that have been found to reproduce the patient's symptoms) in order to establish the effect of the accessory movements on the patient's signs and symptoms. Accessory movements can then be tested for other regions suspected to be a source of, or contributing to, the patient's symptoms. Again, following accessory movements to any one region, the clinician reassesses all the asterisks. Regions likely to be examined are the lumbar spine, sacroiliac joint, knee, foot and ankle (see Table 15.3).

KNOWLEDGE CHECK

1. What might a limitation in internal rotation of the hip indicate?
2. In general terms, tests for FAI are specific but not sensitive: TRUE or FALSE?
3. What are the triad of features which might lead to the diagnosis of FAI according the Warwick consensus?
4. Which physical tests might be helpful in the diagnosis of gluteal tendinopathy?
5. Inguinal hernia is much more common in men: TRUE or FALSE?

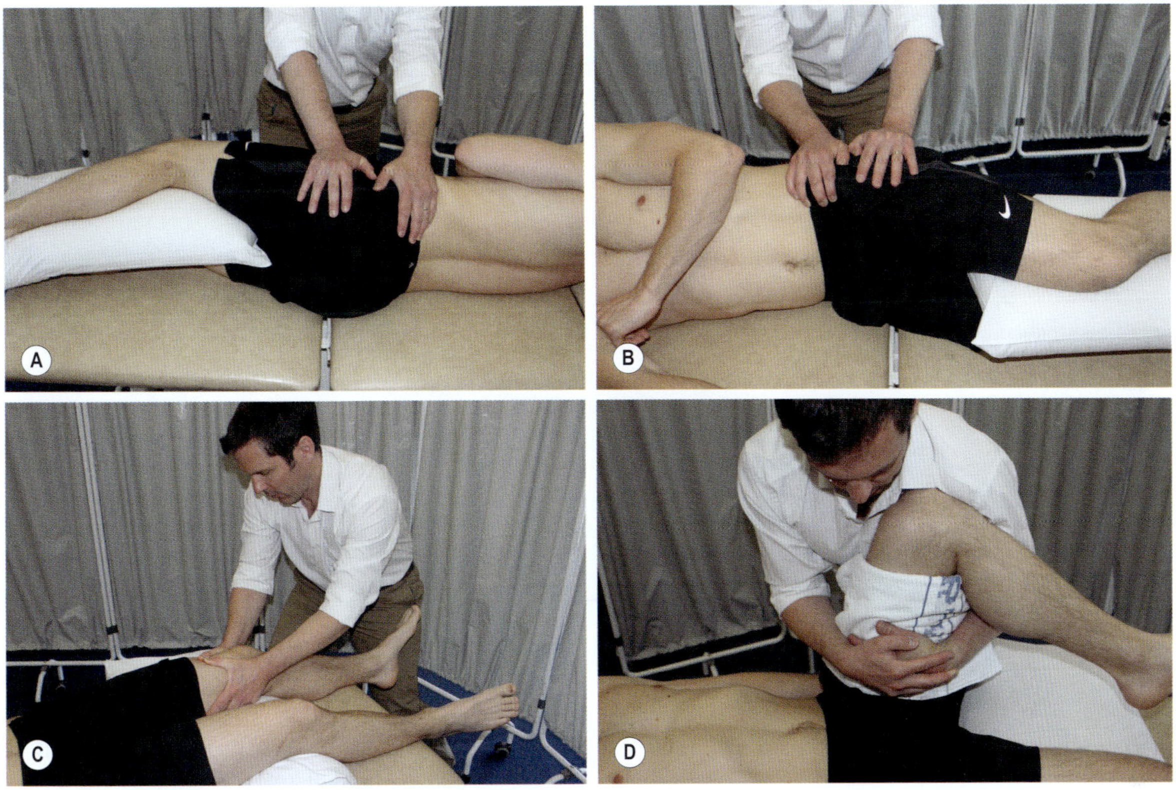

Fig. 15.12 Hip Joint Accessory Movements. (A) Anteroposterior. With the patient in side-lying, pillows are placed between the patient's legs to position the hip joint in neutral. The left hand is then placed posterior on the iliac crest to stabilize the pelvis while the heel of the right hand applies an anteroposterior pressure over the anterior aspect of the greater trochanter. (B) Posteroanterior. With the patient in side-lying, pillows are placed between the patient's legs to position the hip joint in neutral. The right hand grips around the anterior aspect of the anterior superior iliac spine to stabilize the pelvis, while the left hand applies a posteroanterior force to the posterior aspect of the greater trochanter. (C) Longitudinal caudad. The hands grip just proximal to the medial and lateral femoral epicondyles and pull the femur in a caudad direction. (D) Lateral transverse. The hip is flexed and a towel is placed around the upper thigh. The clinician clasps the hands together on the medial aspect of the thigh and pulls the leg laterally.

COMPLETION OF THE EXAMINATION

Once all of the above tests have been carried out, the examination of the hip region is complete. The subjective and physical examinations produce a large amount of information which needs to be recorded accurately and quickly. It is vital at this stage to highlight important findings from the examination with an asterisk (*). These findings are reassessed at, and within, subsequent treatment sessions to evaluate the effects of treatment on the patient's condition.

The physical testing procedures which specifically indicate joint, nerve or muscle tissues, as a source of the patient's symptoms, are summarized in Table 4.9.

TABLE 15.3 Accessory Movements, Choice of Application and Reassessment of the Patient's Asterisks

Accessory Movements	Modifications	Identify Any Effect of Accessory Movements on Patient's Signs and Symptoms
Hip joint ↕ Anteroposterior ↕ Posteroanterior ←•→ Caud longitudinal caudad —•→ Lat lateral transverse	Start position, e.g. • In flexion • In extension • In medial rotation • In lateral rotation (medial or lateral) • In flexion and medial rotation • In extension and lateral rotation Speed of force application Direction of the applied force Point of application of applied force	Reassess all asterisks
Lumbar spine Sacroiliac joint Knee Foot and ankle	As above	Reassess all asterisks

On completion of the physical examination, the clinician:

- warns the patient of possible exacerbation up to 24–48 hours following the examination
- requests the patient to report details on the behaviour of the symptoms following examination at the next attendance
- explains the findings of the physical examination and how these findings relate to the subjective assessment. Any misconceptions patients may have regarding their illness or injury need to be addressed
- evaluates the findings, formulates a clinical diagnosis and writes up a problem list
- determines the objectives of treatment
- devises an initial treatment plan.

In this way, the clinician will have developed the following hypotheses categories (adapted from Jones & Rivett, 2004):

- function: abilities and restrictions
- patient's perspective on his/her experience
- source of symptoms. This includes the structure or tissue that is thought to be producing the patient's symptoms, the nature of the structure or tissues in relation to the healing process and the pain mechanisms
- contributing factors to the development and maintenance of the problem: they may be environmental, psychosocial, behavioural, physical or heredity factors
- precautions/contraindications to treatment and management: this includes the severity and irritability of the patient's symptoms and the nature of the patient's condition
- management strategy and treatment plan
- prognosis: this can be affected by factors such as the stage and extent of the injury as well as the patient's expectations, personality and lifestyle.

For guidance on treatment and management principles, the reader is directed to the companion textbook (Barnard and Ryder, 2024).

REVIEW AND REVISE QUESTIONS

1. Give an example of an acute and a degenerative hip pathology.
2. How might an osteoarthritic hip present subjectively and objectively?
3. What anatomical structures might refer to the groin?
4. What are the morphological changes that are thought to lead to FAI?
5. Catching in the groin might indicate FAI: TRUE or FALSE?
6. Name triad of features leading to a possible diagnosis of FAI:
   a. ____________
   b. ____________
   c. ____________
7. Which two tendons are commonly affected in gluteal tendinopathy?
   a. Gluteus minimus
   b. Gluteus medius
   c. Gluteus maximus
8. Describe an evidence-based approach to the management of tendinopathy.
9. A single leg stance has high specificity for gluteal tendinopathy: TRUE or FALSE?
10. Describe a physical test that might be helpful in the assessment of sports-related groin pain.

Case Study

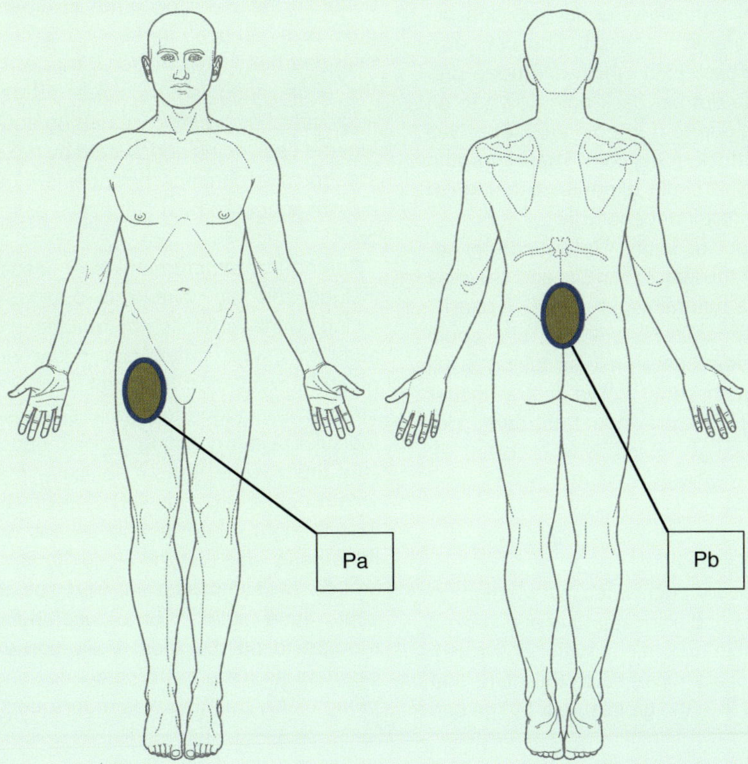

Continued

Case Study—cont'd

16-year-old gymnast

Pa—intermittent catching pain

Aggravating factors—immediate onset of pain with twisting, squatting and landing on the right leg. Able to continue.

Easing factors—rest but could ache at rest after long training session.

Pb—Intermittent ache

Aggravating factors—immediate onset in flexion, e.g. tying shoelaces or unloading dishwasher.

Easing factors—neutral position, immediate relief.

24-h pattern—Both her groin pain and back pain were activity-related throughout the day. Symptoms were no worse first thing in the morning. Occasionally she woke with groin pain when turning in bed at night.

PMH/DH—Fit and well. No significant past medical history and no medicines.

No symptoms anywhere else.

Subjective Examination

History of Present Condition

A 16-year-old county level gymnast presented to the clinic with a 5-month history of right-sided groin pain and occasional catching sensations in the groin. She was also complaining of some low back pain which had been present for a few weeks. She put her back pain down to an alteration in her technique due to her groin pain. She was not complaining of any buttock or leg pain. There were no neurological symptoms. She could experience her groin pain and low back discomfort independently.

She could not recall a specific injury. Unfortunately, her pain had become worse in the last 2 months, and she was now unable to complete a full training session. Typically, she would train four sessions per week, but she could now only complete two sessions as it was taking a full 2 days for the groin pain to settle down following her training. She had not had any previous treatment. Her doctor had organized an x-ray which was reported as normal.

Aggravating and Easing Factors

The groin pain was specifically aggravated by twisting on the hip during floor routines and also squatting and landing on the right leg. She was able to continue with her training, but the groin pain did gradually increase to the point that she would have some aching in the groin at rest by the end of the session. At home she had noticed her groin became sore when sitting cross-legged on the floor.

She noticed her low back ache in flexed positions such as when tying her shoelaces or helping her parents unload the dishwasher. When she moved out of the flexed position her back pain settled within a few seconds.

Twenty-Four-Hour Pattern

Both her groin pain and back pain were activity-related throughout the day. Her symptoms were no worse first thing in the morning. Occasionally she woke with groin pain when turning in bed at night.

Past Medical History and Drug History

She was fit and well and took no medications.

Hypothesis After Subjective Examination

The low back pain and right-sided groin pain were not thought to be directly related, although altered movement patterns as a result of groin pain could be contributing the generation of mechanical back pain. The pains were not thought to be directly related for three reasons: Firstly, the onset of the pains occurred at different times; the right groin pain had been present for 5 months, whilst the back pain had been present for a matter of weeks. Secondly, the aggravating factors were different: the groin being aggravated by twisting, squatting and landing on the right leg, the back being aggravated by flexed positions. Thirdly, she could experience both pains independently so there did not appear to be a subjective association between the two.

Anatomical structures closely associated with the groin include the hip joint and pubic symphysis, muscles including the iliopsoas, the quadricep complex and the hip adductors, and cutaneous nerve supply including the genitofemoral and femoral nerve. Possible referring structures include the lumbar spine and sacroiliac joint, or radicular pain emanating from an upper lumbar nerve root.

As there were no neurological symptoms, and as there was no clear relationship between the back and groin, it was thought a central source was unlikely. The working hypothesis was that the hip joint itself was the most likely source of symptoms in view of the distribution and aggravating factors. Femoroacetabular impingement was thought to be the most likely pathology in view of the catching and discomfort into flexion and rotation. Even though x-ray imaging was reported as normal, the patient

Case Study—cont'd

had not had MRI which is a more accurate modality to assess the labrum and articular cartilage (Griffin et al., 2016).

It was though the groin symptoms would be easy to reproduce with low severity and irritability as even though symptoms would flair as a result of a training session, she was able to continue, and a physical examination was thought unlikely to be as provocative as a full training session.

The pain mechanisms were thought to be mainly nociceptive without evidence of central sensitization or maladaptive output mechanisms such as fear avoidance. The priority at clinical examination was to assess the hip joint and to rule in or out FAI as a potential pathology. Functional testing and hip range of movement were to be performed, together with tests which may be clinically useful in the diagnosis of FAI, namely IROP, FADDIR and FABER. It was expected that there would be discomfort and possibly a reduced range into flex and internal rotation findings with positive impingement tests. It was thought there may also be a lack of control around the hip during functional tasks. Other tests which may have proved valuable for future consideration include examination of the lumbar spine and examination of gluteal strength and control.

There were not thought to be any contraindications or precautions.

Physical Examination

Functional Testing

Stance, gait and one leg control are important considerations in the diagnosis of FAI (Griffin et al., 2016). The patient stood in a small degree of genu valgum. The gait examination was unremarkable; however, during a one leg squat there was a valgus movement pattern. This pattern was accentuated when asked the replicated provocative gymnastics movements involving jumping and landing on one leg. When landing on one leg there was reproduction of symptoms in the right groin. The groin pain proved modifiable and marginally improved when the patient was asked to concentrate on their knee position on landing and to try to avoid falling into valgus.

ROM

Range of movement was full with discomfort at end of range flexion and IROP.

Faddir

When flexion, adduction and internal rotation were combined (FADDIR), groin pain was strongly reproduced with a feeling of catching in the groin.

Faber

FABER test was also positive.

Accessories

As the condition was non-severe and non-irritable, accessory movements were explored through the range and, in particular, in the provocative position of supine and end of range flexion with some internal rotation. It was established that in this provocative position, a lateral transverse accessory glide through the hip joint reduced groin pain and 30 seconds of grade III mobilization with the aid of a fixation belt reduced the intensity of groin pain when testing for hip impingement with the FADDIR test.

Clinical Diagnosis and Plan

Despite the absence of confirmatory MRI, the symptoms and clinical signs supported the clinical diagnosis of FAI in line with the Warwick Consensus document (Griffin et al., 2016).

Accessory mobilization was shown to provide some relief from groin discomfort in the provocative position of flex and internal rotation, and it was decided to trial a course of accessory and physiological movements with the aid of a fixation belt with the aim of modifying groin pain through range.

It was thought that a valgus movement pattern when landing on the right leg might be contributing to the maintenance of the condition as modifying the knee position on landing altered symptoms modestly. It was decided therefore to explore this movement pattern further by attempting to modify this task whilst closely monitoring the symptomatic response and to look at gluteal strength, as well as foot position on the second session.

If after the second session it was thought that gluteal weakness and poor hip control causing a valgus movement pattern could be contributing to the maintenance of the condition, a graded exercise programme to strengthen the gluteal muscles could be a useful starting point with the aim of progressing to more challenging functions and sports-specific tasks.

REFERENCES

Allison, K., Wrigley, T.V., Vicenzino, B., Bennell, K.L., Grimaldi, A., Hodges, P.W., 2016. Kinematics and kinetics during walking in individuals with gluteal tendinopathy. Clin. Biomech. (Bristol, Avon). 32, 56–63.

Barnard, K.J., Ryder, D., 2024. Principles of Musculoskeletal Treatment and Management: A Handbook for Therapists, third ed. Churchill Livingstone, Edinburgh.

Berstock, J.R., Blom, A.W., Beswick, A.D., 2015. A systematic review and meta-analysis of complications following the posterior and lateral surgical approaches to total hip arthroplasty. Ann. R. Coll. Surg. Engl. 97, 11–16.

Cannon, J., Weber, A.E., Park, S., Mayer, E.N., Powers, C.M., 2020. Pathomechanics underlying femoroacetabular impingement syndrome: theoretical framework to inform clinical practice. Phys. Ther. 100 (5), 788–797.

Cyriax, J., 1982. Textbook of Orthopaedic Medicine—Diagnosis of Soft Tissue Lesions, eighth ed. Baillière Tindall, London.

Gifford, L.S., 1998. Pain, the tissues and the nervous system: a conceptual model. Physiotherapy 84, 27–36.

Griffin, D.R., Dickenson, E.J., O'donnell, J., Awan, T., Beck, M., Clohisy, J.C., et al., 2016. The Warwick agreement on femoroacetabular impingement syndrome (FAI syndrome): an international consensus statement. Br. J. Sports Med. 50 (19), 1169–1176.

Grimaldi, A., Fearon, A., 2015. Gluteal tendinopathy: integrating pathomechanics and clinical features in its management. J. Orthop. Sports Phys. Ther. 45, 910–922.

Grimaldi, A., Mellor, R., Hodges, P., Bennell, K., Wajswelner, H., Vicenzino, B., 2015. Gluteal tendinopathy: a review of mechanisms, assessment and management. Sports Med. 45, 1107–1119.

Grimaldi, A., Mellor, R., Nicolson, P., Hodges, P., Bennell, K., Vicenzino, B., 2016. Utility of clinical tests to diagnose MRI-confirmed gluteal tendinopathy in patients presenting with lateral hip pain. Br. J. Sports Med. 51 (6), 519–524.

Janda, V., 1994. Muscles and motor control in cervicogenic disorders: assessment and management. In: Grant, R. (Ed.), Physical Therapy of the Cervical and Thoracic Spine, second ed. Churchill Livingstone, New York, p. 195.

Janda, V., 2002. Muscles and motor control in cervicogenic disorders. In: Grant, R. (Ed.), Physical Therapy of the Cervical and Thoracic Spine, third ed. Churchill Livingstone, New York, p. 182.

Jomaa, G., Kwan, C.K., Fu, S.C., Ling, S.K.K., Chan, K.M., Yung, P.S.H., Rolf, C., 2020. A systematic review of inflammatory cells and markers in human tendinopathy. BMC Musculoskelet. Disord. 21 (1), 1–13.

Jones, M.A., Edwards, I., Gifford, L., 2002. Conceptual models for implementing biopsychosocial theory in clinical practice. Man. Ther. 7, 2–9.

Jones, M.A., Rivett, D.A., 2004. Clinical Reasoning for Manual Therapists. Butterworth-Heinemann, Edinburgh.

Jull, G.A., Janda, V., 1987. Muscles and motor control in low back pain: assessment and management. In: Twomey, L.T., Taylor, J.R. (Eds.), Physical Therapy of the Low Back. Churchill Livingstone, New York, p. 253.

Lack, S., Barton, C., Malliaras, P., Twycross-Lewis, R., Woledge, R., Morrissey, D., 2014. The effect of anti-pronation foot orthoses on hip and knee kinematics and muscle activity during a functional step-up task in healthy individuals: a laboratory study. Clin. Biomech. (Bristol, Avon). 29, 177–182.

Ladurner, A., Fitzpatrick, J., O'Donnell, J.M., 2021. Treatment of gluteal tendinopathy: a systematic review and stage-adjusted treatment recommendation. Orthop. J. Sports Med. 9 (7), 23259671211016850.

LeBlanc, K.E., Aparicio, K., Barta, E., Munez, K., 2013. Inguinal hernias: diagnosis and management. Am. Fam. Phys. 87 (12), 844–848.

Lequesne, M., Mathieu, P., Vuillemin-Bodaghi, V., Bard, H., Djian, P., 2008. Gluteal tendinopathy in refractory greater trochanter pain syndrome: diagnostic value of two clinical tests. Arthritis Rheum. 59, 241–246.

Magee, D.J., 2014. Orthopedic Physical Assessment. Elsevier Health Sciences, Philadelphia.

Magee, D.J., Manske, R., 2021. Orthopedic Physical Assessment. Elsevier Health Sciences, Philadelphia.

Maslowski, E., Sullivan, W., Forster Harwood, J., 2010. The diagnostic validity of hip provocation maneuvers to detect intra-articular hip pathology. PM&R 2, 174–181.

Mellor, R., Bennell, K., Grimaldi, A., Nicolson, P., Kasza, J., Hodges, P., et al., 2018. Education plus exercise versus corticosteroid injection use versus a wait and see approach on global outcome and pain from gluteal tendinopathy: prospective, single blinded, randomised clinical trial. BMJ [online] p.k1662.

Pacheco-Carrillo, A., Medina-Porqueres, I., 2016. Physical examination tests for the diagnosis of femoroacetabular impingement. A systematic review. Phys. Ther. Sport 21, 87–93.

Ramon, S., Russo, S., Santoboni, F., Lucenteforte, G., Di Luise, C., de Unzurrunzaga, R., et al., 2020. Focused shockwave treatment for greater trochanteric pain syndrome: a multicenter, randomized, controlled clinical trial. JBJS 102 (15), 1305–1311.

Reid, D., 2016. The management of greater trochanteric pain syndrome: a systematic literature review. J. Orthop. 13 (1), 15–28.

Reiman, M.P., Goode, A.P., Cook, C.E., Hölmich, P., Thorborg, K., 2015a. Diagnostic accuracy of clinical tests for the diagnosis of hip femoroacetabular impingement/labral tear: a systematic review with meta-analysis. Br. J. Sports Med. 49, 811.

Reiman, M.P., Goode, A.P., Hegedus, E.J., Cook, C.E., Wright, A.A., 2013. Diagnostic accuracy of clinical tests of the hip: a systematic review with meta-analysis. Br. J. Sports Med. 47, 893–902.

Reiman, M.P., Mather, R.C., Cook, C.E., 2015b. Physical examination tests for hip dysfunction and injury. Br. J. Sports Med. 49, 357–361.

Reiman, M.P., Thorborg, K., 2014. Invited clinical commentary. Clinical examination and physical assessment of hip-related pain in athletes. Int. J. Sports Phys. Ther. 9, 737–755.

Sahrmann, S.A., 2002. Diagnosis and Treatment of Movement Impairment Syndromes. Mosby, St Louis.

Shakil, A., Aparicio, K., Barta, E., Munez, K., 2020. Inguinal hernias: diagnosis and management. Am. Fam. Phys. 102 (8), 487–492.

Thacker, M., 2015. Louis Gifford—revolutionary: the mature organism model, an embodied cognitive perspective of pain. Psychother. Priv. Pract. 152, 4–9.

van den Berg, J.C., De Valois, J.C., Go, P.M., Rosenbusch, G., 1999. Detection of groin hernia with physical examination, ultrasound, and MRI compared with laparoscopic findings. Invest Radiol. 34 (12), 739–743.

White, S.G., Sahrmann, S.A., 1994. A movement system balance approach to musculoskeletal pain. In: Grant, R. (Ed.), Physical Therapy of the Cervical and Thoracic Spine, second ed. Churchill Livingstone, Edinburgh, p. 339.

Zuckerbraun, B.S., Cyr, A.R., Mauro, C.S., 2020. Groin pain syndrome known as sports hernia: a review. JAMA Surg. 155 (4), 340–348.

16

Examination of the Knee Region

Andrew Kemp and Kieran Barnard

LEARNING OUTCOMES

After studying this chapter, you should be able to:

- List the key constituents of a thorough subjective examination.
- Know the difference between mechanical and non-mechanical pathology and look out for clues in the subjective examination which might lead you to suspect a non-mechanical cause.
- Understand the value of special questions in relation to knee pathology.
- Be able to hypothesize which structures might be at fault based on the location of symptoms and the aggravating factors.
- List the key constituents of a thorough physical examination.
- Have an appreciation of the sensitivity and specificity of key physical tests.
- Start to develop an appreciation of the value of functional testing and symptom modification when considering the aggravating factors, whilst understanding that such tests lack the validity and reliability of more traditional physical tests.

CHAPTER CONTENTS

Introduction, 431
Subjective Examination/Taking the Patients' History, 431
Patient's Perspectives on Their Experiences, 431
Body Chart, 431
Behaviour of Symptoms, 432
Special/Screening Questions, 433
History of the Present Condition, 433
Past Medical History, 434
Plan of the Physical Examination, 434
Physical Examination, 436
Observation, 436
Active Physiological Movements, 438
Passive Physiological Movements, 439
Joint Effusion Tests, 439
Joint Integrity Tests, 440
Meniscal Tests, 445
Patellofemoral Tests, 446
Muscle Tests, 447
Neurological Tests, 448
Miscellaneous Tests, 449
Palpation, 449
Accessory Movements, 450
Symptom Modification, 453
Assessment of Return to Play/Performance, 455
Physical Examination for Return to Sport, 456
Assessment of Quadriceps Activation, 456
Perturbation Control, 458
Hop Testing Battery, 459
Star Excursion Balance Test SEBT, 459
Completion of the Examination, 459
Case Study, 461
References, 463

INTRODUCTION

The knee is a large and complex region made up of the tibiofemoral, patellofemoral and superior tibiofibular joints with their surrounding soft tissues. It is a common site for traumatic injury. For example, significant varus or valgus force to the knee may cause injury to the collateral ligaments, forceful pivoting over a fixed foot may cause injury to the anterior cruciate ligament (ACL) or menisci and acute pain behind the knee on rapid acceleration may be due to a musculotendinous hamstring injury. Traumatic knee injuries often occur, although not exclusively, during sport.

The knee may also become symptomatic in the presence of overuse or biomechanical stresses such as anterior knee pain or patella tendinopathy. For example, persistent medial torsion of the femur due to reduced endurance of the hip abductors and lateral rotators may in time cause anterior knee symptoms as a result of a valgus knee pattern during walking or running.

Other symptomatic conditions may be more insidious. The knee is a common site for osteoarthritis which may become symptomatic over time. A degenerative meniscal lesion is also a common problem seen within musculoskeletal practice. The clinician must also be mindful of other less common conditions such as inflammatory or infective pathologies, for example rheumatoid or septic arthritis.

This chapter will outline the key subjective information and the core physical tests necessary to perform a thorough examination of the knee. The order of the subjective questioning and the physical tests described below can be altered as appropriate for the patient being examined. The reader is directed to Chapters 3 and 4, respectively, as required pre-reading to further support for further details on the principles of the subjective and physical examinations.

SUBJECTIVE EXAMINATION/TAKING THE PATIENTS' HISTORY

Patient's Perspectives on Their Experiences

The patient's perspectives and experiences may be relevant to the onset and progression of their problem and are therefore recorded. In order to treat the patient appropriately, it is important that the condition be managed within the context of the patient's social and work environment. Therefore the patient's age, employment, home situation and details of any leisure activities are also recorded. Particular factors derived from this information may indicate direct and/or indirect mechanical influences on the knee. The reader is directed to Chapter 3 for further information.

Body Chart

The following information concerning the type and area of the current symptoms can be recorded on a body chart (see Fig. 3.2).

Area of Current Symptoms

Pain may be described as generally at the knee; however, pain emanating from structures local to the knee complex is most frequently felt as a localized area of pain. For example, patellofemoral pain is frequently described in the retro or peripatellar regions, and a medial meniscus tear will most frequently be described as medially located pain. Ascertain which is the worst symptom and record where the patient feels the symptoms are coming from.

Areas Relevant to the Region Being Examined

Symptoms around the knee complex may be referred from more proximal anatomy, including arthrogenic, myogenic or neurogenic structures in the region of the lumbar spine, pelvis or hip. For example, anterior knee pain may be referred from the lumbar spine or may result from a peripheral neuropathy affecting the femoral nerve. Readers should note that the hip joint is a common source of referred pain to the location of the knee, which may or may not also be associated with pain above and below the knee (Dibra et al., 2017).

Symptoms may also arise as a result of contributing factors affecting the foot and/or ankle complex, for example, pronation of the foot may cause excessive medial rotation of the tibia and femur which may in turn lead to increased stress on the lateral patella (Barton et al., 2010).

The reader is directed to Chapter 3 to fully appreciate other aspects of the body chart to be considered, including the quality, intensity and depth of the pain; whether the symptoms are constant or intermittent; or indeed, whether there are any abnormal sensations which could, for example, be referred from the lumber nerve roots.

Relationship of Symptoms

Determine the subjective relationship between symptomatic areas—do they come on together or separately? For example, the patient could have knee pain without back pain, or both types of pain may always be present together. Consider clarifying questions as explored in Chapter 3.

Behaviour of Symptoms

Aggravating Factors

For each symptomatic area, establish what movements and/or positions aggravate the patient's symptoms. If the knee is suspected, specific knee structures may be implicated by correlating the area of symptoms with certain aggravating factors. For example, anterior knee pain which is aggravated by climbing up and down stairs may implicate the patellofemoral joint (Petersen et al., 2014), whereas medial or lateral knee pain whilst squatting may implicate the menisci (McHale et al., 2014).

It is important for the clinician to be as specific as possible when hunting for aggravating factors. Where possible, break the movement or activity down as this may provide clues for what to expect during the physical examination. 'What is it about…?' is a useful question to ask. Knee pain aggravated by 'driving' does not offer as much information as knee pain aggravated by 'pushing the clutch' (extension), 'changing pedals' (twisting) or 'long distances on a motorway' (sustained flexion). Aggravating factors for other regions may need to be queried if they are suspected to be a source of the symptoms.

The clinician ascertains how the symptoms affect function, such as static and active postures, e.g. sitting, standing, lying, bending, walking, running, walking on uneven ground and up and down stairs, driving, work, sport and social activities. Note details of the training regimen for any sports activities. The clinician finds out if the patient is left- or right-handed as there may be increased stress on the dominant side.

Detailed information on each of the above activities is useful in order to help determine the structure(s) at fault and identify functional restrictions. This information can be used to determine the aims of treatment and any advice that may be required.

Easing Factors

For each symptomatic area, the clinician asks what movements and/or positions ease the patient's symptoms to help confirm the relationship between the symptoms as well as determine the level of irritability. Further details can be found in Chapter 3.

Occasionally, particularly with symptoms that are irritable or with a patient who is catastrophizing, it is difficult to establish clear and distinct aggravating factors. When this is the case, it may be worth starting with the easing factors and working backwards. For example, if knee extension eases symptoms, it may be worth asking: 'Does that mean that bending your knee makes your pain worse?'

At this point, the clinician synthesizes the information gained from the aggravating and easing factors and has a working hypothesis of the structure/s which might be at fault. Beware of, and do not dismiss, symptoms which do not conform to a mechanical pattern, as this may be a sign of serious pathology.

Twenty-Four-Hour Behaviour of Symptoms

The clinician determines the 24-hour behaviour of symptoms by asking questions about night, morning and evening symptoms. See Chapter 3 for more details.

Night symptoms. It is important to establish whether the patient has pain at night. Pain at night which is position dependent is typically mechanical, whereas pain which is non-mechanical and not position dependent and unremitting should arouse suspicion of more serious pathology. The clinician may ask: 'Can you find a comfortable position in which to sleep?' or 'What is the most/least comfortable position for you?'

Position-dependent pain may also give clues as to the structure/s at fault; for example, patients with an injury to the medial meniscus often have trouble sleeping and lying with the symptomatic side uppermost as it compresses that side.

Morning and evening symptoms. The clinician determines the pattern of the symptoms first thing in the morning, through the day and at the end of the day. This information may provide clues as to the pain mechanisms driving the condition and the type of pathology present. For example, early-morning pain and stiffness lasting for more than half an hour may indicate inflammatory-driven pain.

Special/Screening Questions

Knee-specific special questions may help in the generation of a clinical hypothesis. Such questions may include the following.

Swelling

Does the knee swell? If so, the clinician needs to establish whether swelling resulted from injury and whether the swelling occurred immediately after the injury (within 2 hours) or whether it took some hours or days to form. Immediate swelling, particularly after a pop or click within the knee, may indicate bleeding (haemarthrosis) suggestive of significant trauma or rupture and is distinct from swelling occurring within hours of an injury, which is more suggestive of the build-up of inflammatory exudate (Wagemakers et al., 2010). Where there is significant acute swelling in the absence of trauma clinicians should be suspicious of non-musculoskeletal causes associated with mono-arthritis including sceptic arthritis and rheumatological disease.

Giving Way

Giving way of the knee may be suggestive of either ligamentous instability or an inability of the surrounding musculature, particularly the quadriceps, to support the knee adequately. Ligamentous instability is normally the result of trauma, whilst giving way of muscular origin is more complex and may be due to weakness as a result of disuse, pain inhibition, joint effusion (Torry et al., 2000) or ligamentomuscular reflex inhibition (Solomonow, 2009). Correlating giving way with the wider clinical picture may therefore provide useful information. For example, falling to the floor without warning and a history of trauma may represent mechanical instability, whilst giving way without trauma and in the presence of pain and/or swelling may represent a muscular cause.

Locking

If locking is present, it is important to distinguish between true and pseudo-locking. True locking might represent an intra-articular derangement such as a meniscal tear, whilst pseudo-locking may simply represent an unwillingness to move the knee due to pain. Qualifying locking by asking: ‘Does your knee get stuck so you can't bend or straighten it?’ may be helpful.

Crepitus

Whilst not considered a special question as such, crepitus with pain may help to build a clinical picture. For example, crepitus anteriorly when descending stairs may suggest chondromalacia patellae.

History of the Present Condition

For each symptomatic area, the clinician needs to know how long the symptom has been present? And have they changed over that time? Whether there was a sudden, possibly as a result of trauma. The mechanism of injury gives the clinician some important clues as to the injured structure in the knee, particularly in the acute stage, when a full physical examination may not be possible. For example, pain on twisting, catching one's foot or rising from a crouched position may indicate a meniscal injury (Drosos & Pozo, 2004; McHale et al., 2014) whilst an ACL rupture may be suspected following an injury that involved rotation of the body on a fixed foot followed by immediate swelling (Wagemakers et al., 2010). Such an injury may be (but not always) accompanied by a pop or cracking sound (Décary et al., 2018). The possible diagnoses suspected from the mechanism of injury are given in Table 16.1.

A slow onset may be related to a change in the patient's lifestyle, e.g. a new job or hobby or a change in sporting activity or training schedule.

Is there a previous history of symptoms? If so, how many episodes has s/he had? When were they? What was the cause? What was the duration of each episode? And did the patient fully recover between episodes? If there is no previous history, has the patient had any episodes of pain and/or stiffness in the lumbar spine, hip, knee, foot, ankle or any other relevant region? What happened to other symptoms when each symptom began? Symptoms which came on at the same time may indicate that the areas of symptoms are related. This evidence is further strengthened if there is a subjective relationship (symptoms come on at the same time or one is dependent on the other) and if the aggravating factors are the same or similar.

TABLE 16.1 The Possible Diagnoses Suspected From the Mechanism of Injury

Mechanism of Injury	Possible Structures Injured	Comments
Hyperflexion	Posterior horn of medial and/or lateral meniscus ACL	May complain of locking
Prolonged flexion	Posterior horn of medial and/or lateral meniscus	Particularly in older patients may complain of locking
Hyperextension	Anterior tibial and/or femoral condyles PCL, ACL, posterior capsule, fat pad	Cruciate injury may result from tibial translation anteriorly (ACL) or posteriorly (PCL)
Valgus	Lateral tibial and/or femoral condyles MCL, ACL, PCL	Cruciate injury with severe force
Varus	Medial tibial and/or femoral condyles LCL, ITB	Uncommon
Flexion valgus without rotation	Lateral tibial and/or femoral condyles MCL, patellar subluxation/dislocation	
Flexion valgus with rotation	Lateral tibial and/or femoral condyles MCL, ACL, medial and/or lateral menisci, patellar subluxation/dislocation	Common injury. Immediate swelling (haemarthrosis) with a pop may suggest ACL rupture, meniscal injury may present with locking
Flexion varus without rotation	Medial tibial and/or femoral condyles ACL, posterolateral corner, medial and/or lateral menisci	Meniscal injury may present with locking
Extension with valgus	Anterolateral tibial and/or femoral condyles MCL, PCL, posteromedial corner	
Extension with varus	Anteromedial tibial and/or femoral condyles ACL Posterolateral corner Popliteal tendon	May lead to unstable posterolateral corner injury
Flexion with posterior tibial translation (dashboard injury)	PCL posterior dislocation with severe force resulting in posterior instability ± patellar, proximal tibial and/or tibial plateau fracture	Most common mechanism for isolated PCL injury

ACL, Anterior cruciate ligament; *ITB*, iliotibial band; *LCL*, lateral collateral ligament; *MCL*, medial collateral ligament; *PCL*, posterior cruciate ligament.
Adapted from Magee & Manske (2020); Hayes et al. (2000).

Has there been any treatment to date? The effectiveness of any previous treatment regime may help to guide patient management. Has the patient seen a specialist or had any investigations which may help with clinical diagnosis, such as blood tests, X-ray or MRI?

Past Medical History

A detailed medical history is vitally important to identify certain precautions or contraindications to the physical examination and/or treatment (see Table 3.3). The medical history includes previous surgery that may be of relevance, such as knee arthroscopy. As mentioned in Chapter 3, the clinician must differentiate between conditions that are suitable for conservative treatment and systemic, neoplastic and other non-musculoskeletal conditions, which require referral to a medical practitioner.

Plan of the Physical Examination

In order to plan the physical examination, the following questions need to be considered:

- How extensive will the physical examination be? Is each area of symptoms severe and/or irritable (see Chapter 3)? Will it be necessary to stop short of symptom reproduction, to reproduce symptoms partially or fully? If symptoms are severe, physical tests are carried out to just short of symptom production or to the very first onset of symptoms; no overpressures will be carried out, as the patient would be unable to tolerate this. If symptoms are irritable, physical tests need to be performed to just short of symptom production or just to the onset of symptoms with fewer physical tests being performed to allow for rest period between tests. Another way to develop the clinician's reasoning is to consider what to expect from each physical test. Will it be easy or hard to reproduce each symptom? Will it be necessary to use combined movements or repetitive movements? Will a particular test prove positive or negative? Will the pain be direction-specific? Synthesizing evidence from the subjective examination and in particular the aggravating and easing factors will provide substantial evidence as to what to expect in the physical examination.

- What are the predominant pain mechanisms which might be driving the patient's symptoms? What are the active 'input mechanisms' (sensory pathways): are symptoms the product of a mechanical, inflammatory or ischaemic nociceptive process? What are the 'processing mechanisms': how has the patient processed this information? What are his or her thoughts and feelings about the pain? Finally, what are the 'output mechanisms': what is the patient's physiological, psychological and behavioural response to the pain? Clearly establishing which pain mechanisms may be causing and/or maintaining the condition will help the clinician manage both the condition and the patient appropriately. The reader is directed to Gifford (1998), Jones et al. (2002) and Thacker (2015) for further reading.
- Are there any precautions and/or contraindications to elements of the physical examination that need to be explored further, such as neurological involvement, recent fracture, trauma, steroid therapy or rheumatoid arthritis? There may also be certain contraindications to further examination and treatment, e.g. symptoms of spinal cord or cauda equina compression.
- What are the possible arthrogenic, myogenic and neurogenic structures which could be causing the patient's symptoms, i.e. what structures could refer to the area of pain and what structures are underneath the area of pain? For example, medial knee pain could theoretically be referred from the lumbar spine, the sacroiliac joint, the hip, the quadriceps and the hip adductors. The structures directly under the medial knee could also be implicated, for example, the medial collateral ligament (MCL), the medial meniscus, the medial compartment joint surfaces, the medial facet of the patellofemoral joint, the pes anserine tendon and the saphenous nerve.
- In addition, are there any contributing factors which could be maintaining the condition? These could be:
  - physical, e.g. weak hip lateral rotators causing medial femoral torsion
  - environmental, e.g. driving for a living
  - psychosocial, e.g. fear of serious pathology
  - behavioural, e.g. excessive rest in an attempt to help the area heal.
- The clinician decides, based on the evidence, which structures are most likely to be at fault and prioritizes the physical examination accordingly. It is helpful to organize structures into ones that 'must, should and could' be tested on day 1 and over subsequent sessions. This will develop the clinician's clinical reasoning and avoid a recipe-based knee assessment. It is advisable where possible to clear an area fully. For example, if the clinician feels the lumbar spine needs to be excluded on day 1, s/he will fully assess this area leaving no stone unturned to implicate or negate this area as a source of symptoms. This approach will avoid juggling numerous potential sources of symptoms for several sessions, which may lead to confusion.
- A physical planning form can be useful for clinicians to help guide them through the clinical reasoning process (see Appendix 3.1).

KNOWLEDGE CHECK

1. What joints make up the knee region?
2. What might unremitting night pain indicate?
3. Anterior knee pain aggravated by descending stairs might indicate what pathology?
4. What might locking indicate?
5. What might giving-way indicate?
6. What might immediate swelling following a twisting injury indicate?

PHYSICAL EXAMINATION

The information from the subjective examination helps the clinician to plan an appropriate physical examination. The severity, irritability and nature of the condition are the major factors that will influence the choice and priority of physical testing procedures. The first and overarching question the clinician might ask is: 'Is this patient's condition suitable for me to manage as a clinician?' For example, a patient presenting with cauda equina compression symptoms may only need neurological integrity testing prior to an urgent medical referral. The nature of the patient's condition has had a major impact on the physical examination. The second question the clinician might ask is: 'Does this patient have a musculoskeletal dysfunction that I may be able to help?' To answer that, the clinician needs to carry out a full physical examination; however, this may not be possible if the symptoms are severe and/or irritable. If the patient's symptoms are severe and/or irritable, the clinician aims to explore movements as much as possible within a symptom-free range. If the patient has constant and severe and/or irritable symptoms, then the clinician aims to find physical tests that ease the symptoms. If the patient's symptoms are non-severe and non-irritable, then the clinician aims to find physical tests that reproduce each of the patient's symptoms.

Each significant physical test that either provokes or eases the patient's symptoms is highlighted in the patient's notes by an asterisk (*) for easy reference. The highlighted tests are often referred to as asterisks or markers.

The order and detail of the physical tests described below need to be appropriate to the patient being examined; some tests will be irrelevant, and some tests will be carried out briefly, while it will be necessary to investigate others fully. It is important for the reader to understand that not all physical tests are equal and that the reliability, sensitivity and specificity will vary markedly between tests (see Chapter 4). The author has chosen to present the most clinically useful tests according to the literature (Table 16.2). None of these physical tests should however take the place of a thorough subjective examination. The clinician needs to have a clear clinical hypothesis after the subjective examination and the purpose of the physical examination is to confirm or refute this hypothesis.

Observation

Informal Observation

The clinician needs to observe the patient in dynamic and static situations; the quality of movement is noted, as are the postural characteristics and facial expression. Informal observation will have begun from the moment

TABLE 16.2 Summary of the Sensitivity and Specificity of the Presented Tests for Structures Associated to the Knee

	Pathology	Test	Sensitivity %	Specificity %	Reference
Articular tests	Knee effusion	Patella tap	High 92	Low 15	Meyer et al., 2021
		Sweep test	85	33	Meyer et al., 2021
	Anterior cruciate ligament rupture	Lachman test	85	94	Benjaminse et al. (2006)
		Pivot shift	24	98	Benjaminse et al. (2006)
		Anterior drawer	92	91	Benjaminse et al. (2006)
	Meniscus tear	McMurray's	61	84	Smith et al. (2015)
		Thessaly	75	87	Smith et al. (2015)
		Joint line tenderness	83	83	Smith et al. (2015)
Extraarticular tests	Patella tendinopathy	Manual palpation	98	94	Maffulli et al. (2017)
		London Hospital	88	98	Maffulli et al. (2017)

the clinician begins the subjective examination and will continue to the end of the physical examination.

Formal Observation

This is particularly useful in helping to determine the presence of intrinsic predisposing factors.

Observation of posture. The clinician examines the patient's lower-limb posture in standing and where necessary in functional positions related to the patient's complaint. Abnormalities include internal femoral rotation, enlarged tibial tubercle (seen in Osgood–Schlatter disease), genu varum/valgum/recurvatum, medial/lateral tibial torsion and excessive foot pronation.

Genu valgum and genu varum are identified by having the patient positioned so that the patellae face forward and the medial aspects of the knees and medial malleoli of both limbs are as close together as possible. If the knees touch and the ankles do not, the patient has a genu valgum. A distance of 9 to 10 cm (3.5 to 4 inches) between the ankles is considered excessive. If two or more fingers (4 cm [1.6 inches]) fit between the knees when the ankles are together, the patient has a varus deformity or genu varum (Magee & Manske, 2020). Normally, medial tibial torsion is associated with genu varum and lateral tibial torsion with genu valgum (Magee & Manske, 2020).

Internal femoral rotation due to insufficient gluteal function is a common finding with patients with patellofemoral pain and can cause squinting of the patella and an increased Q angle. There may be abnormal positioning of the patella from the normal forwards-facing position. Abnormal positioning may include as a medial/lateral glide, a lateral tilt, an anteroposterior tilt, a medial/lateral rotation or any combination of these positions. Rotation or tilting of the patella may be caused by tight myofascial tissues. An enlarged fat pad is usually associated with hyperextension of the knees and poor quadriceps control, particularly eccentric inner range (0 to 20 degrees of flexion).

The clinician can palpate the talus medially and laterally; both aspects will normally be equally prominent in the mid-position of the subtalar joint. If the medial aspect of the talus is more prominent, this suggests that the subtalar joint is in pronation. The position of the calcaneus and talus can be examined: if the subtalar joint is pronated the calcaneus would be expected to be everted. Any abnormality will require further examination, as described in the section on palpation, below. In addition, the clinician notes whether there is even weight-bearing through the left and right legs. The clinician passively corrects any asymmetry to determine its relevance to the patient's problem.

It is worth remembering that pure postural dysfunction rarely influences one region of the body in isolation, and it may be necessary to observe the patient more fully for a full postural examination.

The clinician examines dynamic postures related to the patient's presenting complaint such as squatting, walking or climbing stairs. If the aggravating factors suggest pain occurs when weight bearing and walking, for example, the clinician observes that particular activity meticulously and if possible tries to establish at which phase of the gait cycle pain occurs. Observation of gait may reveal, for example, excessive pelvic rotation (about a horizontal plane) associated with anterior pelvic tilt. This may be due to hyperextension of the knees and limited extension and external rotation of the hip. It may be possible at this stage to modify the activity to see if symptoms change, for example, by adjusting pelvic rotation. The reader is directed to the section on symptom modification to further explore this concept.

Observation of muscle form. The clinician observes the muscle bulk and muscle tone of the patient, comparing left and right sides. In particular, the clinician should look for wasting of the oblique fibres of the vastus medialis muscle (VMO) which is implicated in patellofemoral pain (Jan et al., 2009). It must be remembered that the level and frequency of physical activity as well as the dominant side may well produce differences in muscle bulk between sides. Some muscles are thought to shorten under stress, while other muscles weaken, producing muscle imbalance.

Observation of soft tissues. The clinician observes the quality and colour of the patient's skin, any area of swelling, joint effusion or presence of scarring, and takes cues for further examination.

Observation of balance. Balance is provided by vestibular, visual and proprioceptive information. This rather crude and non-specific test is conducted by asking the patient to stand on one leg with the eyes open and then closed. If the patient's balance is as poor with the eyes open as with the eyes closed, this suggests a vestibular or proprioceptive dysfunction

TABLE 16.3 Active Physiological Movements With Possible Modifications

Active Physiological Movements	Modifications
Knee flexion	Repeated
Knee extension	Speed altered
Medial rotation of the knee	Combined, e.g. • flexion with internal rotation
Lateral rotation of the knee	Compression or distraction
*+?Lumbar spine	Sustained
?Sacroiliac joint	Injuring movement
?Hip	Differentiation tests
?Foot and ankle	Function

(rather than a visual dysfunction). The test is carried out on the affected and unaffected side; if there is greater difficulty maintaining balance on the affected side, this may indicate some proprioceptive dysfunction.

Observation of gait. Analyze gait on even/uneven ground, slopes, stairs and running. Note the stride length and weight-bearing ability. Inspect the feet, shoes and any walking aids.

Active Physiological Movements

Active physiological movements of the knee include flexion, extension, medial rotation of the tibia and lateral rotation of the tibia (Table 16.3). The primary movements of flexion and extension are tested bilaterally with the patient in supine. Movements of flexion and extension are overexpressed if symptoms allow (Fig. 16.1). Tibial rotation can be readily tested with the patient in sitting, although clinically it is unusual to find an isolated rotation dysfunction.

The clinician establishes the patient's symptoms at rest, prior to each movement and passively corrects any movement deviation to determine its relevance to the patient's symptoms. The following are noted:

- quality of movement
- range of movement
- behaviour of pain through the range of movement
- resistance through the range of movement and at the end of the range of movement
- provocation of any muscle spasm.

In a similar way to the manipulation of a symptomatic physical task (see the section on symptom modification), the thoughtful clinician may be able to manipulate physiological movements to help differentiate between tissues. For example, when knee flexion in prone reproduces the patient's anterior knee pain, differentiation between knee joint, anterior thigh muscles and neural tissues may be required. Adding a compression force through the lower leg will stress the knee joint without particularly altering the muscle length or neural tissue. If symptoms are increased, this would suggest that the knee joint (patellofemoral or tibiofemoral joint) may be the source of the symptoms.

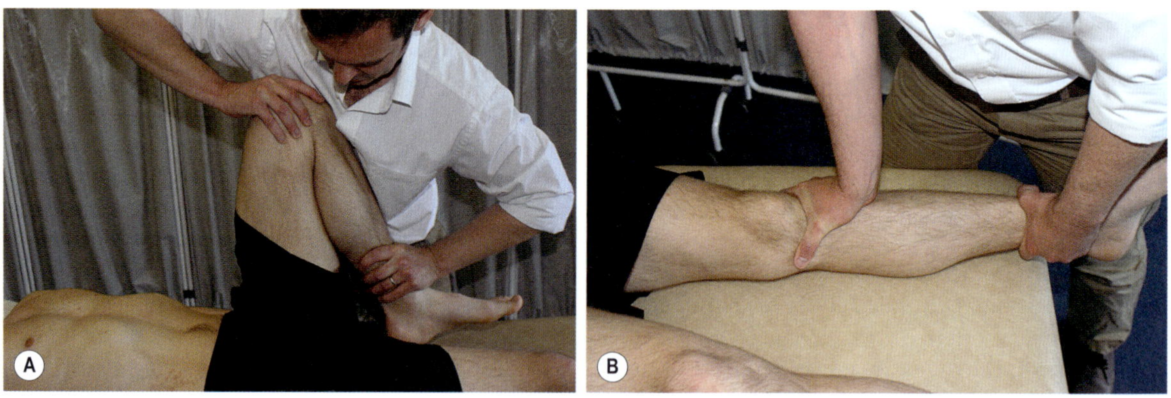

Fig. 16.1 Active Physiological Movements/Overpressures to the Knee. (A) Flexion. One hand supports the knee while the other hand applies overpressure to flexion. (B) Extension. One hand stabilizes the tibia while the other hand lifts the lower leg into extension.

It may be necessary to examine other regions to determine their relevance to the patient's symptoms; they may be the source of the symptoms, or they may be contributing to the symptoms. A screening examination of the hip is most frequently indicated. Hip pathology masquerading as knee pain is well described in paediatric literature, however, the prevalence of knee pain caused by hip pathology in adults is unclear. In patients with knee pain and who are dependent on a walker for ambulation or who are wheelchair dependent, the suspicion for a more proximal source of pain should be high (Dibra et al., 2017).

The other most likely regions are the lumbar spine, sacroiliac joint, foot and ankle. These regions can be quickly screened; see Chapter 4 for further details. Contrary to what their name might suggest, however, performing a clearing test on the lumbar spine, for example, does not fully negate this region as a source of symptoms, and if there is any doubt the clinician is advised to assess the suspected area fully (see relevant chapter).

Passive Physiological Movements

All of the active movements described above can be examined passively with the patient in supine, comparing left and right sides. Comparison of the response of symptoms to the active and passive movements can help to determine whether the structure at fault is non-contractile (articular) or contractile (extra-articular) (Cyriax, 1982). If the lesion is non-contractile, such as ligament, then active and passive movements will be painful and/or restricted in the same direction. If the lesion is in a contractile tissue (i.e. muscle) then active and passive movements are painful and/or restricted in opposite directions. For example, a quadriceps strain may be painful during active extension and passive flexion. Such patterns are however theoretical, and a muscle strain may be more readily assessed by contracting muscle isometrically, where there will be little or no change in the length of non-contractile tissue.

To assess the patient's symptoms passively it may be useful to explore the primary movements of flexion and/or extension with varying degrees of varus or valgus force (Fig. 16.2). It is also possible to add a degree of medial or lateral tibial rotation when exploring these movements. The key is for the clinician to search for the patient's symptoms and not feel constrained by a recipe-based knee assessment. Often it is helpful to refer back to the patient's aggravating factors for clues. For example, if the patient's pain is in knee flexion, the clinician may need to hunt in a similar range of flexion combining different movement components.

As with active physiological movements, it may be necessary to examine other regions such as the lumbar spine, sacroiliac joint, hip, foot and ankle, which may be the source or contributing to the patient's symptoms.

Joint Effusion Tests

The clinician first checks for a knee joint effusion, which may not be necessary if a large effusion is obvious. It is important to distinguish between soft-tissue swelling, which may be localized and superficial, for example in the presence of a low-grade MCL sprain, and swelling within the joint, which may represent a more significant intraarticular injury, e.g. an ACL rupture.

Patellar Tap Test

With the patient lying supine, the clinician adds pressure across the suprapatellar pouch with one hand which will squeeze fluid under the patella. With the other hand the clinician applies a light downward force to the patella which, in the presence of an effusion, will feel as if it is floating and may tap against the underlying femoral condyles. Data on the reliability of the patella tap is conflicting, so the test needs to be used with caution; inter-observer reliability ranges from poor to good, whilst intra-observer reliability appears to be poor (Maricar et al., 2015). Comparing the patellar tap sign to MRI, summary sensitivity and specificity values for diagnostic accuracy of detecting an effusion has been calculated as 0.15, 95% CI (0.04, 0.44) and 0.92, 95% CI (0.79, 0.97), respectively, with a positive predictive value of 0.60 and negative predictive value of 0.58 (Meyer et al., 2021).

Sweep Test (Bulge Sign)

This test is also known as the brush or stroke test. Inter-observer reliability of this test for the presence or absence of an effusion appears to be moderate to

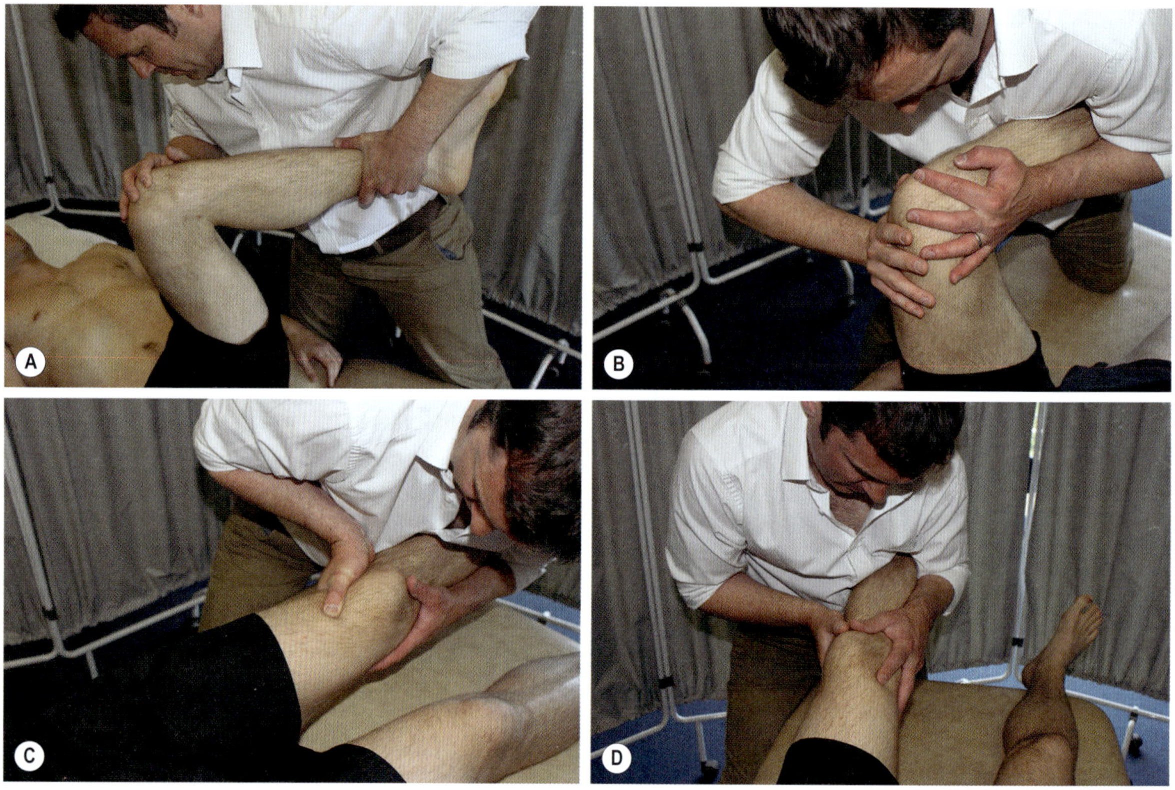

Fig. 16.2 Passive Physiological Joint Movements to the Knee. (A) Flexion/valgus. The patient's knee is flexed passively whilst a valgus force is applied. (B) Flexion/varus. The patient's knee is flexed passively whilst a varus force is applied. (C) Extension/valgus. The patient's knee is extended passively whilst a valgus force is applied. (D) Extension/varus. The patient's knee is extended passively whilst a varus force is applied.

excellent (Maricar et al., 2015). With the patient lying supine, the clinician uses the palm of one hand to sweep fluid proximally up the medial side of the knee into the suprapatellar pouch. The other hand is then used to sweep distally down the lateral side of the knee. In the presence of an effusion, a small bulge of fluid appears on the medial side of the knee. When this test to detect effusion is compared to MRI, summary sensitivity and specificity has been calculated as 0.33, 95% CI (0.26, 0.42) and 0.85, 95% CI (0.80, 0.90), respectively. Positive predictive value has also been calculated as 0.63 and the negative predictive value as 0.62 (Meyer et al., 2021).

Joint Integrity Tests

For all of the joint integrity tests below, a positive test is indicated by excessive movement relative to the unaffected side.

Collateral Stability Tests

The collateral stability tests examine the integrity of the medial and lateral structures of the knee. They comprise the valgus and varus stress tests.

Valgus Stress Tests

With the patient supine, the clinician palpates the medial joint line of the knee and applies a valgus force to gap the medial aspect of the knee. The clinician may perform this test with the knee in full extension and in 20 to 30 degrees flexion (Fig. 16.3); the clinician compares the left and right knee range of movement; excessive movement would be considered a positive test. If the test is positive in slight flexion but negative in full extension, a partial MCL tear is suspected, whilst a test which is positive in both flexion and extension may suggest a complete MCL rupture with possible posteromedial corner and anterior and/or posterior cruciate

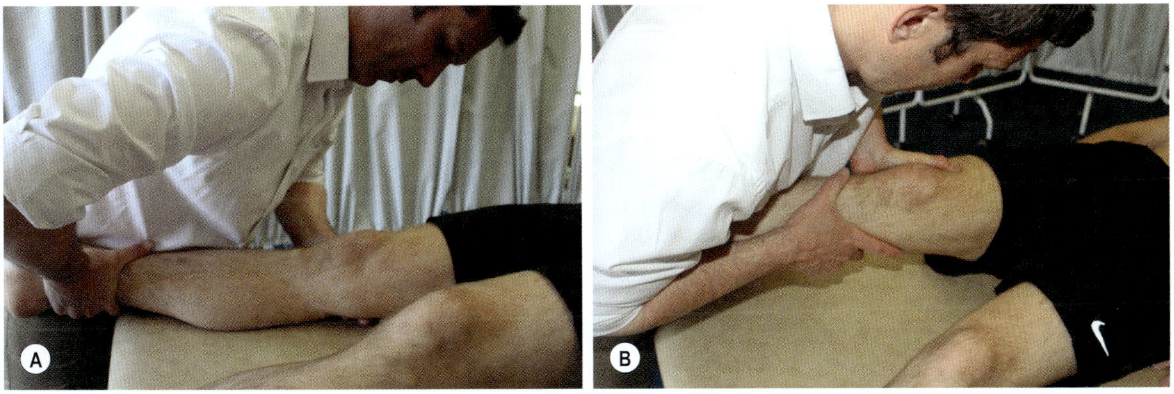

Fig. 16.3 Valgus stress test with the knee in (A) extension and (B) some flexion.

ligament (PCL) injury (Kurzweil & Kelley, 2006). The valgus stress test has previously demonstrated moderate interrater reliability (McClure et al., 1989).

As well as the pure tests described above, it may be beneficial to explore valgus stress testing with and/or through varying degrees of flexion, extension and rotation. Although moving away from the more standardized tests may reduce the validity and reliability of the technique, in some patients, thinking outside the narrow confines of the tests as described may help the clinician reproduce mild symptoms or establish a physical marker. Such variations may even be helpful as treatment techniques.

Varus Stress Tests

With the patient supine, the clinician palpates the lateral joint line and applies a varus force to gap the lateral aspect of the knee. The clinician may perform this test with the knee in full extension and in 20 to 30 degrees flexion (Fig. 16.4). The clinician compares the left and right knee range of movement; excessive movement would be considered a positive test. If the test is positive in slight flexion, as well as the lateral collateral ligament (LCL), the test may suggest injury to the posterolateral capsule, arcuate–popliteus complex, iliotibial band (ITB) and biceps femoris tendon. A positive test in full extension may implicate the LCL, posterolateral capsule, the arcuate–popliteus complex, anterior and PCLs, ITB and lateral gastrocnemius muscle (Magee & Manske, 2020).

Again, as with the valgus stress test, in some patients it may be helpful to explore this test with and/or through varying degrees of flexion, extension and rotation.

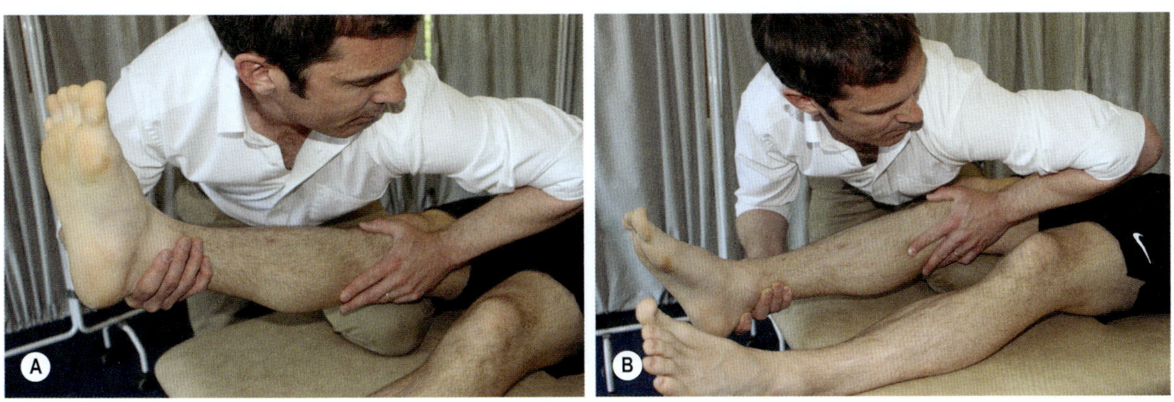

Fig. 16.4 Varus stress test with the knee in (A) extension and (B) some flexion.

Anterior Stability Tests

The anterior stability tests principally examine the integrity of the ACL. ACL injuries range from small, partial tears to complete ruptures and are common injuries in athletes. They can be classified as contact or noncontact injuries with noncontact injuries most frequently occurring in sports that require pivoting (e.g. football, downhill skiing). Female athletes tend to have a higher incidence rate than males and risk factors include knee joint geometry and lower extremity dynamic biomechanics (Hewett et al., 2005).

The ACL is the primary restraint to anterior tibial translation, but it is also a restraint to tibial rotation, varus and valgus knee angulation. The typical noncontact mechanism of an ACL injury is during a sudden change in direction when the foot is firmly planted.

Treatment of an ACL injury is either conservative rehabilitation or a combination of rehabilitation and surgery. Outcomes for conservative and surgical treatment in the nonelite sporting population are similar (Frobel et al., 2010). However, ACL reconstruction surgery is indicated in those with persistent instability and those who are unable to return to sports requiring pivoting or cutting movements despite rehabilitation. Following an ACL injury there should be a progressive and structured rehabilitation program aimed and restoration of the preinjury level of function. Rehabilitation should follow similar principles in both nonsurgically and surgically treated ACL injuries.

Several recent systematic reviews have examined the literature pertaining to the diagnostic accuracy and reliability of physical tests for the integrity of the ACL (Swain et al., 2014; Lange et al., 2015; Leblanc et al., 2015; Anderson et al., 2016; Décary et al., 2016). The tests presented include the Lachman test, the anterior drawer test and the pivot shift. Because these tests have different strengths and weaknesses, the clinician is advised to use the tests in combination.

Lachman Test

The Lachman test is primarily a test for the integrity of the ACL, although the posterior oblique ligament and the arcuate–popliteus complex may also be stressed (Magee & Manske, 2020). With the patient in supine and with the knee flexed (0 to 30 degrees), the clinician stabilizes the femur and applies a posteroanterior force to the tibia along the plane of the joint (Fig. 16.5A). A positive test is indicated by a soft end-feel and excessive motion. The Lachman test can be considered a reliable test (Lange et al., 2015; Décary et al., 2016) and has consistently been shown to be the strongest physical indicator of ACL rupture (Jonsson et al., 1982; Katz & Fingeroth, 1986; Mitsou & Vallianatos, 1988; Ostrowski, 2006; Swain et al., 2014; Leblanc et al., 2015; Anderson et al., 2016). The sensitivity of the test appears reasonable in the detection of partial ruptures (68%), good in the detection of all rupture types (up to 89%) and excellent in the detection of complete ruptures (96%, Leblanc et al., 2015; Décary et al., 2017). A recent systematic review reports specificity to range between 81% and 100% (Décary et al., 2017). The test has its disadvantages, however, as it can be technically

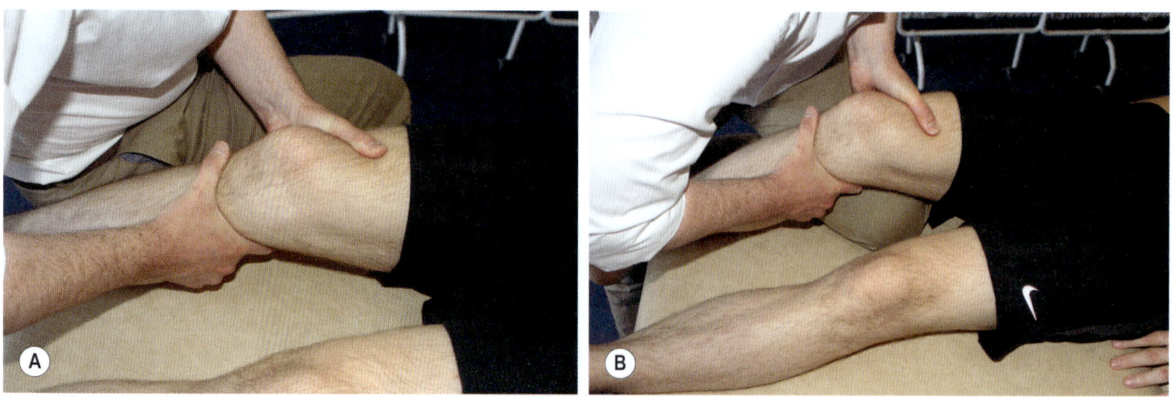

Fig. 16.5 (A) Lachman test. The clinician stabilizes the femur with the left hand and with the right hand applies a posteroanterior force to the tibia. (B) Modified Lachman test. The patient's knee rests over the clinician's thigh and is stabilized by the left hand. The right hand applies a posteroanterior force to the tibia.

difficult, especially if the clinician has small hands or the patient has a particularly large leg. In such circumstances, one modification which may help is for the patient to rest the knee over the clinician's thigh, as shown in Fig. 16.5B. This will stabilize the knee, take some of the leg's weight and allow the patient's muscles to relax fully.

Anterior Drawer Test

The anterior drawer test is similar to the Lachman test but is carried out with the knee flexed to 90 degrees. This test is easier to perform than the Lachman test but appears inferior. The reliability of the test is uncertain, with low-quality studies reporting moderate to excellent interrater reliability (Lange et al., 2015; Décary et al., 2016); the sensitivity appears poor compared to the Lachman at 55%, although the specificity appears good at 92% (Benjaminse et al., 2006). The clinician applies the same posteroanterior force to the tibia along the plane of the joint, feeling the movement of the tibia anteriorly and any contraction of the hamstring muscle group, which may oppose the movement (Fig. 16.6). Sitting on the patient's foot may help to stabilize the leg. A positive test, indicated by a soft end-feel and excessive motion, may indicate injury to the ACL, posterior oblique ligament, arcuate–popliteus complex, posteromedial and posterolateral joint capsules, MCL and the ITB (Magee & Manske, 2020). Again, exploring this test with other angles of knee flexion, and with internal or external tibial rotation, may be relevant and necessary for some patients. Varying the anterior drawer test to include internal and external tibial rotation is known as the Slocum test. With the addition of internal tibial rotation, excessive movement on the lateral aspect of the knee is thought to indicate anterolateral instability, whilst excessive movement of the medial aspect of the knee with the addition of lateral rotation may represent anteromedial instability.

Pivot Shift Test

A further test for anterolateral stability and ACL integrity is the pivot shift test. This test exploits the fact that the ITB acts as a flexor in flexion and an extensor in extension. The patient lies supine with the hip slightly flexed and medially rotated and with the knee flexed. In the first part of the test, the lower leg is medially rotated at the knee and the clinician moves the knee into extension while applying a posteroanterior force to the fibula. The tibia subluxes anteriorly when there is anterolateral instability as the ITB draws the tibia anteriorly. In the second part of the test, the clinician applies an adduction stress to the lower leg and passively moves the knee from extension to flexion while maintaining the medial rotation of the lower leg (Fig. 16.7). A positive test is indicated if at about 20 to 40 degrees of knee flexion the tibia jogs backwards as the ITB draws the tibia posteriorly (reduction of the subluxation). This will often reproduce the patient's feeling of the knee giving way.

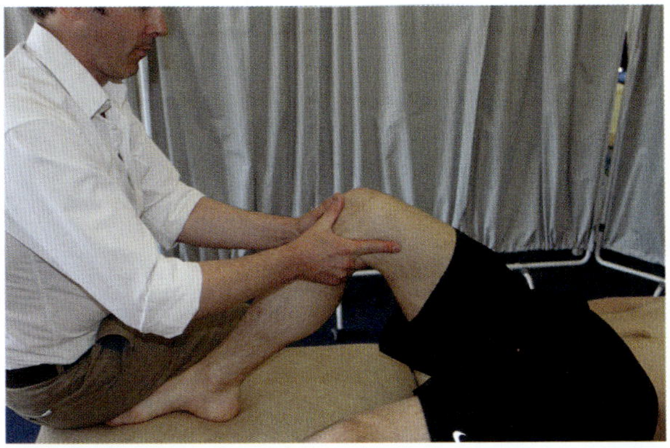

Fig. 16.6 Anterior Drawer Test. With the knee around 90 degrees flexion the clinician sits lightly on the patient's foot to stabilize the leg. The fingers grasp around the posterior aspect of the calf to apply the posteroanterior force, while the thumbs rest over the anterior joint line to feel the movement.

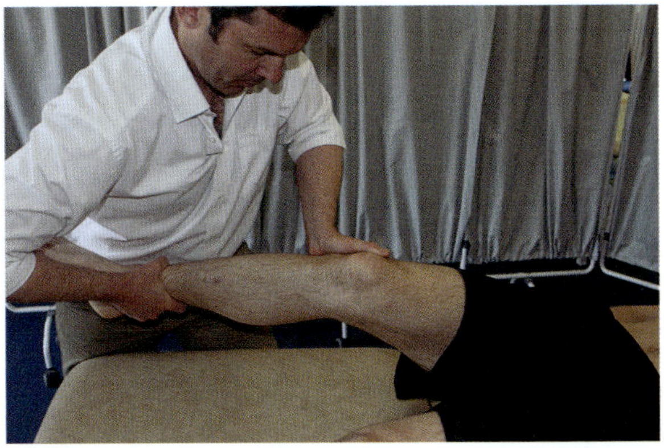

Fig. 16.7 Lateral Pivot Shift. The clinician applies an adduction stress to the lower leg with the left hand, and the right hand passively moves the knee from extension to flexion, whilst maintaining the medial rotation of the lower leg.

Although a difficult test to master, the pivot shift test is the most specific of all ACL integrity tests. In the awake patient, the specificity has been reported at 81%, and when the patient is anaesthetized, the specificity may be as high as 98% (van Eck et al., 2013; Décary et al., 2017). The sensitivity is reasonable but inferior to the Lachman at 86% for complete ruptures (Leblanc et al., 2015). The interrater reliability of the test across low-quality studies is difficult to determine ranging from moderate to excellent (Lange et al., 2015; Décary et al., 2016).

Posterior Stability Tests

The posterior stability tests examine the integrity of the posterior structures of the knee including the PCL and the posterolateral corner (PLC). The typical mechanism of injury for a PCL tear is posteriorly directed force at the anterior aspect of the proximal tibia termed as a 'dashboard injury'. Landing on a flexed knee with the ankle plantar flexed, hyperflexion and hyperextension injuries are also reported (Pache et al., 2018). Tears may be partial or complete ruptures; however, it should be noted that isolated PCL injuries and PLC are uncommon. The aim of rehabilitation is to restore stability and function, and surgery would be indicated for those with ongoing instability or loss of function. The tests presented are the posterior drawer test and the dial test.

Posterior Drawer Test

Although a commonly performed test, the true diagnostic accuracy of the posterior drawer test is yet to be established (Kopkow et al., 2013). The test is typically carried out with the knee flexed to 90 degrees. The clinician first inspects the knee to check if the tibia is not sagging posteriorly and then applies an anteroposterior force to the tibia (Fig. 16.8). A positive test is indicated by excessive motion due to injury of one or more of the following structures: PCL, arcuate–popliteus complex, posterior oblique ligament and ACL (Magee & Manske, 2020). If the clinician inadvertently performs the test on a tibia which is already sagging posteriorly, due to injury of the aforementioned structures, the test may appear falsely negative.

As mentioned in previous tests, exploring the posterior drawer test in different angles of knee flexion, and with internal or external tibial rotation, may be relevant and necessary for some patients. The addition of external tibial rotation during the posterior drawer test may be useful to check for posterolateral instability, which would be indicated by excessive movement at the lateral aspect of the tibia (Bonadio et al., 2014).

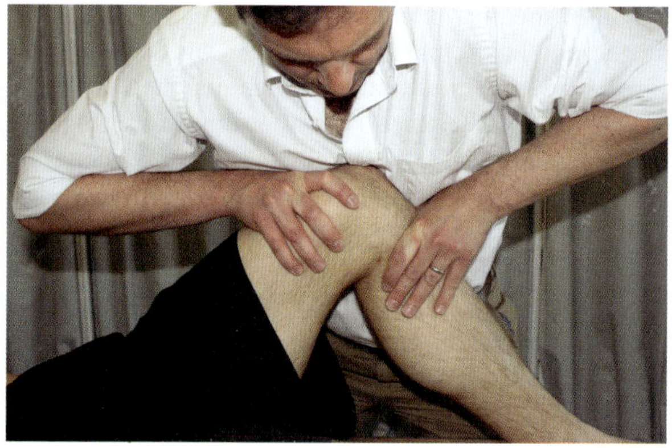

Fig. 16.8 Posterior Drawer Test. With the knee around 90 degrees flexion, the right hand supports the knee, and the web space of the left hand applies an anteroposterior force to the tibia.

Dial Test

A further test to assess for posterolateral instability is the dial test (Fig. 16.9). During this test the patient may lie supine or prone, and the clinician externally rotates the tibia at both 30 and 90 degrees. Increased rotation compared with the uninjured side at 30 degrees but not 90 degrees may indicate PLC instability, whilst increased rotation at 30 and 90 degrees may indicate injury to both the PLC and PCL (Weiler et al., 2021).

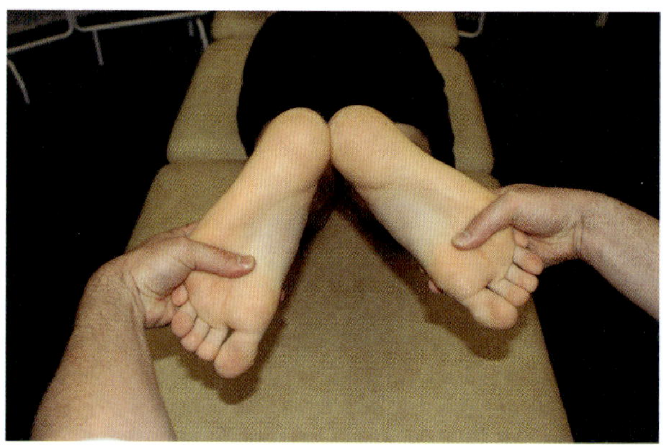

Fig. 16.9 Dial Test. The clinician externally rotates both tibia at 30 and 90 degrees.

The reliability and validity of the dial test is uncertain so the test should be used with caution and reference should be made to the subjective history when diagnosing posterolateral instability.

Meniscal Tests

The medial and lateral menisci perform vital biomechanical functions including load transmission, shock absorption and joint stability (Fox et al., 2015). The menisci transmit between 50% and 95% of the loads acting upon the knee (Rao et al., 2015). Tears to the meniscus are a common problem, and tears disrupt load transmission across the knee increasing the risk of subsequent knee osteoarthritis (Smith et al., 2015). However, not all meniscal tears are the same. Radial tears, meniscal root tears and flap tears can have a devastating effect on meniscal function, yet degenerate tears, particularly in the middle aged or older person, appear to be an entirely normal finding in asymptomatic knees (Englund et al., 2008).

An acute painful locked knee is an uncommon consequence of a meniscus tear and requires referral for a surgical opinion. In an otherwise healthy knee, meniscus repair surgery for a painful meniscus tear constitutes optimal treatment as it aims to preserve meniscal function and reduce the risk of developing subsequent osteoarthritis. However, not all meniscus tears are suitable for repair surgery. In middle aged and older adults with meniscus tears, randomized controlled trials comparing keyhole surgery to remove the damaged part of the meniscus (arthroscopic partial meniscectomy) to either sham surgery or physiotherapy and exercise rehabilitation show similar outcomes (Moseley et al., 2002; Kirkley et al., 2008; Herrlin et al., 2013; Katz et al., 2013; Sihvonen et al., 2013; Yim et al., 2013; van de Graaf et al., 2018), even in the presence of mechanical symptoms (Sihvonen et al., 2016). In those not suitable for meniscus repair surgery and without significant mechanical symptoms, clinical practice guidelines now recommend rehabilitation as the first line intervention (Beaufils & Becker, 2016; Siemieniuk et al., 2018; Abram et al., 2019).

Although the following tests may be useful in detecting meniscal lesions, a degree of caution is advised because not all meniscal tears are symptomatic. The tests presented are the Thessaly test, the McMurray test and joint line tenderness test.

McMurray Test

During the McMurray test, the medial meniscus is typically tested using a combination of knee flexion/extension with lateral rotation of the tibia whilst compressing the medial compartment. The clinician palpates the medial joint line and passively flexes and then laterally rotates the knee so that the posterior part of the medial meniscus is rotated with the tibia—a snap of the joint may occur if the meniscus is torn. The knee is then moved from this fully flexed position to 90 degrees flexion, so the whole of the posterior part of the meniscus is tested (Fig. 16.10). A positive test occurs if the clinician feels a click, which may be heard, indicating a tear of the medial meniscus (McMurray, 1942). The test is then repeated to bias the lateral meniscus, this time using a combination of knee flexion/extension with medial rotation of the tibia whilst compressing the lateral compartment (Fig. 16.11). A recent systematic review has calculated the sensitivity of the McMurray test to be 61% with a specificity of 84% (Smith et al., 2015). Interrater reliability has however been calculated as low to moderate (Décary et al., 2016).

Clinicians vary in performing this test; they may, for example, internally and externally rotate the tibia while moving the knee from full flexion to extension. The key is to explore both the medial and lateral compartments fully. It is worth noting that tears most commonly occur at the posterior horns of the menisci. Most positive findings during the McMurray test therefore occur towards end-of-range flexion when the menisci are maximally loaded.

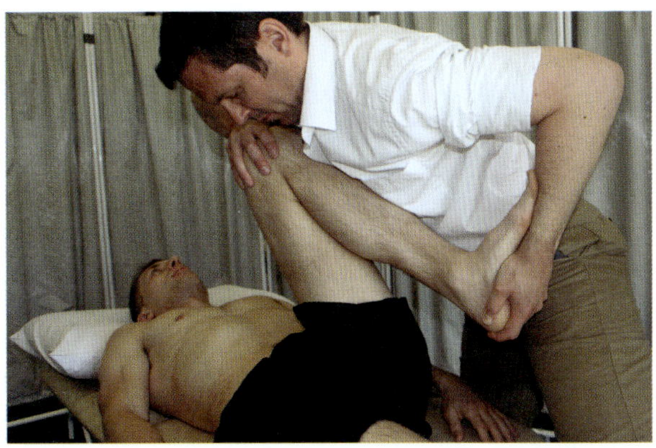

Fig. 16.10 Medial Meniscus. The right hand supports the knee and palpates the medial joint line. The left hand laterally rotates the lower leg and moves the knee from full flexion to extension.

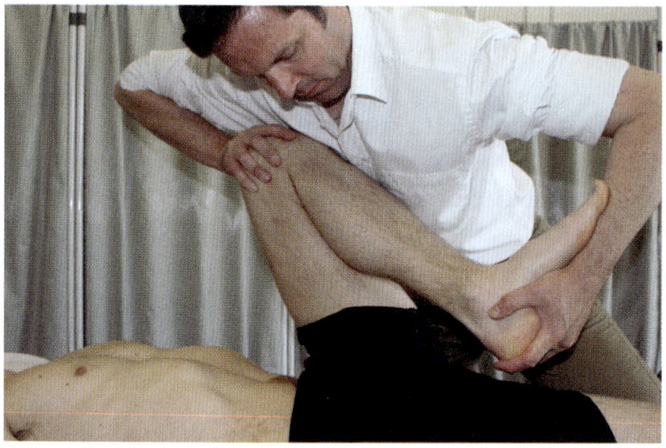

Fig. 16.11 Lateral Meniscus. The right hand supports the knee and palpates the lateral joint line. The left hand medially rotates the lower leg and moves the knee from full flexion to extension.

Thessaly Test

The Thessaly test is a relatively new orthopaedic test (Karachalios et al., 2005) with a fairly high sensitivity (75%) and specificity (87%, Smith et al., 2015). Interrater reliability of the test is moderate (Décary et al., 2016). The Thessaly test is performed at 5 degrees and 20 degrees of flexion. The patient is asked to stand on their symptomatic leg with their arms outstretched and support from the clinician at the hands. The clinician guides the patient around to full external rotation and then full internal rotation at the knee (Fig. 16.12). This movement is repeated three times at 5 degrees of flexion and three further times at 20 degrees of flexion. A positive test is indicated by the reproduction of medial or lateral joint line pain, or a sense of locking or catching (Karachalios et al., 2005). The Thessaly test is a valid, quick and easy test that does not require significant skill to perform on the part of the clinician.

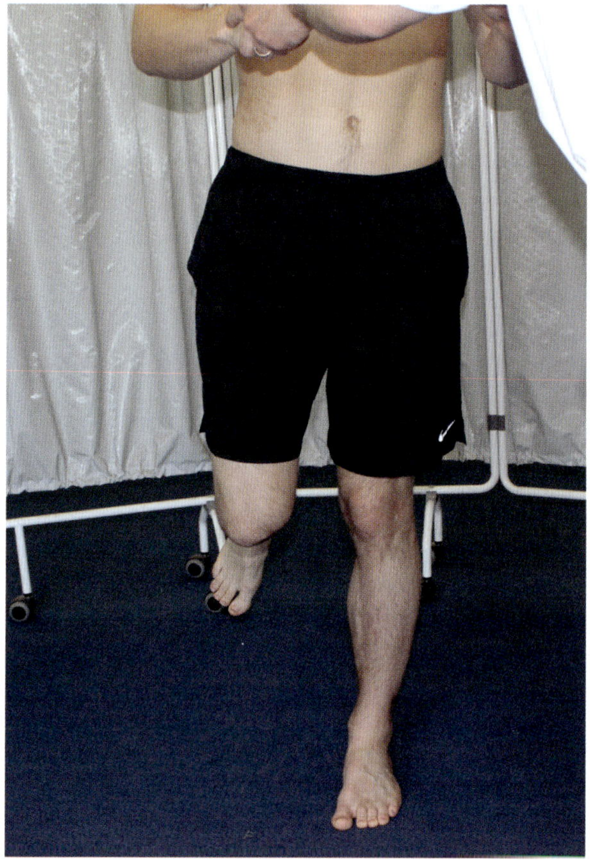

Fig. 16.12 Thessaly Test. With the patient standing on one leg with support at the hands for balance, the clinician guides the patient around to full external rotation and then full internal rotation at the knee. This movement is repeated three times at 5 degrees of flexion and three further times at 20 degrees for flexion.

Joint Line Tenderness

Palpation of the medial and lateral joint lines should not be overlooked when suspicious of a meniscal tear. Although joint line palpation is used as an adjunct to, and not a replacement for, the McMurray or the Thessaly test, it is of note that joint line tenderness in itself has a sensitivity of 83% and a specificity of 83% (Smith et al., 2015). Such tenderness could of course also be emanating from structures other than the meniscus, e.g. the MCL, but the index of suspicion may be heightened if, for example, valgus stress testing was negative and the MCL proximal and distal to the joint line was pain free.

Patellofemoral Tests

Unfortunately, no patellofemoral tests have demonstrated significant diagnostic accuracy (Nijs et al., 2006; Cook et al., 2012; Papadopoulos et al., 2015). The Clarke and Fairbank tests are presented below for completeness, but patellofemoral pain is primarily a diagnosis made during the subjective assessment and through the reproduction of pain during functional testing such as squatting and stair climbing when other causes of anterior knee pain have been excluded (Willy et al., 2019). The clinician is also encouraged to explore symptom modification in the diagnosis and management of patellofemoral pain as the condition is invariably multi-factorial (see the section on symptom modification).

Clarke Test

The Clarke test is of limited value as this test is often provocative to some degree in the asymptomatic population. Thankfully, patellofemoral pain usually offers the clinician strong subjective clues from which to build a clinical hypothesis such as pain descending stairs and provocation tests should be seen as the icing on the cake of the assessment.

The Clarke test is possibly the most widely used patellofemoral provocation test together with palpation of the patella facets which can be partially palpated by gliding the patella medially and laterally. With the patient lying supine or in long sitting and the knee in full extension, the clinician places the web space of one hand just superior to the patella and applies a gentle downward and caudad force (Fig. 16.13). The patient is then instructed to contract the quadriceps by pushing the back of their knee into the bed. The test is positive if pain is reproduced. As the test is often painful in the absence of patellofemoral dysfunction, the clinician needs to be aware of the falsely positive test and when positive it is helpful to ask the patient, 'Was that your pain?'

Fairbank's Apprehension Test

This is considered a test for patellar subluxation or dislocation. It is typically carried out with the patient's knee in 30 degrees of flexion; the clinician passively moves the patella laterally, and a positive test is indicated by pain, apprehension of the patient and/or excessive movement (Nijs et al., 2006). There may also be a reflex contraction of the quadriceps in the presence of instability. It may be necessary and relevant for some patients to test the patellar glide with the knee in other angles of knee flexion.

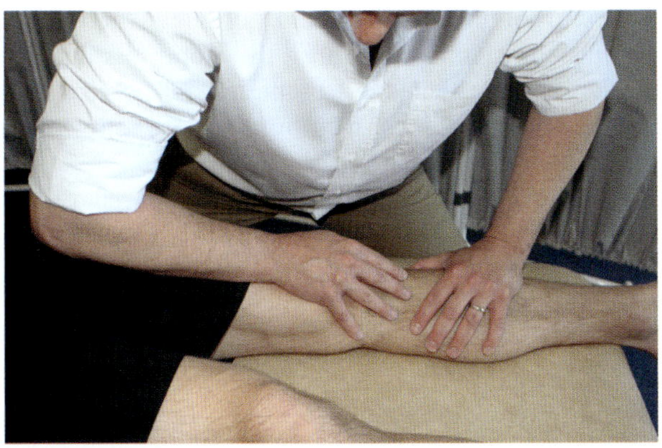

Fig. 16.13 Clarke Test. The clinician places the web space of the right hand just superior to the patella and applies a gentle downward and caudad force. The patient then contracts the quadriceps.

Patella Tendinopathy Test

Patella tendinopathy is a chronic overuse condition, relatively frequent in sports such as volleyball and basketball where jumping is a key activity. It can present as a stubborn injury. Treatment for chronic patella tendinopathy includes progressive tendon loading exercise (Everhart et al., 2017). Manual palpation of the patella tendon has been shown to have 98% sensitivity and 94% specificity for diagnosing patella tendinopathy (Maffulli et al., 2017).

London Hospital Test

The test is performed with the patient lying supine and the knee extended. The patella tendon is gently palpated starting at its attachment on the inferior pole of the patella, along its length from proximal to distal whilst the patient is asked to report tenderness. Once tenderness has been elicited on palpation in knee extension, the tender area of the knee is again palpated with the knee flexed to 90 degrees. The test is considered positive if pain on palpation in extension is significantly less on palpation in the flexed position (Maffulli et al., 2017).

Muscle Tests

Muscle tests include examining muscle strength, control, length and isometric muscle testing.

Muscle Strength

For a true appreciation of a muscle's strength, the clinician tests the muscle isotonically through the available range. During the physical examination of the knee, it may be appropriate to test the knee flexors/extensors and the ankle dorsiflexors/plantarflexors and any other relevant muscle groups.

Strength tests for lower-limb muscles thought particularly prone to becoming weak—gluteus maximus, medius and minimus, vastus lateralis, medialis and intermedius, tibialis anterior and the peronei

(Jull & Janda, 1987; Sahrmann, 2002)—are described in Chapter 4.

Muscle Length

The clinician may test the length of muscles, in particular those thought prone to shorten (Janda 1994, 2002), that is, erector spinae, quadratus lumborum, piriformis, iliopsoas, rectus femoris, tensor fasciae latae, hamstrings, tibialis posterior, gastrocnemius and soleus (Jull & Janda, 1987; Sahrmann, 2002). Testing the length of these muscles is described in Chapter 3.

Isometric Muscle Testing

Isometric muscle testing may help to differentiate whether symptoms are arising from contractile or non-contractile tissue. Isometric testing is described in detail in Chapter 3.

It may be appropriate to test the isometric strength of the knee flexors (with tibia medially and laterally rotated to stress, in particular, the lateral and medial hamstrings, respectively), extensors and ankle dorsiflexors and plantarflexors in resting position and, if indicated, in different parts of the physiological range. The clinician notes the strength and quality of the contraction, as well as any reproduction of the patient's symptoms.

Muscle Control

The single-leg squat is a particularly useful test of lower-limb dynamic alignment and muscle control. A greater frontal plane projection angle (a measure of dynamic knee valgus), ipsilateral trunk lean, pelvis drop, hip adduction and knee abduction have been shown in studies of subjects with patellofemoral pain (Warner et al., 2019). Impaired proximal muscle strength and endurance (Baldon et al., 2012; Lack et al., 2015) and a pronated foot posture (Barton et al., 2010, 2011) have also been associated with the development and maintenance of patellofemoral pain by causing excessive medial rotation of the tibia and femur which may in turn lead to increased stress on the lateral patella. These dysfunctions may lead to the phenomenon of 'medial collapse', where the whole knee is seen to deviate medially during the single-leg squat. This seemingly simple task requires significant control of the pelvis, hip and knee, and foot. If the test is performed poorly and reproduces the patient's symptoms, the clinician may attempt to correct the lower-limb alignment to see if this changes the patient's symptoms (see the section on symptom modification).

Neurological Tests

Neurological examination includes neurological integrity testing and neurodynamic tests.

Integrity of the Nervous System

The integrity of the nervous system is tested if the clinician suspects the symptoms are emanating from the spine or from a peripheral nerve.

Dermatomes/peripheral nerves. Light touch and pain sensation of the lower limb are tested using cotton wool and pinprick, respectively, as described in Chapter 4. Knowledge of the cutaneous distribution of nerve roots (dermatomes) and peripheral nerves enables the clinician to distinguish the sensory loss due to a root lesion from that due to a peripheral nerve lesion. The cutaneous nerve distribution and dermatome areas are shown in Chapter 4.

Myotomes/peripheral nerves. The following myotomes are tested and are shown in Chapter 4.

- L2: hip flexion
- L3: knee extension
- L4: foot dorsiflexion and inversion
- L5: extension of the big toe
- S1: eversion of the foot, contract buttock, knee flexion
- S2: knee flexion, toe standing
- S3–S4: muscles of pelvic floor, bladder and genital function.

A working knowledge of the muscular distribution of nerve roots (myotomes) and peripheral nerves enables the clinician to distinguish the motor loss due to a root lesion from that due to a peripheral nerve lesion. The peripheral nerve distributions are shown in Chapter 4.

Reflex testing. The following deep tendon reflexes are tested and are shown in Chapter 4.

- L3/4: knee jerk
- S1: ankle jerk.

Neurodynamic Tests

The following neurodynamic tests may be carried out in order to ascertain the degree to which neural tissue is responsible for the production of the patient's symptom(s):

- passive neck flexion

- straight-leg raise
- passive knee bend
- slump.

  These tests are described in detail in Chapter 4.
- Palpable nerves around the knee region are as follows:
  - The common peroneal nerve can be palpated medial to the tendon of biceps femoris and also around the head of the fibula.
  - The tibial nerve can be palpated centrally over the posterior knee crease medial to the popliteal artery; it can also be felt behind the medial malleolus, which is more noticeable with the foot in dorsiflexion and eversion.

Miscellaneous Tests

Vascular Tests

If the circulation is suspected of being compromised, the clinician palpates the pulses of the femoral, tibial, popliteal and dorsalis pedis arteries. The clinician then checks for skin and temperature changes as well as capillary refill of the nail beds. The state of the vascular system can also be determined by the response of symptoms to positions of dependence and elevation of the lower limbs. Refer to Chapter 8 in the companion text (Barnard & Ryder, 2024) for further information.

Leg Length

True leg length which tends to be congenital is measured from the anterior superior iliac spine to the medial or lateral malleolus. Apparent leg length, which results from compensatory changes such as pronated foot or spinal scoliosis, is measured from the umbilicus to the medial or lateral malleolus. A difference in leg length of up to 1 to 1.5 cm is considered normal (Magee & Manske, 2020.).

Palpation

The clinician palpates the knee region and any other relevant areas. It is useful to record palpation findings on a body chart (see Fig. 3.2) and/or palpation chart (see Fig. 4.34).

The clinician notes the following:

- The temperature of the area.
- Localized increased skin moisture.
- The presence of oedema or effusion—the clinician examines with the patellar tap and sweep test to assess if joint effusion is present. The circumference of the limb or joint can be measured with a tape measure and the left and right sides compared.
- Mobility and feel of superficial tissues, e.g. ganglions, nodules, scar tissue.
- The presence or elicitation of any muscle spasm.
- Tenderness of bone (the upper pole of the patella and the femoral condyle may be tender in plica syndrome, while the undersurface of the patella may be tender with patellofemoral joint problems), bursae (prepatellar, infrapatellar), ligaments, muscle, tendon, tendon sheath, trigger points and nerve.
- Increased or decreased prominence of bones—observe the position of the patella in terms of glide, lateral tilt, anteroposterior tilt and rotation on the femoral condyles (see below). The quadriceps (Q) angle can be measured. It is the angle formed by the intersection of the line of pull of the quadriceps muscle and the patellar tendon measured through the centre of the patella. The normal outer value is considered to be in the region of 15 degrees. An increased Q angle has been proposed to lead to an increased lateralization force on the patella which may lead to pain or dislocation; however, this measure does not appear as useful as once thought. Indeed, the literature suggests an increased Q angle does not adequately 'distinguish between pathological and non-pathological knees' (Smith et al., 2013).
- Pain provoked or reduced on palpation.

Increased or decreased prominence of bones. The optimal position of the patella is thought to be one in which the patella is parallel to the femur in the frontal and sagittal planes, and the patella is midway between the two condyles of the femur when the knee is slightly flexed (Grelsamer & McConnell, 1998). Patellofemoral pain has been linked to increased lateralization of the patella leading to increased stress on the lateral facet (Heino Brechter & Powers, 2002; Farrokhi et al., 2011; Lack et al., 2015). Often these stresses result from biomechanical causes such as a pronated foot or weak proximal musculature causing internal rotation of the femur and tibia. Such forces may alter the tracking of the patella causing increased lateral translation, tilt and rotation (Herrington, 2008; Draper et al., 2009; Wilson et al., 2009; Souza et al., 2010; Lack et al., 2015). The reader is directed to the section on symptom modification to further explore the assessment of patellofemoral pain. There is evidence to suggest that assessment of patella position, particularly by an experienced clinician has variable intratester reliability with moderate to good criterion validity when compared to MRI (McEwan et al., 2007; Smith et al., 2009; Décary et al., 2016).

In terms of the position of the patella, the following may be noted:

- The base of the patella normally lies equidistant (±5 mm) from the medial and lateral femoral epicondyles when the knee is flexed 20 degrees. If the patella lies closer to the medial or lateral femoral epicondyle, it is considered to have a medial or lateral glide, respectively. The clinician also needs to test for any lateral glide of the patella on quadriceps contraction. The clinician palpates the left and right base of the patella and the VMO and vastus lateralis with thumbs and fingers, respectively, while the patient is asked to extend the knee. In some cases the patella is felt to glide laterally, indicating a dynamic problem, and VMO may be felt to contract after vastus lateralis; VMO is normally thought to be activated simultaneously with, or slightly earlier than, vastus lateralis. Quite a large difference will be needed to enable the clinician to feel a difference in the timing of muscle contraction.
- The lateral tilt is calculated by measuring the distance of the medial and lateral borders of the patella from the femur. The patella is considered to have a lateral tilt, for example, when the distance is decreased on the lateral aspect and increased on the medial aspect such that the patella faces laterally. A lateral tilt is considered to be due to a tight lateral retinaculum (superficial and deep fibres) and ITB. When a passive medial glide is first applied (see below), the patellar tilt may be accentuated, indicating a dynamic tilt problem implicating a tight lateral retinaculum (deep fibres). Validity of the physical assessment of patella tilt and medio-lateral positioning compared to MRI has been demonstrated (McEwan et al., 2007).
- The anteroposterior tilt is calculated by measuring the distance from the inferior and superior poles of the patella to the femur. Posterior tilt of the patella occurs if the inferior pole lies more posteriorly than the superior pole and may lead to fat pad irritation and inferior patellar pain. Dynamic control of a posterior patellar tilt is tested by asking the patient to brace the knee back and observing the movement of the tibia. With a positive patellar tilt the foot moves away from the couch and the proximal end of the tibia is seen to move posteriorly; this movement is thought to pull the inferior pole of the patella into the fat pad.
- Rotation is the relative position of the long axis of patella to the femur and is normally parallel. The patella is considered to be laterally rotated if the inferior pole of the patella is placed laterally to the long axis of the femur. A lateral or medial rotation of the patella is considered to be due to tightness of part of the retinaculum. The most common abnormality seen in patellofemoral pain is both a lateral tilt and a lateral rotation of the patella, which is thought to be due to an imbalance of the medial (weakness of VMO) and lateral structures (tightness of the lateral retinaculum and/or weakness of vastus lateralis) of the patella (McConnell, 1996).
- Testing the length of the lateral retinaculum. With the patient in side-lying position and the knee flexed approximately 20 degrees, the clinician passively glides the patella in a medial direction. The patella will normally move sufficiently to expose the lateral femoral condyle; if this is not possible then tightness of the superficial retinaculum is suspected. The deep retinaculum is tested as above, but with the addition of an anteroposterior force to the medial border of the patella. The lateral border of the patella is normally able to move anteriorly away from the femur; inability may suggest tightness of the deep retinaculum.

Accessory Movements

It may be useful to use the palpation chart and movement diagrams (or joint pictures) to record findings. These are explained in detail in Chapter 4.

The clinician notes the following:

- quality of movement
- range of movement
- resistance through the range and at the end of the range of movement
- behaviour of pain through the range
- provocation of any muscle spasm.

Patellofemoral joint (Fig. 16.14), tibiofemoral joint (Fig. 16.15) and superior tibiofibular joint (Fig. 16.16) accessory movements are listed in Table 16.4. All movements can be explored in various degrees of flexion/extension and medial/lateral tibial rotation. The clinician reassesses all the physical asterisks (movements

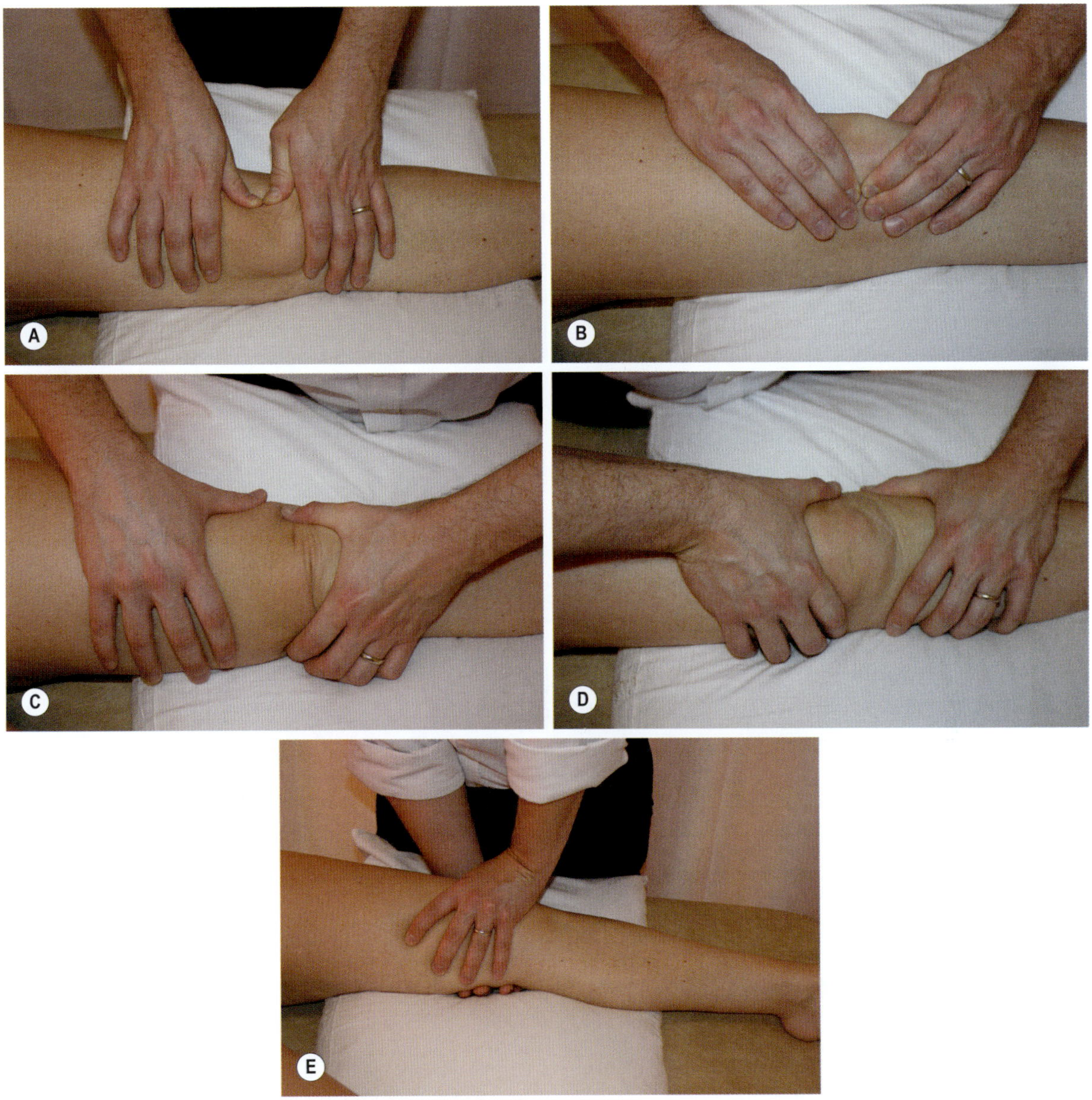

Fig. 16.14 Patellofemoral Joint Accessory Movements. (A) Medial transverse. The thumbs move the patella medially. (B) Lateral transverse. The fingers move the patella laterally. (C) Longitudinal cephalad. The left hand pushes the patella in a cephalad direction. (D) Longitudinal caudad. The right hand pushes the patella in a caudad direction. (E) Compression. The left hand rests over the anterior aspect of the patella and pushes the patella towards the femur.

or tests that have been found to reproduce the patient's symptoms) following accessory movements, in order to establish the effect of the accessory movements on the patient's signs and symptoms. Accessory movements can then be tested for other regions suspected to be a source of, or contributing to, the patient's symptoms. Again, following accessory movements, the clinician reassesses all the asterisks. Regions likely to be examined are the lumbar spine, sacroiliac joint, hip, foot and ankle (see Table 16.4).

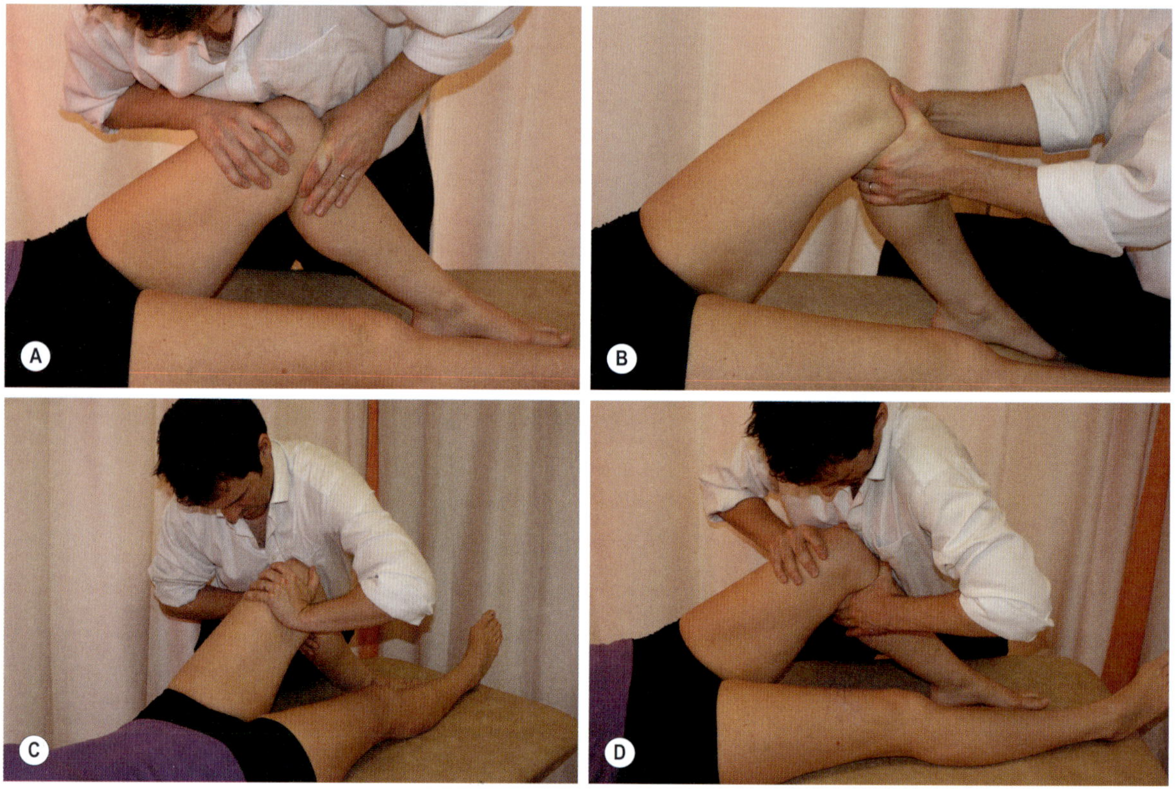

Fig. 16.15 Tibiofemoral Joint Accessory Movements. (A) Anteroposterior. The knee is placed in flexion. With the right hand stabilizing, the web space of the left hand is placed around the anterior aspect of the tibia and applies an anteroposterior force to the knee. (B) Posteroanterior. The knee is placed in flexion, and the clinician lightly sits on the patient's foot to stabilize this position. The fingers grasp around the posterior aspect of the calf to apply the force, while the thumbs rest over the anterior joint line to feel the movement. (C) Medial transverse. The left hand stabilizes the medial aspect of the thigh while the right hand applies a medial force to the tibia. (D) Lateral transverse. The right hand stabilizes the lateral aspect to the thigh while the left hand applies a lateral force to the tibia.

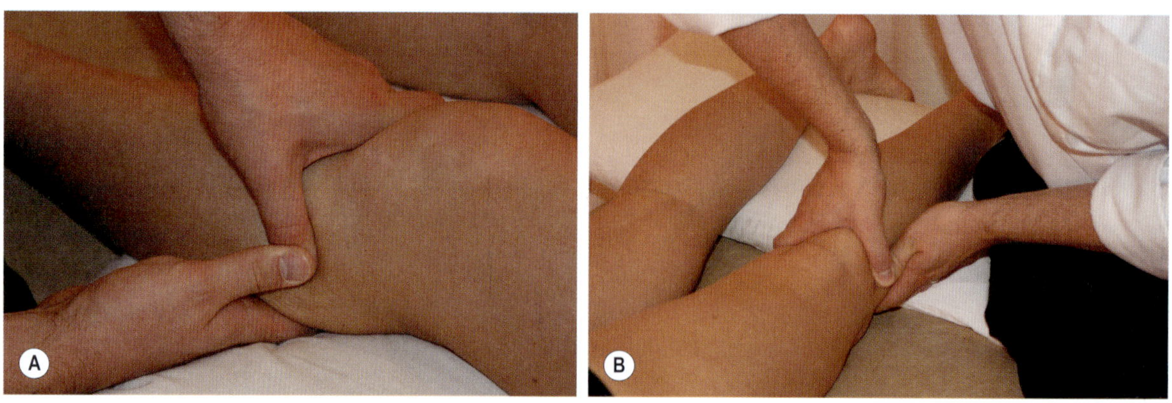

Fig. 16.16 Superior Tibiofibular Joint Accessory Movements. (A) Anteroposterior. Thumb pressures are used to apply an anteroposterior force to the anterior aspect of the head of the fibula. (B) Posteroanterior. Thumb pressures are used to apply a posteroanterior force to the posterior aspect of the head of the fibula.

TABLE 16.4 Accessory Movements, Choice of Application and Reassessment of the Patient's Asterisks

Accessory Movements	Choice of Application	Identify Any Effect of Accessory Movements on Patient's Signs and Symptoms
Patellofemoral Joint		
Med medial transverse	Start position, e.g.	Reassess all asterisks
Lat lateral transverse	• in flexion	
Ceph longitudinal cephalad	• in extension	
Medial rotation	• in medial rotation	
Medial tilt	• in lateral rotation	
Lateral rotation	• in flexion and lateral rotation	
Lateral tilt	• in extension and medial rotation	
Comp compression	Speed of force application Direction of the applied force	
Distr distraction	Point of application of applied force	
Tibiofemoral Joint		
Anteroposterior	As above	Reassess all asterisks
Posteroanterior		
Med medial transverse		
Lat lateral transverse		
Superior Tibiofibular Joint		
Anteroposterior	As above	Reassess all asterisks
Posteroanterior		
Ceph longitudinal cephalad by eversion of the foot		
Caud longitudinal caudad by inversion of the foot		
Other Regions to Consider		
?Lumbar spine	As above	Reassess all asterisks
?Sacroiliac joint		
?Hip		
?Foot and ankle		

Symptom Modification

It can be extremely useful to examine a symptomatic physical task specific to the patient's complaint. This functional task can then be modified, and the patient's symptomatic response can be closely monitored. A suitable functional task may be replicated in the clinical setting and can often be identified when asking the patient about the aggravating factors. It may be useful to examine a functional task early in the assessment; this is for three reasons:

1. The task will provide a useful initial snapshot of the patient's problem.
2. It may be possible to manipulate the task to aid the clinical diagnosis and highlight possible treatment options (see the worked example below).
3. The task will provide a useful physical marker (*).

By manipulating the functional task in various ways to bias different tissues (which need not be time-consuming) useful information may be gleaned as to the likely clinical diagnosis as well as the most appropriate way to manage the condition. Although the worked example below highlights the art of clinical reasoning in practice, it is important to emphasize that modifications to symptomatic functional tasks are not standardized tests and will therefore lack a degree of validity and reliability. There is a trade-off here: on the one hand, the clinician is being very patient focused and examining the specific problem that prompted the patient to seek help in the first place, but on the other hand, there is lack of standardization. It is worth noting, however, that even well-known orthopaedic tests may lack robust diagnostic accuracy or reliability. It may be wise to use both approaches in a clinical context as both have relative strengths and add to the clinical picture. As always, the clinician is encouraged to synthesize information from the whole subjective and physical examination to reach a reasoned view of the patient's condition, rather than placing too much emphasis on any one test.

A worked example of symptom modification: anterior knee pain.

Anterior knee pain is multi-factorial (Lankhorst et al., 2012; Barton et al., 2015) leading to abnormal patella stresses during functional tasks (Wilson, 2009; Draper et al., 2009; Souza et al., 2010; Farrokhi et al., 2011). Factors which may contribute the generation of anterior knee pain may include the following:

- Local factors—these may include, for example, tight retinacular tissue or altered timing of the VMO (Herrington, 2008; Draper et al., 2009; Wilson, 2009; Souza et al., 2010; Giles et al., 2013, 2015).
- Proximal factors—these may include reduced hip strength, endurance and control leading to medial femoral torsion and lateralization of the patella (Meira & Brumitt, 2011; Noehren et al., 2012).
- Distal factors—These may include pronation of the foot leading to internal tibial rotation and altered patellofemoral mechanics (Barton et al., 2011).

Because of the multi-factorial nature of anterior knee pain, therefore a multi-modal approach to its assessment and management should be adopted (Barton et al., 2015). For further information on current recommendations for the treatment of patellofemoral pain, clinicians are recommended read the 2018 consensus statement for the 5th International Patellofemoral Pain Research Retreat (Collins et al., 2018). If the patient complains of pain during stair climbing then a one-leg squat or step up may be a useful functional task during which to explore the impact of altering local, proximal and distal factors.

The clinician closely monitors the symptomatic response to the functional task. If the task reproduces symptoms immediately then symptom modification may begin. If not, the clinician may need to think of ways of provoking the symptoms, for example a deeper squat, higher step or repeated movements.

Once the task has been observed and confirmed to be symptomatic, the clinician may attempt to modify the task whilst closely monitoring the symptomatic response. It may help for the clinician to think systematically and ask themselves 'How can I influence the local/proximal/distal structures to see if those structures are playing a role in the maintenance of this condition?'

In relation to the local structures, the clinician may wish to explore gliding of the patella in varying directions during the movement to see the symptomatic response. Some directions may reduce pain and some may increase it. As the patella may become lateralized in the presence of patellofemoral pain, the clinician may find that gliding the patella medially during the movement (Fig. 16.17) reduces symptoms. If symptoms improve then this technique in itself may be employed therapeutically or symptoms may be modified with the addition of tape (Barton et al., 2014) to allow rehabilitation. It is worth noting that mobilization techniques in themselves lack level 1 evidence in the management of patellofemoral pain (Barton et al., 2015).

In relation to the proximal structures, the clinician may wish to activate the abductors and lateral rotators of the hip during the movement which may correct a dynamic adducted and medially rotated femoral position. This could be done either manually by asking the patient to abduct/laterally rotate against resistance

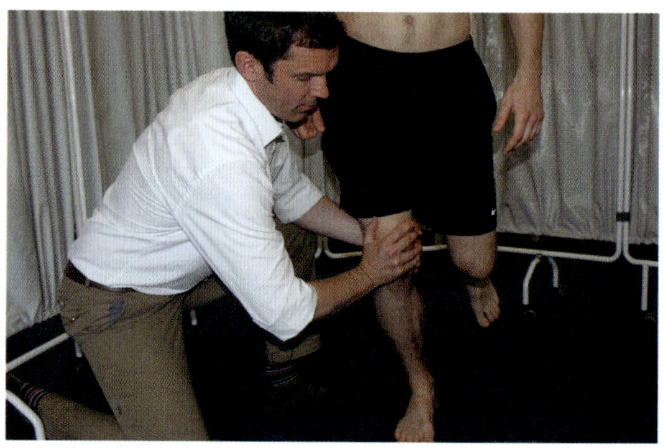

Fig. 16.17 Manual application of a medial glide of the patella during a single leg squat to modify symptoms.

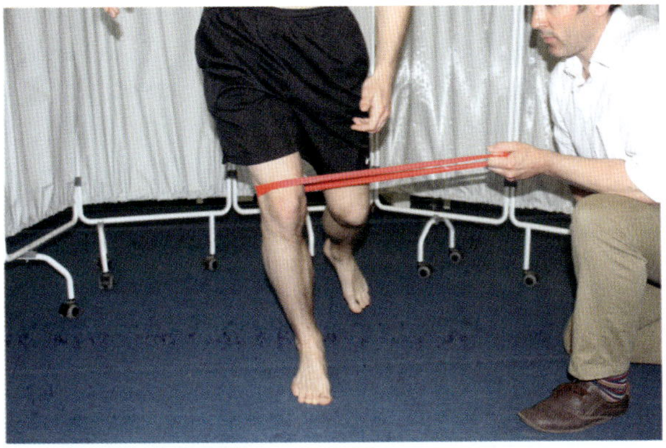

Fig. 16.18 Activation of the hip lateral rotators using resistance to modify symptoms.

applied to the lateral knee or it could be done with the application of a resistance band (Fig. 16.18). If symptoms improve then the clinician may consider a graded strengthening programme for the proximal muscles which can be effective in the management of patellofemoral pain (Baldon et al., 2012; Peters & Tyson, 2013; Lack et al., 2015).

In relation to the distal structures, the clinician may wish to alter the position of the patient's foot as foot pronation has been linked to patellofemoral pain (Barton et al., 2011). The clinician may wish to correct foot position manually or by placing a block or orthotic under the foot if the foot pronates during movement (Fig. 16.19). If changing foot position positively influences symptoms, the clinician may wish to trial the addition of an orthotic to control foot motion. The use of foot orthotics has been shown to improve functional performance in individuals with patellofemoral pain (Barton et al., 2009).

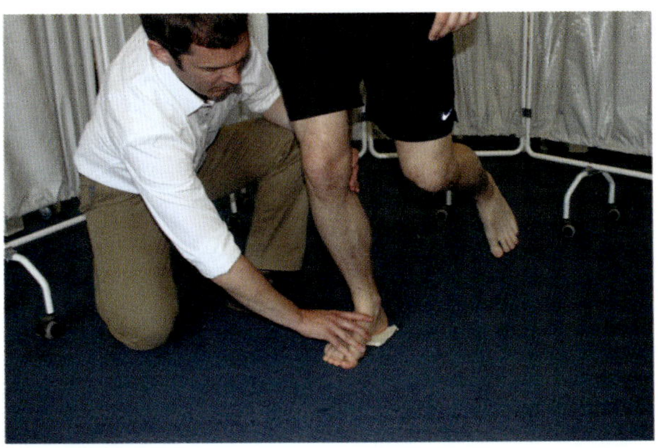

Fig. 16.19 Correction of pronation using a block or orthotic to modify symptoms.

This example has sought to demonstrate how methodically manipulating a functional task in various ways may bias different tissues and help to determine the tissues which may be contributing to symptoms. Symptom modification may also help to direct appropriate management strategies. In practice, a multi-factorial problem requires a multi-factorial management approach, and it may be that several strategies may need to be combined into one coherent management plan. Other strategies not mentioned may also need to be employed; for example, does contracting the deep abdominal muscles to control pelvic movement make a difference? Or do mobilizations to the head of fibula, the tibia or the femur during the movement alter symptoms? When thinking about symptoms modification, it may be helpful for the clinician to ask themselves 'which myogenic, arthrogenic or neurogenic structures may be contributing to this patient's problem?' The clinician is encouraged to think functionally, methodically and creatively, whilst at the same time closely monitoring the patient's symptomatic response to the intervention.

Assessment of Return to Play/Performance

For a comprehensive review of decision-making with return play, readers are directed to Chapter 10 in the companion text (Barnard & Ryder, 2024). Return to play whether it be sport or normal daily activities is a primary goal for rehabilitation of any injury and a key consideration with management of injuries of the knee.

Decision-making around return to play can present a significant challenge to clinicians. Clinicians will frequently be required to advise when it is safe for a patient to return to sport or provide information based on factors including the risk of injury and potential consequences to enable patients to make informed decisions about the advantages and disadvantages about returning to sports. A precise risk/consequence calculation is impossible, and great care is required when determining readiness. The clinician needs to provide a reasoned hypothesis based upon available knowledge and experience in order to avoid re-injury (please refer to chapter 10 in the companion text, Barnard & Ryder, 2024).

Due to differences in healing rates, resolution of impairments, recovery of neuromuscular control, functional skills and psychological readiness, the period of time for return to sport is going to be variable between individuals with the same injury and a purely time-based return to play following injury or surgery is therefore going to be insufficient and inappropriate. A criterion-based rehabilitation process whereby the patient reaches set milestones in order to progress to the next activity level, inclusive of return to play or sport is necessary.

Physical testing provides integral information that will be necessary in the decision-making upon readiness for the return to sport and can be used alongside questionnaires to determine the athletes' readiness for returning to sport from knee injury or surgery. Common questionnaires include Psychological Readiness to Return to Sport scale (I-PRRS) (Glazer, 2009) and the IKDC questionnaire (Irrgang et al., 2001).

Physical Examination for Return to Sport

No one set criteria or system has been determined to assess an individual's readiness for return to sport, and clinicians should incorporate the appropriate assessment techniques already included within this chapter to inform a decision on readiness. Below are further factors which may be useful in the decision on readiness for return to play/sport.

Limb Symmetry Index

For an evaluation of strength and function, clinicians should consider the limb symmetry index (LSI) and quadriceps/hamstrings ratio measurement. Poor quadriceps strength has been associated with poor outcome following injury such as ACL reconstruction and a quadriceps LSI of less than 90% increases the risk of re-injury. Indeed, in those who are recovering (Herrington et al., 2021) from ACL injury, for every 1% point increase in strength symmetry there is a 3% less re-injury rate (Grindem et al., 2016). The LSI is calculated by taking the average of any test scores for the affected limb, divided by the unaffected limb, which is then multiplied by 100 to obtain a percentage difference between limbs.

The quadriceps/hamstrings ratio (H:Q) is a measure of the quadriceps strength compared to the hamstring strength and has been used to in both lower extremity rehabilitation and injury prevention. Debate exists over normative values however a ratio of 0.6 (hamstring strength should be 60% of the quadriceps) has previously been proposed (Ruas et al., 2019). However, clinicians should note that factors such as fatigue may significantly affect the quadriceps/hamstrings ratio and limit the usefulness of this test.

Assessment of Quadriceps Activation

A quadriceps lag (weakness of terminal knee extension) is common after knee injury or surgery and needs to be corrected. This can be evident during an active straight leg raise technique and indicates that the quadriceps are not strong enough to fully extend the knee. The lag results from loss of mechanical advantage, muscle atrophy, decreasing power of the muscle as it shortens adhesion formation, effusion, or reflex inhibition (Magee & Manske, 2020).

Objective strength testing using an isokinetic dynamometer is reliable but not freely available to many clinicians. In patients who have undergone ligament reconstruction surgery, clinicians are encouraged to consider strength testing that does not risk graft integrity. Although not specific for the quadriceps, strength testing using the leg press LSI will provide the clinician with a measure of strength.

Functional Testing

Single-leg squat test and qualitative analysis of single-leg loading (QASL) (Herrington et al., 2013) involve dichotomous scoring of movement strategies in individual body regions (arms trunk, pelvis, thigh, knee and foot), with a score 0 for an appropriate strategy and a 1 for an inappropriate strategy, with 0 being the best overall score and 10 being the worst score. The score sheet is shown below and the photos demonstrate both the appropriate and inappropriate movement strategies. In patients who have undergone surgery, the dynamic valgus pattern of movement should be avoided to avoid strain upon the graft and risking further injury. Good control should also include a good range of knee flexion to around 90 degrees, which has been shown to have excellent validity when compared to 3D motion capture during single-leg squatting and landing (Herrington & Munro, 2014). Almangoush et al. (2014) has shown this to have excellent intra- and intertester reliability (kappa score ranging $k = .63$ to 1.0). Fig. 16.20 demonstrates the suboptimal and optimal strategies in the QASLS assessment.

QASLS		Optimal	Sub-optimal
Arm strategy	Excessive arm movement to balance	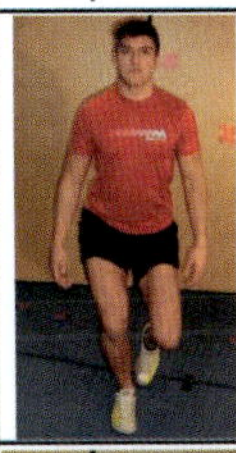	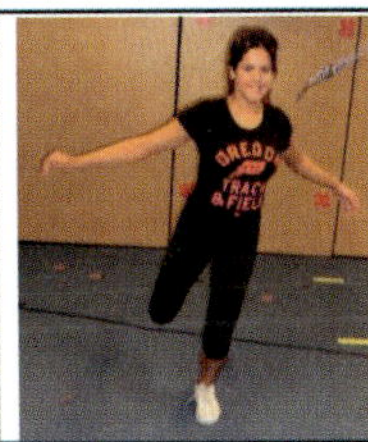
Trunk alignment	Leaning in any direction	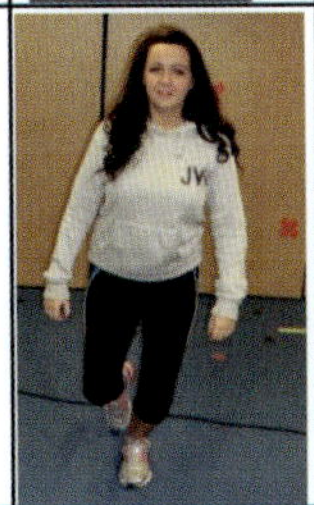	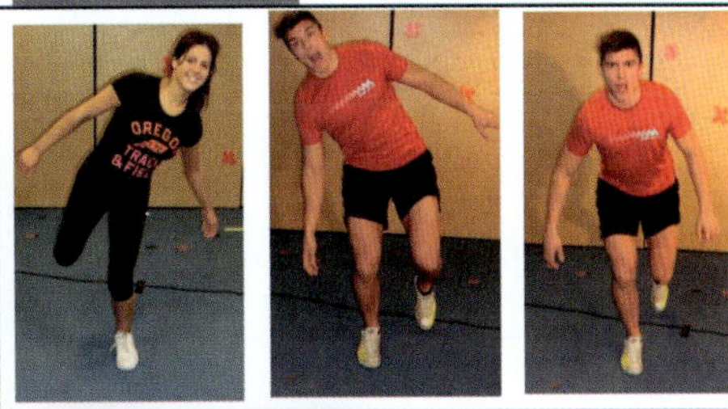
Pelvic plane	Loss of horizontal plane	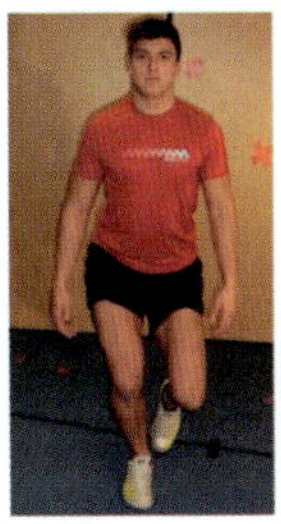	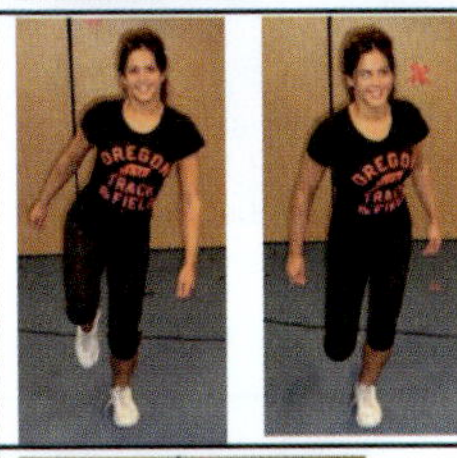
	Excessive tilt or rotation		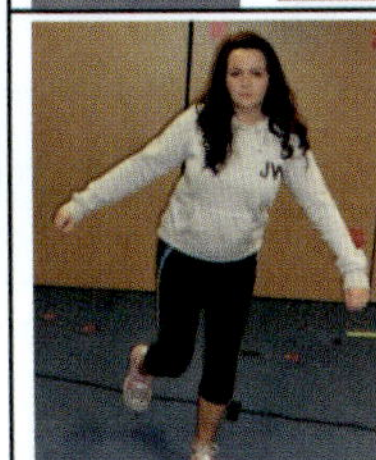
Thigh motion	WB thigh moves into hip adduction	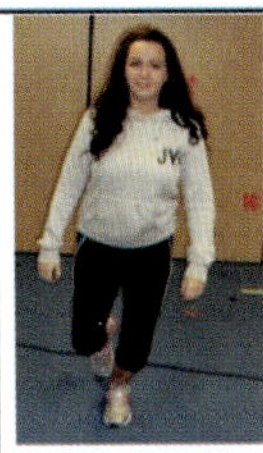	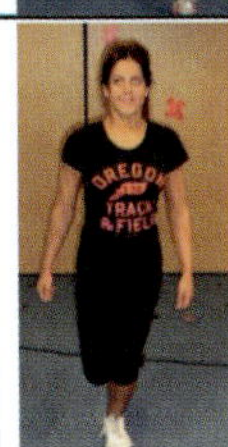

Fig. 16.20 QASLS (Qualitative Analysis of Single leg Loading). (From Herrington et al. 2013.)

Step Down/Single Leg Landing/Load Acceptance

When assessing readiness for return to sport, the clinician will want to assess the patient's ability to appropriately control landing and loading through the injured leg in a progressive way, gradually increasing the challenge in an appropriate manner for their sport. Appropriate control would be able to complete the movement by maintaining good alignment of the leg, avoiding the dynamic valgus position, with a range of good knee flexion which avoids a stiff leg landing. The clinician can progress the difficulty from stepping down in a straight line off of a set 30 cm box. This can initially be progressed by increasing the height of the box. Inability to adequately control the landing means that further cued practice is required before progression to more challenging levels of load acceptance.

	NWB thigh not held in neutral		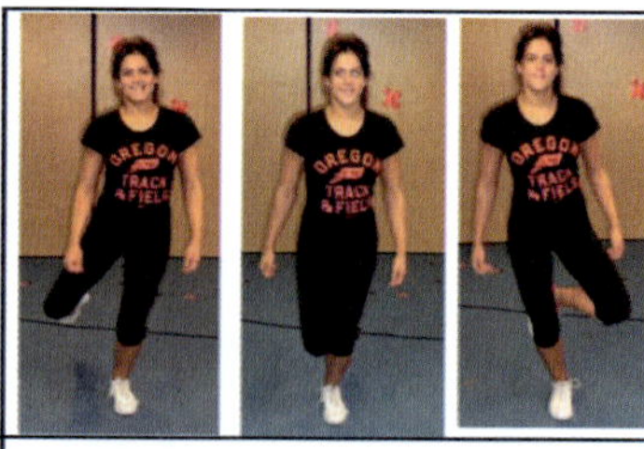
Knee position	Patella pointing towards 2nd toe (noticeable valgus)	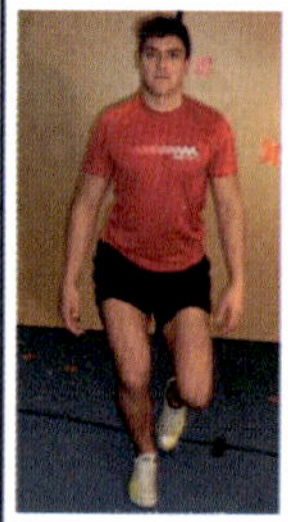	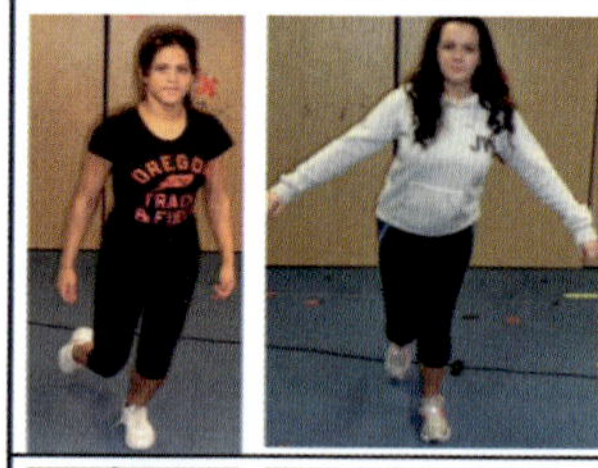
	Patella pointing past inside of foot (significant valgus)		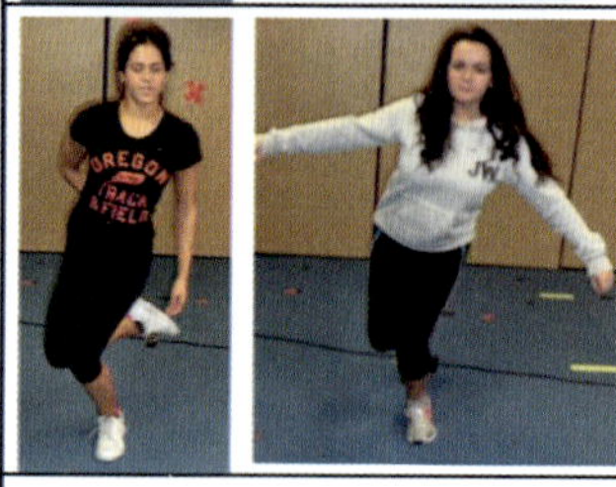
Steady stance	Touches down with NWB foot		
	Stance leg wobbles noticeably		

Fig. 16.20, cont'd

Oblique or Sideways Step Down/Landing

To assess the patient's ability to control single leg landing more progressively the clinician can ask the patient to step down at an angle rather than straight. The patient may start standing facing forwards off of the step aiming to land at an angle such as 45 degrees from the starting position. This can be progressed to 90 degrees. The clinician observes the patient for their ability to balance and control the landing that would control against going into the dynamic valgus position or a stiff leg landing. Inability to adequately control the landing means that further cued practice is required.

Landing on an Unstable Surface (Soft Mat)

The clinician can assess the patient's ability to control landing on to an unstable surface by asking the patient to step down onto a soft mat. The clinician observes the patient's ability to balance and control the landing that would control against going into the dynamic valgus position or a stiff leg landing. Inability to adequately control the landing means that further cued practice is required.

Perturbation Control

The clinician can assess the patient's ability to control landing with the challenge of balance perturbation. The patient steps down whilst the therapist adds perturbation either manually or by gently pulling on resistance band attached to the patient. The clinician observes the patient's ability to balance and control the landing that would control against going into the dynamic valgus position or a stiff leg landing. Inability to adequately control the landing means that further cued practice is required.

Hop Testing Battery

A battery of four hop tests has been used successfully in return to sport rehabilitation with success for each test being deemed as a performance of 90% LSI for the affected limb (Kyritsis et al., 2016; Grindem et al., 2016). These tests are shown to have good test-retest reliability (ICC range 0.92 to 0.97) (Ross et al., 2002). Caution however should be applied when interpreting these tests, as they may not account for fatigue and or transverse plane (rotational) movement.

A single hop for distance: In this test the aim is to hop as far as possible on a single leg without losing balance. The distance is measured from the start line to the heel of the landing foot.

Triple hop for distance: In this test the aim is to hop as far as possible on a single leg three consecutive times without losing balance. The distance is measured from the start line to heel of the landing foot.

Cross-over hop for distance: The aim is to hop as far as possible on a single leg three consecutive times without losing balance. The athlete has to hop across the midline for each consecutive hop. The distance is measured from the start line to heel of the landing foot.

Six-meter hop for time: The aim is to hop as fast as possible on a single leg over a distance of 6 m without losing balance and landing firmly.

Star Excursion Balance Test SEBT

This test is a series of single-limb squats using the non-stance limb to reach maximally to touch a point along one of eight designated lines on the ground. The eight lines extend from the centre point of a grid with each line set 45 degrees from the other (Gribble et al., 2012). The goal of the task is to have the individual remain stable at the centre of the star on the stance limb. The individual maintains stability on the stance limb whilst attempting to reach as far as possible with the reaching limb along the line. The individual lightly touches the line with the reaching foot without needing to rest or shift weight to this limb. The individual returns to the centre of the grid to stand on both feet. Scoring of the test is by measuring how far the participants can reach along each line and is compared between the injured or noninjured limb (Gribble et al., 2012). The SEBT has excellent test-retest reliability in healthy individuals in each direction (0.84 to 0.92 95% CI) (Munro & Herrington, 2010).

KNOWLEDGE CHECK

- Patellofemoral tests lack sensitivity and specificity: TRUE or FALSE?
- Which physical test has consistently been shown to be the strongest physical indicator of ACL rupture?
- Which types of meniscal tears have a particularly detrimental effect on meniscal function?
- What are the pros and cons of symptom modification?

COMPLETION OF THE EXAMINATION

Having carried out all the above tests, the examination of the knee region is now complete. The subjective and physical examination produces a large amount of information, which needs to be recorded accurately and quickly. The outline subjective and physical examination charts in Chapters 3 and 4 may be useful for some clinicians. It is important, however, that the clinician does not examine in a rigid manner, simply following the suggested sequence outlined in the chart. Each patient presents differently, and this needs to be reflected in the examination process. It is vital at this stage to highlight important findings from the examination with an asterisk (*). These findings are to be reassessed at, and within, subsequent treatment sessions to evaluate the effects of treatment on the patient's condition.

The physical testing procedures which specifically indicate joint, nerve or muscle tissues, as a source of the patient's symptoms, are summarized in Table 4.9.

On completion of the physical examination the clinician:

- warns the patient of possible exacerbation up to 24 to 48 hours following the examination
- requests the patient to report details on the behaviour of the symptoms following examination at the next attendance
- explains the findings of the physical examination and how these findings relate to the subjective assessment. Any misconceptions patients may have regarding their illness or injury should be addressed
- evaluates the findings, formulates a clinical diagnosis and writes up a problem list
- determines the objectives of treatment
- devises an initial treatment plan.

In this way, the clinician will have developed the following hypotheses categories (adapted from Jones & Rivett 2004):

- function—abilities and restrictions
- patient's perspective on his/her experience
- source of symptoms—this includes the structure or tissue that is thought to be producing the patient's symptoms, the nature of the structure or tissues in relation to the healing process and the pain mechanisms
- contributing factors to the development and maintenance of the problem—they may be environmental, psychosocial, behavioural, physical or heredity factors
- precautions/contraindications to treatment and management—these include the severity and irritability of the patient's symptoms and the nature of the patient's condition
- management strategy and treatment plan
- prognosis—this can be affected by factors such as the stage and extent of the injury as well as the patient's expectation, personality and lifestyle.

For guidance on treatment and management principles, the reader is directed to the companion textbook (Barnard & Ryder, 2024).

REVIEW AND REVISE QUESTIONS

1. Complete the following
   The knee is a large and complex region made up of the ___________, ___________ and ___________ joints.
2. A forced valgus injury may injure which of the following structures?
   a. Collateral ligaments
   b. Anterior cruciate ligament
   c. Menisci
3. Immediate swelling following an acute twisting injury with a popping sensation suggests a meniscal tear: TRUE or FALSE?
4. Name three factors that might cause the knee to give way?
   a. ___________
   b. ___________
   c. ___________
5. The Thessaly test is a useful sensitive and specific test for:
   a. Meniscal pathology
   b. A posterolateral corner injury
   c. A cruciate ligament rupture
   d. Patellofemoral pathology
6. A positive Clarke and Fairbank test in isolation indicates a strong possibility that symptoms are patellofemoral in origin: TRUE or FALSE?
7. Which of the following might accessory movements NOT be useful in the assessment of?
   a. Quality of movement
   b. Range of movement
   c. Resistance through the range and at the end of the range of movement
   d. Degree of effusion
   e. Behaviour of pain through the range
   f. Provocation of any muscle spasm.
8. Describe how you might functionally explore lateral knee pain which is aggravated by getting into a car. Think about what structures are local to the lateral knee or may refer to the lateral knee and how you might differentiate between these structures using symptom modification.

Case Study

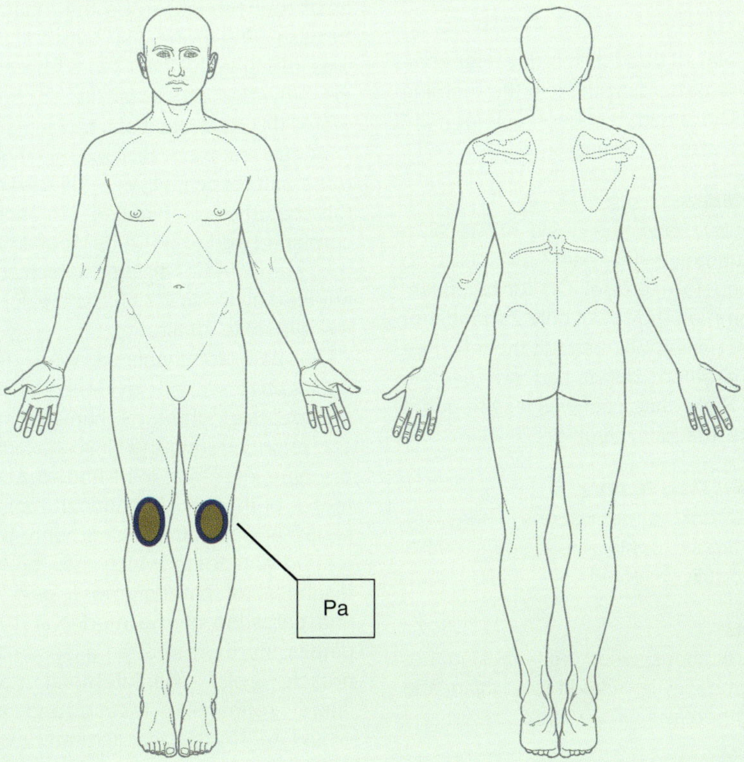

24-year-old netball player.

Pa—L=R. Intermittent pain, ache, occasionally sharp with occasional crepitus.

Aggravating factors—immediate onset of pain when landing from a jump, after running, descending stairs.

Easing factors—rest. Pain could last the rest of the day if aggravated by exercise.

24-h pattern—activity related through the day. Generally better first thing in the morning with no knee stiffness.

Sleep—There had only been pain at night on a couple of occasions after a training session.

PMH/DH—Fit and well, no medications.

No symptoms elsewhere

Subjective Examination

History of Present Condition

A 24-year-old accountant and club netball player presented to the clinic with a 5-month history of bilateral vague anterior knee pain located in the retro and peripatellar regions that was occasionally felt as sharp. There were no symptoms of locking or giving way, and the patient had not noticed any significant swelling. She did report symptoms of crepitus which was particularly noticeable when descending stairs. She denied any spinal, groin or leg pain and there were no neurological symptoms.

Aggravating and Easing Factors

The knee pain was typically most aggravated when landing from a jump whilst playing netball. It was also felt during and after running, and the pain could be felt for the rest of the day when going down stairs following netball or running. She would also notice pain occasionally when sitting and working, which would soon ease with straightening the knee.

Twenty-Four-Hour Pattern

Knee pain was activity related through the day. Her knee symptoms were generally better first thing in the morning with no knee stiffness. There had only been pain at night on a couple of occasions after a training session.

History of Present Condition

Pain had started insidiously, and she could not recall a specific injury. Unfortunately, her pain continued to worsen as she continued to exercise. On further questioning she had run a half marathon with only 2 months of training and 5 months for earlier. She had felt the left knee pain during the half marathon, but it had not been a problem during training. Right knee pain was less frequent and had developed since the half marathon.

Past Medical History and Drug History

She was fit and well and took no medications. There was history of a left ankle sprain sustained 2 years earlier during netball which had fully resolved.

Beliefs and Expectations

The patient was unsure about what was causing her problem and thought that it may be related to an injury she sustained whilst playing netball.

Hypothesis After Subjective Examination

The knee pain was thought to be related to the patellofemoral joint for multiple reasons. The location of pain was in the retro and peripatella regions. The aggravating factors were typical for patellofemoral pain and the fact that symptoms were felt bilaterally is also an indicator that the patellofemoral joint is more likely to be implicated. The fact that there was also no history of trauma and that patellofemoral pain is a common problem in the sporting all provide the clinician with a high index of suspicion that symptoms are patellofemoral.

Local anatomical structures that may cause anterior knee pain in a similar location to the patellofemoral joint include the patella and quadriceps tendons and fat pad. Whilst it is less likely, the clinicians should also not overlook a meniscus tear. The infrapatellar branch of the saphenous nerve was considered an unlikely source of symptoms as there were no neurological symptoms and no other indicators of a neurogenic cause for the pain. Possible referring structures also considered unlikely to be causing pain include the hip joint and sacroiliac joint, or radicular pain emanating from an upper lumbar nerve root.

The working hypothesis was that the patellofemoral joint itself was thought to be the most likely source of symptoms in view of the distribution and aggravating factors. It was thought the pain would be easy to reproduce with low severity and irritability as even though symptoms would flair as a result of a training session, she was able to continue and a physical examination was thought unlikely to be as provocative as a full training session. It was also felt that the combination of running the half marathon combined added on to her regular netball had overloaded the patellofemoral joint which may also have been affected by the loss of full ankle dorsiflexion resulting from the old ankle sprain.

The pain mechanisms were thought to be mainly nociceptive without evidence of central sensitization or maladaptive output mechanisms such as fear avoidance. The priority during the clinical examination was to assess the patellofemoral joint and to rule it in or out as a potential pathology. Functional testing including single-leg squat and landing along with symptom modification testing and tests which may be clinically useful in the diagnosis of patellofemoral pain, namely Clarke's test and palpation of the medial and lateral margins of the patella. Furthermore, an assessment of limb alignment, muscle bulk, patellofemoral positional assessment, lateral retinacular testing and accessory movement would inform the assessment. It was thought there may also be a lack of single leg dynamic stability during function tasks and with the history of a previous ankle sprain on the most symptomatic side possible loss of ankle dorsiflexion ROM. Other tests which may have proved valuable for consideration included examination of passive hip range of movement, ITB length and examination of gluteal strength and control as well as foot and ankle biomechanical assessment.

There were not thought to be any contraindications of precautions.

Physical Examination

Functional Testing

The patient stood in a small degree of genu valgum. There was good muscle bulk bilaterally. During a one-leg squat, there was a valgus movement pattern on both legs with less ankle dorsiflexion on the left side. The knee pain proved modifiable and marginally improved when the patient was asked to concentrate on their knee position on landing and to try to avoid falling into

Continued

Case Study—cont'd

valgus. There was a significant improvement with a medial glide applied to the patella. Single-leg squat felt easier when performed with a heel raise.

ROM

Range of movement was full with no discomfort at end of range or extension.

Passive ROM

Screening of the hip showed this fully mobile and pain free when fully flexed and on examination of medial and lateral rotation in 90 degrees.

Clarke's Test

There was clear discomfort bilaterally on Clarke's testing which was worse on the left side.

Palpation

There was tenderness on palpation of both the medial and lateral margins of the patella bilaterally. There was no tenderness palpating the medial and lateral tibiofemoral joint lines and no pain on palpation of the patella or quadriceps tendons.

Patella Position Assessment and Patella Accessory Movements

The patella was well positioned; however, there was a slight lateral tilt which was accentuated on medial glide of the patella indicating tightness of the lateral retinaculum.

McMurray's Test

This was negative on both sides.

Clinical Diagnosis and Plan

The examination supported the diagnosis of patellofemoral pain. As pain during single-leg squat improved with a medial glide it was decided to trial a course of taping the patella with a medial glide. It was thought that a valgus movement pattern when landing on the right leg might be contributing to the maintenance of the condition as modifying the knee position on landing improved pain. Furthermore, loss of full ankle dorsiflexion was also felt to be a contributing factor and treatment was also targeted at this. It was decided therefore to explore this movement pattern further by attempting to modify this task whilst closely monitoring the symptomatic response and to look at gluteal strength, Craig's test for femoral anteversion as well as foot position on the second session. Treatment to reduce the effect of the tight lateral retinaculum was also considered an appropriate next step depending upon the outcome from the first session.

If after the second session it was thought that gluteal weakness and poor hip control were causing a valgus movement pattern as opposed to femoral anteversion contributing to the maintenance of the condition, a graded exercise programme to strengthen the gluteal muscles could be a useful starting point with the aim of progressing to more challenging function and sports-specific tasks.

REFERENCES

Abram, S.G.F., Beard, D.J., Price, A.J., BASK Meniscus Working Group, 2019. Arthroscopic meniscal surgery: a national society treatment guideline and consensus statement. Bone Jt. J. 101-B, 652–659.

Almangoush, A., Herrington, L., Jones, R., 2014. A preliminary reliability study of a qualitative scoring system of limb alignment during single leg squat. Phys. Ther. Rehabil. 1, 2.

Anderson, M.J., Browning 3rd, W.M., Urband, C.E., Kluczynski, M.A., Bisson, L.J., 2016. A systematic summary of systematic reviews on the topic of the anterior cruciate ligament. Orthop. J. Sports Med. 4 (3), 2325967116634074.

Baldon, R.M., Lobato, D.F., Carvalho, L.P., Wun, P.Y., Santiago, P.R., Serrao, F.V., 2012. Effect of functional stabilization training on lower limb biomechanics in women. Med. Sci. Sports Exerc. 44, 135–145.

Barnard, K.J., Ryder, D., 2024. Principles of Musculoskeletal Treatment and Management: A Handbook for Therapists, third ed. Churchill Livingstone, Edinburgh.

Barton, C.J., Balachandar, V., Lack, S., Morrissey, D., 2014. Patellar taping for patellofemoral pain: a systematic review and meta-analysis to evaluate clinical outcomes and biomechanical mechanisms. Br. J. Sports Med. 48 (6), 417–424.

Barton, C.J., Bonanno, D., Levinger, P., Menz, H.B., 2010. Foot and ankle characteristics in patellofemoral pain syndrome: a case control and reliability study. J. Orthop. Sports Phys. Ther. 40, 286–296.

Barton, C.J., Lack, S., Hemmings, S., Tufail, S., Morrissey, D., 2015. The 'best practice guide to conservative management of patellofemoral pain': incorporating level 1 evidence with expert clinical reasoning. Br. J. Sports Med. 49, 923–934.

Barton, C.J., Levinger, P., Crossley, K.M., Webster, K.E., Menz, H.B., 2011. Relationships between the Foot Posture Index and foot kinematics during gait in individuals with and without patellofemoral pain syndrome. J. Foot Ankle Res. 4, 10.

Beaufils, P., Becker, R., 2016. ESSKA Meniscus Consensus Project. ESSKA, Luxembourg.

Benjaminse, A., Gokeler, A., van der Schans, C.P., 2006. Clinical diagnosis of an anterior cruciate ligament rupture: a meta-analysis. J. Orthop. Sports Phys. Ther. 36, 267–288.

Bonadio, M.B., Helito, C.P., Gury, L.A., Demange, M.K., Pécora, J.R., Angelini, F.J., 2014. Correlation between magnetic resonance imaging and physical exam in assessment of injuries to posterolateral corner of the knee. Acta Ortop. Bras. 22, 124–126.

Collins, N.J., Barton, C.J., van Middelkoop, M., Callaghan, M.J., Rathleff, M.S., Vicenzino, B.T., et al., 2018. 2018 Consensus statement on exercise therapy and physical interventions (orthoses, taping and manual therapy) to treat patellofemoral pain: recommendations from the 5th international patellofemoral pain research retreat, Gold Coast, Australia, 2018. Br. J. Sports Med. 52, 1170–1178.

Cook, C., Mabry, L., Reiman, M.P., Hegedus, E.J., 2012. Best tests/clinical findings for screening and diagnosis of patellofemoral pain syndrome: a systematic review. Physiotherapy 98, 93–100.

Cyriax, J., 1982. Textbook of Orthopaedic Medicine—Diagnosis of Soft Tissue Lesions, eighth ed. Baillière Tindall, London.

Décary, S., Fallaha, M., Belzile, S., Martel-Pelletier, J., Pelletier, J.P., Feldman, D., et al., 2018. Clinical diagnosis of partial or complete anterior cruciate ligament tears using patients' history elements and physical examination tests. PLoS One 13 (6), e0198797.

Décary, S., Ouellet, P., Vendittoli, P.A., Desmeules, F., 2016. Reliability of physical examination tests for the diagnosis of knee disorders: evidence from a systematic review. Man. Ther. 26, 172–182.

Décary, S., Ouellet, P., Vendittoli, P.-A., Roy, J.-S., Desmeules, F., 2017. Diagnostic validity of physical examination tests for common knee disorders: an overview of systematic reviews and meta-analysis. Phys. Ther. Sport. 23, 143–155.

Dibra, F.F., Prieto, H.A., Gray, C.F., Parvataneni, H.K., 2017. Don't forget the hip! Hip arthritis masquerading as knee pain. Arthroplast. Today 4 (1), 118–124.

Draper, C.E., Besier, T.F., Santos, J.M., Jennings, F., Fredericson, M., Gold, G.E., et al., 2009. Using real-time MRI to quantify altered joint kinematics in subjects with patellofemoral pain and to evaluate the effects of a patellar brace or sleeve on joint motion. J. Orthop. Res. 27, 571–577.

Drosos, G.I., Pozo, J.L., 2004. The causes and mechanisms of meniscal injuries in the sporting and non-sporting environment in an unselected population. Knee 11 (2), 143–149.

Englund, M., Guermazi, A., Gale, D., Hunter, D.J., Aliabadi, P., Clancy, M., et al., 2008. Incidental meniscal findings on knee MRI in middle-aged and elderly persons. N. Engl. J. Med. 359 (11), 1108–1115.

Everhart, J.S., Cole, D., Sojka, J.H., Higgins, J.D., Magnussen, R.A., Schmitt, L.C., et al., 2017. Treatment options for patellar tendinopathy: a systematic review. J. Arthr. Relat. Surg. 33 (4), 861–872.

Farrokhi, S., Keyak, J.H., Powers, C.M., 2011. Individuals with patellofemoral pain exhibit greater patellofemoral joint stress: a finite element analysis study. Osteoarthr. Cartil. 19, 287–294.

Fox, A.J., Wanivenhaus, F., Burge, A.J., Warren, R.F., Rodeo, S.A., 2015. The human meniscus: a review of anatomy, function, injury, and advances in treatment. Clin. Anat. 28 (2), 269–287.

Frobell, R.B., Roos, E.M., Roos, H.P., Ranstam, J., Lohmander, L.S., 2010. A randomized trial of treatment for acute anterior cruciate ligament tears. N. Engl. J. Med. 363 (4), 331–342.

Gifford, L.S., 1998. Pain, the tissues and the nervous system: a conceptual model. Physiotherapy 84 (1), 27–36.

Giles, L.S., Webster, K.E., McClelland, J.A., Cook, J., 2013. Does quadriceps atrophy exist in individuals with patellofemoral pain? A systematic literature review with meta-analysis. J. Orthop. Sports Phys. Ther. 43, 766–776.

Giles, L.S., Webster, K.E., McClelland, J.A., Cook, J., 2015. Can ultrasound measurements of muscle thickness be used to measure the size of individual quadriceps muscles in people with patellofemoral pain? Phys. Ther. Sport 16, 45–52.

Glazer, D.D., 2009. Development and preliminary validation of the injury-psychological readiness to return to sport (I-PRRS) scale. J. Athl. Train. 44 (2), 185–189.

Grelsamer, R., McConnell, J., 1998. The Patella in a Team Approach. Aspen, Gaithersburg.

Gribble, P.A., Hertel, J., Plisky, P., 2012. Using the star excursion balance test to assess dynamic postural-control deficits and outcomes in lower extremity injury: a literature and systematic review. J. Athl. Train. 47 (3), 339–357.

Grindem, H., Snyder-Mackler, L., Moksnes, H., Engebretsen, L., Risberg, M.A., 2016. Simple decision rules can reduce reinjury risk by 84% after ACL reconstruction: the Delaware-Oslo ACL cohort study. Br. J. Sports Med. 50 (13), 1–6.

Hayes, C.W., Brigido, M.K., Jamadar, D.A., Propeck, T., 2000. Mechanism-based pattern approach to classification of complex injuries of the knee depicted at MR imaging. Radiographics a review publication of the Radiological Society of North America, Inc, 20 Spec No, S121-S134. https://doi.org/10.1148/radiographics.20.suppl_1.g00oc21s121.

Heino Brechter, J., Powers, C.M., 2002. Patellofemoral stress during walking in persons with and without patellofemoral pain. Med. Sci. Sports Exerc. 34, 1582–1593.

Herrington, L., 2008. The difference in a clinical measure of patella lateral position between individuals with patellofemoral pain and matched controls. J. Orthop. Sports Phys. Ther. 38, 59–62.

Herrington, L., Meyer, G., Horsley, I., 2013. Task based rehabilitation protocol for elite athletes following anterior cruciate ligament reconstruction: a clinical commentary. Phys. Ther. Sport. 14, 188–198.

Herrington, L., Munro, A., 2014. A preliminary investigation to establish the criterion validity of a qualitative scoring system of limb alignment during single-leg squat and landing. J. Ex. Sports Orthop. 1 (3), 1–6.

Herrington, L., Hussain, G., Comfort, P., 2021. Quadriceps strength and functional performance after anterior cruciate ligament reconstruction in professional soccer players at time of return to sport. J. Strength Cond. Res., 35 (3), 769–775.

Herrlin, S.V., Wange, P.O., Lapidus Gunilla, G., Hållander, M., Werner, S., Weidenhielm, L., 2013. Is arthroscopic surgery beneficial in treating non-traumatic, degenerative medial meniscal tears? A five year follow-up. Knee Surg. Sports Traumatol. Arthrosc. 21, 358–364.

Hewett, T.E., Myer, G.D., Ford, K.R., Heidt Jr., R.S., Colosimo, A.J., McLean, S.G., et al., 2005. Biomechanical measures of neuromuscular control and valgus loading of the knee predict anterior cruciate ligament injury risk in female athletes: a prospective study. Am. J. Sports Med. 33 (4), 492–501.

Irrgang, J.J., Anderson, A.F., Boland, A.L., Harner, C.D., Kurosaka, M., Neyret, P., et al., 2001. Development and validation of the international knee documentation committee subjective knee form. Am. J. Sports Med. 29 (5), 600–613.

Jan, M.-H., Lin, D.-H., Lin, J.-J., Lin, C.-H., Cheng, C.-K., Lin, Y.-F., 2009. Differences in sonographic characteristics of the vastus medialis obliquus between patients with patellofemoral pain syndrome and healthy adults. Am. J. Sports Med. 37 (9), 1743–1749.

Janda, V., 1994. Muscles and motor control in cervicogenic disorders: assessment and management. In: Grant, R. (Ed.), Physical Therapy of the Cervical and Thoracic Spine, second ed. Churchill Livingstone, New York, p. 195.

Janda, V., 2002. Muscles and motor control in cervicogenic disorders. In: Grant, R. (Ed.), Physical Therapy of the Cervical and Thoracic Spine, third ed. Churchill Livingstone, New York, p. 182.

Jones, M.A., Edwards, I., Gifford, L., 2002. Conceptual models for implementing biopsychosocial theory in clinical practice. Man. Ther. 7 (1), 2–9.

Jonsson, T., Althoff, B., Peterson, L., Renström, P., 1982. Clinical diagnosis of ruptures of the anterior cruciate ligament: a comparative study of the Lachman test and the anterior drawer sign. Am. J. Sports Med. 10, 100–102.

Jull, G.A., Janda, V., 1987. Muscles and motor control in low back pain: assessment and management. In: Twomey, L.T., Taylor, J.R. (Eds.), Physical Therapy of the Low Back. Churchill Livingstone, New York, p. 253.

Karachalios, T., Hantes, M., Zibis, A.H., Zachos, V., Karantanas, A.H., Malizos, K.N., 2005. Diagnostic accuracy of a new clinical test (the Thessaly test) for early detection of meniscal tears. J. Bone Jt. Surg. Am. 87, 955–962.

Katz, J.N., Brophy, R.H., Chaisson, C.E., de Chaves, L., Cole, B.J., Dahm, D.L., et al., 2013. Surgery versus physical therapy for a meniscal tear and osteoarthritis. N. Engl. J. Med. 368 (18), 1675–1684.

Katz, J.W., Fingeroth, R.J., 1986. The diagnostic accuracy of ruptures of the anterior cruciate ligament comparing the Lachman test, the anterior drawer sign, and the pivot shift test in acute and chronic knee injuries. Am. J. Sports Med. 14 (1), 88–91.

Kirkley, A., Birmingham, T.B., Litchfield, R.B., Giffin, J.R., Willits, K.R., Wong, C.J., et al., 2008. A randomized trial of arthroscopic surgery for osteoarthritis of the knee. N. Engl. J. Med. 359, 1097–1107.

Kopkow, C., Freiberg, A., Kirschner, S., Seidler, A., Schmitt, J., 2013. Physical examination tests for the diagnosis of posterior cruciate ligament rupture: a systematic review. J. Orthop. Sports Phys. Ther. 43, 804–813.

Kurzweil, P.R., Kelley, S.T., 2006. Physical examination and imaging of the medial collateral ligament and posteromedial corner of the knee. Sports Med. Arthrosc. Rev. 14 (2), 67–73.

Kyritsis, P., Bahr, R., Landreau, P., Miladi, R., Witvrouw, E., 2016. Likelihood of ACL graft rupture: not meeting six clinical discharge criteria before return to sport is associated with a four times greater risk of rupture. Br. J. Sports Med. 50, 946–951.

Lack, S., Barton, C., Sohan, O., Crossley, K., Morrissey, D., 2015. Proximal muscle rehabilitation is effective for patellofemoral pain: a systematic review with meta-analysis. Br. J. Sports Med. 49 (21), 1365–1376.

Lange, T., Freiberg, A., Dröge, P., Lützner, J., Schmitt, J., Kopkow, C., 2015. The reliability of physical examination tests for the diagnosis of anterior cruciate ligament rupture—a systematic review. Man. Ther. 20, 402–411.

Lankhorst, N.E., Bierma-Zeinstra, S.M., van Middelkoop, M., 2012. Factors associated with patellofemoral pain syndrome: a systematic review. Br. J. Sports Med. 47, 193–206.

Leblanc, M.C., Kowalczuk, M., Andruszkiewicz, N., Simunovic, N., Farrokhyar, F., Turnbull, T.L., et al., 2015.

Diagnostic accuracy of physical examination for anterior knee instability: a systematic review. Knee Surg. Sports Traumatol. Arthrosc. 23, 2805–2813.

Maffulli, N., Oliva, F., Loppini, M., Aicale, R., Spiezia, F., King, J.N., 2017. The Royal London Hospital test for the clinical diagnosis of patellar tendinopathy. Muscles Ligaments Tendons J. 7 (2), 315–322.

Magee, D.J., Manske, R.C., 2020. Orthopedic Physical Assessment, seventh ed. Elsevier.

Maricar, N., Callaghan, M.J., Parkes, M.J., Felson, D.T., O'Neill, T.W., 2015. Clinical assessment of effusion in knee osteoarthritis—a systematic review. Semin. Arthritis Rheum. 45, 556–563.

McClure, P.W., Rothstein, J.M., Riddle, D.L., 1989. Intertester reliability of clinical judgments of medial knee ligament integrity. Phys. Ther. 69 (4), 26–33.

McConnell, J., 1996. Management of patellofemoral problems. Man. Ther. 1 (2), 60–66.

McEwan, I., Herrington, L., Thom, J., 2007. The validity of clinical measures of patella position. Man. Ther. 12, 226–230.

McHale, K.J., Park, M.J., Tjoumakaris, F.P., 2014. Physical examination for meniscus tears. In: Kelly, I.V.J.D. (Ed.), Meniscal Injuries. Springer, New York, pp. 9–20 (Chapter 2).

McMurray, T.P., 1942. The semilunar cartilages. Br. J. Surg. 29 (116), 407–414.

Meira, E.P., Brumitt, J., 2011. Influence of the hip on patients with patellofemoral pain syndrome: a systematic review. Sports Health 3, 455–465.

Meyer, R., Lin, C., Yenokyan, G., Ellen, M., 2021. Diagnostic utility of ultrasound versus physical examination in assessing knee effusions: a systematic review and meta-analysis. J. Ultrasound Med. 41, 17–31.

Mitsou, A., Vallianatos, P., 1988. Clinical diagnosis of ruptures of the anterior cruciate ligament: a comparison between the Lachman test and the anterior drawer sign. Injury 19, 427–428.

Moseley, J.B., O.'Malley, K., Petersen, N.J., Menke, T.J., Brody, B.A., Kuykendall, D.H., et al., 2002. A controlled trial of arthroscopic surgery for osteoarthritis of the knee. N. Engl. J. Med. 347, 81–88.

Munro, A.G., Herrington, L.C., 2010. Between-session reliability of the star excursion balance test. Phys. Ther. Sport. 11 (4), 128–132.

Nijs, J., Van Geel, C., Van der auwera, C., Van de Velde, B., 2006. Diagnostic value of five clinical tests in patellofemoral pain syndrome. Man. Ther. 11, 69–77.

Noehren, B., Pohl, M.B., Sanchez, Z., Cunningham, T., Lattermann, C., 2012. Proximal and distal kinematics in female runners with patellofemoral pain. Clin. Biomech. 27, 366–371.

Ostrowski, J.A., 2006. Accuracy of 3 diagnostic tests for anterior cruciate ligament tears. J. Athl. Train. 41 (1), 120–121.

Pache, S., Aman, Z.S., Kennedy, M., Nakama, G.Y., Moatshe, G., Ziegler, C., et al., 2018. Posterior cruciate ligament: current concepts review. Arch. Bone Jt. Surg. 6 (1), 8–18.

Papadapoulos, K., Stasinopoulos, D., Ganchev, D., 2015. A systematic review of reviews on patellofemoral pain syndrome. Exploring the risk factors, diagnostic tests, outcome measurements and exercise treatment. Open Sports Med. J. 9, 7–19.

Peters, J.S.J., Tyson, N.L., 2013. Proximal exercises are effective in treating patellofemoral pain syndrome: a systematic review. Int. J. Sports Phys. Ther. 8 (5), 689–700.

Petersen, W., Ellermann, A., Gösele-Koppenburg, A., Best, R., Rembitzki, I.V., Brüggemann, G.P., et al., 2014. Patellofemoral pain syndrome. Knee Surg. Sports Traumatol. Arthrosc. 22, 2264–2274.

Rao, A.J., Erickson, B.J., Cvetanovich, G.L., Yanke, A.B., Bach Jr., B.R., Cole, B.J., 2015. The meniscus-deficient knee: biomechanics, evaluation, and treatment options. Orthop. J. Sports Med. 3 (10), 1–14.

Ross, M.D., Langford, B., Whelan, P.J., 2002. Test-retest reliability of 4 single-leg horizontal hop tests. J. Strength Cond. Res. 16 (4), 617–622.

Ruas, C.V., Pinto, R.S., Haff, G.G., Lima, C.D., Pinto, M.D., Brown, L.E., 2019. Alternative methods of determining hamstrings-to-quadriceps ratios: a comprehensive review. Sports Med. Open. 5 (11), 1–14.

Sahrmann, S.A., 2002. Diagnosis and Treatment of Movement Impairment Syndromes. Mosby, St Louis.

Siemieniuk, R.A.C., Harris, I.A., Agoritsas, T., Poolman, R.W., Brignardello-Petersen, R., Van de Velde, S., et al., 2018. Arthroscopic surgery for degenerative knee arthritis and meniscal tears: a clinical practice guideline. Br. J. Sports Med. 52 (5), 313.

Sihvonen, R., Englund, M., Turkiewicz, A., Järvinen, T.L., 2016. Mechanical symptoms and arthroscopic partial meniscectomy in patients with degenerative meniscus tear: a secondary analysis of a randomized trial. Ann. Intern. Med. 164, 449–455.

Sihvonen, R., Paavola, M., Malmivaara, A., Itälä, A., Joukainen, A., Nurmi, H., et al., 2013. Arthroscopic partial meniscectomy versus sham surgery for a degenerative meniscal tear. N. Engl. J. Med. 369, 2515–2524.

Smith, B.E., Thacker, D., Crewesmith, A., Hall, M., 2015. Special tests for assessing meniscal tears within the knee: a systematic review and meta-analysis. Evid. Based Med. 20, 88–97.

Smith, N.A., Costa, M.L., Spalding, T., 2015. Meniscal allograft transplantation: rationale for treatment. Bone Jt. J. 97-B (5), 590–594.

Smith, T.O., Davies, L., Donell, S.T., 2009. The reliability and validity of assessing medio-lateral patellar position: a systematic review. Man. Ther. 14, 355–362.

Smith, T.O., McNamara, I., Donell, S.T., 2013. The contemporary management of anterior knee pain and patellofemoral instability. Knee 20, S3–S15.

Solomonow, M., 2009. Ligaments: a source of musculoskeletal disorders. J. Bodyw. Mov. Ther. 13 (2), 136–154.

Souza, R.B., Draper, C.E., Fredericson, M., Powers, C.M., 2010. Femur rotation and patellofemoral joint kinematics: a weight-bearing magnetic resonance imaging analysis. J. Orthop. Sports Phys. Ther. 40, 277–285.

Swain, M.S., Henschke, N., Kamper, S.J., Downie, A.S., Koes, B.W., Maher, C.G., 2014. Accuracy of clinical tests in the diagnosis of anterior cruciate ligament injury: a systematic review. Chiropr. Man. Ther. 22, 25.

Thacker, M., 2015. Louis Gifford–revolutionary: the mature organism model, an embodied cognitive perspective of pain. Priv. Pract. 152, 4–9.

Torry, M.R., Decker, M.J., Viola, R.M., O'Connor, D.D., Steadman, J.R., 2000. Intra-articular knee joint effusion induces quadriceps avoidance gait patterns. Clin. Biomech. 15, 147–159.

van de Graaf, V.A., Noorduyn, J.C.A., Willigenburg, N.W., Butter, I.K., de Gast, A., Mol, B.W., et al., 2018. Effect of early surgery vs physical therapy on knee function among patients with nonobstructive meniscal tears: the ESCAPE randomized clinical trial. JAMA 320 (13), 1328–1337.

van Eck, C.F., van den Bekerom, M.P., Fu, F.H., Poolman, R.W., Kerkhoffs, G.M., 2013. Methods to diagnose acute anterior cruciate ligament rupture: a meta-analysis of physical examinations with and without anaesthesia. Knee Surg. Sports Traumatol. Arthrosc. 21, 1895–1903.

Wagemakers, H.P., Luijsterburg, P.A., Boks, S.S., Heintjes, E.M., Berger, M.Y., Verhaar, J.A., et al., 2010. Diagnostic accuracy of history taking and physical examination for assessing anterior cruciate ligament lesions of the knee in primary care. Arch. Phys. Med. Rehabil. 91, 1452–1459.

Warner, M.B., Wilson, D.A., Herrington, L., Dixon, S., Power, C., Jones, R., et al., 2019. A systematic review of the discriminating biomechanical parameters during the single leg squat. Phys. Ther. Sport. 36, 78–91.

Weiler, A., Frosch, K.H., Gwinner, C., Strobel, M.J., Lobenhoffer, P., 2021. The posterolateral Instability Score (PoLIS) of the knee joint: a guideline for standardized documentation, classification, and surgical decision-making. Knee Surg. Sports Traumatol. Arthrosc. 29 (3), 889–899.

Willy, R.W., Hoglund, L.T., Barton, C.J., Bolgla, L.A., Scalzitti, D.A., Logerstedt, D.S., et al., 2019. Patellofemoral pain. J. Orthop. Sports Phys. Ther. 49 (9), CPG1–CPG95.

Wilson, N.A., Press, J.M., Koh, J.L., Hendrix, R.W., Zhang, L. Q., 2009. In vivo noninvasive evaluation of abnormal patellar tracking during squatting in patients with patellofemoral pain. J. Bone Jt. Surg. Am. 91, 558–566.

Yim, J.-H., Seon, J.-K., Song, E.-K., Choi, J.-I., Kim, M.-C., Lee, K.-B., et al., 2013. A comparative study of meniscectomy and nonoperative treatment for degenerative horizontal tears of the medial meniscus. Am. J. Sports Med. 41 (7), 1565–1570.

17

Examination of the Foot and Ankle

Andrea Moulson

LEARNING OUTCOMES

After studying this chapter, you should be able to:

- Outline the anatomy and key functions of the foot and ankle complex.
- Discuss common pathological presentations for this region.
- Outline pertinent comorbidities and conditions which may affect the foot and ankle region.
- Describe the subjective and physical assessment for this region.
- Using clinical reasoning, justify the selection of tests and interpretation of findings related to common pathological presentations of the foot and ankle.

CHAPTER CONTENTS

Introduction to the Foot and Ankle Complex, 469
Anatomical and Functional Overview, 469
Subjective Examination/Taking the Patient's History, 470
Patient's Perspectives on Their Experience, 470
Outcome Measures, 470
Social History, 470
Body Chart, 471
Behaviour of Symptoms, 472
Special/Screening Questions and General Health, 472
Past Medical History, 473
History of the Present Condition, 473
Plan of the Physical Examination, 474
Physical Examination, 475
Observation, 475
Functional Testing, 476
Active Physiological Movements, 477
Passive Physiological Movements, 477
Weight-Bearing Lunge Test, 477
Joint Integrity Tests, 477
Muscle Tests, 481
Neurological Tests, 482
Tests for Circulation and Swelling, 482
Further Tests of the Foot and Ankle, 483
Palpation, 484
Accessory Movements, 484
Symptom Modification and Mobilizations With Movements, 486
Completion of the Examination, 488
Case Study, 494
References, 497

INTRODUCTION TO THE FOOT AND ANKLE COMPLEX

Anatomical and Functional Overview

The foot and ankle normally consist of a complex of 28 bones (tibia, fibula, calcaneus, talus, navicular, cuboid, medial/intermediate/lateral cuneiforms, 5 meta-tarsals, 14 phalanges), a variable number of sesamoids, with 34 joints and over 100 muscles, tendons and ligaments, all supplied by three different peripheral nerves—the tibial, common peroneal and saphenous. The main blood supply for the area originates from the peroneal, posterior tibial and anterior tibial arteries. Anatomically the foot is classically divided into the forefoot, midfoot and hindfoot, with specific joints associated with each area (Table 17.1).

Function

The foot and ankle form part of the whole-body kinetic chain and combine flexibility with stability to facilitate two principal functions: propulsion and support. For propulsion, the foot and ankle act as a complex flexible lever; for support, it acts as a rigid structure that supports the entire body weight. Aligned with these functions the foot and ankle must also adapt to uneven terrain and act as a shock absorber during the gait cycle as well as provide sensory information for balance (Nyland et al., 2018).

Foot and Ankle Dysfunction

There are many musculoskeletal (MSK) pathologies that can impact on the normal function of the foot and ankle; symptoms can arise from local anatomical sources, can be referred from other areas of the body or may be the result of systemic or genetic conditions. Trauma is common and can be problematic; for example, the reported pooled prevalence of lateral ankle sprains (LAS) is 11.88% in the general population (Doherty et al., 2014), and LAS can cause (amongst other injuries) fractures of the lateral malleolus, fractures of the fifth metatarsal, osteochondral defects of the talus, disruption of the inferior tibiofibular joint and lateral ligamentous complex with resultant ankle instability (Miller et al., 2017). Patients with foot and ankle dysfunction can also present with tendinopathies associated with acute overload or degenerative changes such as tibialis posterior tendon dysfunction or mid-substance/insertional Achilles tendinopathy (Chimenti et al., 2017; Ling & Liu, 2017). Neural tissue sensitization can be associated with trauma, surgery, increased pressure, degenerative changes or entrapment; examples of this include tarsal tunnel syndrome and Morton's neuroma (Pomeroy et al., 2015). Other insidious-onset conditions, such as plantar fasciopathy and osteoarthritis can significantly impact activities of daily living, whilst systemic inflammatory conditions, such as rheumatoid arthritis (RA), ankylosing spondylosis (AS) and gout, can also result in pain and deformities (Helliwell et al., 2019). Metabolic disorders such as diabetes may affect the foot, causing peripheral neuropathy, vascular compromise and specific disease such as Charcot disease (Dewi & Hinchcliffe, 2020). Hereditary predisposition to certain conditions is recognized, including a familial link to hallux valgus and lesser-toe deformities (Hannan et al., 2013). Less commonly encountered upper motor neuron and lower motor neuron conditions, such as traumatic brain injury, stroke, spinal cord injury, cerebral palsy and Charcot–Marie–Tooth disease, can also have a significant impact on foot and ankle function. These examples are by no means exhaustive but highlight the diversity of conditions which can affect the region. In recognition of the foot and ankle's functional significance and complexity patients with specific conditions (or postsurgery) may be managed by a dedicated foot and ankle therapy team which could include orthopaedic doctors, physiotherapists, chiropodists, podiatrists, nurses and radiologists.

TABLE 17.1 Functional Units of the Foot

Rearfoot	Midfoot	Forefoot
Talocrural joint	Talonavicular joint	Tarsometatarsal joints
Subtalar joint	Calcaneocuboid joint	Metatarsophalangeal joint Interphalangeal joints

A thorough knowledge of functional anatomy and biomechanics will inform clinical reasoning, ensuring the initial examination is efficient and management strategies seek to optimize all aspects of functional restoration.

KNOWLEDGE CHECK

1. What are the four key functions of the foot and ankle?
2. Name the main joints which make up the foot and ankle complex.
3. Name the three main nerves and arteries which supply the foot and ankle complex.
4. Name four common musculoskeletal conditions that can affect the foot and ankle.
5. Name four health care professions commonly involved with the management of patients with foot and ankle conditions.

SUBJECTIVE EXAMINATION/TAKING THE PATIENT'S HISTORY

This chapter will focus on questions asked and tests utilized in the physical examination of the foot and ankle complex; these should be individualized to the patient. Details on the principles of the subjective and physical examinations can be found in Chapters 3 and 4, respectively.

Patient's Perspectives on Their Experience

Most patients will seek treatment because they have symptoms and/or functional limitations which are impacting their activities of daily living, for example, pain, paraesthesia, swelling and/or difficulty with weight-bearing activities. Sometimes patients experience difficulty finding comfortable footwear or the aesthetic appearance of the foot alone or in combination with other symptoms is troublesome, this may affect the patient's psychological well-being. Examples of this include progressive hallux valgus or claw/hammer-toe deformities (Souza Júnior et al., 2020) (Fig. 17.1).

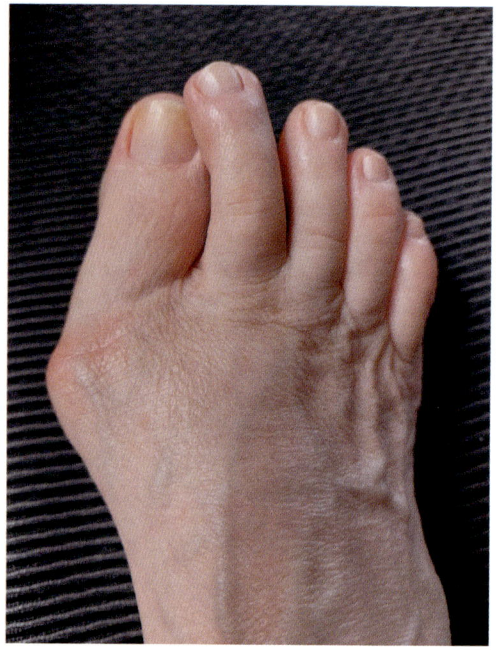

Fig. 17.1 Right hallux valgus with associated lesser toe deformity.

Outcome Measures

There are a number of self-reported outcome tools that can be used to measure patients' perception of disability, the impact of symptoms/surgery on function and to measure the effect of interventions over time, e.g.

- American Orthopaedic Foot and Ankle Score (AOFAS)
- Foot and Ankle Ability Measure (FAAM)
- Foot and Ankle Disability Index (FADI)
- Foot Function Index (FFI)
- Foot Health Status Questionnaire (FHSQ)
- Lower Extremity Function Scale (LEFS)
- Manchester-Oxford Foot Questionnaire (MOFQ)

See Shazadeh Safavi et al. (2019) and Jia et al. (2017) for an overview of the properties of these and similar outcome measures.

Social History

Social history that is relevant to the onset and progression of the patient's problem is important to explore. For example, an increased training load may result in symptoms related to conditions such as plantar fasciopathy or Achilles tendinopathy (Martin et al., 2014; Silbernagel et al., 2020). Early identification of psychosocial and behavioural risk factors is important as these may play a role in the development of symptoms and persistent disability. For example, chronic alcohol consumption can result in foot and lower limb paraesthesia/anaesthesia, pain, hyporeflexia, reduced proprioception and gait ataxia (Thomas et al., 2019), whereas smoking and depression have been linked to the development of chronic regional pain syndrome following elective foot surgery (Rewhorn et al., 2014).

Body Chart

The following information concerning the type and area of current symptoms can be recorded on a body chart (see Fig. 3.2 for an example of a typical body chart).

Area of Current Symptoms

Be exact. It is often useful to ask the patient to use one finger to point to the location of predominant symptoms. Dysfunction in the foot and ankle tends to produce local symptoms and follow recognizable patterns. For example, with stress fractures of the foot and lower limb, the area of pain tends to be localized, can be exercise-induced and improves with rest (Welck et al., 2017), whilst plantar fasciopathy is the most common cause of medial plantar heel pain, is often worse on initial weight bearing after periods of rest and can get worse with prolonged weight-bearing activities (Martin et al., 2014).

Areas Relevant to the Region Being Examined

Symptoms in the foot and ankle may be referred from more proximal sources such as the lumbosacral spine, sacroiliac and hip structures (Slipman et al., 2000; Lesher et al., 2008; Nelson & Hall, 2011). Symptoms may also arise as a result of poor proximal control of the pelvis, hip or knee or as a result of dysfunctional foot biomechanics, which may result in compensatory pathological loads on tendons at the foot and ankle (Sueki et al., 2013).

Quality of Symptoms

The quality of symptoms informs clinical reasoning; paraesthesia supports a hypothesis of neural tissue dysfunction, especially if associated with burning, shooting or electric shock-type pain (Pomeroy et al., 2015). Following LAS, functional or mechanical ligamentous instability may result in 'giving way' of the ankle, ankle stiffness and complaints of weakness (Remus et al., 2018; Hertel & Corbett, 2019). Descriptions of stiffness and locking may indicate degenerative changes, for example, hallux rigidus of the first metatarsophalangeal joint (MTPJ) or OA of the talocrural joint (Adukia et al., 2020; Chan & Sakellariou, 2020). Prolonged joint stiffness, especially in the morning, may indicate systemic disorders particularly if associated with other signs and symptoms of inflammatory/reactive disease, e.g. RA, Reiter's, gout, psoriasis, AS (NICE, 2017). It is important to check for any altered sensation such as paraesthesia, anaesthesia, hypoaesthesia, hyperaesthesia and allodynia throughout the lower limb and locally around the foot. The distribution of any sensory changes will help to differentiate between dermatomal distribution from spinal nerve roots, symptoms of peripheral nerve origin and upper motor neuron lesions (see Chapter 3). For example, bilateral paraesthesia/anaesthesia in both hands and feet associated with weakness/heaviness in the legs, difficulty walking and difficulties with fine-motor activities, e.g. writing, could indicate the serious condition of cervical myelopathy (Cook & Cook, 2016).

Determine whether symptoms are felt on the surface or deep inside. Deep anterolateral or anteromedial ankle pain after LAS in conjunction with pain on weight bearing may indicate the presence of an osteochondral lesion, whilst more superficial symptoms may support purely soft-tissue involvement (Wodicka et al., 2016; Kerkhoffs & Karlsson, 2019).

Intensity of Pain

The intensity of pain can be measured (as explained in Chapter 3) and contributes to clinical reasoning of severity, alongside the use of analgesic medication, sleep disturbance and limitation in activities. Severity and irritability will guide the extent and vigour of the physical examination.

Constant or Intermittent Symptoms

Ascertain the frequency of symptoms. Progressive unremitting pain may require investigation to exclude serious pathology such as neoplastic disease (Kennedy et al., 2016; Darcey, 2017). Whilst cancer is uncommon in the foot and ankle constant pain may indicate inflammatory disorders such as gout and RA (NICE. 2017). Incapacitating pain associated with sensory, motor, vasomotor and/or trophic changes, could highlight the development of chronic regional pain syndrome, which can be a complication following fractures, minor injury and surgery (Kim, 2016; Cowell et al., 2019).

Relationship of Symptoms

If the patient has proximal and distal symptoms, determine the relationship between the areas. This information will assist with reasoning the most likely source of symptoms and so focus the physical examination.

Behaviour of Symptoms

Aggravating Factors

For each symptomatic area, ask what functional activities, movements and/or positions aggravate the patients' symptoms, if they are able to maintain an activity or position or whether they have to stop (severity)? How long does it take for symptoms to ease once the position or movement is stopped (irritability)? Irritability and severity are explained in Chapter 3. The clinician should clinically reason how symptoms impact function and lifestyle. For example, patients with Morton's neuroma or hallux valgus tend to dislike tight, narrow shoe wear and prefer to be barefoot or use flipflops, etc. (Alrabai et al., 2016). Validated clinical prediction rules are useful to diagnose specific pathologies. For example, anterolateral ankle impingement demonstrates the following features: anterolateral joint tenderness and recurrent swelling, pain with forced dorsiflexion and eversion, pain with single-leg squat, pain with activities and the possible absence of ankle instability (Liu et al., 1997).

Easing Factors

For each symptomatic area, the clinician assesses irritability by exploring what eases symptoms, how long symptoms take to ease and to what extent. Collating this information with a thorough knowledge of specific pathologies and typical presentations helps to refine hypothesis generation, guide further history taking and determine reasoned physical examination. If the patient's symptoms do not fit an MSK presentation, then the clinician needs to be alert to other, possibly more serious causes and refer on.

Behaviour of Symptoms Over Time

How do symptoms behave over 24 hours?

Night symptoms. Whilst night pain may raise suspicions of serious pathology, it is useful to consider alternative hypotheses as well. For example, patients with OA may describe night pain as the disease progresses (Khlopas et al., 2019), and night pain in this group may be one indication for surgery.

Morning and evening symptoms. The clinician determines the pattern of the symptoms throughout the day. Early-morning pain and stiffness for an hour or more may be suggestive of inflammatory conditions such as RA or AS (NICE, 2017). Patients with plantar fasciopathy or tendinopathy describe classic 'start-up' pain on initial weight bearing in the morning which can continue in the day with prolonged weight bearing or repetitive activity (Lancaster & Madhaven, 2021).

Special/Screening Questions and General Health

As discussed in Chapter 3, the clinician must differentiate between conditions that are suitable for conservative treatment and other systemic, neoplastic and nonmusculoskeletal conditions, which may require referral elsewhere. Chapter 3 discusses special questions in detail; hence, only examples relevant to the foot and ankle are highlighted below.

Serious Pathology

Malignant tumours in this area are rare (Kennedy et al., 2016), and the foot and ankle are also atypical sites for MSK tuberculosis; if suspected, patients should be asked about possible exposure to tuberculosis (Faroug et al., 2018).

Osteoporosis

Associations between low bone mineral density and ankle fractures in the elderly have been established (So et al., 2020), and if osteoporosis is suspected the vigour of the physical examination will need to be modified.

Inflammatory Arthritis

Patients should be asked if they or a member of their family has been diagnosed with an inflammatory condition. Overall, the lifetime risk of foot involvement in patients with RA is 90%, and this condition can initially present in the small joints of the feet (Yano et al., 2018; Walker et al., 2019).

Cardiovascular Disease

Does the patient have a history of cardiovascular disease, e.g. hypertension, angina, previous myocardial infarction, stroke? Patients who develop symptoms of peripheral vascular disease may present with intermittent claudication—an aching muscle pain in the calf or foot that is brought on by exercise and rapidly relieved by rest (Spannbauer et al., 2019).

Diabetes Mellitus

The foot and ankle are targets of this complex multisystem disease, which is a result of chronic hyperglycaemia caused by insulin deficiency. The effects of diabetes can manifest from mild neuropathy to severe ulcerations, infections, vasculopathy, Charcot arthropathy, neuropathic fractures and ultimately amputation (Walker et al., 2019; Dewi & Hinchcliffe, 2020). As a result of vascular deficits, tissue healing is likely to be slower. Patients with the disease have been shown to have significantly higher rates of postoperative complication, infection, Charcot arthropathy, nonunion and amputation after ankle fracture compared to patients without diabetes (Lavery et al., 2020). Diabetic neuropathy affecting the feet and hands typically presents with a stocking-and-glove distribution, beginning distally and spreading proximally, and can demonstrate a combination of diminished light touch sensation, proprioception, temperature awareness and pain perception (Oji & Schon, 2013).

Neurological Symptoms If a Spinal Lesion Is Suspected

See Chapter 3 for discussions related to spinal cord compression, cauda equina syndrome and neuropathic pain presentations. Of note, spinal cord compression may also result in bilateral tingling in the hands or feet (Cook & Cook, 2016). Pes cavus (clawing of the feet) can be the result of a number of hereditary, neurological and idiopathic conditions (Seaman & Ball, 2021) but new onset, unilateral progressive pes cavus warrants urgent further neurosurgical investigation as this may indicate the present of a spinal cord or brain tumour (Grice et al., 2016).

Past Medical History

A detailed medical history will identify contraindications and precautions to the physical examination and may help explain the development of current symptoms. For example, a history of endocrine abnormalities, in particular, vitamin D deficiency has been associated with nonunion after elective foot and ankle reconstruction (Moore et al., 2017). Other relevant disorders have been outlined above in special questions and general health.

History of the Present Condition

For each symptomatic area, the clinician asks how long symptoms have been present, whether there was a sudden or slow onset and whether there was a clear cause. If the patient can recall a traumatic onset, such as a fall, closer questioning of the mechanism of injury is imperative. Under the Ottawa ankle rules, patients should be referred for radiographic examination (or other medical imaging) to exclude fractures if they have pain and tenderness in the malleolar area/s, the base of the fifth metatarsal, navicular or an inability to weight bear four steps immediately after injury and when admitted to an emergency department. These rules have a sensitivity of almost 100% and a modest specificity and are used for adults and children over the age of 5 (Beckenkamp et al., 2017). Alternatively, if there has been an insidious onset of symptoms, the clinician questions for change in the patient's lifestyle, e.g. a new job or hobby, or a change in existing sporting activities, including alterations in footwear, equipment, surface or intensity. Sensitively determining recent or chronic weight gain can assess the impact of additional biomechanical stresses; increased body mass index in the nonathletic population has been associated with conditions such as plantar fasciopathy (Martin et al., 2014). The goal is to establish what has happened or to build a picture of what has changed to understand fully why a patient is presenting with symptoms.

Is this the first episode or is there a history of foot or ankle problems? If so, how many episodes? When were they? What was the cause? What was the duration of each episode? Did the patient fully recover between episodes? It may be that injuries sustained years previously are relevant, for example, previous ankle sprains or fractures have been associated with the development of osteochondral lesions and posttraumatic arthritis (Ewalefo et al. 2018; Lee et al., 2021). If there have been no previous episodes, has the patient had incidences of stiffness in the lumbar spine, hip or knee or any other relevant region? In addition, the clinician needs to ask if the patient has sought treatment to date, what it was and whether it helped. What has the patient been told and by whom? What does the patient believe is going on? Collaboratively clarifying the patient's journey can help the clinician to understand the patient's context and inform patient-centred clinical reasoning.

Radiography and Medical Imaging

Has the patient undergone any radiological investigations? Radiographs are the cornerstone of diagnostic imaging and provide an often essential screening tool for many foot and ankle problems. When trauma is involved the Ottawa ankle rules provide guidelines for patients who should be x-rayed (Beckenkamp et al. 2017). Magnetic resonance imaging (MRI) is used to evaluate soft-tissue pathology of the foot and ankle and is particularly useful for imaging osteochondral lesions, bony and soft-tissue tumours, stress reactions, bone bruising, ligamentous damage, bursitis, fasciopathy, tendinopathy/tendon tears and the diabetic foot (Mohan et al., 2010; Pedowitz, 2012). Ultrasound is used to examine soft tissues, such as tendons, ganglions and neuromas, and is the preferred imaging modality when Morton's neuroma or Achilles tendinosis is suspected (Beard & Gousse, 2018). It is also useful for guiding aspirations and specific injections. Computed tomography (CT) provides rapid imaging to help evaluate complex anatomy and pathology and is used primarily for evaluating bone as opposed to soft tissue. The multiplanar nature of CT enhances its ability to detect disease not appreciable on plain radiographs (Haapamäki et al., 2005). SPECT-CT, a radionuclide bone scan with single-photon emission CT and CT, is a relatively new imaging modality which combines highly detailed CT with the functional information from a triple-phase radionuclide bone scan. SPECT-CT is increasingly recognized as having high diagnostic accuracy and is recommended for use in foot and ankle cases of diagnostic uncertainty and for the evaluation of chronic foot/ankle pain, especially in patients with previous surgery or in-situ metal work (Eelsing et al., 2021).

Other tests may include blood tests, required if systemic inflammatory conditions such as RA, AS or gout are suspected.

Results from additional investigations will provide information to inform clinical reasoning and may help indicate a likely prognosis.

KNOWLEDGE CHECK

1. Name four non-MSK comorbidities which may have an impact on the assessment and management of patients with MSK foot and ankle conditions.
2. Describe how diabetes might affect the foot and ankle.
3. What rules are used to determine if a patient needs an x-ray to exclude fracture in the ankle and midfoot after trauma?
4. How does plantar fasciopathy typically present?

KNOWLEDGE CHECK—cont'd

5. Name four types of medical imaging which may be used in the management of foot and ankle dysfunction and what these are typically used for.

Plan of the Physical Examination

The information from the subjective examination helps the clinician identify an initial primary hypothesis, alternative hypotheses and to plan the physical examination. The severity, irritability and nature of the condition are key factors that influence the choice and priority of physical testing procedures. Initially, the clinician might ask: 'Is this patient's condition suitable for me to manage as a therapist?' For example, a patient presenting with progressive unilateral pes cavus symptoms may only need neurological testing prior to an urgent medical referral. Hence the nature of the patient's condition has a major impact on the physical examination. Following this, the clinician might question: 'Does this patient have a musculoskeletal dysfunction that I may be able to help?' To answer that, a full physical examination is required; however, this may not be possible if the symptoms are severe and/or irritable. If this is the case, the clinician aims to explore movements as much as possible, within a symptom-free range. If the patient has constant and severe and/or irritable symptoms, then it is wise to use physical tests that ease symptoms; it may be that the patient will require rest periods between tests to avoid build-up in symptoms. Alternatively, for patients with symptoms judged to be of low severity and irritability, physical testing will need to be more searching and may require the use of overpressures, and repeated and combined movements to reproduce symptoms. In addition to symptom reproduction and easing, contributing factors such as foot posture and biomechanics may need to be examined for relevance. A planning form can help guide the clinician's reasoning in the selection of physical examination procedures (see Fig. 3.7). An understanding of the sensitivity and specificity (see Chapter 4) of the tests applied should also be considered so that findings can be interpreted appropriately. Each significant physical test that either provokes or eases the patient's symptoms is highlighted in the patient's notes by an asterisk (*) for easy reference. The clinician needs to have a clear clinical hypothesis after the subjective examination, the purpose of the physical examination is to confirm or refute this hypothesis.

It is important for readers to understand that the physical examination approaches included in this chapter are some of many and that those chosen are clinically useful and include an indication of their level of support in the literature.

PHYSICAL EXAMINATION

Observation

Informal Observation

Throughout the subjective and physical examination, the clinician notices the patient's behaviours. Has the patient been able to weight bear easily on the foot and ankle coming into the clinic, what footwear is being used, is the patient distressed, etc.?

Formal Observation

Observation of posture. The patient should be suitably dressed so that the clinician can observe the patient's bony and soft-tissue contours in standing and non-weight bearing, noting the posture of the feet, lower limbs, pelvis and spine. General lower-limb abnormalities include uneven weight bearing through the legs and feet, internal femoral rotation and genu varum/valgum or recurvatum (hyperextension). It is worth noting whether the foot has a particularly flattened or exaggerated medial longitudinal arch, as these may indicate pes planus or pes cavus respectively. The toes may be deformed, for example, claw toes, hammer toes, mallet toes and hallux valgus/rigidus. Further details of these abnormalities can be found in a standard orthopaedic textbook (Thordarson, 2013; Magee, 2021).

Observation of foot and ankle alignment. Impaired alignment of the foot and ankle may result in suboptimal movement patterns, impacting on function. Multiple theories and approaches to the assessment of foot and lower-limb biomechanics have developed over time (Root et al., 1977; Dananberg, 1986; McPoil & Hunt, 1995; Kirby, 2001; Vicenzino, 2004; Redmond et al., 2006; Fuller & Kirby, 2013). Preferencing one method over another is controversial (Kirby, 2015; Harradine et al., 2018); however, it is useful when beginning to assess foot and ankle biomechanics to use a systematic approach.

The Foot Posture Index (FPI) (Redmond et al., 2006) is one such approach and consists of six validated, criterion-based observations of the rearfoot and forefoot with a patient standing in a relaxed position. The rearfoot is assessed via palpation of the head of the talus, observation of the curves above and below the lateral malleoli and the extent of the inversion/eversion of the calcaneus. Observations of the forefoot consist of assessing the bulge in the region of the talonavicular joint, the congruence of the medial longitudinal arch and the extent of abduction/adduction of the forefoot on the rearfoot. The FPI has demonstrated concurrent and internal construct validity as well as high intra-rater reliability and moderate interrater reliability (Redmond et al. 2006; Keenan et al., 2007; Fraser et al., 2017), and results in a score between -12 and $+12$ (where -12 indicates a highly supinated foot posture and $+12$ indicates a highly pronated foot posture; normative values of $+4$ in the adult population have been suggested) (Redmond et al., 2008). Research has linked FPI scores to lower-limb pathologies such as medial compartment knee OA, hip OA, chronic plantar heel pain, medial tibial stress syndrome and midfoot OA (Yates & White, 2004; Irving et al., 2007; Reilly et al. 2009; Levinger et al., 2010; Lithgow et al., 2020), although this relationship is unclear and not fully established (Neal et al., 2014). The use of such tools can assist clinicians in supporting or refuting clinically reasoned hypotheses, communicating with colleagues, educating patients and can assist in management decision making such as the use of/referral for orthotics.

Observation of muscle form. The clinician observes the muscle bulk and muscle tone of the lower limb, comparing the left and right sides for relevant differences, remembering that level and frequency of physical activity as well as leg dominance may produce differences in muscle bulk between sides.

Observation of soft tissues. The clinician observes the quality of the patient's skin, any area of swelling, redness, exostosis, callosities or presence of scarring or infection.

Common observations in the foot and ankle include the following:

- pes planus (flatfoot)
- pes cavus (high arch)
- hallux valgus: valgus alignment of the hallux at the MTPJ with prominent medial eminence $\pm$ pronation

of the big toe. Often referred to as a 'bunion' (see Fig. 17.1)
- hallux rigidus: OA of the first MTPJ which may result in palpable bony osteophytes over the dorsal aspect of the first MTPJ
- hammer-toe deformity: affecting the lesser toes, the proximal interphalangeal joint has a flexion contracture with secondary extension at the MTPJ and distal interphalangeal joint. Can be fixed or flexible
- claw-toe deformity: affecting the lesser toes, the MTPJ is hyperextended, with flexion contracture at the proximal interphalangeal and distal interphalangeal joints. Can be fixed or flexible
- mallet-toe deformity: flexion contracture of the distal interphalangeal joint. Can be fixed or flexible
- bunionette (tailor's bunion): characterized by the prominence of the lateral aspect of the fifth metatarsal head and medial deviation of the fifth toe at the MTPJ, often with associated callus
- Haglund's deformity: a bony exostosis located on the posterolateral or posteromedial aspect of the calcaneus. Aetiology is unclear but may be the result of overuse, hereditary factors or biomechanical stresses (Vaishya et al., 2016)
- fusiform swelling locally in the Achilles tendon may indicate a reactive tendinopathy (Cook et al., 2016), usually observed in the midportion of the Achilles tendon.
- intractable plantar keratosis (IPK): hyperkeratotic tissue proliferation (callus) on the plantar aspect of the foot, usually under the metatarsal head(s), occurs as a result of excessive mechanical load.
- posteromedial pitting oedema along the course of the tibialis posterior: this observation has been associated with tibialis posterior tendon dysfunction; a condition more common in mid to later-aged women often with comorbidities (DeOrio et al. 2011; Ross et al., 2018)
- adult acquired flatfoot deformity: secondary to tibialis posterior tendon dysfunction, this ranges from a flexible deformity to a rigid deformity with advanced arthritis. Clinical observations can include hindfoot valgus, medial arch collapse, forefoot abduction with 'too-many-toes' sign and inability to perform double and single heel-rise tests (Zaw & Calder, 2010; Ross et al., 2017).
- oedema as a result of trauma/ankle sprain—swelling observed proximally to the ankle mortise may indicate syndesmotic injury of the inferior tibiofibular joint, whereas swelling distal to the lateral malleolus may indicate a lateral ligament complex injury, although this may spread into the foot if the capsule has been damaged (Dubin et al., 2011)

Functional Testing

Functional testing can be carried out early in the examination. Clues for appropriate tests can be obtained from the subjective examination, particularly aggravating factors; these might include activities such as walking, ascending/descending stairs, squatting, walking on uneven surfaces, hopping or running.

Observation of Gait

Gait analysis is important. Observe gait in a logical manner from head to toe, or vice versa, observing each body segment for variations in the normal range. Look for asymmetries, e.g. uneven arm swing, trunk rotation, stride length and differences in weight bearing. Each variation may indicate tight musculature, structural anomalies or functional movement patterns which may have altered through habit or dysfunction. The gait cycle is defined as 'the time interval between two successive occurrences of one of the repetitive events of walking' (Whittle et al. 2012, p. 32). The gait cycle consists of the following events:

1. initial contact (often heel strike)
2. opposite toe-off
3. heel rise
4. opposite initial contact
5. toe-off
6. feet adjacent
7. tibial vertical
8. initial contact—the gait cycle begins again.

The angle of heel contact with the ground is usually slightly varus. Marked variations from this may cause abnormal foot function, with compensation attained either across the midtarsal joint and first and fifth rays or more proximally in the ankle, knee and hip joints. Early heel lift may indicate tight posterior leg muscles which can be a cause of functional ankle equinus (Pascual Huerta, 2014), where the range of dorsiflexion required for normal gait is lacking.

The degree of pronation of the foot during midstance is noted. Pronation is a normal part of gait that allows the foot to become a shock absorber and mobile adapter. Prolonged pronation or failure/delayed supination of the subtalar joint during mid to late stance (often indicated by a prolonged or rigid valgus of the calcaneum and collapse of the medial longitudinal arch) may indicate tibialis posterior tendon dysfunction (Zaw & Calder, 2010; Stein & Schon, 2015). At heel lift the foot changes to a more rigid lever for toe-off. Limitation of normal function at the MTPJs may affect toe-off and result in more proximal compensations (Nix et al. 2013).

Active Physiological Movements

Active physiological movements of the foot and ankle and possible modifications are shown in Table 17.2. Movements can be tested with the patient in prone, supine or sitting with the right and left sides compared. The range of movement for the foot and ankle can be measured using a goniometer. For active physiological movements, the clinician notes the following:

- willingness of the patient to move
- range of movement available
- quality of movement, e.g. coordination, muscle activation patterns
- behaviour of pain through the range of movement.

Active movements with overpressure to the foot and ankle are shown in Fig. 17.2. Overpressure at the end of the range can be applied to the whole foot. For differentiation purposes, the foot may be considered in functional units: the rearfoot, midfoot and forefoot (see Table 17.1). Using a knowledge of the joint lines the various regions may be individually examined with localized overpressure at the end of the range. The clinician establishes the patient's symptoms at rest, prior to each movement, and notes the effect of passively correcting any movement deviation to determine its relevance to the patient's symptoms.

TABLE 17.2 Active Physiological Movements and Possible Modifications

Active Physiological Movements	Modifications
Ankle dorsiflexion	Repeated
Ankle plantarflexion	Speed altered
Inversion	Combined, e.g.
Eversion	• Inversion with plantarflexion
Metatarsophalangeal	Compression or distraction
• Flexion	Sustained
• Extension	Injuring movement
Interphalangeal joints:	Differentiation tests
• Flexion	Function
• Extension	

Passive Physiological Movements

All of the active movements can be examined passively with the patient in prone with the knee at 90 degrees flexion, or supine with the knee flexed over a pillow, comparing the left and right sides. Comparison of the response of symptoms/range of movement to the active and passive movements can help to determine whether the structures contributing to symptoms/restriction are noncontractile (articular) or contractile (myogenic).

Weight-Bearing Lunge Test

This is a test to measure the range of functional dorsiflexion of the ankle joint. The patient is in weight-bearing and is asked to place one foot perpendicular to a wall, and then lunge the ipsilateral knee to the wall, keeping the hips in a neutral position. The foot is then progressively moved away from the wall until the knee barely touches the wall; however, the foot should remain flat to the floor, without the heel lifting and should not deviate laterally or medially (Fig. 17.3). The distance from the wall to the big toe is then measured in centimetres. Left and right sides are compared for differences; normative studies on healthy adults suggest a 2 cm or greater lunge distance asymmetry can delineate subjects with clinically relevant impairments in ankle/subtalar dorsiflexion (Hoch & McKeon, 2011). Research also indicates this test is both reliable and valid and has reasonable responsiveness to detect a true change in range of motion (Powden et al., 2015; Hall & Docherty, 2017).

Joint Integrity Tests

Osseous congruency, static ligamentous and capsular restraints and myofascial structures are the major contributors to stability at the ankle. LAS are the most common injury, followed by syndesmotic disruption and then medial ankle sprain (Doherty et al., 2014), with significant rates of persistent symptoms and disability following acute ankle sprain (Martin et al., 2021). LAS consist of partial or complete disruption of the lateral ankle ligaments (anterior talofibular ligament

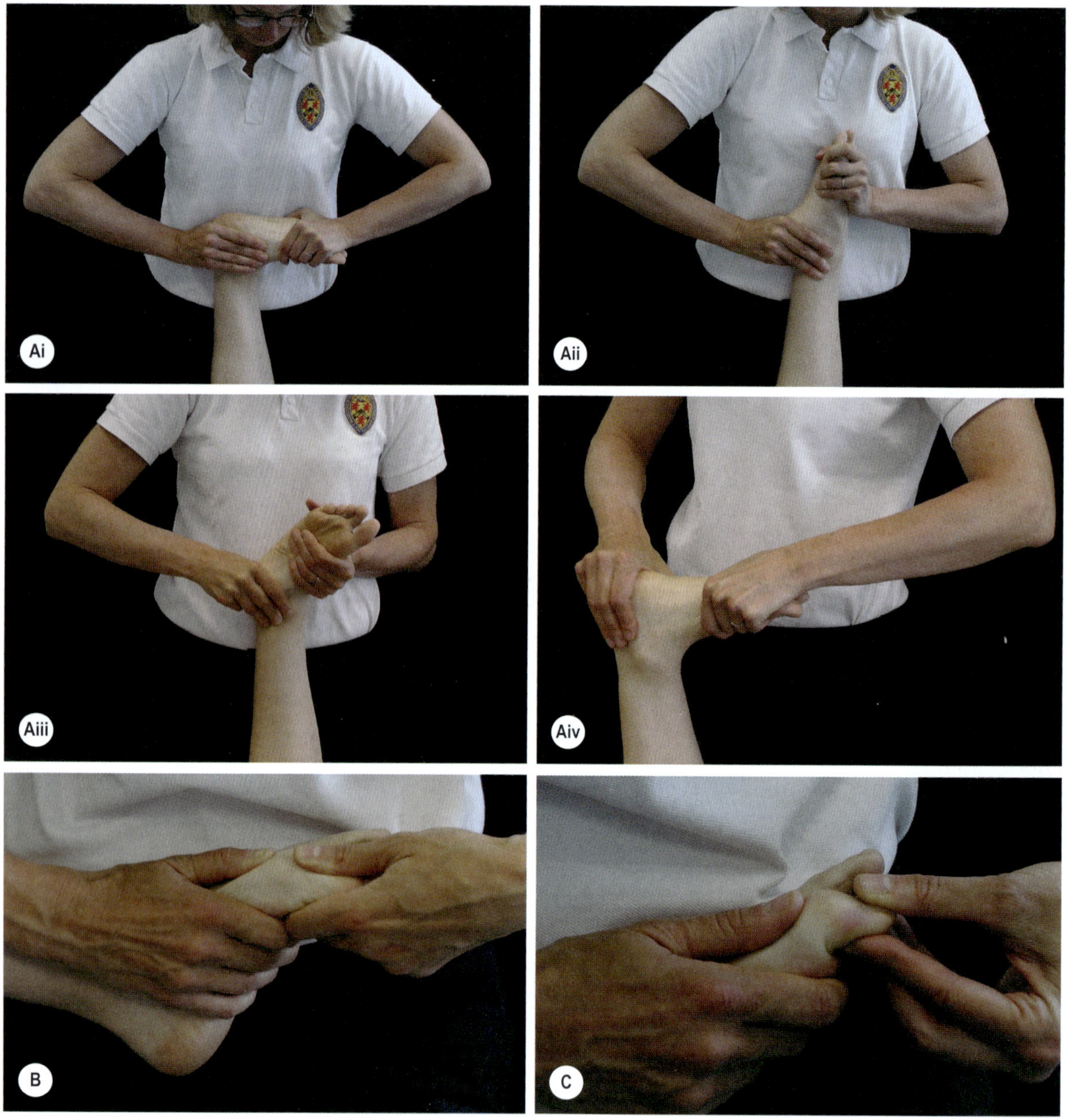

Fig. 17.2 Overpressures to the foot and ankle. (Ai) Dorsiflexion. The right hand tips the calcaneus into dorsiflexion while the left hand and forearm apply overpressure to dorsiflexion through the forefoot. (Aii) Plantarflexion. The left hand grips the forefoot, and the right hand grips the calcaneus, and together they move the foot into plantarflexion. (Aiii) Inversion. The right hand adducts the calcaneus and reinforces the plantarflexion movement while the left hand plantarflexes the hindfoot and adducts, supinates and plantarflexes the midfoot and forefoot. (Aiv) Eversion. The right hand abducts the calcaneus and reinforces the dorsiflexion while the left hand dorsiflexes the hindfoot and abducts, pronates and dorsiflexes the midfoot and forefoot. (B) Metatarsophalangeal joint flexion (demonstrated) and extension. The right hand stabilizes the metatarsal while the left hand flexes and extends the proximal phalanx. (C) Interphalangeal joint flexion and extension. The right hand stabilizes the proximal phalanx while the left hand flexes (demonstrated) and extends the distal phalanx.

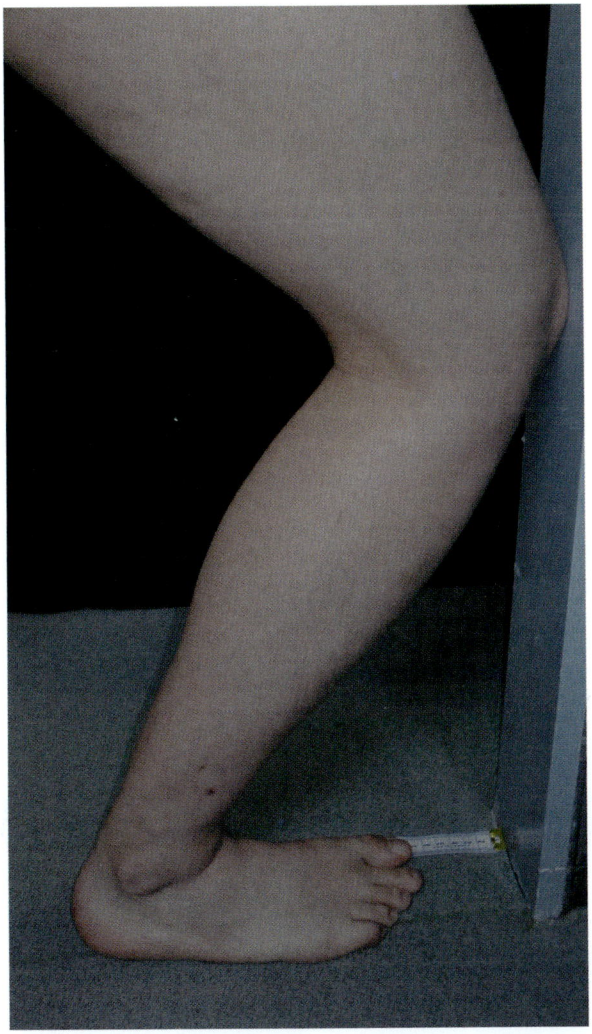

Fig. 17.3 Weight-bearing lunge test. Ankle fully dorsiflexed and knee against the wall. Note the heel is firmly on the floor and perpendicular to the wall, with measurement of the distance of the big toe from the wall.

[ATFL], calcaneofibular ligament [CFL] and posterior talofibular ligament [PTFL]), but the majority of injuries involve ATFL disruption (Martin et al., 2021). Differing mechanisms of injury are suggested for different ligamentous structures. For example, the ATFL is most likely to be injured in positions of ankle plantarflexion and inversion, whereas the CFL is vulnerable in positions of ankle dorsiflexion and inversion. Conversely, the most common position for syndesmotic injuries is ankle dorsiflexion and external rotation (Sman et al., 2013; Delahunt et al., 2018). For a comprehensive review of anatomical considerations see Medina McKeon & Hoch (2019). Subjective information can be combined with physical examination tests to support the clinical reasoning process. Joint integrity tests then form part of a reasoned examination.

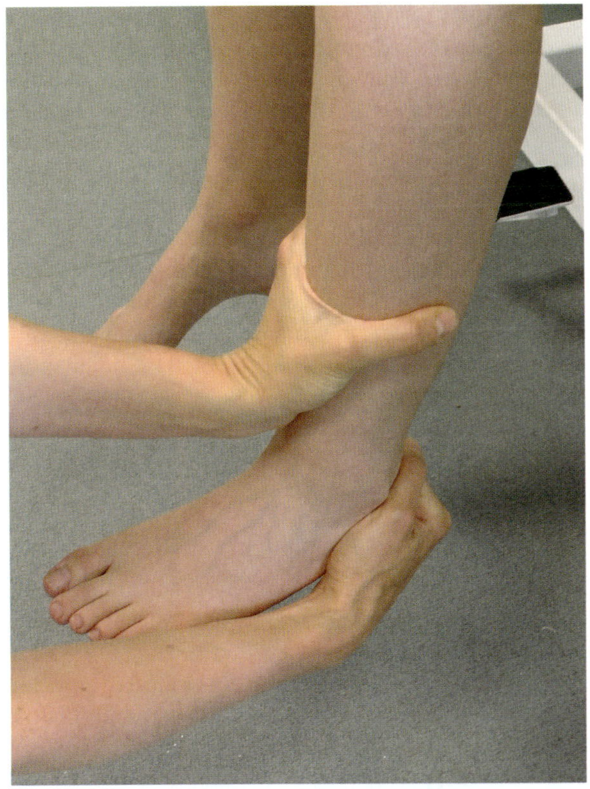

Fig. 17.4 Anterior drawer sign. The left hand stabilizes the lower leg while the right hand applies a posteroanterior force to the talus via the calcaneus.

Anterior Drawer Sign

This is a test of anterior talar translation with respect to the ankle mortise. The patient is usually positioned in sitting with 90 degrees of knee flexion and ankle plantarflexion between 10 and 20 degrees. The leg should be relaxed and unsupported. One hand of the examiner is placed on the anterior aspect of the distal tibia and fibula. The second hand grasps the posterior aspect of the calcaneus. The test is performed by applying a firm posteroanterior force to the calcaneus (and hence the talus) while the distal tibia/fibula is stabilized (Fig. 17.4). The test can also be performed in other positions, such as supine or prone, with slight flexion of the knee. Excessive anterior translation of the talus, compared to the uninvolved side, with a loose end-feel, indicates a reduction in the passive stabilizing function of the medial and lateral ligaments (Martin et al., 2021). Observation of a dimple or sulcus sign near the region of the ATFL may also indicate a rupture of the ATFL (Cook & Hegedus, 2011; Delahunt et al., 2018). The combination of pain with palpation of the ATFL, lateral haematoma and a positive anterior drawer on examination 5 days after the injury has demonstrated a sensitivity of 96% and specificity of 84% to identify lateral ligament rupture (van Dijk et al. 1996) and is recommended in several clinical guidelines (Delahunt et al., 2018; Vuurberg et al. 2018; Martin et al., 2021) to assess ATFL integrity.

Talar Tilt

The talar tilt is a test of the amount of talar inversion occurring within the ankle mortise. The patient is usually positioned in sitting with 90 degrees of knee flexion, with the leg relaxed and unsupported and the ankle in a plantigrade position. One hand of the examiner is placed on the distal tibia and fibula while the second hand grasps the calcaneus and slowly moves it into inversion; a small amount of traction can be applied (Fig. 17.5). Increased adduction movement of the calcaneus on the involved side compared to the uninvolved side, a reduced or absent end-feel and clicks/clunks suggest injury to the lateral ligament complex or that the calcaneofibular ligament (CFL) is injured. The test can also be performed in other positions, such as supine or prone. Sensitivity ranges between 17% and 66% and specificity ranges between 82% and 100% have been reported for this test which predominantly biases the CFL (Netterström-Wedin et al. 2021; Schweitzerian et al., 2013).

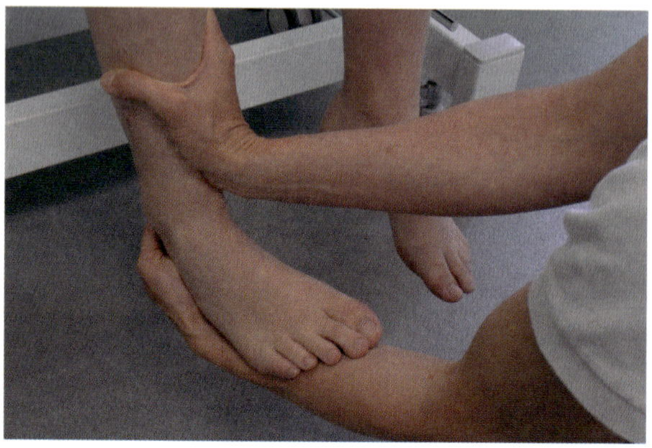

Fig. 17.5 Talar tilt. The left hand grips around the calcaneum and talus and moves it into a small amount of inversion whilst the other hand stabilizes the lower leg.

External Rotation Stress Test (Kleiger Test)

This is a test of the integrity of the inferior tibiofibular syndesmosis; it is pain provocative. The patient is usually positioned in sitting with 90 degrees of knee flexion. The examiner stabilizes the tibia and fibula with one hand in a manner which does not compress the distal tibiofibular syndesmosis. With the other hand, the examiner holds the foot in plantigrade and applies a passive lateral rotation stress to the foot and ankle (Fig. 17.6). The test can also be performed in other positions, such as supine or prone. A positive test is indicated if pain is produced over the anterior or

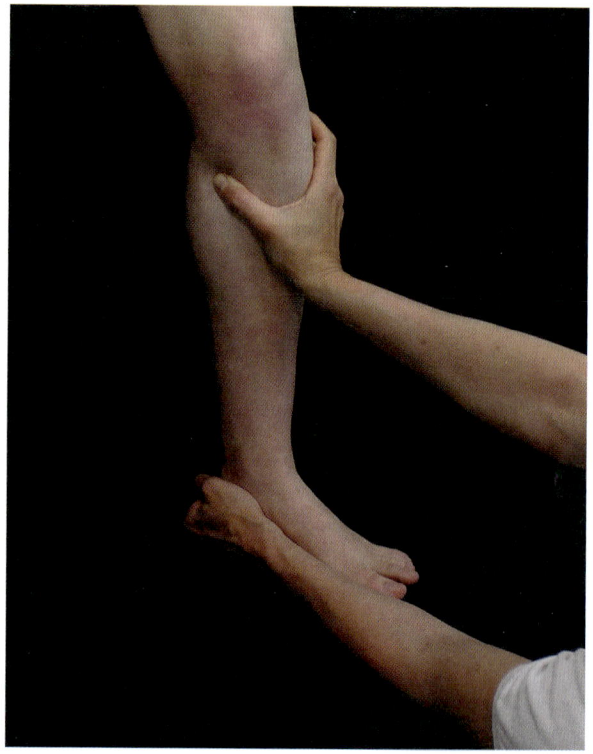

Fig. 17.6 External rotation stress test. The right hand stabilizes the lower leg while the left hand holds the foot in plantigrade and applies a passive external rotation stress to the foot and ankle.

posterior tibiofibular ligaments and the interosseous membrane and is indicative of a syndesmosis 'high ankle' injury. The specificity for this test has been reported at 78% with a sensitivity of 70% (Netterström-Wedin & Bleakley, 2021).

Squeeze Test

The squeeze test is a test of the integrity of the inferior tibiofibular syndesmosis; it is pain provocative. The patient is usually positioned in sitting with 90 degrees of knee flexion or in supine with the knee in a small degree of flexion. The examiner applies a manual squeeze, pushing the fibula and tibia together, and applying a force at the midpoint of the calf. The examiner then applies the same load at more distal locations moving toward the ankle (Fig. 17.7). Pain in the lower leg may indicate a syndesmotic injury (provided fracture and compartment syndrome have been ruled out). Pooled specificity data for this test was reported at 85% in a systematic review with the meta-analysis by Netterström-Wedin and Bleakley (2021), who promote the use of this test as, not/part of a cluster to include syndesmotic palpation, dorsiflexion lunge test and the external rotation stress test to help diagnose syndesmotic injuries.

Muscle Tests

Muscle system examination is based on the patient's subjective history as well as observations of posture and movement (Kendall et al. 2010). See Chapter 4 for details of muscle testing which may include isometric, isotonic and eccentric muscle testing in various parts of the range of the muscle group being tested, e.g. inner range, outer range and through range.

Muscle Strength

Manual muscle testing may be carried out for the following muscle groups:

- ankle dorsiflexors, plantarflexors
- foot inverters, evertors
- toe flexors, extensors, abductors and adductors.

For details of these tests, readers are directed to Kendall et al. (2010).

Muscle Length

The clinician tests the length of muscles that may have an impact on lower-limb function, in particular, those thought prone to shorten, that is, piriformis, iliopsoas, rectus femoris, tensor fasciae latae, hamstrings, gastrocnemius and soleus (Janda 1994, 2002). Testing the length of these muscles is described in Chapter 4.

Other Muscle Tests

Thompson's test for Achilles tendon rupture. With the patient prone and the feet over the end of the plinth or kneeling with the foot unsupported, the clinician squeezes the calf muscle; the absence of ankle plantarflexion indicates a positive test (Fig. 17.8). Sensitivity and specificity for this test to detect a subcutaneous Achilles tendon rupture have been reported as 96% and 93% respectively (Maffulli 1998; Schweitzerian et al., 2013).

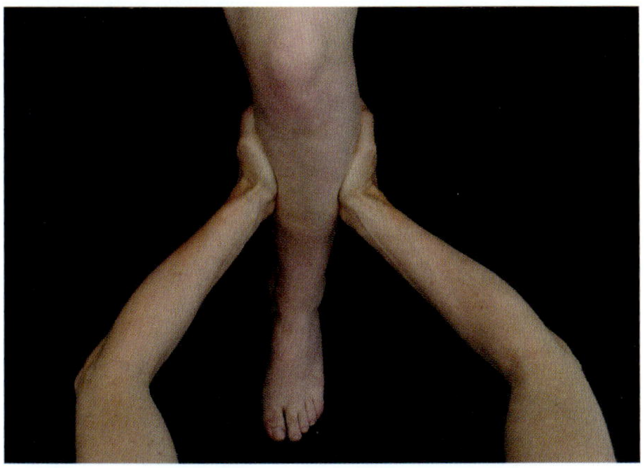

Fig. 17.7 Squeeze test. Both hands apply a manual squeeze, pushing the tibia and fibula together at the midpoint of the calf.

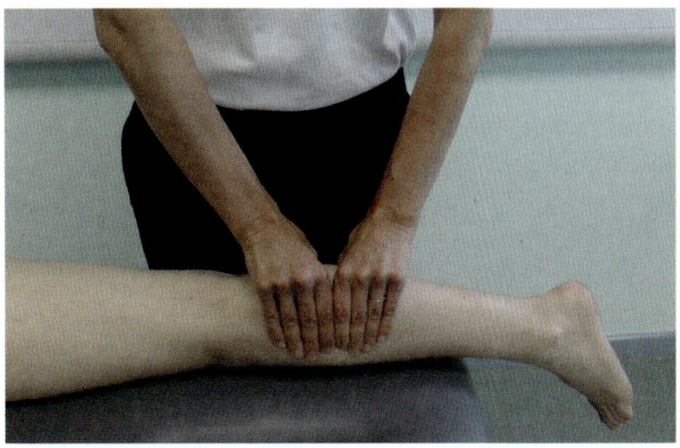

Fig. 17.8 Thompson's test. The therapist's hands squeeze the calf while observing plantarflexion movement of the foot.

Matles test for Achilles tendon rupture. The patient is positioned in prone lying and is asked to actively flex the knees to 90 degrees. The position of the ankles and feet is observed during flexion of the knee. If the foot on the affected side falls into neutral or into dorsiflexion, an Achilles tendon tear is suspected. On the uninjured side, the foot remains in slight plantarflexion when the knee is flexed to 90 degrees (Matles, 1975). Sensitivity and specificity values of 88% of 85% respectively have been reported for this test (Maffulli, 1998; Reiman et al., 2014).

Neurological Tests

The clinician will use clinical reasoning from the reported distribution and quality of symptoms, to justify a neurological examination.

Integrity of the Nervous System

Dermatomes/peripheral nerves. Sensory testing of the lower limb can be done as described in Chapter 4. Knowledge of the cutaneous distribution of spinal nerve roots (dermatomes) and peripheral nerves enables the clinician to distinguish sensory loss due to a spinal root lesion from that due to a peripheral nerve lesion. The cutaneous nerve distribution and dermatome areas are shown in Chapter 4.

Myotomes/peripheral nerves. A working knowledge of the myotomes of spinal nerve roots and peripheral nerves enables the clinician to distinguish motor loss due to a root lesion from that due to a peripheral nerve lesion. The peripheral nerve distributions are shown in Chapter 4.

Reflex testing. The following deep tendon reflexes can be tested (see Chapter 4):

- L3–L4: knee jerk
- S1: ankle jerk.

Neurodynamic Tests

Lower limb neurodynamic tests (SLR, Slump and PKB) may be used to assess for a possible neural tissue contribution to the patient's ankle and foot symptoms, see review in Chapter 4.

Variations in foot position have been suggested to stress different peripheral nerves. For example, ankle plantarflexion/inversion may bias the common peroneal nerve, ankle dorsiflexion/eversion may bias the tibial (and consequently the medial and lateral plantar nerves and the medial calcaneal nerve), whilst dorsiflexion/inversion may bias the sural nerve (Alshami et al., 2008).

Nerve Palpation

- Palpable nerves in the lower limb are as follows:
  - The tibial nerve can be palpated behind the medial malleolus, which may be more noticeable with the foot in dorsiflexion and eversion and may even produce symptoms if percussed, e.g. in tarsal tunnel syndrome (McSweeney & Cichero, 2015).
  - The common peroneal nerve can be palpated medial to the tendon of the biceps femoris and also around the head of the fibula.
  - The superficial peroneal nerve can be palpated on the dorsum of the foot along an imaginary line over the fourth metatarsal; it is more noticeable with the foot in plantarflexion and inversion.
  - The deep peroneal nerve can be palpated between the first and second metatarsals, lateral to the extensor hallucis tendon.
  - The sural nerve can be palpated on the lateral aspect of the foot behind the lateral malleolus, lateral to the Achilles.

For a review of foot and ankle entrapment neuropathies, see Pomeroy et al. (2015).

Tests for Circulation and Swelling

Vascular Tests

The vascular evaluation of the foot and ankle includes palpation of the dorsalis pedis and posterior tibial pulses and peripheral testing of capillary refill (Thordarson, 2013; King et al. 2014). The state of the vascular system can also be determined by the response of symptoms to positions of dependence and elevation of the lower limbs and response to exercise, e.g. in intermittent claudication.

Wells score for suspected deep-vein thrombosis. If an adult patient presents with signs or symptoms of deep-vein thrombosis (DVT), such as a painful warm, swollen leg, clinicians are advised to carry out an assessment of their general medical history and a physical examination to exclude other causes. National Institute for Health and Care Excellence (NICE) guidelines recommend the use of a two-level DVT Wells score to estimate the clinical probability of DVT (NICE, 2020). From this, the patient is given a score of between −2 and +9. A simplified scoring system of two points or more indicates a likely DVT, whilst a score of one point or less indicates this is unlikely. In both situations further investigation is required; this may include a D-dimer blood test, proximal leg vein ultrasound or parenteral anticoagulant. Readers are referred to the most current NICE guidelines for further information on this topic, including details of the two-level Wells score and exceptions to these recommendations (Wells et al. 2003; NICE, 2020; NICE CKS, 2020).

Figure-of-eight ankle measurement. This test measures the size and swelling of an ankle. The patient is positioned in long sitting with both feet extended over the end of a plinth. The ankle should be in approximately 20 degrees of plantarflexion. A 6-mm (1/4-inch)-wide plastic tape measure is placed midway between the tendon of the tibialis anterior and the lateral malleolus. The tape is pulled medially toward the instep, just distal to the tuberosity of the navicular. The tape is then drawn across the arch of the foot to just proximal to the base of the fifth metatarsal, then continues across the tibialis anterior tendon, around the ankle joint just distal to the medial malleolus and then across the Achilles tendon. From here the tape circles around the ankle, ending just distal to the lateral malleolus, before returning to the start position (Fig. 17.9). The figure-of-eight method has been demonstrated to be a reliable and valid method of measuring ankle oedema (Mawdsley et al., 2000; Rohner-Spengler et al., 2007; Devoogdt et al., 2019).

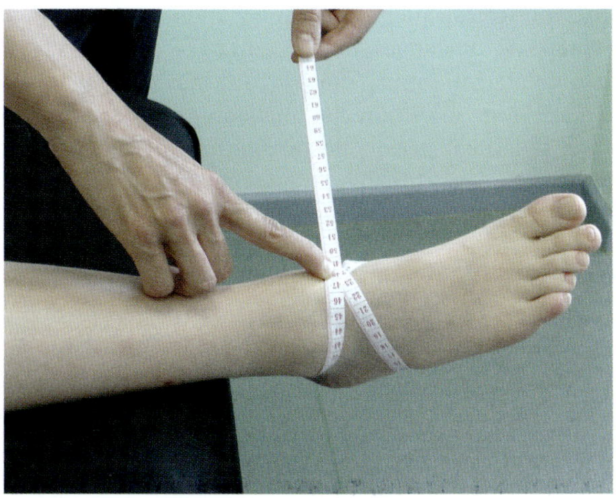

Fig. 17.9 Figure-of-eight ankle measurement for swelling.

Further Tests of the Foot and Ankle

Anterior Impingement Sign of the Talocrural Joint

This is a pain provocation test for anterior impingement of the talocrural joint (bony and/or soft tissue). The patient is usually positioned in sitting with 90 degrees of knee flexion, with the leg relaxed and unsupported. The test can also be performed with the patient supine or prone. One hand of the examiner is placed with the thumb palpating the anterolateral ankle and applying localized pressure whilst the other hand moves the ankle from a plantarflexed to dorsiflexed position (Fig. 17.10). Reproduction of symptoms signifies a positive test. Research suggests a sensitivity of 95% and a specificity of 88% for this sign (Molloy et al., 2003).

Mulder's Test for Morton's Neuroma

This is a pain provocation test for Morton's neuroma between the metatarsal heads. The patient is normally positioned in supine with the foot relaxed. This test is performed with the thumb and index finger on the plantar and dorsal aspect of the painful intermetatarsal space, exerting local pressure. The forefoot is then further compressed with the opposite hand by squeezing together the metatarsal heads. The test is considered positive if a palpable click is felt with the reproduction of pain. Mahadevan et al. (2015) report a

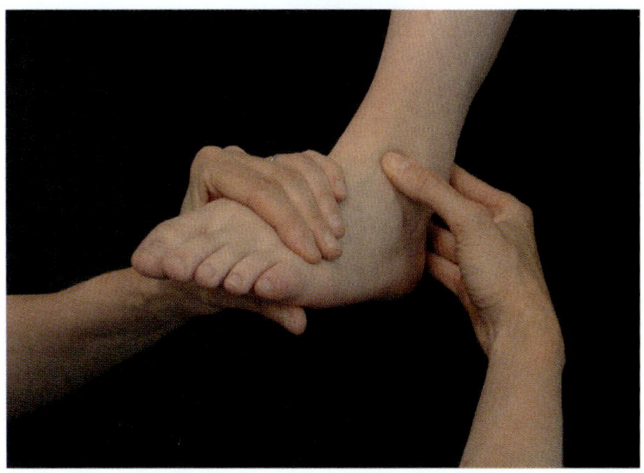

Fig. 17.10 Anterior impingement sign of the talocrural joint. The thumb of the right hand palpates the anterolateral aspect of the ankle joint, applying a localized pressure whilst the left hand moves the ankle from a plantarflexed to dorsiflexed position.

sensitivity of 62% and a specificity of 100% for this test compared with ultrasonography.

Star Excursion Balance Test

This is a measurement of dynamic balance of the lower limb. The Star Excursion Balance Test (SEBT) layout consists of eight lines set out from a central point, arranged at 45 degree angles (Fig. 17.11). The patient is asked to maintain balance on the lower limb to be tested while reaching as far as possible in eight different directions with the other foot, lightly touching the ground with that foot and then returning to centre. The distance achieved is measured in centimetres along each line. Patients should not move their supporting foot and keep their hands on their hips. The patient is allowed six practice and three test trials in each of the eight directions.

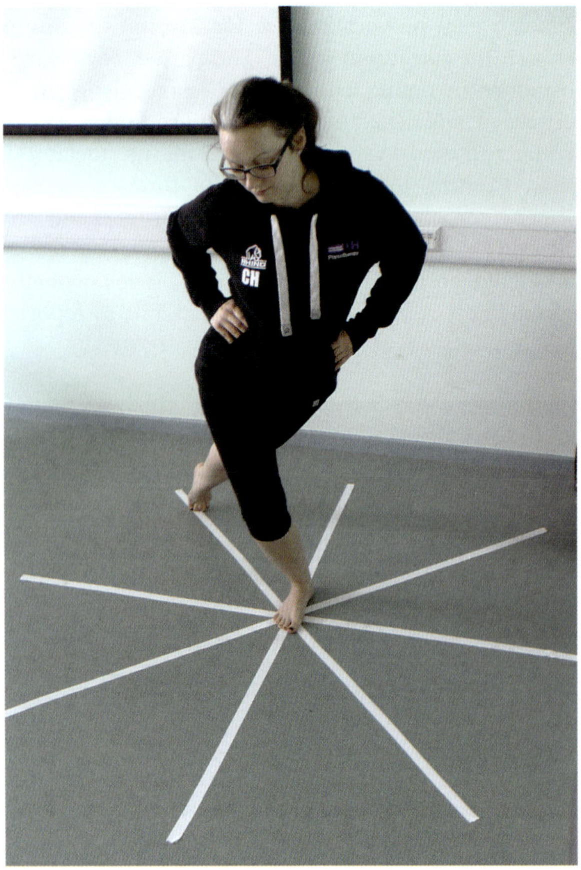

Fig. 17.11 Star excursion balance test (SEBT).

The SEBT has been shown to be a valid and reliable measure which can predict the risk of lower-extremity injury, identify dynamic balance deficits in patients with a variety of lower-extremity conditions, and is responsive to training programmes in healthy and injured populations (Gribble et al., 2012; Powden et al., 2019). Modifications to the test include a reduction of the number of practice tests to four (Robinson & Gribble, 2008) and simplifying the SEBT to three directions only (anterior, posterolateral and posteromedial); this is known as the Y-balance test (Hertel et al., 2006; Neves et al. 2017).

Palpation

Clinical reasoning will determine which structures the clinician palpates in the foot and ankle; however, it is useful to have a systematic approach to this so that nothing is missed (Alazzawi et al., 2017). Palpation findings can be recorded on a body chart (see Fig. 3.2) and/or palpation chart (see Fig. 4.34).

Suggested Approach to Systematic Palpation

Palpate bones, tendons and soft tissues for tenderness, crepitus, swelling, temperature, presence of ganglions/lumps, muscle spasm and any additional variations from the expected.

Palpate proximally to distally, starting from the proximal fibula and moving distally along the fibula to the syndesmosis, distal fibula, Achilles tendon (note if there is an intrasubstance gap which may indicate a tendon rupture), peroneal tendons laterally, PTFL, CFL, ATFL, anterior talocrural joint line, sinus tarsi, dorsalis pedis pulse, calcaneum, calcaneocuboid joint, cuboid, metatarsals, phalanges, first IP and MTP joint, first ray, tarsometatarsal joints, cuneiforms, navicular, talonavicular joint, talus, medial malleolus, posterior tibial pulse, tibialis posterior, flexor digitorum longus, flexor hallucis longus, tibialis anterior, toe extensors and flexors and the plantar fascia.

Accessory Movements

A selection of accessory movements for the foot and ankle joints are shown in Fig. 17.12 and listed in Table 17.3; however, it will not be necessary to test all of those listed, as selection will be based on clinical reasoning of findings so far in the physical examination. For example, if ankle dorsiflexion is limited then

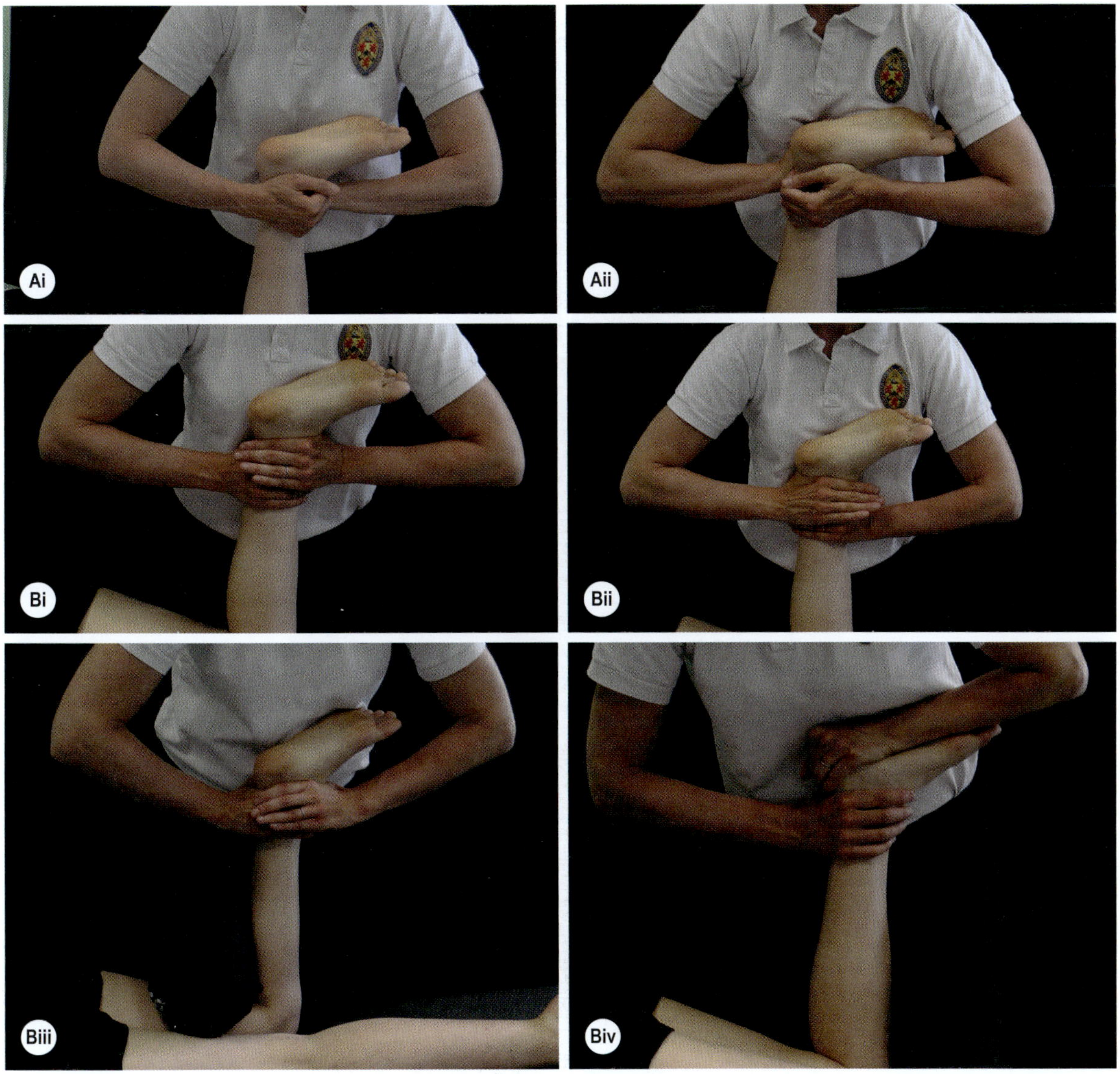

Fig. 17.12 Accessory movements for the foot and ankle joints. (A) Inferior tibiofibular joint. (Ai) Anteroposterior. The heel of the right hand applies a posteroanterior force to the tibia while the left hand applies an anteroposterior force to the fibula. (Aii) Posteroanterior. The left hand applies an anteroposterior force to the tibia while the right hand applies a posteroanterior force to the fibula. (B) Talocrural joint. (Bi) Anteroposterior. The right hand stabilizes the calf while the left hand applies an anteroposterior force to the anterior aspect of the talus. (Bii) Posteroanterior. The left hand stabilizes the tibia/fibula while the right hand applies a posteroanterior force to the posterior aspect of the talus. (Biii) Longitudinal caudad. The clinician lightly rests their leg on the posterior aspect of the patient's thigh to stabilize and then grasps around the talus to pull upwards. (Biv) Longitudinal cephalad. The right hand supports the foot in dorsiflexion while the left hand applies a longitudinal cephalad force through the calcaneus.

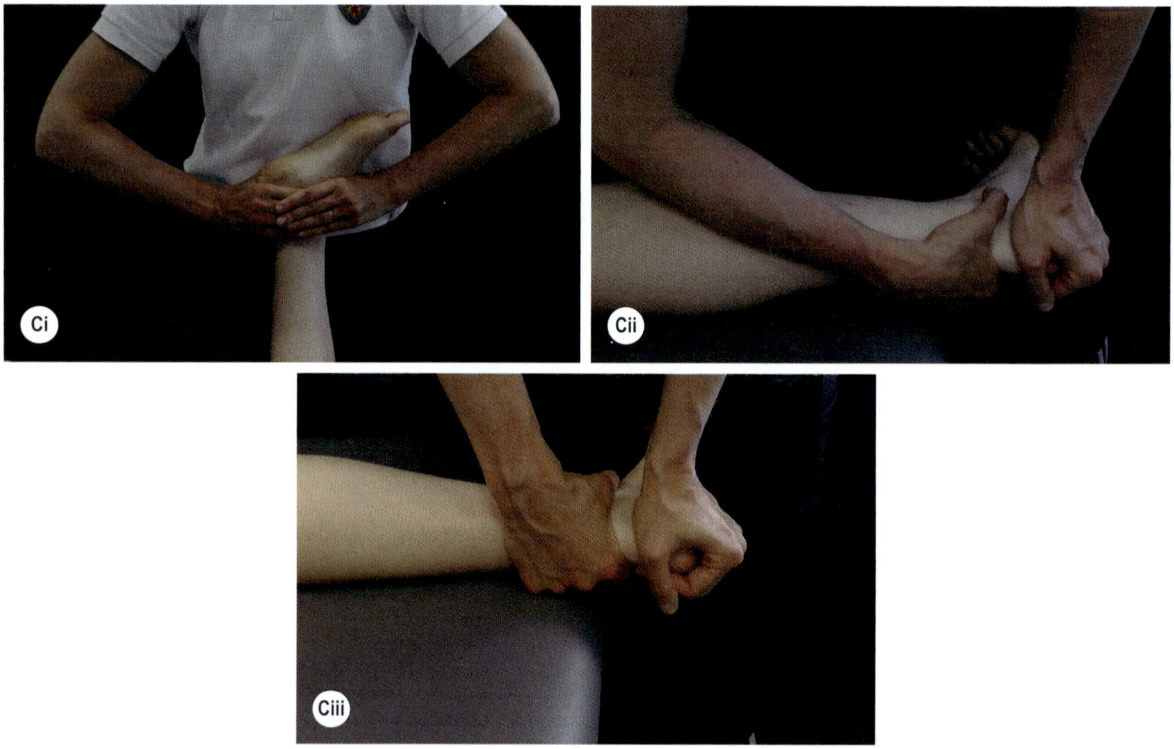

Fig. 17.12, cont'd (C) Subtalar joint. (Ci) Longitudinal caudad. The clinician lightly rests their leg on the posterior aspect of the patient's thigh to stabilize it and then grasps around the calcaneus with the right hand and the forefoot with the left hand, and pulls the foot upwards. (Cii) Transverse medial glide. The patient is in side-lying. The therapist's right hand stabilizes the talus and distal tibia with the second and third fingers in a 'V' formation, while the left hand cups around the calcaneus. The forearms are directed opposite each other, and transverse medial glide of the calcaneus relative to the talus is produced mainly via the left hand whilst the right hand maintains the position of the talus. (Ciii) Transverse lateral glide. The patient is in side-lying. The therapist's right hand stabilizes the talus and distal tibia with the second and third fingers in a 'V' formation while the left hand cups around the calcaneus. The forearms are directed opposite each other, and movement is produced mainly via the left hand whilst the right hand maintains the position of the talus.

examination may initially focus on the talocrural joint, where the majority of dorsiflexion occurs. An accessory examination can be further refined, using the Kaltenborn tests to explore joints in more detail (Kaltenborn, 2002). It is not necessary to complete all ten parts of the test. For example, if the patient's symptoms were focused around the medial aspect of the midfoot the clinician may choose to explore parts 3, 4 and 5 of the Kaltenborn test (Table 17.4).

Although joint play movement is limited, a small study comparing the judgements of two clinicians found there to be fair to good intra- and interrater reliability in identifying hyper and hypomobile joints using joint play testing test (Fraser et al., 2017).

Symptom Modification and Mobilizations With Movements

Mobilizations with movements (MWMs) are accessory movements applied during an active movement and were developed by physiotherapist Brian Mulligan (Hing et al., 2019). These techniques can be used to assess symptom modification and changes in ROM in response to MWMs; this may strengthen hypotheses relating to the structures contributing to symptoms and be considered as treatment options.

Inferior Tibiofibular Joint

The patient lies supine and is asked to actively invert the foot while the clinician applies an anteroposterior

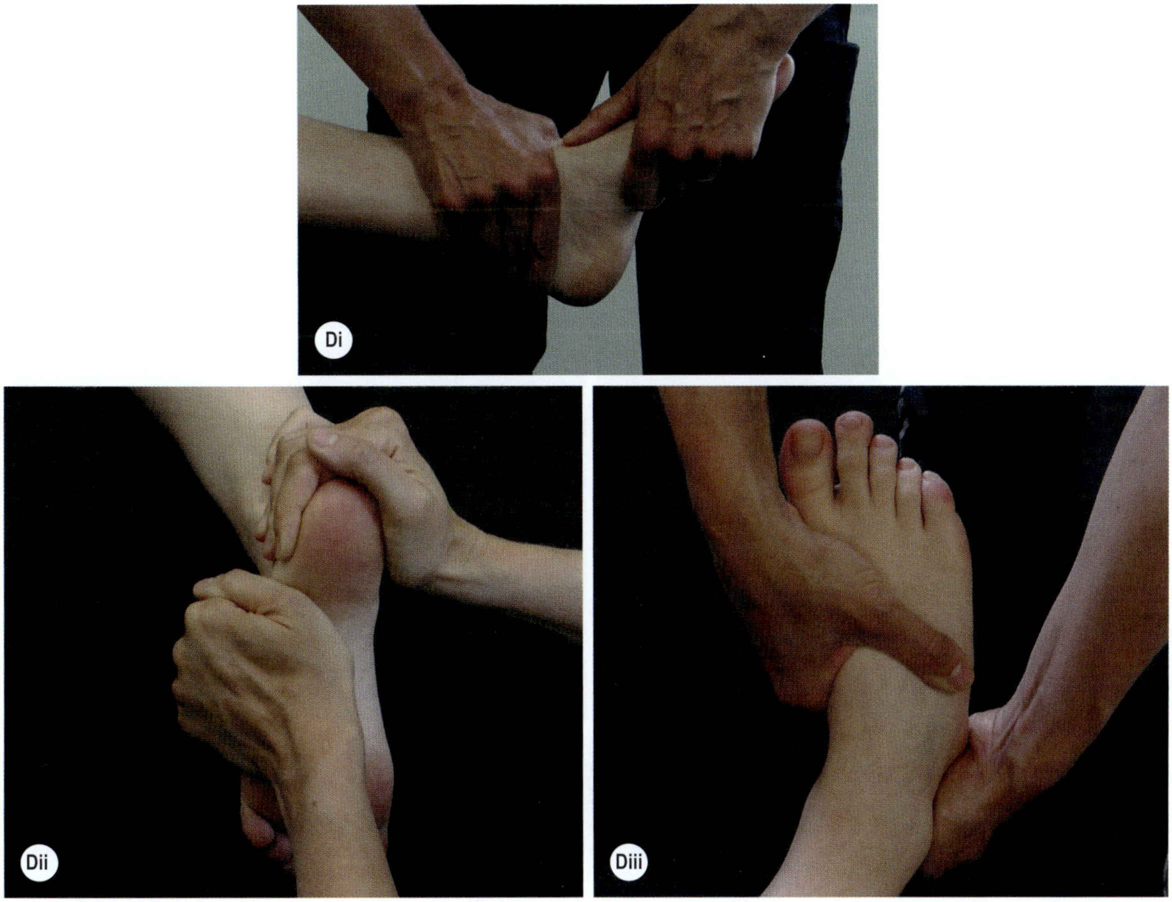

Fig. 17.12, cont'd (D) Midfoot. (Di) Anteroposterior to the navicular. Pressure is applied to the anterior aspect of the navicular through a key grip or the thenar eminence. The other hand stabilizes the talus. (Dii) Posteroanterior to the cuboid. Pressure is applied to the posterior aspect of the cuboid through the thenar eminence whilst the other hand stabilizes the calcaneum. (Diii) Abduction/adduction. The left hand grasps and stabilizes the heel while the right hand grasps the forefoot. The right hand then applies an abduction force to the foot. The foot does not evert. Hands swapped over for adduction.

glide to the fibula (Fig. 17.13). An increase in range and no/reduced pain are positive examination findings indicating a possible mechanical joint problem.

Plantarflexion of the Ankle Joint

The patient lies supine with the knee flexed and the foot over the end of the plinth. With one hand the clinician applies an anteroposterior glide to the lower end of the tibia and fibula and with the other hand rolls the talus anteriorly while the patient is asked actively to plantarflex the ankle (Fig. 17.14A). An increase in range and no/reduced pain are positive examination findings potentially indicating a possible mechanical joint problem.

Dorsiflexion of the Ankle Joint

The patient lies supine with the foot over the end of the plinth, and knee slightly flexed over a rolled towel. The clinician uses one hand to hold the calcaneus, whilst the web space of the other hand contacts the anterior talus. Both hands contribute to the anteroposterior glide of the talus, while the patient is asked to actively dorsiflex the ankle (see Fig. 17.14B). Since the extensor tendons lift the examiner's hand away from the talus,

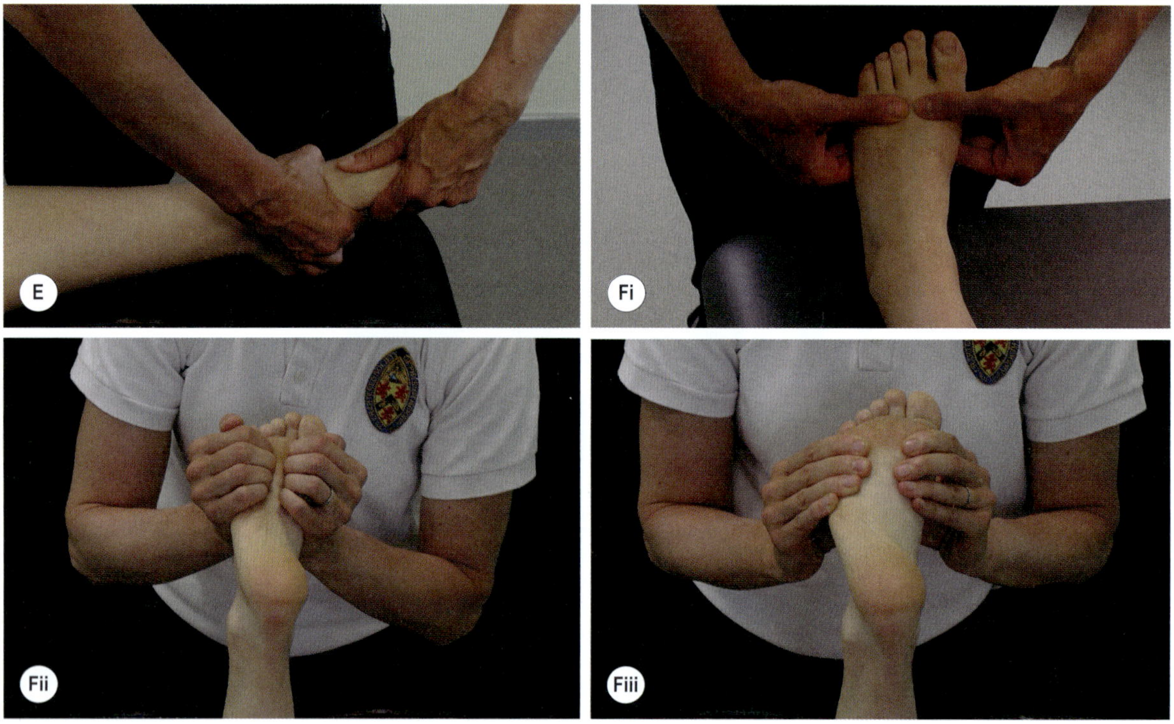

Fig. 17.12, cont'd (E) Anteroposterior and posteroanterior movement of the first tarsometatarsal joint. The right hand stabilizes the medial cuneiform while the left hand applies an anteroposterior and posteroanterior force to the base of the metatarsal. (F) Proximal and distal intermetatarsal joints. (Fi) Anteroposterior and posteroanterior movement. The hands grasp adjacent metatarsal heads and apply a force in opposite directions to produce an anteroposterior and a posteroanterior movement at the distal intermetatarsal joint. (Fii) Horizontal flexion. The fingers are placed in the centre of the foot at the level of the metatarsal heads. The metatarsal heads are then curved around the fingertips to produce horizontal flexion. You might think of folding the foot over. (Fiii) Horizontal extension. The fingers are placed in the centre of the foot at the level of the metatarsal heads. The metatarsal heads are then opened out, curving over the thumbs on the dorsum of the foot to produce horizontal extension. You might think of fanning the foot out.

the patient is asked to contract repetitively and then relax. With relaxation, the clinician moves the ankle into the further range of dorsiflexion gained during the contraction.

For further guidance on the use of mobilizations with movements, see Mulligan (2019) and Hing et al. (2019).

COMPLETION OF THE EXAMINATION

On completion of the physical examination, the clinician will need to collate the information to evaluate and revisit how findings compare with expected findings, based on the clinician's initial primary hypothesis and alternative hypotheses. Information needs to be accurately recorded. Significant findings from the subjective and physical examination can be highlighted with an asterisk* as reassessment markers for use within subsequent sessions to evaluate the effects of treatment on the patient's presentation.

It is good practice that the clinician:

- explains the findings of the physical examination and how these findings relate to the subjective assessment, offering some initial advice if appropriate.

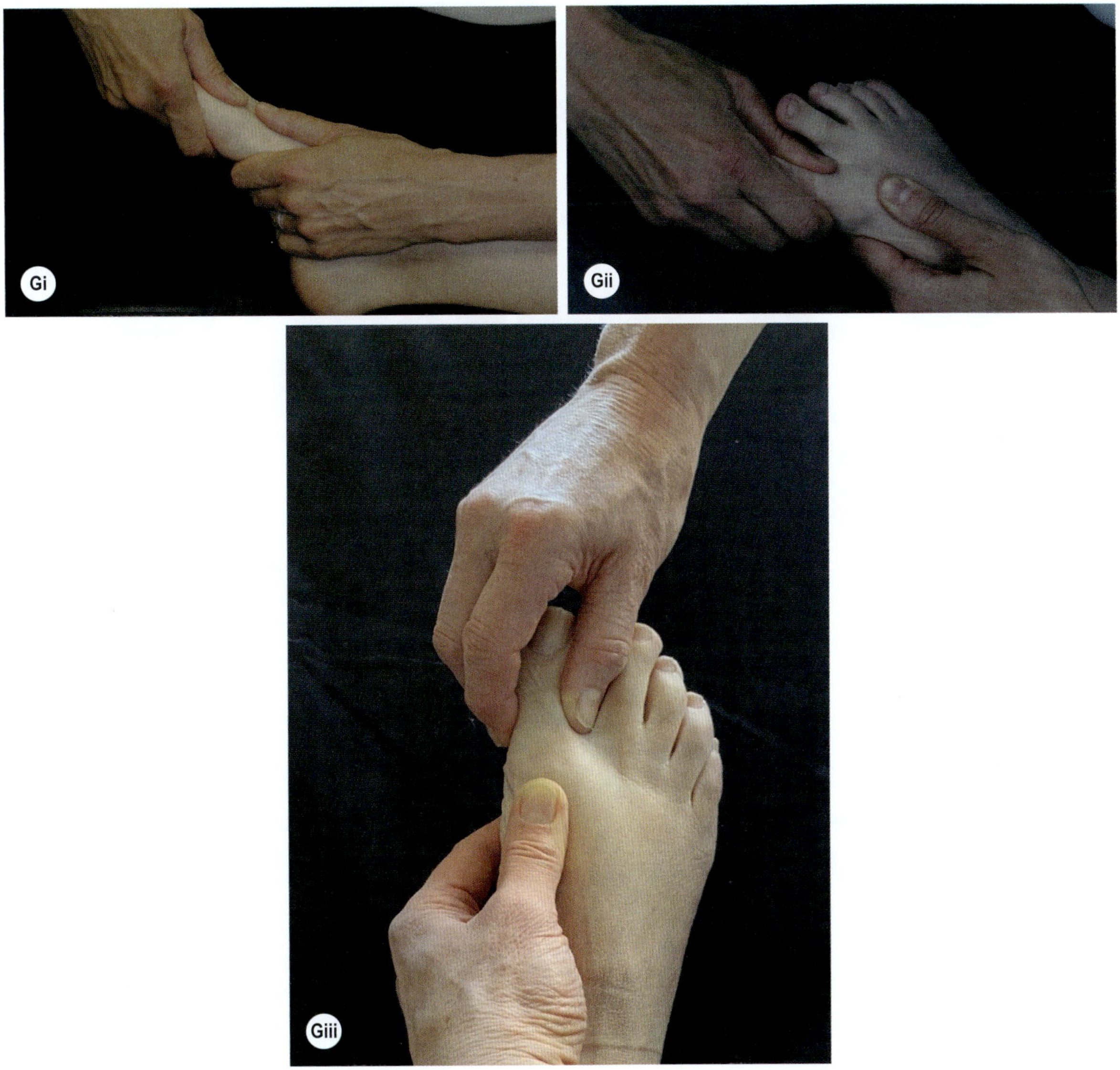

Fig. 17.12, cont'd (G) First metatarsophalangeal joint. For all these movements, one hand stabilizes the metatarsal head while the other hand moves the proximal phalanx. (Gi) Anteroposterior and posteroanterior movement. The proximal phalanx is moved anteriorly and posteriorly. (Gii) Medial and lateral transverse movement. The proximal phalanx is glided medially and laterally. (Giii) Medial and lateral rotation. The proximal phalanx is moved into medial and lateral rotation.

- allows the patient sufficient opportunity to discuss thoughts and beliefs which may well have changed over the course of the examination.
- revisits the patient's initial expectations and through collaboration with the patient identifies an agreed treatment strategy in order to achieve agreed goals.
- requests the patient to report details on the behaviour of the symptoms following examination at the next attendance.

For guidance on treatment and management principles, the reader is directed to the companion textbook (Barnard & Ryder, 2024).

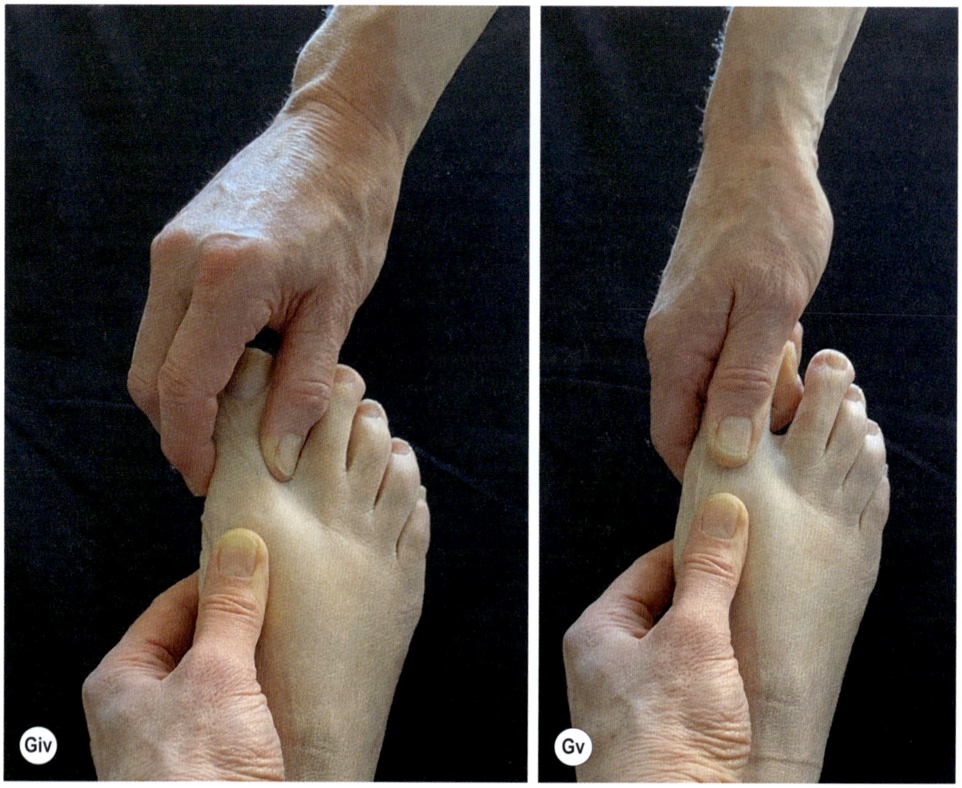

Fig. 17.12, cont'd (Giv) Abduction and adduction. The proximal phalanx is moved into abduction and adduction. (Gv) Longitudinal caudad and cephalad. The proximal phalanx is moved in a cephalad and caudad direction.

TABLE 17.3 Accessory Movements, Choice of Application and Reassessment of the Patient's Asterisks

Accessory Movements	Choice of Application	Identify Any Effect of Accessory Movements on Patient's Signs and Symptoms
Accessory Movements for the Foot and Ankle Joints Inferior tibiofibular joint Anteroposterior Posteroanterior	Start position, e.g. • In dorsiflexion • In plantarflexion • In inversion • In eversion	Reassess all asterisks
Talocrural Joint Anteroposterior Posteroanterior Med-Medial rotation Lat-Lateral rotation Caud-Longitudinal caudad Ceph-Longitudinal cephalad	Speed of force application Direction of applied force Point of application of applied force	

TABLE 17.3 Accessory Movements, Choice of Application and Reassessment of the Patient's Asterisks—cont'd

Accessory Movements	Choice of Application	Identify Any Effect of Accessory Movements on Patient's Signs and Symptoms
Subtalar Joint		
Anteroposterior		
Posteroanterior		
Med-Transverse medial glide		
Lat-Transverse lateral glide		
Med-Medial rotation		
Lat-Lateral rotation		
Caud-Longitudinal caudad		
Ceph-Longitudinal cephalad		
Midtarsal Joints		
Anteroposterior		
Posteroanterior		
Med-Medial rotation		
Lat-Lateral rotation		
Abd Abduction		
Add Adduction		
Med-Medial glide		
Lat-Lateral glide		
Intertarsal Joints		
Anteroposterior		
Posteroanterior		
Med-Medial rotation		
Lat-Lateral rotation		
Abd Abduction		
Add Adduction		
Tarsometatarsal Joints		
Anteroposterior		
Posteroanterior		
Med-Medial rotation		
Lat-Lateral rotation		
Med-Medial glide		
Lat-Lateral glide		

Continued

TABLE 17.3 Accessory Movements, Choice of Application and Reassessment of the Patient's Asterisks—cont'd

Accessory Movements	Choice of Application	Identify Any Effect of Accessory Movements on Patient's Signs and Symptoms
Proximal and Distal Intermetatarsal Joints		
Anteroposterior		
Posteroanterior		
HF Horizontal flexion		
HE Horizontal extension		
Metatarsophalangeal and Interphalangeal Joints		
Anteroposterior		
Posteroanterior		
Med-Medial transverse		
Lat-Lateral transverse		
Med-Medial rotation		
Lat-Lateral rotation		
Abd Abduction		
Add Adduction		
Caud-Longitudinal caudad		
Ceph-Longitudinal cephalad		
?Lumbar spine	As above	Reassess all asterisks
?Sacroiliac joint	As above	Reassess all asterisks
?Hip	As above	Reassess all asterisks
?Tibiofemoral joint	As above	Reassess all asterisks
?Patellofemoral joint	As above	Reassess all asterisks

TABLE 17.4 Ten Accessory Movements of the Tarsal Bones

Movements in the Middle of the Foot
1. Fix second and third cuneiform bones and mobilize second metatarsal bone
2. Fix second and third cuneiform bones and mobilize third metatarsal bone
Movements on the Medial Side of the Foot
3. Fix first cuneiform bone and mobilize first metatarsal bone
4. Fix the navicular bone and mobilize the first, second and third cuneiform bones
5. Fix the talus and mobilize the navicular bone
Movements on the Lateral Side of the Foot
6. Fix the cuboid bone and mobilize the fourth and fifth metatarsal bones
7. Fix the navicular and third cuneiform bones and mobilize the cuboid bone
8. Fix the calcaneus and mobilize the cuboid bone
Movement Between Talus and Calcaneus
9. Fix the talus and mobilize the calcaneus
Movements in the Ankle Joint
10. Fix the tibia/fibula and move the talus or fix the talus and move the tibia/fibula

Kaltenborn (2002).

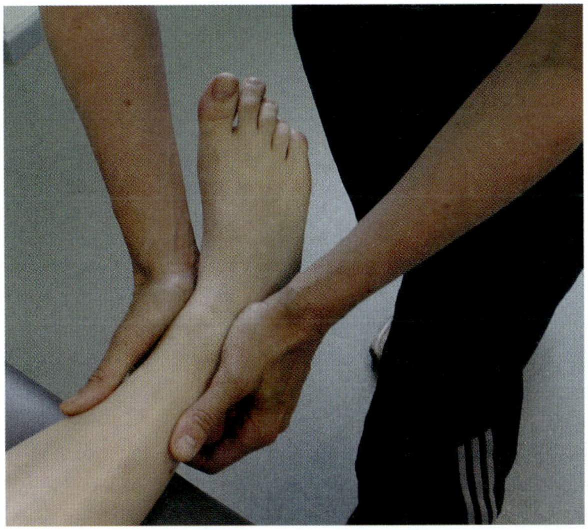

Fig. 17.13 Mobilizations with movement for the inferior tibiofibular joint. The right hand supports the ankle while the heel of the left hand applies an anteroposterior and superior glide to the fibula as the patient inverts the foot.

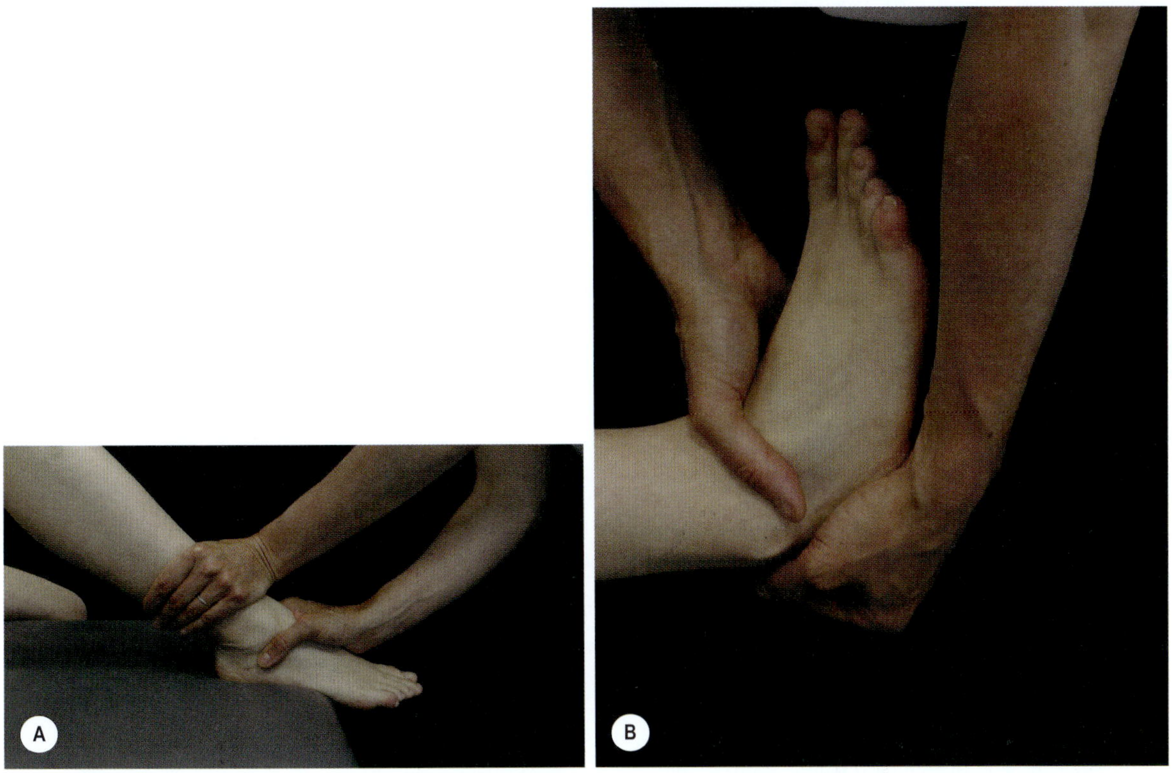

Fig. 17.14 Mobilizations with movement for the ankle joint. (A) Plantarflexion. The left hand applies an anteroposterior glide to the tibia and fibula while the other hand rolls the talus anteriorly as the patient actively plantarflexes. (B) Dorsiflexion. The left hand holds the posterior aspect of the calcaneus, and the right hand grips the anterior aspect of the talus. Both hands apply an anteroposterior glide as the patient actively dorsiflexes.

REVIEW AND REVISE QUESTIONS

1. What measurement tool is useful for the assessment of foot posture?
2. How might a patient with hallux rigidus typically present both subjectively and on physical examination?
3. 'Giving way' of the ankle is a typical symptom included in a clinical prediction rule for anterolateral ankle impingement. TRUE or FALSE?
4. Name three physical examination tests you might consider using if you suspected a patient had an acute Achilles rupture:
   a. ____________
   b. ____________
   c. ____________
5. Which tendon is commonly associated with a pathology resulting in posteromedial pitting oedema of the ankle?
   a. Peroneus longus
   b. Tibialis posterior
   c. Achilles
6. The weight-bearing lunge test is a valid and reliable measure of ankle dorsiflexion. TRUE or FALSE?
7. How would a patient with a syndesmosis injury typically present both subjectively and on physical examination?
8. What is the name of the scoring system that aids in the diagnosis of DVTs?
9. Name one pulse you are able to palpate on the dorsal aspect of the foot and one pulse at the posteromedial aspect of the ankle.
10. Describe an evidenced-based approach to the assessment and management of an acute LAS.

Case Study

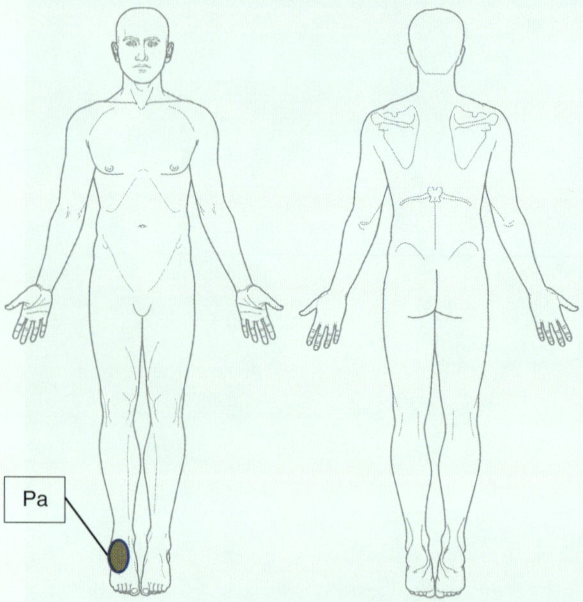

Pa—intermittent pain, generally achy but sharp with foot movements. 6/10

Aggravating factors—walking without boot, squatting activities and descending stairs; sharper pain with plantarflexing and inverting the foot. Can continue.

Easing factors—rest, settles within a few mins.

24-h pattern—activity related throughout the day. No worse first thing in the morning. Ankle swelling was better in the morning. Swelling and ankle 'ache' worsens as the day goes on if doesn't rest and elevate her leg.

Sleep—Occasionally wakes with sharp ankle pain when turning in bed at night.

No symptoms anywhere else

Subjective Examination

History of Present Condition

A 34-year-old marketing director presented to the clinic with a 6-day history of moderately severe, lateral ankle pain (VAS 6/10), swelling and haematoma affecting her right ankle, following a trauma. The pain was described as intermittent and generally achy but sharp with foot movements. She denied knee, hip or low back pain. There were no neurological symptoms.

Six days previously she had landed awkwardly when coming down the stairs and had 'rolled over' on her right ankle and heard a 'pop'. There was immediate local ankle pain and swelling, and she was unable to walk. Her husband drove her to Accident and Emergency, where she had an x-ray. She was told by medics there was no obvious fracture and was given a walking boot and elbow crutches to use. She was advised to rest as she had a 'nasty ankle sprain' and told not to drive.

Case Study—cont'd

Beliefs and Expectations

She was frightened to touch her ankle. She was concerned that she had 'ripped her ankle ligaments' and that she would not be able to return to work for a long time or to her usual gym activities, which included two classes of step aerobics per week. Her husband was supportive, but she felt she was becoming a burden as she was so restricted. She had no previous treatment or MSK problems and was trying to work from home. She hoped physiotherapy would improve her pain and help restore her normal activity levels but was concerned that she had done 'long lasting damage' to her ankle.

Aggravating and Easing Factors

The lateral ankle pain was specifically aggravated by walking without the boot, squatting activities and descending stairs; the pain also became sharper with plantarflexing and inverting the foot, e.g. when trying to put the walking boot on. She was able to continue these activities but was afraid she was doing more damage so rested frequently by elevating her leg on the sofa. After a few minutes of this, her pain settled.

24 Hour Pattern

Her ankle symptoms were activity related throughout the day and no worse first thing in the morning. The ankle swelling was better in the morning. The swelling and ankle 'ache' worsened as the day went on if she didn't rest and elevate her leg. Occasionally she woke with sharp ankle pain when turning in bed at night.

Past Medical History and Drug History

She was fit and well. She had a BMI of 23. She did not drink alcohol and had never smoked.

She took paracetamol (500 mg) irregularly up to three times a day when the ankle pain was 'really bad'.

Hypothesis After Subjective Examination

There was a clear traumatic episode which initiated the patient's symptoms. The history was suggestive of a plantarflexion and inversion mechanism of injury with associated soft tissue damage and inflammation, typical of an LAS. Local anatomical structures associated with this type of injury include the ATFL, CFL, PTFL, syndesmosis joint and ligaments, peroneals, sinus tarsi, talocrural/subtalar and calcaneocuboid joints and cutaneous nerve supply including the superficial common peroneal and sural nerve. Possible referring structures include the lumbar spine, sacroiliac joint, hip and knee joint or radicular pain emanating from a lower lumbar nerve root; however, these referred sources were unlikely given there was no previous or current history of MSK symptoms in these areas. A neuropathic cause of symptoms was unlikely given the lack of neurological symptoms. The history of ankle swelling, haematoma and a 'pop' following trauma made Achilles rupture a relevant differential diagnosis to consider.

The primary working hypothesis was that the lateral ankle ligament structures, particularly the ATFL, were the most likely source of symptoms in view of the mechanism of injury, distribution of symptoms and aggravating factors. An acute LAS (grade II or III) was thought to be the most likely pathology in view of the swelling, haematoma and exclusion of bony injury via x-ray. Being female is also a risk factor for LAS (Martin et al., 2021). Syndesmotic injury was considered less likely as symptoms were not distributed in the high ankle area and the mechanism of injury did not involve dorsiflexion or external rotation forces.

The pain mechanisms were thought to be predominantly mechanical nociception due to the intermittent nature of symptoms with clear mechanical aggravating features. In addition, there was an inflammatory component as evidenced by swelling, haematoma, symptoms easing with rest and the timeline from trauma (Watson, 2021). She displayed some catastrophization and fear-avoidant behaviours which may have impacted on her pain perception and upregulated her sympathetic nervous system. She was concerned about work, the impact of her injury on her husband and was less physically active, all of which may have reduced the resilience of her tissues and influenced her wellbeing.

The priorities for the clinical examination were to check the x-ray (in case of a missed fracture), assess the ankle joint and rule in or out LAS as a potential pathology and exclude a syndesmosis injury or missed Achilles rupture as the latter may require surgical intervention. Functional testing, measurement of swelling and ankle range of movement were to be performed, together with tests which may be clinically useful in the diagnosis of LAS; namely anterior drawer, palpation and talar tilt test (Delahunt et al., 2018; Vuurberg et al., 2018; Martin et al., 2021).

To rule out Achilles rupture the following tests were included: Thompson test, Matles test and palpation for a gap in the Achilles tendon (Boyd et al., 2015; Singh, 2017), and the squeeze test was used to assess the syndesmosis (Delahunt et al., 2018; Netterström-Wedin & Bleakley, 2021).

It was expected that there would be discomfort and possibly a reduced range of movement in all directions of

Case Study—cont'd

ankle movement but particularly into dorsiflexion, plantarflexion and inversion.

Other tests which may have proved valuable for future consideration included examination for balance function, e.g. single leg balance, SEBT, ability to jump and land and examination of gluteal strength and control (Martin et al., 2021). A review of the ankle and foot x-ray confirmed no bony injury. There were not thought to be any significant contraindications or precautions.

Physical Examination

Functional Testing

Stance, gait and one-leg control are important considerations for patients with LAS (Martin et al., 2021). Although the patient was apprehensive, she was able to stand with equal weight bearing on both feet without the walking boot on or the use of elbow crutches. She was able to mobilize without aids for short distances although had a reduced stance time and terminal stance phase due to limited dorsiflexion; there was some discomfort with walking (VAS 4/10). She was unable to single-leg stand or single-leg squat due to apprehension and discomfort in the right ankle (VAS 6/10). With double-leg squat, there was reduced dorsiflexion of the right ankle to half ROM and a valgus movement pattern at the knee.

ROM

ROM of the right knee was full and pain-free. Ankle ROM was limited to ½ for plantarflexion and inversion with movement stopped short of sharp anterolateral ankle pain. Dorsiflexion was ½ range with anterolateral ankle aching increased. The weight-bearing lunge test was limited to 2 cm on the right and 5 cm on the left.

Selective Tests

Thompson test, Matles test and palpation for a gap in the Achilles tendon were all negative. Squeeze test for, and palpation of, the syndesmosis was negative.

There was local bruising on the lateral side of the right ankle. Figure of eight measurement of swelling revealed a 30 mm difference between the left and right ankle indicating a moderate level of oedema (Rohner-Spengler et al., 2007). Local palpation of the ATFL reproduced the patient's sharp pain, but palpation of CFL did not. The talar tilt test was uncomfortable but did not reproduce the patient's specific symptoms and had a firm, stable end-feel similar to the left side. The right anterior drawer test was positive with a visible sulcus.

Accessories

As the condition was moderately severe and irritable, accessory movements were limited. There was noted increased ankle ROM and reduced pain with a mini trial of MWMs for the talocrural joint into plantarflexion in nonweight-bearing and a small increase in pain-free ankle ROM with the use of posterior-anterior talocrural mobilization. Weight-bearing MWMs were not undertaken at assessment but were planned for follow-up.

Clinical Diagnosis and Plan

Symptoms and physical signs supported the clinical diagnosis of acute LAS with probable rupture of the ATFL (Vuurberg et al., 2018). The initial plan was to explain examination findings with nonthreatening language and use a patient-centred approach to explore the patient's beliefs and expectations after the examination. Evidence-informed explanation of expected time scales for recovery was essential as was a discussion regarding the importance of completing a comprehensive exercise-based rehabilitation programme to help avoid chronic ankle dysfunction. Initial management included weaning the patient off the walking boot and elbow crutches, use of an ankle brace for up to 10 days and progressive weight bearing on the right side. The use of intermittent cryotherapy was encouraged but only in conjunction with her exercise programme. A progressive multimodal rehabilitation programme was planned to include supervised and home-based ankle and foot ROM exercises, gait re-education, neuromuscular training, coordination and balance exercises and manual therapy with encouragement to undertake a graded and scheduled return to work and sport (Vuurberg et al. 2018; Martin et al., 2021). The patient-reported FAAM outcome tool was used to evaluate treatment. If anticipated recovery was not achieved as expected, onward referral for further investigation could be considered to rule out coexisting pathologies such as osteochondral lesions, talar dome injuries, syndesmotic injuries, etc. (Polzer et al., 2012; Vuurberg et al., 2018; Martin et al., 2021). For guidance on treatment and management principles, the reader is directed to the companion textbook (Barnard & Ryder, 2024).

REFERENCES

Adukia, V., Mangwani, J., Issac, R., Hussain, S., Parker, L., 2020. Current concepts in the management of ankle arthritis. J. Clin. Orthop. Trauma. 11 (3), 388–398.

Alazzawi, S., Sukeik, M., King, D., Vemulapalli, K., 2017. Foot and ankle history and clinical examination: a guide to everyday practice. World J. Orthop. 8 (1), 21–29.

Alrabai, H.M., Alrashidi, Y., Valderrabano, V., Delmi, M., 2016. Morton's neuroma in sports. In: Valderrabano, V., Easley, M. (Eds.), Foot and Ankle Sports Orthopaedics. Springer, Switzerland, pp. 391–396.

Alshami, A.M., Souvlis, T., Coppieters, M.W., 2008. A review of plantar heel pain of neural origin: differential diagnosis and management. Man. Ther. 13, 103–111.

Barnard, K., Ryder, D., 2024. Principles of Musculoskeletal Treatment and Management: A Handbook for Therapists, fourth ed. Churchill Livingstone, Edinburgh.

Beard, N.M., Gousse, R.P., 2018. Current ultrasound application in the foot and ankle. Orthop. Clin. 49 (1), 109–121.

Beckenkamp, P.R., Lin, C.W.C., Macaskill, P., Michaleff, Z.A., Maher, C.G., Moseley, A.M., 2017. Diagnostic accuracy of the Ottawa ankle and midfoot rules: a systematic review with meta-analysis. Br. J. Sports Med. 51 (6), 504–510.

Boyd, R.P., Dimock, R., Solan, M.C., Porter, E., 2015. Achilles tendon rupture: how to avoid missing the diagnosis. Br. J. Gen. Pract. 65 (641), 668–669.

Chan, O., Sakellariou, A., 2020. Hallux rigidus: a review. Orthop. Trauma. 34, 23–29.

Chimenti, R., Cychosz, C.C., Hall, M.M., Phisitkul, P., 2017. Current concepts review update: insertional Achilles tendinopathy. Foot Ankle Int. 38 (10), 1160–1169.

Cook, C., Cook, A., 2016. Differential diagnosis and treatment of cervical myelopathy, cervical radiculopathy and cervical myeloradiculopathy. In: Fernandez-de-las-Penas, C., Cleland, J., Dommerholt, J. (Eds.), Manual Therapy for Musculoskeletal Pain Syndromes: An Evidence and Clinical Informed Approach. Elsevier, UK, pp. 118–2008.

Cook, C., Hegedus, E., 2011. Orthopedic Physical Examination Tests: An Evidence-Based Approach, second ed. Prentice Hall, New Jersey.

Cook, J.L., Rio, E., Purdam, C.R., Docking, S.I., 2016. Revisiting the continuum model of tendon pathology: what is its merit in clinical practice and research? Br. J. Sports Med. 50 (19), 1187–1191.

Cowell, F., Gillespie, S., Narayan, B., Goebel, A., 2019. Complex regional pain syndrome (CRPS) in orthopaedics: an overview. Orthop. Trauma. 33, 217–223.

Dananberg, H., 1986. Functional hallux limitus and its relationship to gait efficiency. J. Am. Podiatr. Med. Assoc. 76, 648–652.

Darcey, S., 2017. Primary lung cancer presenting as foot pain. Can. Fam. Phys. 63, 453–454.

Delahunt, E., Bleakley, C.M., Bossard, D.S., Caulfield, B.M., Docherty, C.L., Doherty, C., et al., 2018. Clinical assessment of acute lateral ankle sprain injuries (ROAST): 2019 consensus statement and recommendations of the International Ankle Consortium. Br. J. Sports Med. 52 (20), 1304–1310.

DeOrio, J.K., Shapiro, S.A., McNeil, R.B., Stansel, J., 2011. Validity of the posterior tibial edema sign in posterior tibial tendon dysfunction. Foot Ankle Int. 32, 189–192.

Devoogdt, N., Cavaggion, C., Van der Gucht, E., Dams, L., De Groef, A., Meeus, M., 2019. Reliability, validity, and feasibility of water displacement method, figure-of-eight method, and circumference measurements in determination of ankle and foot edema. Lymphat. Res. Biol. 17 (5), 531–536.

Dewi, F., Hinchliffe, R.J., 2020. Foot complications in patients with diabetes. Surgery 38 (2), 108–113.

Doherty, C., Delahunt, E., Caulfield, B., Hertel, J., Ryan, J., Bleakley, C., 2014. The incidence and prevalence of ankle sprain injury: a systematic review and meta-analysis of prospective epidemiological studies. Sports Med. 44, 123–140.

Dubin, J.C., Comeau, D., McClelland, R.I., Dubin, R.A., Ferrel, E., 2011. Lateral and syndesmotic ankle sprain injuries: a narrative literature review. J. Chiropr. Med. 10, 204–219.

Eelsing, R., Hemke, R., Schepers, T., 2021. The added value of SPECT/CT in the painful foot and ankle: a review of the literature. Foot Ankle Surg. 27 (7), 715–722.

Ewalefo, S.O., Dombrowski, M., Hirase, T., Rocha, J.L., Weaver, M., Kline, A., 2018. Management of posttraumatic ankle arthritis: literature review. Curr. Rev. MSK Med. 11 (4), 546–557.

Faroug, R., Psyllakis, P., Gulati, A., Makvana, S., Pareek, M., Mangwani, J., 2018. Diagnosis and treatment of tuberculosis of the foot and ankle – a literature review. Foot 37, 105–112.

Fraser, J.J., Koldenhoven, R.M., Saliba, S.A., Hertel, J., 2017. Reliability of ankle-foot morphology, mobility, strength, and motor performance measures. Int. J. Sports Phys. Ther. 12 (7), 1134–1149.

Fuller, E.A., Kirby, K.A., 2013. Subtalar joint equilibrium and tissue stress approach to biomechanical therapy of the foot and lower extremity. In: Albert, S.F., Curran, S.A. (Eds.), Biomechanics of the Lower Extremity: Theory and Practice, Vol. 1. Bipedmed, Denver, pp. 205–264.

Gribble, P.A., Hertel, J., Plisky, P., 2012. Using the star excursion balance test to assess dynamic postural-control deficits and outcomes in lower extremity injury: a literature and systematic review. J. Athl. Train. 47, 339–357.

Grice, J., Willmott, H., Taylor, H., 2016. Assessment and management of cavus foot deformity. Orthop. Trauma. 30 (1), 68–74.

Haapamäki, V.V., Kiuru, M.J., Mustonen, A.O., Koskinen, S.K., 2005. Multidetector computed tomography in acute joint fractures. Acta. Radiol. 46, 587–598.

Hall, E.A., Docherty, C.L., 2017. Validity of clinical outcome measures to evaluate ankle range of motion during the weight-bearing lunge test. J. Sci. Med. Sport. 20 (7), 618–621.

Hannan, M.T., Menz, H.B., Jordan, J.M., Cupples, L.A., Cheng, C.H., Hsu, Y.H., 2013. High heritability of hallux valgus and lesser toe deformities in adult men and women. Arthritis Care Res. 65 (9), 1515–1521.

Harradine, P., Gates, L., Bowen, C., 2018. If it doesn't work, why do we still do it? The continuing use of subtalar joint neutral theory in the face of overpowering critical research. J. Orthop. Sports Phys. Ther. 48, 130–132.

Helliwell, P.S., Backhouse, M.R., Siddle, H.J., 2019. The Foot and Ankle in Rheumatology. Oxford University Press, Oxford.

Hertel, J., Braham, R.A., Hale, S.A., Olmsted-Kramer, L.C., 2006. Simplifying the star excursion balance test: analyses of subjects with and without chronic ankle instability. J. Orthop. Sports Phys. Ther. 36, 131–137.

Hertel, J., Corbett, R.O., 2019. An updated model of chronic ankle instability. J. Athl. Train. 54, 572–588.

Hing, W., Hall, T., Mulligan, B., 2019. The Mulligan Concept of Manual Therapy: Textbook of Techniques, second ed. Churchill Livingstone, Chatswood, NSW, Australia.

Hoch, M.C., McKeon, P.O., 2011. Normative range of weight-bearing lunge test performance asymmetry in healthy adults. Man. Ther. 16, 516–519.

Irving, D.B., Cook, J.L., Menz, H.B., 2007. Factors associated with chronic plantar heel pain: a systematic review. J. Sci. Med. Sport. 9, 11–22.

Janda, V., 1994. Muscles and motor control in cervicogenic disorders: assessment and management. In: Grant, R. (Ed.), Physical Therapy of the Cervical and Thoracic Spine, second ed. Churchill Livingstone, New York, p. 195.

Janda, V., 2002. Muscles and motor control in cervicogenic disorders. In: Grant, R. (Ed.), Physical Therapy of the Cervical and Thoracic Spine, second ed. Churchill Livingstone, New York, p. 182.

Jia, Y., Huang, H., Gagnier, J.J., 2017. A systematic review of measurement properties of patient-reported outcome measures for use in patients with foot or ankle diseases. Qual. Life Res. 26 (8), 1969–2010.

Kaltenborn, F.M., 2002. Manual Mobilisation of the Joints, Vol. I, sixth ed. The extremities. Norli, Oslo.

Keenan, A.M., Redmond, A.C., Horton, M., Conaghan, P.G., Tennant, A., 2007. The foot posture index: Rasch analysis of a novel, foot-specific outcome measure. Arch. Phys. Med. Rehabil. 88, 88–93.

Kendall, F.P., McCreary, E.K., Provance, P.G., 2010. Muscles: Testing and Function with Posture and Pain, fifth ed. Lippincott, Williams & Wilkins, Baltimore.

Kennedy, J.G., Ross, K.A., Smyth, N.A., Hogan, M.V., Murawski, C.D., 2016. Primary tumors of the foot and ankle. Foot Ankle Spec. 9, 58–68.

Kerkhoffs, G.M., Karlsson, J., 2019. Osteochondral lesions of the talus. Knee. Surg. Sports. Traum. Arthros. 27, 2719–2720.

Khlopas, H., Khlopas, A., Samuel, L.T., Ohliger, E., Sultan, A.A., Chughtai, M., et al., 2019. Current concepts in osteoarthritis of the ankle. Surg. Technol. Int. 35, 1–15.

Kim, J.H., 2016. Complex regional pain syndrome in the foot and ankle. In: Jung, H.G. (Ed.), Foot and Ankle Disorders – an Illustrated Reference. Springer, Berlin, pp. 606–630.

King, D., Morton, R., Bevan, C., 2014. How to use capillary refill time. Arch. Dis. Child Educ. Pract. Ed. 99, 111–116.

Kirby, K., 2001. Subtalar joint axis location and rotational equilibrium, theory of foot function. J. Am. Podiatr. Med. 91, 465–487.

Kirby, K., 2015. Prescribing orthoses: has tissue stress theory supplanted root theory? Podiatry Today 28 (4). Available online at: https://www.hmpgloballearningnetwork.com/site/podiatry/prescribing-orthoses-has-tissue-stress-theory-supplanted-root-theory.

Lancaster, S.T., Madhaven, D., 2021. Current concepts review: management of Achilles tendinopathy overview. J. Arthrosc. Jt. Surg. 8, 216–221.

Lavery, L.A., Lavery, D.C., Green, T., Hunt, N., La Fontaine, J., Kim, P.J., et al., 2020. Increased risk of nonunion and Charcot arthropathy after ankle fracture in people with diabetes. J. Foot Ankle Surg. 59 (4), 653–656.

Lee, S., Song, K., Lee, S.Y., 2022. Epidemiological study of post-traumatic ankle osteoarthritis after ankle sprain in 195,393 individuals over middle age using the National Health Insurance Database: A retrospective design. J. Sci. Med. Sport. 25 (2), 129–133.

Lesher, J.M., Dreyfuss, P., Hager, N., Kaplan, M., Furman, M., 2008. Hip joint pain referral patterns: a descriptive study. Pain Med. 9 (1), 22–25.

Levinger, P., Menz, H.B., Fotoohabadi, M.R., Feller, J.A., Bartlett, J.R., Bergman, N.R., 2010. Foot posture in people with medial compartment knee osteoarthritis. J. Foot Ankle Res. 3 (1), 1–8.

Ling, S.K., Lui, T.H., 2017. Posterior tibial tendon dysfunction: an overview. Open Orthop. J. 11 (7), 14–723.

Lithgow, M.J., Munteanu, S.E., Buldt, A.K., Arnold, J.B., Kelly, L.A., Menz, H.B., 2020. Foot structure and lower limb function in individuals with midfoot osteoarthritis: a systematic review. Osteoarthritis. Cartilage. 20 (12), 1514–1524.
Liu, S.H., Nuccion, S.L., Finerman, G., 1997. Diagnosis of anterolateral ankle impingement. Comparison between magnetic resonance imaging and clinical examination. Am. J. Sports Med. 25, 389–393.
Maffulli, N., 1998. The clinical diagnosis of subcutaneous tear of the Achilles tendon. Am. J. Sports Med. 26, 266–270.
Magee, D.J., 2021. Orthopedic Physical Assessment, seventh ed. Elsevier, St Louis.
Mahadevan, D., Venkatesan, M., Bhatt, R., Bhatia, M., 2015. Diagnostic accuracy of clinical tests for Morton's neuroma compared with ultrasonography. J. Foot Ankle Surg. 54, 549–553.
Martin, R.L., Davenport, T.E., Reischl, S.F., McPoil, T.G., Matheson, J.W., Wukich, D.K., et al., 2014. Heel pain-plantar fasciitis: revision. J. Orthop. Sports Phys. Ther. 44, A1–A33.
Martin, R.L., Davenport, T.E., Fraser, J.J., Sawdon-Bea, J., Carcia, C.R., Carroll, L.A., et al., 2021. Ankle Stability and Movement Coordination Impairments: Lateral Ankle Ligament Sprains Revision 2021. J. Orthop. Sports Phys. Ther. 51 (4), CPG1–CPG80.
Matles, A.L., 1975. Rupture of the tendo Achilles. Another diagnostic sign. Bull. Hosp. Joint Dis. 36, 48–51.
Mawdsley, H.R., Hoy, D.K., Erwin, P.M., 2000. Criterion-related validity of the figure-of-eight method of measuring ankle edema. J. Orthop. Sports Phys. Ther. 30, 49–153.
McPoil, T.G., Hunt, G.C., 1995. Evaluation and management of foot and ankle disorders: present problems and future directions. J. Orthop. Sports Phys. Ther. 21, 381–388.
McSweeney, S.C., Cichero, M., 2015. Tarsal tunnel syndrome – a narrative literature review. Foot 25 (4), 244–250.
Medina McKeon, J.M., Hoch, M.C., 2019. The ankle-joint complex: a kinesiologic approach to lateral ankle sprains. J. Athl. Train. 54 (6), 589–602.
Miller, J., Dunn, K.W., Ciliberti Jr., L.J., Eldridge, S.W., Reed, L.D., 2017. Diagnostic value of early magnetic resonance imaging after acute lateral ankle injury. J. Foot Ankle Surg. 56 (6), 1143–1146.
Mohan, H.K., Gnanasegaran, G., Vijayanathan, S., Fogelman, I., 2010. SPECT/CT in imaging foot and ankle pathology – the demise of other coregistration techniques. Semin. Nucl. Med. 40, 41–51.
Molloy, S., Solan, M.C., Bendall, S.P., 2003. Synovial impingement in the ankle: a new physical sign. J. Bone Joint Surg. 85-B, 330–333.
Moore, K.R., Howell, M.A., Saltrick, K.R., Catanzariti, A.R., 2017. Risk factors associated with nonunion after elective foot and ankle reconstruction: a case-control study. J. Foot Ankle Surg. 56 (3), 457–462.
Mulligan, B.R., 2019. Manual Therapy 'NAGs', 'SNAGs', 'MWMs' Etc, seventh ed. Plane View Services, New Zealand.
Neal, B.S., Griffiths, I.B., Dowling, G.J., Murley, G.S., Munteanu, S.E., Franettovich Smith, M.M., et al., 2014. Foot posture as a risk factor for lower limb overuse injury: a systematic review and meta-analysis. J. Foot Ankle Res. 7, 55.
Nelson, R., Hall, T., 2011. Bilateral dorsal foot pain in a young tennis player managed by neurodynamics treatment techniques. Man. Ther. 16, 641–645.
Netterström-Wedin, F., Bleakley, C., 2021. Diagnostic accuracy of clinical tests assessing ligamentous injury of the ankle syndesmosis: a systematic review with meta-analysis. Phys. Ther. Sport. 49, 214–226.
Netterström-Wedin, F., Matthews, M., Bleakley, C., 2021. Diagnostic accuracy of clinical tests assessing ligamentous injury of the talocrural and subtalar joints: A systematic review with meta-analysis. Sports Health, 19417381211029953.
Neves, L.F., Souza, C.Q.D., Stoffel, M., Picasso, C.L.M., 2017. The Y balance test–how and why to do it. Int. Phys. Med. Rehab. J. 2 (4), 58–59.
NICE, 2017. Spondyloarthritis in over 16s: Diagnosis and Management. Available online at: https://www.nice.org.uk/guidance/ng65.
NICE, 2020. Venous Thromboembolic Diseases: Diagnosis, Management and Thrombophilia Testing. Available online at: https://www.nice.org.uk/guidance/ng158.
NICE Clinical Knowledge Summaries, 2020. Deep Vein Thrombosis. Available online at: https://cks.nice.org.uk/topics/deep-vein-thrombosis.
Nix, S.E., Vicenzino, B.T., Collins, N.J., Smith, M.D., 2013. Gait parameters associated with hallux valgus: a systematic review. J. Foot Ankle Res. 6 (9), 1–12.
Nyland, J., Franklin, T., Short, A., Calik, M., Kaya, D., 2018. Posture, kinesthesia, foot sensation, balance, and proprioception. In: Kaya, D., Yosmaoglu, B., Doral, M.N. (Eds.), Proprioception in Orthopaedics, Sports Medicine and Rehabilitation. Springer, Cham, pp. 13–24. https://doi.org/10.1007/978-3-319-66640-2_2.
Oji, D.E., Schon, L.C., 2013. The diabetic foot. In: Thordarson, D.B. (Ed.), Foot and Ankle, second ed. Lippincott Williams and Wilkins, Philadelphia, pp. 104–124.
Pascual Huerta, J., 2014. The effect of the gastrocnemius on the plantar fascia. Foot Ankle Clin. 26, 701–718.
Pedowitz, D.I., 2012. General imaging of the adult foot and ankle. In: Hurwitz, S.R., Parekh, S.G. (Eds.), Musculoskeletal Examination of the Foot and Ankle. Slack, New Jersey.
Polzer, H., Kanz, K.G., Prall, W.C., Haasters, F., Ockert, B., Mutschler, W., et al., 2012. Diagnosis and treatment of

acute ankle injuries: development of an evidence-based algorithm. Orthop. Rev. 4, e5.

Pomeroy, G., Wilton, J., Anthony, S., 2015. Entrapment neuropathy about the foot and ankle: an update. J. Am. Aca Orthop. Surg. 23, 58–66.

Powden, C.J., Dodds, T.K., Gabriel, E.H., 2019. The reliability of the star excursion balance test and lower quarter Y-balance test in healthy adults: a systematic review. Int. J. Sports Phys. Ther. 14 (5), 683–694.

Powden, C.J., Hoch, J.M., Hoch, M.C., 2015. Reliability and minimal detectable change of the weight-bearing lunge test: a systematic review. Man. Ther. 20, 524–532.

Redmond, A.C., Crane, Y.Z., Menz, H.B., 2008. Normative values for the foot posture index. J. Foot Ankle Res. 1 (6), 1–9.

Redmond, A.C., Crosbie, J., Ouvrier, R.A., 2006. Development and validation of a novel rating system for scoring standing foot posture: the Foot Posture Index. Clin. Biomech. (Bristol, Avon) 21, 89–98.

Reilly, K.K., Barker, K., Shamley, D., Newman, M., Oskrochi, G.R., Sandall, S., 2009. The role of foot and ankle assessment of patients with lower limb osteoarthritis. Physiotherapy. 95, 164–169.

Reiman, M., Burgi, C., Strube, E., Prue, K., Ray, K., Elliott, A., et al., 2014. The utility of clinical measures for the diagnosis of Achilles tendon injuries: a systematic review with meta-analysis. J. Athl. Train. 49 (6), 820–829.

Remus, A., Caulfield, B., Doherty, C., Crowe, C., Severini, G., Delahunt, E., 2018. A laboratory captured 'giving way' episode in an individual with chronic ankle instability. J. Biomech. 76, 241–246.

Rewhorn, M.J., Leung, A.H., Gillespie, A., Moir, J.S., Miller, R., 2014. Incidence of complex regional pain syndrome after foot and ankle surgery. J. Foot Ankle Surg. 53, 256–258.

Richards, J., Levine, D., Whittle, M., 2012a. Normal gait. In: Levine, D., et al. (Eds.), Whittle's Gait Analysis, fifth ed. Churchill Livingstone, Edinburgh (Chapter 2).

Robinson, R.H., Gribble, P.A., 2008. Support for a reduction in the number of trials needed for the star excursion balance test. Arch. Phys. Med. Rehabil. 89, 364–370.

Rohner-Spengler, M., Mannion, A.F.,, Babst, R., 2007. Reliability and minimal detectable change for the figure-of-eight-20 method of measurement of ankle edema. J. Orthop. Sports Phys. Ther. 37, 199–205.

Root, M.L., Orien, W.P., Weed, J.H., 1977. Clinical Biomechanics. Normal and Abnormal Function of the Foot, Vol. II. Los Angeles. Clin. Biomech. (Bristol, Avon).

Ross, M.H., Smith, M., Plinsinga, M.L., Vicenzino, B., 2018. Self-reported social and activity restrictions accompany local impairments in posterior tibial tendon dysfunction: a systematic review. J. Foot Ankle Res. 11, 49–60.

Ross, M.H., Smith, M.D., Vicenzino, B., 2017. Reported selection criteria for adult acquired flatfoot deformity and posterior tibial tendon dysfunction: are they one and the same? A systematic review. PLoS One. 12 (12), e0187201.

Schweitzerian, B., Haas, D., Columber, K., Knupp, D., Cook, C., 2013. Diagnostic accuracy of physical examination tests of the ankle/foot complex: a systematic review. Int. J. Sports Phys. Ther. 8, 416–426.

Seaman, T.J., Ball, T.A., 2021. Pes Cavus. [Updated 11 Aug 2021]. in: StatPearls [Internet]. StatPearls Publishing, Treasure Island (FL). Available online from: https://www.ncbi.nlm.nih.gov/books/NBK556016/.

Shazadeh Safavi, P., Janney, C., Jupiter, D., Kunzler, D., Bui, R., Panchbhavi, V.K., 2019. A systematic review of the outcome evaluation tools for the foot and ankle. Foot Ankle Spec. 12 (5), 461–470.

Silbernagel, K.G., Hanlon, S., Sprague, A., 2020. Current clinical concepts: conservative management of Achilles tendinopathy. J. Athl. Train. 55 (5), 438–447.

Singh, D., 2017. Acute Achilles tendon rupture. Br. J. Sports Med. 51 (15), 1158–1160.

Slipman, C.W., Jackson, H.B., Lipetz, J.S., Chan, K.T., Lenrow, D., Vresilovic, E.J., 2000. Sacroiliac joint pain referral zones. Arch. Phys. Med. Rehab. 81, 334–338.

Sman, A., Hiller, C.E., Refshauge, K.M., 2013. Diagnostic accuracy of clinical tests for diagnosis of ankle syndesmosis injury: a systematic review. Br. J. Sports Med. 47, 620–628.

So, E., Rushing, C.J., Simon, J.E., Goss Jr., D.A., Prissel, M. A., Berlet, G.C., 2020. Association between bone mineral density and elderly ankle fractures: a systematic review and meta-analysis. J. Foot Ankle Surg. 59 (5), 1049–1057.

Souza Júnior, E., Vieira, M.C.T., Baumfeld, T.S., Baumfeld, D.S., 2020. Patients' perspective on the surgical treatment of hallux valgus. J. Foot Ankle 14 (1), 36–40.

Spannbauer, A., Chwała, M., Ridan, T., Berwecki, A., Mika, P., Kulik, A., et al., 2019. Intermittent Claudication in Physiotherapists' Practice. Biomed Res. Int. 1–10.

Stein, B.E., Schon, L.C., 2015. Posterior tibial tendon dysfunction in the adult: current concepts. Instr. Course Lect. 64, 441–450.

Sueki, D.G., Cleland, J.A., Wainner, R.S., 2013. A regional interdependence model of musculoskeletal dysfunction: research, mechanisms, and clinical implications. J. Man. Manip. Ther. 21, 90–102.

Thomas, J., Glascow, N., Syeed, R., Zis, P., 2019. Alcohol-related peripheral neuropathy: a systematic review and meta-analysis. J. Neurol. 266 (12), 2907–2919.

Thordarson, D.B., 2013. Foot and Ankle, second ed. Lippincott Williams and Wilkins, Philadelphia.

Vaishya, R., Agarwal, A.K., Azizi, A.T., Vijay, V., 2016. Haglund's syndrome: a commonly seen mysterious condition. Cureus. 8 (10), e820.

van Dijk, C.N., Lim, L.S.L., Bossuyt, P.M.M., Marti, R.K., 1996. Physical examination is sufficient for the diagnosis of sprained ankles. J. Bone Joint Surg. 78-B, 958–962.
Vicenzino, B., 2004. Foot orthotics in the treatment of lower limb conditions: a musculoskeletal physiotherapy perspective. Man. Ther. 9, 185–196.
Vuurberg, G., Hoorntje, A., Wink, L.M., Van Der Doelen, B.F., Van Den Bekerom, M.P., Dekker, R., 2018. Diagnosis, treatment and prevention of ankle sprains: update of an evidence-based clinical guideline. Br. J. Sports Med. 52 (15), 956–956.
Walker, R., Wong, F., Singh, S., Ajuied, A., 2019. The foot in systemic disease: management of the patient with rheumatoid arthritis or diabetes mellitus. Orthop. Trauma. 33, 249–262.
Watson, T., 2022. Soft Tissue Repair and Healing Review. Available online at: http://www.electrotherapy.org/modality/soft-tissue-repair-and-healing-review.
Welck, M.J., Hayes, T., Pastides, P., Khan, W., Rudge, B., 2017. Stress fractures of the foot and ankle. Injury 48 (8), 1722–1726.
Wells, P.S., Anderson, D.R., Rodger, M., Forgie, M., Kearon, C., Dreyer, J., et al., 2003. Evaluation of d-dimer in the diagnosis of suspected deep-vein thrombosis. NEJM. 349, 1227–1235.
Whittle, M., Levine, D., Richards, J., 2012. Normal gait. In: Levine, D., Richards, J., Whittle, M.W. (Eds.), Whittle's Gait Analysis, fifth ed. Churchill Livingstone, Edinburgh (Chapter 2).
Wodicka, R., Ferkel, E., Ferkel, R., 2016. Osteochondral lesions of the ankle. Foot Ank. Int. 37, 1023–1034.
Yano, K., Ikari, K., Inoue, E., Sakuma, Y., Mochizuki, T., Koenuma, N., et al., 2018. Features of patients with rheumatoid arthritis whose debut joint is a foot or ankle joint: a 5479-case study from the IORRA cohort. PLoS One. 13 (9), e0202427.
Yates, B., White, S., 2004. The incidence and risk factors in the development of medial tibial stress syndrome among naval recruits. Am. J. Sports Med. 32, 772–780.
Zaw, H., Calder, J.D., 2010. Operative management options for symptomatic flexible adult acquired flatfoot deformity: a review. Knee Surg. Sports Traumatol. Arthrosc. 18, 135–142.

INDEX

Note: Page numbers followed by "f" indicate figures, "t" indicate tables and "b" indicate boxes.

A
A-A segment, 197
A-O joint, 197
ABCDEFW acronym, 156, 158b
Abdomen, lumbar region and, 365
Abdominal aortic aneurysm, 378
Abnormal end-feels, 75t
Abnormal sensation, 44
in cervicothoracic region, 231
in elbow region, 310
in shoulder, 285
in temporomandibular joint, 177
in thoracic region, 260
Accessory movements, 67t, 126–129, 127f, 128b, 160–162, 161t
analytical assessment of, 128f
of elbow region, 326, 326b, 327f–329f, 329t
of foot and ankle, 484–486, 485f, 490t–492t
of hip region, 422, 422b, 423f, 424t
of knee region, 450–451, 451f–452f, 453t, 454f–455f
modifications to, 129, 129b
of shoulder region, 300f, 302
of temporomandibular joint, 188, 189f, 189t
of upper cervical region, 211–214
as combined technique, 213–214, 214t
of wrist and hand, 351–353, 352f, 355t–357t, 357b
Acromioclavicular joint, in joint clearing tests, 77t
Active compression test, 294–295, 295f
Active listening, 12, 12f
Active movements, 67
examination on, 158
of muscle, 161t
Active physiological movements, 67t, 72–75, 161t
of cervicothoracic region, 236, 237f, 240t
combined movements and, 75–77, 76f, 77t
differentiation tests for, 78
in elbow region, 316–317, 316t, 317f
in hip region, 412–414, 413f, 414t
injuring movement and, 78
of knee region, 438–439, 438f, 438t
of lumbar region, 370–372, 371f–372f
modifications to examination of, 75–78, 75b
overpressure and, 74–75
of pelvis, 393–395, 394f–395f
repeated movements and, 77
in shoulder, 287–289, 288f
speed of movements and, 77
standard active testing in, 73–74
sustained movements and, 77
in thoracic region, 267–271, 269f–270f, 270t
differentiation and symptom modification for, 268–271, 271f–272f
in upper cervical region, 208, 209f
of wrist and hand, 340–341, 341t
Active range of motion (AROM), 183
Active straight-leg raise (ASLR) test, for pelvis, 394–395, 395f
Active trigger point, 44
Adaptation of techniques, 1–2
Adaptive coping strategies, 46
Adson's manoeuvre, 301–302
Adson's test, 249
Advanced cognitive skills, 144
Advice, offering, in assessment findings, 28–29
Affective touch, 23
Aggravating factors, of symptoms, 45–46, 49t–50t
in cervicothoracic region, 231
in elbow region, 310–311
in foot and ankle, 472
in hip region, 408–409
in knee region, 432, 437
in lumbar region, 365
in pelvis, 391
in shoulder, 286
in temporomandibular joint, 177
in thoracic region, 260
in upper cervical region, 205
in wrist and hand, 336–337
Alar ligaments, 198f
Allen test, 351
Allodynia, 376
Analgesia, 376
Ankle jerk, 105f, 377
Ankle joint
in joint clearing tests, 77t
measurement of, using figure-of-eight, 483, 483f
mobilizations with movement
dorsiflexion, 487–488, 493f
plantarflexion, 487, 493f
pain in, 477
Ankylosing spondylitis, 262t–264t, 312, 367
Antalgic gait, 71–72
Anterior drawer test
for foot and ankle, 479–480, 479f
for knee region, 443, 443f
Anterior gapping test, for pelvis, 395
Anterior impingement sign, of talocrural joint, 483, 483f
Anterior interosseous syndrome, 325
Anterior stability tests, 442
Anteroposterior glide, of sacroiliac joint, 389f
Anticoagulant therapy, 158
Aortic aneurysm, 378
Apprehension test, for shoulder instability, 298, 298f

Arcuate-popliteus complex, injury to, 441
Arthritic conditions, in elbow region, 312
Arthrogenic gait, 72
'Ask-Offer-Ask' approach, 28
Assessment, 143–172
  activity and participation capabilities and restrictions and, 151
  clinical impression in, 163b
  clinical reasoning and, 144–146
  contributing factors to development and maintenance of problem in, 156–157
  decision-making and, development in, 146–149
  management strategy and treatment planning of, 160–166
  pathobiological mechanisms of, 152–154
    pain, 153–154, 154b
    tissue responses and healing, 152–153
  patient's perspectives on their experience in, 152
  person's story and, entering into, 150–151
  physical examination in, precautions/contraindications to, 157–158
  physical impairments and associated structure/tissue sources of, 154–155
  prognosis of, 166
  severity and irritability in, 158–160
  source of symptoms and, 161t
Atlantoaxial joint, 197f, 214t
Atlantooccipital joint, 197f, 214t
Attitude, patient's, observation of, 236
Audio-recording consultations, 12
Auscultation, 193b
Automatic motivation, 27
Axial compression test (grind test), 346–347, 348f
Axillary nerve, of upper arm, 98f
Axioscapular muscles, 218

B
Babinski response, 98, 105f
Babinski sign
  in cervicothoracic region, 245
  in thoracic region, 273
Baer's point, 422
Balance
  for hip region examination, 412
  for knee region examination, 437–438
Behaviour change wheel, 27, 27f
Behaviour of symptoms
  in cervicothoracic region, 231–232
  in elbow region, 310–311
  in foot and ankle, 472
  in hip region, 408–409
  in knee region, 432–433
  in lumbar region, 365–367, 366t
  in shoulder, 286
  in temporomandibular joint, 177–178
  in thoracic region, 260–261
  in upper cervical region, 205
  in wrist and hand, 336–337
Beighton 9-point score, 73
Biceps femoris tendon, injury to, 441
Biceps jerk, 105f
Biceps load tests I and II, 294, 295f
Biceps tests, for shoulder region, 293
Bicipital tendinopathy, Speed's test for, 293, 294f
Biopsychosocial model, of health, 149f
Bite test, for temporomandibular joint, 189, 191f
Black flags, 48t
Blood pressure
  cervical arterial dysfunction and, 218
  cervicothoracic region and, 249
Blood tests, 155
Blue flags, 48t
Body, division of, 1
Body chart, 37–44, 37t, 38f, 43f, 49t–50t
  of abnormal sensations, 44
  of area of current symptoms, 37–38
  of areas relevant to the region being examined, 38
  of cervicothoracic region, 230–231
  of elbow region, 310
  of foot and ankle, 471–472
    area of current symptoms, 471
    area relevant to region being examined, 471
  of hip region, 408
Body chart (*Continued*)
  of knee region, for examination, 431–432
  of lumbar region, 365, 367, 378
    area of current symptoms, 365
    area relevant to region being examined, 365
    constant or intermittent symptoms in, 365–367
    intensity of pain, 365
    relationship of symptoms in, 365
  of shoulder, 285–286
  of temporomandibular joint, 176–177, 176f
  of thoracic region, 259–260
  of upper cervical region, 204–205
  of wrist and hand, 336, 336f
Bones, prominence of, palpation and, 449–450
Bony alignment, observation of, 315, 315f
Bouchard's nodes, 340
Boutonnière deformity of fingers or thumb, 339, 340f
Brachial plexus, 90f, 311
  palpation of, 301
Bruising, observation of, in elbow region, 315–316
Bruxism, temporomandibular joint and, 179, 185b
Building strong relationship, in communication, 6–9
Bunionette (tailor's bunion), 476
Bursitis, in elbow region, 309t
Buttock pain, mechanism of injury in, 410

C
C-reactive protein (CRP), 55
C1, 197
  nerve roots, 197
C2, 197
C2-3, 197
CAD. *See* Cervical arterial dysfunction
Call, starting the, in remote consultations, 19–20, 20f, 21t–22t
Cancer
  history of, 52
  in thoracic region, 262t–264t
Capsular pattern, of glenohumeral joint, 296

Cardiovascular disease, 472
history of, 51–52
lumbar region and, 368
Carpal bone
palpation of, 351
ten-point movement test for, 357t
Carpal compression test, modified, 350
Carpal tunnel syndrome (CTS)
in median nerve compression, 350
as night symptoms, 337
Carpometacarpal joints, 335
accessory movements of, 355t–356t
active physiological movements of, 340, 341t
movement at, 337f
osteoarthritis of, 335
Cauda equina compression, 367, 370, 410, 435
Cauda equina syndrome (CES), 367
screening for, 53–54, 54b
CCS. *See* Craniocervical spine
Central nervous system testing
for cervicothoracic region, 245
for thoracic region, 273
Central sensitization, 39b, 153
Cervical arterial dysfunction (CAD), 198–208
cranial-nerve examination for, 219
early features of, 157–158
history of, 54
ischaemic presentation of, 207t
preischaemic stage of, 207t
risk factors for, 207t
temporomandibular joint and, 179–180
testing for, 218–219, 249
blood pressure, 218
functional positional testing, 218
proprioception tests, 219
pulse palpation, 219
Cervical arterial system, 199f
Cervical joint position error tests, 247
Cervical plexus, 197, 199f
Cervical spine
combined movement to, 239f
definition of, 230
fracture, 232
in joint clearing tests, 77t
overpressure to, 237f
red-flag screening for, 205, 206t
Cervical spine (*Continued*)
symptoms from, in elbow region, 309t
wrist and hand symptoms referred to, 338
Cervical traction, 215f
Cervicogenic dizziness (CGD), 203
Cervicogenic headache (CGH), 200t, 201
clinical assessment in, 202–203
supportive criteria in, 201t
Cervicothoracic region, 229–256
abnormal sensation in, 231
active physiological movements of, 236, 237f, 240t
aggravating factors in, 231
area of current symptoms in, 230
areas relevant to region being examined, 230–231
behaviour of symptoms in, 231–232
body chart of, 230–231
case study, 253b–254b
completion of examination of, 250–251, 251b
constant or intermittent symptoms in, 231
definition of, 230
differential diagnosis in, 233–234
drug history and, 234
easing factors of, 231–232
family history and, 233
general health in, 233
history of current complaint in, 233
integrity of nervous system and, 243–245
intensity of pain in, 231
investigations, injections and imaging in, 234
isometric muscle testing of, 241–243, 247f–248f
movement control of, 241, 245t, 246f
muscle tests in, 241–243
natural apophyseal glides in, 240–241, 244f
neurodynamic tests of, 245
neurological symptoms in, 234
neurological tests of, 243–245
observation of, 235–236
formal, 235–236
informal, 235
Cervicothoracic region (*Continued*)
palpation of, 236–241
passive accessory intervertebral movements of, 239–240, 242f, 243t, 244f
passive intervertebral examination of, 239, 240t
past medical history in, 233–234
pattern recognition in, 233–234
physical examination of, 235–249
plan of, 234–235
presenting condition in, 233
quality of pain in, 231
relationship of symptoms in, 231
reversed natural apophyseal glides in, 241, 244f
sensorimotor tests for, 245–247, 249f
special questions about, 232–233
state of condition of, 232
subjective examination of, 230–235
sustained natural apophyseal glides in, 241, 244f
twenty-four-hour behaviour of symptoms in, 232
vascular symptoms in, 234, 234b
CES. *See* Cauda equina syndrome
CGD. *See* Cervicogenic dizziness
CGH. *See* Cervicogenic headache
Chair push-up test, 321
Chronic regional pain syndrome, 336
Chronicity, risk factors for, 48, 48t
Circulation, of wrist and hand, tests for, 351
Clarke test, 447, 447f
Clavicular fibres, length testing of, 84f
Claw hand, 340
Claw-toe deformity, 476
Clenching, temporomandibular joint and, 179
Clicking, temporomandibular joint and, 178
Clinical prediction rules (CPRs), of spinal manipulation, criteria for, 147–148, 148t
Clinical reasoning, 1, 35, 143–172, 146b
activity and participation capabilities and restrictions and, 151
clinical impression in, 163b

Clinical reasoning (*Continued*)
complex process of, 144
contributing factors to development and maintenance of problem in, 156–157
form of, using hypothesis categories, 59, 59f
management strategy and treatment planning of, 160–166
pathobiological mechanisms of, 152–154
pain, 153–154, 154b
tissue responses and healing, 152–153
patient's perspectives on their experience in, 152
person's story and, entering into, 150–151
for physical examination, 335
physical examination in, precautions/contraindications to, 157–158
physical impairments and associated structure/tissue sources of, 154–155
process of, 147f
prognosis of, 166
severity and irritability in, 158–160
source of symptoms and, 161t
in working hypotheses, 309
Clinical stage, of cancer, 50
Clinicians, additional, in building strong relationship, 7
Clonus
in cervicothoracic region, 245
in nerve tests, 377
in reflex testing, 98–100
in thoracic region, 273
Cognitive functional therapy, 148
Collaborative reasoning, 35
Collateral ligament testing
lateral, in elbow region, 319–321, 320f
medial, in elbow region, 318–319
Collateral stability tests, 440
Colles fracture, 351
Combined movements, 75–77, 76f, 77t
to cervical spine, 239f
Comfort of performance of technique, 2
Common peroneal nerve palpation, 422, 449
Communication, 3–33
active listening, 12, 12f
of assessment findings, 23–29
changing behaviour, 26–27, 27f
decision-making, shared, 24–26, 25t–26t
goal setting, 26
motivational interviewing, 27
offering advice, 28–29, 29f
perceptions of diagnosis, 23–24, 23t
treatment options, 27–28
in building strong relationship, 6–9
additional companions, 6–7
clinicians, additional, 7
first impressions, 7–9
meeting and greeting, 6, 7t
effective, skills for, 144
empathy, 12–13, 13f
environment preparation, 5, 5b, 6f
hand and, 335
initial contact, 4–5
in negotiating an exit, 29–30, 30b
opening questions and agenda setting, 9, 10t
in person-focused (patient-centered care), 18, 18b, 19f
in physical examination, 20–23
providing feedback, 22
role of touch in communication, 22–23
signposting, 20
undress negotiation, 20–22
in physiotherapy consultations, 13–18, 15t–16t
challenging conversations, 16–17
documenting psychological distress, 17–18
interruptions, 14–16, 14f, 16b, 17t
question styles, 9–12
in remote consultations, 18–20
clear signposting, 18
gaining consent, 20, 21t–22t
starting the call, 19–20, 20f, 21t–22t
technology concerns, 19
self preparation, 5
suggestions when assessing patient with irritable conditions, 159b
Communication (*Continued*)
with severe conditions, 159b
Communication skills, 4
practical guides to, 12
Companions, in building strong relationship, 6–7
Complex classification systems, 148
Complex regional pain syndrome 1 (CRPS 1), 71
Compression
to cervical spine, 237f
pattern, regular, 76
Compression neuropathy, testing for, in elbow region, 324–325
Compression test/posterior gapping, for pelvis, 396, 396f
Computed tomography (CT), for foot and ankle, 473–474
Concave-convex rule, 127, 127f
Consent, in remote consultations, 20, 21t–22t
Constant pain, 44
Constant symptoms, 44, 158
in cervicothoracic region, 231
in elbow region, 310
in foot and ankle, 471
in hip region, 408
in temporomandibular joint, 177
in thoracic region, 260
Contact, initial, 4–5
Contract buttock, 103f
Contraindications, to physical examination
in elbow region, 313
in lumbar region, 367, 369
to physical examination, 157–158
in wrist and hand, 338
Contributing factors, for patient's symptoms, 156–157
Conversations, challenging, in physiotherapy consultations, 16–17
Coordination, in nerve tests, 100, 100b, 106f, 377
Coping strategies, 46
Cord compression, red-flag screening for, 206t
Cortical spreading depression (CSD), 201
Costochondral joints, accessory movements in, 277t
Cozen's test, 322
CPRs. *See* Clinical prediction rules

Cranial nerve disorders, temporomandibular joint and, 179
Cranial nerve examination, of cervicothoracic region, 249
Craniocervical extension test, 217
Craniocervical flexion test, 217f
Craniocervical spine (CCS), 197
  muscle group, 198f
  neurological conductivity testing for, 210t–211t
  stability, 197
  symptoms associated with, 198–204
Crepitus
  with groin pain, 409t, 411b
  in knee region, 433
CRP. *See* C-reactive protein
CSD. *See* Cortical spreading depression
CTS. *See* Carpal tunnel syndrome
Cubital tunnel syndrome, elbow flexion test for, 324–325
Cubital valgus, 315
Cubital varus, 315
Cutaneous nerve
  supply to face, head, and neck, 91f
  supply to trunk, 92f

D

DASH. *See* Disabilities of the Arm, Shoulder and Hand
De Quervain disease
  area of current symptoms in, 335
  tests for, 349, 349f
Decision-making
  development in, 146–149
  shared, 24–26, 25t–26t
Deep cervical extensors, 217
  test, 217, 218f
Deep cervical flexors, strength testing of, 80f
Deep cervical muscle testing
  for cervicothoracic region, 241
  for upper cervical region, 216
Deep craniocervical flexors, 216
Deep occipital muscles, length testing of, 84f, 218
Deep-vein thrombosis, suspected, Wells score for, 482–483
Degenerative conditions, of ankle, 469
Demonstration, 22
Dental disorders, temporomandibular joint and, 179
Dental occlusion, temporomandibular joint and, 174
Dermatomes
  associated with thoracic spinal nerves, 92f
  of cervicothoracic region, 243
  of elbow region, 323–324
  of head and neck, 91f
  of lower limb nerves, 94f
  test for
    for foot and ankle, 482
    for hip region, 421
    for lumbar region, 376
    for temporomandibular joint, 186
  of thoracic region, 271
  of upper cervical region, 209–211
  of upper limb nerves, 94f
  of wrist and hand examination, 349
Dexterity tests, 340
Diabetes mellitus, 311, 473
  history of, 52
  lumbar region and, 368
  red flag and, 157
  wrist and hand examination and, 339
Dial test, 444–445, 444f
Differentiation testing
  for active physiological movements, 78
  in elbow region, 317, 318f
  for thoracic region, 268–271, 271f
Disabilities of the Arm, Shoulder and Hand (DASH), 335–336
Disability, health and, hypothesis categories framework of, 35, 35f, 36b
Distraction, to cervical spine, 237f
Distraction/anterior gapping test, for pelvis, 395
Dizziness
  from cervicothoracic region, 230–231
  differential diagnosis of, 203f
  upper cervical spine, 203
  whiplash-related, 203–204
Dorsal horn, pathways of, underlying referred pain, 41–42, 42f
Dorsal scapular nerve, palpation of, 301
Double adductor test, for hip region, 419, 419f
Drawer test
  anterior
    for foot and ankle, 479–480, 479f
    for knee region, 443, 443f
  posterior
    for knee region, 444, 444f
    for shoulder instability, 298, 298f
Drop-foot gait, 72
Drug history, 495b–496b
Drug therapy
  lumbar region and, 368–369
  in subjective examination, 55
Dupuytren's contracture, of palmar fascia, 340
Dynamic loading and distraction, in temporomandibular joint, 189
Dysaesthesia, 44

E

Ear symptoms, temporomandibular joint and, 180
Ease of performance, of technique, 2
Easing factors, 45–46
  in cervicothoracic region, 231–232
  in elbow region, 311
  in foot and ankle, 472
  in hip region, 409
  in knee region, 432
  in lumbar region, 366, 366t
  in pelvis, 391
  in shoulder, 286
  in temporomandibular joint, 177–178
  in thoracic region, 260
  in upper cervical region, 205
  in wrist and hand, 337
EAST. *See* Elevated arm stress test
EBP. *See* Evidence-based practice
Effective communication skills, 144
Effectiveness of technique performance, 1–2
Effusion, palpation and, 449
Ehlers-Danlos syndrome, 73
Eichhoff test, 349
Elbow flexion test, for cubital tunnel syndrome, 324–325
Elbow joint, in joint clearing tests, 77t
Elbow ligamentous injuries, 312

Elbow region, examination of, 307–333, 308b
accessory movements in, 326, 326b, 327f–329f, 329t
active physiological movements in, 316–317, 316t
behaviour of symptoms in, 310–311
aggravating factors, 310–311
easing factors, 311
stage of the condition, 313, 313b
twenty-four-hour, 311
body chart in, 310
abnormal sensation, 310
area of current symptoms, 310
areas relevant to the region being examined, 310
constant or intermittent symptoms, 310
intensity of pain, 310
quality of pain, 310
relationship of symptoms, 310
case study on, 330b–332b
causes of pain and/or limitation of movement in, 309t
completion of, 326–329
functional testing in, 316
joint integrity tests in, 318–321
muscle strength testing in, 347
muscle tests in, 321–323
observation in, 315–316
palpation in, 325–326
passive physiological movements in, 318
patients' perspective, on experience, 309–310
physical, 315–326
accessory movements in, 326, 326b, 327f–329f, 329t
active physiological movements in, 316–317, 316t, 317f
completion of, 326–329
developing working and alternative hypotheses in, 313, 314t
functional testing in, 316
joint integrity tests in, 318–321
muscle tests in, 321–323
palpation in, 325–326
passive physiological movements in, 318, 318f
plan of, 313–314
Elbow region, examination of (*Continued*)
precautions and contraindications for, 313
predominant pain mechanism in, 313–314
sequence and extent of, 314
vascular considerations in, 325
present condition, history of, 312–313
special questions for, 311–312
drug history in, 312
elbow stiffness or arthritic conditions in, 312
past medical and family history in, 312
radiography and medical imaging in, 312
sudden swelling in, 312
subjective, 309–314
behaviour of symptoms in, 310–311
body chart in, 310
drug history in, 312
patients' perspective, on experience, 309–310
present condition, history of, 312–313
special/screening questions in, 311
vascular considerations in, 325
Elbow tendinopathy
lateral, symptom modification for, 323, 324f
medial, 323
Elevated arm stress test (EAST), 301
Empathy, 12–13, 13f
Empty-can test, for supraspinatus tear or tendinopathy, 292, 293f
End-feels
abnormal, 75t
normal, 75t
Epilepsy, history of, 52
Erector spinae
length testing of, 84f
muscle length of, 448
Erythrocyte sedimentation rate (ESR), 55
ESR. *See* Erythrocyte sedimentation rate
Evening symptoms, 47
in cervicothoracic region, 232
Evening symptoms (*Continued*)
in elbow region, 311
in foot and ankle, 472
in hip region, 409
in knee region, 432–433
in lumbar region, 366–367
in pelvis, 391–392
in shoulder region, 286
in wrist and hand, 337
Evidence-based practice (EBP), 163f
Extension, to cervical spine, 237f
Extensor carpi radialis brevis, 322
External rotation stress test, 480–481, 480f
Extrinsic muscle tightness, of wrist and hand, 348
Eye contact, in nonverbal behaviours, 8–9

F

FABER test. *See* Flexion abduction external rotation (FABER) test
FABQ. *See* Fear avoidance belief questionnaire
Face, symmetry of, test of, 181f
Facet joint, in thoracic region, 262t–264t
Facial chart, for recording head and facial symptoms, 176f
FADDIR. *See* Flexion adduction internal rotation
FAI. *See* Femoroacetabular impingement
Fairbank's apprehension test, 447
Family history
in cervicothoracic region examination, 233
in elbow region examination, 312
in lumbar region examination, 367–369
in subjective examination, 37t, 56
FBC. *See* Full blood count
FDS. *See* Flexor digitorum superficialis
Fear avoidance behaviours, 359b–360b
Fear avoidance belief questionnaire (FABQ), 148, 149b
Feedback, during physical examination, 22
Feelings, patient's, observation of, 236

Femoral nerve slump test, 108–110, 109f
Femoral nerve tension test in side-lying, 377
Femoroacetabular impingement (FAI), 407–408, 411b, 414
Fibromyalgia syndrome, in thoracic region, 262t–264t
Figure-of-eight measurement
  of ankle, 483, 483f
  of wrist and hand, 351
Finger-nose tests, 377
Fingers
  in joint clearing tests, 77t
  muscle strength testing in, 347
Finkelstein test, for De Quervain's disease, 349, 349f
First impressions, in building strong relationship, 7–9
  good consultation as, 8
  handshakes as, 7–8
  nonverbal behaviours as, 8–9
  prosody as, 8
  small talk as, 8
Flat-back posture, 68, 69f
Flatfoot deformity, 476
Flexion, to cervical spine, 237f
Flexion abduction external rotation (FABER) test, for hip region, 416–417, 416f
Flexion adduction internal rotation (FADDIR), 416, 416f
Flexion-extension PPIVM, 211, 212f
Flexion-rotation test, 202, 202f, 211
Flexor digitorum superficialis (FDS), test for, 349
Foot and ankle, 468–501, 469t
  accessory movements of, 484–486, 485f, 490t–492t
  anatomical and functional overview, 469–470, 469t, 470b
  body chart, 471–472
    area of current symptoms, 471
    area relevant to region being examined, 471
  case study on, 495b–496b
  completion of examination, 488–489
  constant or intermittent symptoms in, 471
  dorsiflexion, 103f
  dysfunction, 469–470
Foot and ankle (*Continued*)
  eversion, 103f
  function of, 469
  functional testing of, 476–477
  history of present condition and, 473–474
  intensity of pain, 471
  joint integrity tests of, 477–481
  mobilizations with movement, symptom modification and, 486–488
  muscle tests for, 481–482
    length, 481
    strength, 481
  neurological symptoms of, 473
  neurological tests for, 482
    integrity of nervous system, 482
    nerve palpation, 482
    neurodynamic tests, 482
    reflex testing, 482
  observation of, 475–476
    alignment, 475
    formal, 475–476
    gait, 476–477
    informal, 475
    of muscle form, 475
    of posture, 475
    of soft tissue, 475–476
  outcome measures of, 470
  palpation, 484
    nerve, 482
  past medical history, 473
  physical examination for, 475–488
    plan, 474–475
  physiological movements of
    active, 469t, 477, 477t, 478f
    passive, 477
  quality of symptoms in, 471
  radiograph and medical imaging for, 473–474, 474b
  relationship of symptoms in, 472
  serious pathology of, 472
  social history and, 470–471
  subjective examination of, 470–475
    patients' perspective, 470, 470f
    special questions, 472–473
  symptoms, referred from, 431
  symptoms behaviour of, 472
    aggravating factors, 472
    easing factors, 472
    twenty-four-hour, 472
  vascular tests of, 482–483
Forearm
  muscle strength testing in, 347
  pronation and supination, in mobilizations with movement, 348–349
Formal observation, 67–72
  in elbow region, 315–316
  in thoracic region, 266–267
  in wrist and hand, 339
Fracture, 420t
Fracture test, for hip region, 417
Froment's sign
  for elbow region, 325
  for ulnar nerve paralysis, 351
Fulcrum test, for hip region, 417, 417f
Full blood count (FBC), 55
Full-can test, for supraspinatus tear or tendinopathy, 292, 293f
Function observation, for hip region, 412
Functional ability, 72, 72b
Functional reach tests, 72
Functional testing
  for elbow region, 316
  for knee region, 456
  for pelvis, 393
  for wrist and hand, 340

G

Gaenslen's/pelvic torsion test, for pelvis, 396, 396f
Gait
  in foot and ankle examination, 476–477
  in hip region examination, 412
  in knee region examination, 438
  observation of, 71–72
Gait analysis, 476
Gait cycle, 476
Gastrocnemius
  length testing of, 84f
  muscle length of, 448
Gaze stability, 204
General health, 51
  in cervicothoracic region, 233
  in foot and ankle, 472–473
  in lumbar region, 368
  in pelvis, 392
  in thoracic region, 261
  in wrist and hand examination, 337–338

Genu valgum, 437
Genu varum, 437
Gerber 'lift-off,' for subscapularis tendinopathy, 292–293, 293f
Gifford's mature organism model of reasoning, 153, 153f
Gillet test, for pelvis, 394, 394f
Glenohumeral joint
accessory movements to, 300f
capsular pattern of, 296
instability, 296–298
Global mobilizers, 79, 83t
Global stabilizer, 79, 83t
Gluteal tendinopathy, 417–418, 420t
Gluteus maximus
gait, 72, 412
strength testing of, 80f
Gluteus medius
gait, 72
posterior, strength testing of, 80f
Gluteus minimus, strength testing of, 80f
Goal setting, in assessment findings, 26
Golfer's elbow, 309t
muscle length in, 321
test for, 323
Good consultation, first impressions and, 8
Gout, 469
Gradual symptom onset, in elbow region, 313
Greeting, in building strong relationship, 6, 7t
Grind test, 346–347, 348f
'Grip and grind' test, 317
Grip strength, 323, 347–348
Groin
hernia, 420t
locking/catching in, 409t
lumbar region and, 365
pain
with crepitus, 409t
mechanism of injury, 410
sports-related, 420t
sports-related chronic, 419
on squatting, 409t
Gut-feeling response, 145–146
Guyon's canal, palpation on, 350–351

H
Haemarthrosis, in knee region, 433
Haglund's deformity, 476
Hallux rigidus, 476
Hallux valgus, 475–476
Hammer-toe deformity, 476
Hamstrings
length testing of, 84f
muscle length of, 448
Hand
deformities of, 339–340
neurological symptoms of, in elbow region, 310
Handling improvement tips, 2
Handshakes, first impressions and, 7–8
Hautant's test, 219
Hawkins-Kennedy test, 296, 296f
Headache, 199–201
cervicogenic, 200t
differential diagnosis of, 200t
sustained natural apophyseal glides for, 215f
in temporomandibular joint, 180
Headache Disability Index Questionnaire, 220, 220f–221f
Healing, tissue response and, 152–153
Health
biopsychosocial model of, 149f
disability and, hypothesis categories framework of, 35, 35f, 36b
Heberden's nodes, 340
Heel-shin sliding tests, 377
Heel-to-knee test, 219
Herpes zoster, in thoracic region, 262t–264t
Hip joint, in joint clearing tests, 77t
Hip region, 407–429
accessory movements in, 422, 422b, 423f, 424t
active physiological movements in, 412–414, 413f, 414t
body chart of, 408
area of current symptoms, 408
areas relevant to region being examined, 408
case study, 425b–427b
completion of examination of, 423–424
constant or intermittent symptoms in, 408

Hip region (*Continued*)
extraarticular structure tests for, 417–420
double adductor test, 419
gluteal tendinopathy, 417–418
resisted external derotation test, 418, 418f
sports-related chronic groin pain, 419
squeeze test, 419–420, 419f, 420t
sustained single-leg stance, 418, 418f
flexion, 103f
history of present condition in, 409–410
impingement, 420t
intraarticular structure tests for, 414–417
flexion abduction external rotation (FABER) test, 416–417, 416f
flexion adduction internal rotation (FADDIR) test, 416, 416f
fracture test, 417
fulcrum test, 417, 417f
hip impingement test, 414–416
internal rotation over pressure (IROP) test, 416, 416f
muscle tests for, 420–421
isometric testing, 421
muscle control, 420–421
muscle length, 421
muscle strength, 420
neurological tests for, 421
integrity of nervous system, 421
neurodynamic, 421
reflex testing, 421
observation of, 411–412
balance, 412
function, 412
gait, 412
muscle form, 412
posture, 412
soft tissues, 412
palpation of, 418–419
passive physiological movements in, 414
past medical history of, 410
physical examination of, 411–422
plan of, 410–411
subjective examination of, 408–411

Hip region (*Continued*)
special questions, 409, 409t
symptom behaviour in, 408–409
aggravating factors, 408–409
easing factors, 409
twenty-four-hour symptoms, 409
symptom relationship with, 408
vascular tests for, 421–422
History of present condition
in elbow region, 312–313
in foot and ankle, 473–474
in hip region, 409–410
in knee region, 433–434, 434t
in lumbar region, 367
in pelvis, 392
in shoulder region, 286–287
in subjective examination, 37t, 56
HIV. *See* Human immunodeficiency virus
Hook test, for distal biceps, 323f
Hop testing battery, 459
Horizontal adduction, shoulder region and, 291, 291f
HSD. *See* Hypermobility spectrum disorder
Human immunodeficiency virus (HIV), history of, 52
Human intersubjectivity, 150
Humeroradial joint, 308
accessory movements in, 326, 328f, 329t
active physiological movements in, 316
aggravating factors in, 310–311
differentiation testing in, 317, 318f
passive physiological movements in, 318
Humeroulnar joint, 308
accessory movements in, 326, 327f, 329t
active physiological movements in, 316
aggravating factors in, 310–311
differentiation testing in, 317, 318f
passive physiological movements in, 318
Humerus, fracture of, in elbow region, 309t
Hyperalgesia, 376
Hypermobility, 73
lumbar region and, 373
temporomandibular joint and, 182
Hypermobility spectrum disorder (HSD), 73
history of, 54
Hypermobility syndrome, in elbow region, 309t
Hyperpathia, 376
Hypomobility, lumbar region and, 373
Hypothenar eminence, muscle strength testing in, 347
Hypothesis categories
clinical reasoning form using, 59, 59f
in framework of health and disability, 35, 36b
Hypothetico-deductive reasoning, 35, 145–146, 160

I

ICAs. *See* Internal carotid arteries
ICF. *See* International Classification of Functioning, Disability and Health
Iliopsoas
length testing of, 84f
muscle length of, 448
Iliotibial band (ITB), injury to, 441
Illness scripts, 144–145, 145f
Impingement test, for hip region, 414–416
Infection
in elbow region, 309t
in lumbar region, 365
Inferior radioulnar joint, 308
accessory movements in, 326, 329f, 329t
active physiological movements in, 316
Inferior tibiofibular joint, 469
mobilizations with movement, 486–487, 493f
Inflammatory arthritis, 312, 472
history of, 53
Inflammatory conditions
of ankle, 469
of elbow region, 309t
of lumbar region, 366
of wrist and hand, 335
Inflammatory pain, 39b
Informal observation
in elbow region, 315
in thoracic region, 266
Informal observation (*Continued*)
in wrist and hand, 339
Infraspinatus, full-thickness tears of, external rotation lag sign for, 293, 294f
Initial observation, 67
Injuring movements, in active physiological movements, 78
Instability, laxity *versus*, 297
Instrumental touch, 22
Intercarpal joints, 335
accessory movements of, 352f, 355t–356t
Interchondral joints, accessory movements in, 277t
Intermetacarpal joints, hand, 335
accessory movements of, 352f, 355t–356t
Intermetatarsal joints, 483–484
Intermittent symptoms, 44, 158
in cervicothoracic region, 231
in elbow region, 310
in foot and ankle, 471
in hip region, 408
in temporomandibular joint, 177
in thoracic region, 260
Internal carotid arteries (ICAs), 198
dissection, pain presentation for, 207f
dysfunction, 207t
typical pain presentation for, 207f
Internal femoral rotation, 437
Internal rotation over pressure (IROP) test, for hip region, 416, 416f
International Classification of Functioning, Disability and Health (ICF), 149
Interphalangeal joints, of foot, 476
Interruptions, in physiotherapy consultations, 14–16, 14f, 16b, 17t
Intervertebral disc disorders, lumbar region and, 364
Interviewing, motivational, 27
Intractable plantar keratosis, 476
Intrinsic muscle tightness, of wrist and hand, 348
Irritability, of symptoms, 45b, 46–47, 143–144, 158–160, 160b
Irritable symptoms
in elbow region, 314
in knee region, 436

Irritable symptoms (*Continued*)
in lumbar region, 370
Ischaemic pain, 39b
Isometric contraction, of muscle, 67t, 161t
Isometric muscle testing, 89, 89b
for cervicothoracic region, 241–243, 247f–248f
for elbow region, 321, 322f
for hip region, 421
for knee region, 448
for upper cervical region, 214–215
for wrist and hand, 348–349
Isotonic testing, for upper cervical region, 214
ITB. *See* Iliotibial band

J
Jendrassik manoeuvre, 97
Joint
effusion tests, 439–440
palpation of, 160–162, 161t
physical examination tests for, 67
as source of symptoms, of upper motor neurone lesion, 219
tests, 67t, 162
Joint clearing tests, 76–77, 77t
Joint integrity tests, 67t, 78
for elbow region, 318–321
for knee region, 440–445
for wrist and hand, 341–347
Joint position error (JPE), 249f
Joint proprioception, 93
JPE. *See* Joint position error

K
Kaltenborn tests, for accessory movements, 351–353, 357t
Kienbock's disease, 336
Kinetic chain, thoracic spine dysfunction and, 258–259
Kleiger test, 480–481
Knee extension, 103f
Knee jerk, 105f, 377, 448, 482
Knee joint, in joint clearing tests, 77t
Knee region, 430–467
accessory movements of, 450–451, 451f–452f, 453t, 454f–455f
active physiological movements of, 438–439, 438f, 438t
Knee region (*Continued*)
assessment of quadriceps activation, 456–458
assessment of return to play/performance, 455–456
behaviour of symptoms and, 432–433
aggravating factors in, 432
easing factors in, 432
twenty-four-hour, 432–433
body chart for, 431–432
area of current symptoms in, 431
areas relevant to the region being examined in, 431–432
case study on, 461b–463b
completion of the examination of, 459–460
contributing factors and, 435
crepitus in, 433
giving way of, 433
history of the present condition of, 433–434, 434t
informal observation, 436–437
irritable symptoms in, 436
joint effusion tests for, 439–440
joint integrity tests for, 440–445
joint line tenderness for, 446
leg length and, 449
locking of, 433
mechanism of injury of, 433, 434t
meniscal test for, 445–446
muscle tests for, 447–448
control, 448
isometric, 448
length, 448
strength, 447–448
neurological tests for, 448–449
integrity of the nervous system and, 448
neurodynamic, 448–449
reflex testing in, 448
observation of, 436–438
balance, 437–438
gait, 438
muscle form, 437
posture, 437
soft tissue, 437
pain in
depth of, 431–432
intensity of, 431–432
mechanisms of, 435
Knee region (*Continued*)
provoked or reduced on palpation, 449
quality of, 431–432
palpation of, 449–450
passive physiological movements of, 439, 440f
past medical history of, 434
patellofemoral tests for, 446–447
physical examination of, 436–459, 436t
plan of, 434–435, 435b
for return to sport, 456
quality of movement in, 438
referred, symptoms in, 431
relationship of symptoms and, 432
source of symptoms in, 435
subjective examination of, 431–435
hypothesis after, 436
special questions in, 433
swelling of, 433
symptom modification and, 453–455
vascular tests for, 449
Knowledge flow diagram, 145f
Kyphosis-lordosis posture, 68, 68f

L
Lachman test, 442–443, 442f
Latent irritability, 47
Lateral collateral ligament injury, 441
Lateral collateral ligament testing, in elbow region, 319–321, 320f
Lateral elbow tendinopathy, symptom modification for, 323, 324f
Lateral epicondylalgia, 309t
Lateral epicondyles, 315, 315f
Lateral flexion, to cervical spine, 237f
Lateral tibial torsion, 437
Lateralis, 216
Latissimus dorsi, length testing of, 84f
Laxity, instability *versus*, 297
Left extension quadrant, to cervical spine, 237f
Leg length, 378
measurement of, 422, 449
Lens model, 145–146
Levator scapulae
length testing of, 84f

Levator scapulae (*Continued*)
muscle length testing, 218
Ligament of Struthers, 325
Ligamentous injuries, in elbow region, 312
Ligamentous instability test, for joints of thumb and fingers, 346
Ligamentous sprain, in elbow region, 309t
Light touch
examination, 91–92
for hip region, 421
for knee region, 448
lower limb and, 376
Likelihood ratios (LRs), in physical examination, 66
Limb symmetry index, 456
Linea alba, 182, 182f
Lingual mandibular reflex (CN V), temporomandibular joint and, 188
Listening, active, 12, 12f
Load and shift test, for shoulder instability, 297, 297f
Local stabilizer muscles, 79, 83t
London Hospital test, 447
Long dorsal ligament, palpation of, 399
Longus capitis, 216
Longus colli, 216
Lordosis, lumbar region and, 376
LOVE acronym, 152–153
Low-back pain, 364
pain diary, 365
Low flexion, shoulder region and, 291, 291f
Lower limb
lumbar region and, 365
nerves of, 100f
pain sensation of, 421
LRs. *See* Likelihood ratios
Lumbar multifidus, 374–375
Lumbar nerve roots
myotome testing for, 103f
Lumbar region, 363–386
compensatory movement strategies for, 372
examination, completion of, 380
irritable symptoms in, 370
neurological symptoms in, 367
pain in
behaviour, 370
Lumbar region (*Continued*)
night symptoms, 366
provoked or reduced on palpation, 378
physical examination for, 370–380
active physiological movements, 370–372, 371f–372f
differentiation or symptom modification, 372–373, 373f
miscellaneous tests, 377–378
muscle tests, 374–376
neurological tests, 376–377
observation, 370
palpation, 378
passive accessory intervertebral movements, 378–380, 379f–380f, 380b
passive physiological movements, 373–374, 374f
plan of, 369
precautions or contraindications to, 367
severe symptoms, 369
subjective examination of, 364–369
behaviour of symptoms in, 365–367, 366t
body chart of, 365, 367
family history and, 367–369
history of present condition in, 367
hypotheses, development of, 369
past medical history in, 367
patient's perspective, 364–365
special questions, 367
Lumbar spine, 364
in joint clearing tests, 77t
pain on, 70, 71f
Lunotriquetral ballottement (Reagan's) test, 342–344

M

Magnetic resonance imaging (MRI)
for foot and ankle, 473–474
for wrist and hand, 338
Maladaptive coping strategies, 46, 47b
Mallet finger, 340
Mallet-toe deformity, 476
Management strategy, of clinical reasoning, 160–166
Mandible, resting position of, 181
Mandibular condyle, palpation of, via external auditory meatus, 191f
Mastication, muscles of, 174, 176b
Matles test, for Achilles tendon rupture, 482
Maudsley test, 322
McKenzie method, of mechanical diagnosis, 148
McMurray test, 445, 445f–446f
Mechanical pain, 39b
Medial collateral ligament testing, in elbow region, 318–319
Medial elbow tendinopathy, 323
Medial epicondylalgia, 309t
Medial epicondyles, 315, 315f
Medial tibial torsion, 437
Median nerve
compression neuropathy tests, 325
palpation of, 301
test for, 350
of upper limb, 99f
upper-limb neurodynamic test for. *See* ULNT 1, ULNT 2a
Medical Communications Behavior System (MCBS), 15t–16t
Medical imaging
for cervicothoracic region, 234
for elbow region, 312
for foot and ankle, 473–474, 474b
for lumbar region, 369
for pelvis, 392–393
in subjective examination, 55
for thoracic region, 261
Medical referral, 232, 370
Meeting, in building strong relationship, 6, 7t
Meniscal tear, 433
Meniscal tests, 445–446
Metacarpophalangeal joints, accessory movements of, 342f, 355t–356t
Metatarsophalangeal joints, 471
Michigan Hand Outcomes Questionnaire, 335–336
Midcarpal joints, 335
Midcarpal shift test, 344
Midtarsal joints, 476
Migraine, 200, 200t
Miscellaneous tests
for lumbar region, 377–378
for temporomandibular joint, 188

Miscellaneous tests (*Continued*)
for thoracic region, 273–274
Modification, progression and regression of treatment, 165f
Morning symptoms, 47
in cervicothoracic region, 232
in elbow region, 311
in foot and ankle, 472
in hip region, 409
in knee region, 432–433
in lumbar region, 366–367
in pelvis, 391–392
in shoulder region, 286
in wrist and hand, 337
Morton's neuroma, Mulder's test for, 483–484
Motivational interviewing, 27
Motor changes, 96, 97t, 98f–100f, 103f
Motor control
definition of, 273b
training, 375–376
Motor loss
in elbow region, 324
in lumbar region, 377
Motor neurone lesion, in upper cervical region, pathological reflex testing for, 211
Movement control, of cervicothoracic region, 241, 245t, 246f
Movement diagrams, 129–132, 129f
knee region and, 450
procedure for drawing, 129–132
muscle spasm, 131–132, 131f–133f
pain, 67, 131
resistance, 129–131, 130f
Movement system balance theory, 73
MRI. *See* Magnetic resonance imaging
Mulder's test, for Morton's neuroma, 483–484
Muscle
active movements of, 161t
classification of, 83t
isometric contraction of, 161t
palpation of, 161t, 162
passive lengthening of, 161t
patterns/reactions of, to stress, 82t
physical examination tests for, 67t
Muscle (*Continued*)
as source of symptoms, of upper motor neurone lesion, 219
Muscle control, 83–84
test
for hip region, 420–421
for knee region, 448
for lumbar region, 375
Muscle endurance, definition of, 273b
Muscle form, observation of, 70–71
in cervicothoracic region, 236
in elbow region, 316
in hip region, 412
in knee region, 437
in wrist and hand examination, 339
Muscle imbalance, 79–82
Muscle length, 84–89, 84f
definition of, 273b
testing
for elbow region, 321
for hip region, 421
for knee region, 448
for pelvis, 399
for upper cervical region, 218
for wrist and hand, 348
Muscle spasm, 74
in elbow region, 316
in knee region, 438, 449
in lumbar region, 370–372
movement diagrams for, 131–132, 131f
Muscle strength, 83t
definition of, 273b
testing
for elbow region, 321
for hip region, 420
for knee region, 447–448
for lumbar region, 374–375
for upper cervical region, 214–218
for wrist and hand, 347–348
Muscle tests, 67t, 78–89, 82t
in cervicothoracic region, 241–243
in elbow region, 321–323
for foot and ankle, 481–482
length, 481
strength, 481
for hip region, 420–421
isometric muscle testing. *See* Isometric muscle testing
for knee region, 447–448
Muscle tests (*Continued*)
for lumbar region, 374–376
muscle length. *See* Muscle length
muscle strength. *See* Muscle strength
for pelvis, 398–399
for shoulder
control in, 298–299, 300f
strength in, 299
temporomandibular joint and, 186
endurance testing, 186
isometric, 186
muscle control, 186
muscle strength, 186, 187f
for thoracic region, 271, 273b
for upper cervical region, 214–218
for wrist and hand, 347–349
Musculocutaneous nerve, 98f
Musculoskeletal condition, examination of patients with, 2
Musculoskeletal dysfunction, process of examination of, 1
Myelopathy, 261
Myogenic pain, in temporomandibular joint, 179
Myositis ossificans, in elbow region, 309t
Myotomes, 97t
in cervicothoracic region, 243–245
in elbow region, 324
in foot and ankle, 482
in hip region, 421
in knee region, 448
in lumbar region, 376–377
in temporomandibular joint, 186
in upper cervical region, 211
in wrist and hand examination, 349–350

N
NAG. *See* Natural apophyseal glides
Narrative reasoning, 35
Natural apophyseal glides (NAGs), in cervicothoracic region, 240–241, 244f
Nature of symptoms, of pelvis, 390–391
area of current symptoms, 390–391, 390f
intensity of pain, 391
quality of symptoms, 391
relationship of symptoms, 391

Neck, vascular pathologies of, 232–233
Neck Disability Index, 230
Neer test, for shoulder impingement syndrome, 296, 296f
Neoplastic conditions, 311
  lumbar region and, 367
Neoplastic disease, temporomandibular joint and, 177
Nerve
  palpation of, 120–126, 161t, 301
  physical examination for, 67t
  as source of symptoms, of upper motor neurone lesion, 219
  tests, 67t
Nervous system, integrity of, 89–100
  in temporomandibular joint, 186
  in upper cervical region, 209
  in wrist and hand, 349–350
Neural sensitization tests, 100–106
  femoral nerve slump test, 108–110, 109f
  for lumbar region, 377
  obturator nerve test, 111
  passive neck flexion, 107–108, 108f
  prone knee bend, 108
  saphenous nerve test, 110, 110f
  straight leg raise, 108, 109f
  testing principles of, 106–120
  upper limb neurodynamic tests, 111–120
Neurodynamic tests, 106
  in cervicothoracic region, 245
  in elbow region, 324
  in knee region, 448–449
  in temporomandibular joint, 186
  in thoracic region, 271–273
  in upper cervical region, 211
  in wrist and hand, 350
Neurological integrity, in thoracic region, 271–273
Neurological symptoms, 53–54
  in foot and ankle, 473
  in lumbar region, 367
  in shoulder, 286
  in thoracic region, 261
Neurological tests, 89–126, 126b
  for cervicothoracic region, 243–245
  for elbow region, 323–325
  for foot and ankle, 482
    integrity of nervous system, 482
Neurological tests (*Continued*)
    nerve palpation, 482
    neurodynamic tests, 482
    reflex testing, 482
  for hip region, 421
  for knee region, 448–449
  for lumbar region, 376–377
    dermatomes/peripheral nerves, 376
    myotomes/peripheral nerves, 376–377
    nervous system, integrity of, 376–377
    neural sensitization tests, 377
    reflex testing, 377
  for shoulder region, 301
  for temporomandibular joint, 186–188
    dermatomes, 186
    integrity of nervous system, 186
    myotomes, 186
    neurodynamic tests, 186
    reflex testing, 186
  for thoracic region, 271
  for upper cervical region, 208–211
  for wrist and hand, 349–351
Neuropathic pain, 160
  symptoms of, 54
Night symptoms, 47
  in cervicothoracic region, 232
  in elbow region, 311
  in foot and ankle, 472
  in hip region, 409
  in knee region, 432
  in lumbar region, 366
  in pelvis, 391
  in shoulder region, 286
  in upper cervical region, 205
  in wrist and hand, 337
Nociceptive pain, 39b, 154b
Nociplastic pain, 39b, 154b
Nonpropositional knowledge, 145, 145f
Nonverbal behaviours, 8–9, 9b
  eye contact in, 8–9
  posture in, 9
  smiling in, 9
Normal end-feels, 75t
NPRS. *See* Numerical pain rating scale
Numerical pain rating scale (NPRS), 41f, 231

O

OA. *See* Osteoarthritis
Objective, in physical examination, 66
Oblique/sideways step down/landing test, 458
Observation, 67–72, 67t
  of cervicothoracic region, 235–236
  of elbow region, 315–316
  of foot and ankle, 475–476
    alignment, 475
    formal, 475–476
    informal, 475
    of muscle form, 475
    of posture, 475
    of soft tissue, 475–476
  formal, 67–72, 235–236
  of gait, 71–72
  of hip region, 411–412
  informal, 235
  initial, 67
  of knee region, 437–438
  of lumbar region, 370
  of muscle form, 70–71
  of pelvis, 393
  of posture, 67–70
  of soft tissues, 71
  of upper cervical region, 208
  of wrist and hand, 339–340
Obstetric history, pelvis and, 392, 393b
Obturator nerve test, 111
Oculomotor function, tests for, 204
Oculomotor tests, of cervicothoracic region, 247, 249f
Oedema, 325, 422, 449, 476
Olecranon, 315, 315f
Olecranon bursitis, 67
Opening question, agenda setting and, 9, 10t
Orange flags, 48t
Osgood-Schlatter disease, 437
Osteoarthritis
  of elbow region, 309t
  stiff shoulder and, 296
  of thoracic region, 262t–264t
  of wrist and hand, 335
Osteochondral defects, affecting talus, 469
Osteoporosis, 157, 472
  history of, 53
  in lumbar region, 368

Osteoporosis (*Continued*)
in thoracic region, 262t–264t
Overlaps, in physiotherapy consultations, 17t
Overpressure, 74–75
active movements with, in shoulder, 288f
to cervical spine, 237f
to elbow complex, 317f
in hip joint, 415f
to temporomandibular joint, 184f
to thoracic spine, 269f–270f

P

Pain
characteristics of, 39b
constant, unremitting, 365
definition of, 38–39, 152
depth of, 431–432
dimensions of, 39f
intensity of, 39–41, 41f
in cervicothoracic region, 231
in elbow region, 310
in foot and ankle, 471
in lumbar region, 365
in pelvis, 391
in temporomandibular joint, 177
in thoracic region, 259–260
ischaemic, nociception, 339
mechanisms of, 153–154, 154b–155b, 435
movement diagrams for, 65, 131
neuropathic, symptoms of, 54
night symptoms, 366
in pelvis, 388
predominant, mechanism of, 313–314
provoked or reduced, on palpation, 378, 449
quality of, 39–44
in cervicothoracic region, 231
in elbow region, 310
in pelvis, 391
in shoulder, 285
in temporomandibular joint, 177
referred, 41–44, 42f, 44b
symptoms of, in knee region, 431
Pain diary, for low-back pain, 365
Pain provocation tests, for pelvis, 395–397, 396f–397f
Pain-rating scale, for intensity of pain, 431–432
PAIVMs. *See* Passive accessory intervertebral movements
Palmaris longus, 325
Palpation, 67t, 126, 126b
of cervicothoracic region, 236–241
of elbow, 325–326
of foot and ankle, 484
nerve, 482
of hip region, 418–419
of joint, 83t, 160–162, 161t
of knee region, 449–450
of lumbar region, 378
of muscle, 83t
of nerve, 120–126
of pelvis, 399
of pulses, 325
of shoulder region, 302
systematic, suggested approach to, 326
of thoracic region, 274
trigger points, 126
of upper cervical region, 211
of wrist and hand examination, 351
systematic, suggested approach to, 351
Palpation chart, 127f, 378, 450, 484
for upper cervical region, 213
Paraesthesia, upper cervical spine examination and, 201
Parafunctional habits, temporomandibular joint and, 178, 178t, 180b
Passive accessory intervertebral movements (PAIVMs), 68–69, 202
in atlantoaxial joint, 214t
in atlantooccipital joint, 214t
in cervicothoracic region, 239, 242f, 243t, 244f
in lumbar region, 378–380, 379f–380f, 380b
in thoracic region, 274, 275f–276f, 277t, 278b
in upper cervical region, 211–212, 213f, 214t
Passive intervertebral examination (PIE)
of cervicothoracic region, 239, 240t
of upper cervical region, 212f
Passive knee bend, 449
Passive lengthening of muscle, 161t
Passive movements, examination on, 158
Passive neck flexion, 107–108, 108f, 377, 448
Passive physiological intervertebral movements (PPIVMs), 68–69, 202
of cervicothoracic region, 239, 241f
of thoracic region, 271, 273f
Passive physiological movements, 67t, 78, 78b, 79f, 160–162
of elbow region, 318, 318f
of hip region, 414
of knee region, 439, 440f
of lumbar region, 373–374, 374f
of shoulder, 289–292
posterior shoulder tightness and, 289–292, 291f
of wrist and hand, 341
Passive sensitizing movement, 110
Past medical history
cervicothoracic region and, 233–234
in pelvis, 392–393
in shoulder, 287
in subjective examination, 37t, 55
in thoracic region, 265
Patella tendinopathy test, 447
Patellar pubic percussion test, for hip region, 417, 417f
Patellar subluxation or dislocation, 447
Patellar tap test, 439
Patellofemoral joint, 432
accessory movements of, 450–451, 453t
in joint clearing tests, 77t
Patellofemoral tests, 446–447
Pathobiological mechanisms, of clinical reasoning, 152–154
pain, 153–154, 154b
tissue responses and healing, 152–153
Pathology, serious, of shoulder, 285, 287b
Patients' perspectives
on hip region, 408

Patients' perspectives (*Continued*)
on knee region, for examination, 431
in subjective examination, 36–37, 36b, 37t
Pattern recognition, 145–146
Pectoralis major, length testing of, 84f
Pectoralis minor, length testing of, 84f
Pelvic floor, 399
Pelvic region, 388–390, 388f, 390b
Pelvic tilt, 69–70, 70f
Pelvic torsion test/Gaenslen's, for pelvis, 396, 396f
Pelvis, 387–406
case study, 401b–404b
examination, completion of, 400
physical examination of, 393–399
active physiological movements, 393–395, 394f–395f
functional testing, 393
muscle tests, 398–399
observation, 393
pain provocation tests, 395–397, 396f–397f
palpation, 399, 399b
passive accessory movements, 397–398, 397f–398f
pelvic floor, 399
plan of, 393
subjective examination of, 390–393
behaviour of symptoms, 391–392
history of the present condition, 392
imaging and investigations, 392–393
nature of symptoms, 390–391
past medical history, 392–393
patient's perspective, 390
special questions, 392
Pelvis girdle, 388, 388f–389f
Peripheral nerves
compression of, 89–90
in elbow region, 323–324
in foot and ankle, 482
formation of, 90f
in hip region, 421
in knee region, 448
in lumbar region, test for, 376
in temporomandibular joint, 186
in thoracic region, 271
Peripheral nerves (*Continued*)
in upper cervical region, 209–211
in wrist and hand examination, 349
Peripheral neuropathic pain, 39b, 154b
Person-focused (patient-centered care), communication in, 18, 18b, 19f
Perturbation control, 458
Pes cavus, 475
Pes planus, 475
Phalen's wrist flexion test, 350
Physical capability, 26
Physical examination, 65–142
accessory movements in, 126–129, 127f–128f, 128b
active physiological movements in, 72–75
aims of, 66
for cervicothoracic region, 235–249
chart, 134f
clinical reasoning in, 65, 136f, 144–146
aims of, 160, 166b
precautions/contraindications to, 157–158
communication in, 20–23
providing feedback, 22
role of touch in communication, 22–23
signposting, 20
undress negotiation, 20–22
completion of, 133–138, 134f–135f
for elbow region, 315–326
completion of, 326–329
plan of, 313–314
sequence and extent of, 314
functional ability/physical performance tests in, 72, 72b
for hip region, 411–422
interpretation of, 66–67
joint integrity tests in, 78
for knee region, 436–459, 436t
for lumbar region, 370–380
management planning form in, 135f
muscle tests in, 78–89, 82t
neurological tests in, 89–126, 126b
observation in, 67–72
palpation in, 126, 126b
Physical examination (*Continued*)
passive physiological movements in, 67t, 78, 78b, 79f
for pelvis, 393–399
performing testing procedures in, 1
plan of
form, 369
for hip region, 410–411
for lumbar region, 369
for pelvis, 393
for thoracic region, 265–274
planning sheet, 56–57, 58f
sensorimotor tests in, 89–126
for shoulder, 287–302
step by step, 67–132
summary of, 67t
for temporomandibular joint, 181–189
tests, 77t
trigger points, 126
for upper cervical region, 208–219
for wrist and hand, 339–353
completion of, 353–357
planning, 338–339
Physical factors, 156–157
Physical impairments, associated structure/tissue sources and, 154–155
Physical opportunity, 27
Physical performance tests, 72, 72b
Physical tests, 155
Physiotherapy consultations, content of, 13–18, 15t–16t
challenging conversations, 16–17
documenting psychological distress, 17–18
interruptions, 14–16, 14f, 16b, 17t
PIE. *See* Passive intervertebral examination
Pinch-grip strengths, measurement of, 347–348
Pinch-grip test, 325
Pink flags, 151
Pinprick sensation, 93
lower limb and, 376
Piriformis
length testing of, 84f
muscle length of, 448
Pisohamate. *See* Guyon's canal
Pisotriquetral joint, accessory movements of, 352f, 355t–356t
Pivot shift test, 443–444, 443f

Planetary model, of reasoning, 149, 150f
Planning sheet, in cervicothoracic region, 234
Plantar response
thoracic region and, 273
for upper motor neurone lesion, 245, 377
Plica syndrome, 449
Poor treatment, outcome of, in subjective examination, 48
Posterior cruciate ligament, injury to, 440–441
Posterior drawer test
for knee region, 444, 444f
for shoulder instability, 298, 298f
Posterior gapping/compression test, for pelvis, 396, 396f
Posterior shear test, for pelvis, 396, 396f
Posterior shoulder tightness (PST), 289–292, 291f
Posterior stability tests, 444
Posterolateral rotatory instability, tests for, in elbow region, 320–321, 320f
Posttraumatic stress reactions, 230
Postural stability, of cervicothoracic region, 247
Posture
of cervicothoracic region, 235
in foot and ankle examination, 475
in hip region examination, 412
ideal alignment, 68, 68f
of lumbar region, 370
in nonverbal behaviours, 9
observation of, 67–70, 315
in knee region examination, 437
in wrist and hand examination, 339
Pott disease, in thoracic region, 262t–264t
PPIVMs. *See* Passive physiological intervertebral movements
Precautions, to physical examination, 157–158
of elbow region, 313
of lumbar region, 367, 369
Predictive values, in physical examination, 66
Predominant pain mechanism, 313–314
Prehension, of hand, 335
Pressure biofeedback unit, 216
Previous history, knee region and, 433
Primary bone tumours, in elbow region, 309t, 311
Prodromal stage, of cancer, 50
Prognosis, of clinical reasoning, 166
Pronator syndrome, test for, 325
Pronator teres, 325
Prone knee bend, 108
Prone push-up test, 320f
Propositional knowledge, 145, 145f
Proprioception
for cervical arterial dysfunction, 219
for cervicothoracic region, 247, 249f
for upper cervical region, 203
Prosody, first impressions and, 8
PST. *See* Posterior shoulder tightness
Psychological capability, 27
Psychological distress, documenting, in physiotherapy consultations, 17–18
Psychosocial factors, 156
in recovery and treatment response, 364
Psychosocial yellow flags, 48
Pubic symphysis, 398
lumbar region and, 369
Pulses, palpation of
for cervical arterial dysfunction, 219
in elbow region, 325
in shoulder, 302
Push-up test, 321

Q

Quadratus lumborum
length testing of, 84f
muscle length of, 448
Qualitative analysis of single-leg loading (QASL), 456, 457f
Quality of movement
in elbow region, 316
in lumbar region, 370
Question
agenda setting and, 9, 10t
styles, 9–12
involve handling over control, 11–12, 12b
sensitive questioning, 11
Socratic questions, 11, 11t
TED questions, 10–11

R

RA. *See* Rheumatoid arthritis
Radial artery, Allen test for, 351
Radial nerve
palpation of, 301
test for, 351
upper-limb neurodynamic test for. *See* ULNT 2b
Radial nerve compression, in elbow region, 325
Radial tunnel syndrome, test for, 325
Radiocarpal joint, 335
accessory movements of, 351–353, 355t–356t
inferior radioulnar joint and, 342f
Radiograph
of elbow region, 312
of foot and ankle, 473–474, 474b
in subjective examination, 55
of wrist and hand examination, 338
Radius, dislocation of the head of, 309t
Range of movement
in elbow region, 316
in knee region, 438
in lumbar region, 370–372
Rapport, with patients, 151
RCRSP. *See* Rotator cuff-related shoulder pain
Reagan's test, 342–344
Reassessment, of patient's asterisks
for cervicothoracic region, 243t
for elbow region, 329t
for foot and ankle, 490t–492t
for hip region, 424t
for knee region, 453t
for temporomandibular joint, 189t
for thoracic region, 277t
for wrist and hand, 353
Rectus capitis anterior, 216
Rectus femoris
muscle length of, 448
Red-flag system, 157
Red flags, 48t, 49
hierarchical list of, 51t
Referred pain, 41–44, 42f, 44b
from viscera, 42f
Reflective motivation, 27
Reflex changes, 96–100, 97t, 105f
Reflex testing, 105f
for cervicothoracic region, 245
for foot and ankle, 482

Reflex testing (*Continued*)
for hip region, 421
for knee region, 448
for lumbar region, 377
for temporomandibular joint, 186
for upper motor neurone lesion, 211
Regional interdependence, definition of, 258–259, 259b
Relationship of symptoms, 44, 45b
in cervicothoracic region, 231
in elbow region, 310
in foot and ankle, 472
in hip region, 408
in knee region, 432
in lumbar region, 365
in pelvis, 391
in shoulder, 286
in temporomandibular joint, 177
in thoracic region, 260
in upper cervical region, 204–205
in wrist and hand, 336
Remote consultations, 18–20
clear signposting, 18
gaining consent, 20, 21t–22t
starting the call, 19–20, 20f, 21t–22t
technology concerns, 19
Repeated movements, 77
Resistance
in elbow region, 316
in knee region, 438
movement diagrams for, 129–131, 130f
Resisted external derotation test, for hip region, 418, 418f
Respiration
rib mechanics during, 275–276, 277f
thoracic region and, 273–274
Respiratory disease, history of, 52
Reversed natural apophyseal glides, in cervicothoracic region, 241, 244f
Rheumatoid arthritis (RA), 309t, 312, 435, 469
lumbar region and, 367–369
of wrist and hand, 335
Ribcage
examination of, 274–276, 276f
during respiration, 275–276, 277f
Ribs
accessory movements to, 276f, 277t
mechanics of, during respiration, 275–276, 277f
Romberg's test, 219
Roos test, 249, 301
Rotation, to cervical spine, 237f
Rotation PPIVM, 212f
Rotator cuff pathology tests, for shoulder, 292–293
empty- and full-can tests, 292, 293f
external rotation lag sign as, 293, 294f
Gerber 'lift-off,', 292–293, 293f
Rotator cuff-related shoulder pain (RCRSP), 295–296

S

Sacral nerve roots, myotome testing for, 103f
Sacral thrust test, for pelvis, 396–397, 397f
Sacroiliac joints (SIJ), 388
active straight-leg raise (ASLR) test for, 394–395, 395f
behaviour of symptoms
aggravating factors, 391–392
easing factors, 391
distraction/anterior gapping test for, 395, 396f
Gaenslen's/pelvic torsion test for, 396, 396f
in joint clearing tests, 77t
lumbar region and, 369
pain provocation tests for, 395–397, 396f–397f
palpation of, 399
posterior gapping/compression test for, 396, 396f
posterior shear test for, 396, 396f
sacral thrust test for, 396–397, 397f
standing hip flexion test (Gillet test) for, 394, 394f
Saphenous nerve test, 110, 110f
SAPS. *See* Sub-acromial pain syndrome
Scalenes
length testing of, 84f
muscle length testing, 218
Scaphoid fractures, 338
Scaphoid shift test, 342, 347f
Scapula, role of, 298
Scapular assistance test, 299, 299f
Scapular dyskinesis, 299
Scapular strength, of cervicothoracic region, 241
Scheuermann's disease, in thoracic region, 262t–264t
Sciatic nerve palpation, 422
SCM. *See* Sternocleidomastoid
Scoliosis, lumbar region and, 370–372
Seated heel lock position, for testing axial rotation, 270f
SEBT. *See* Star excursion balance test
Semispinalis capitis, 217
Semispinalis cervicis, 217
Sensation, abnormal
in cervicothoracic region, 231
in elbow region, 310
in shoulder, 285
in temporomandibular joint, 177
in thoracic region, 260
Sensitive questioning, 11
Sensitivity, in physical examination, 66
Sensorimotor control, in upper cervical region, 215–216
Sensorimotor testing, 89–126
for cervicothoracic region, 245–247, 249f
Sensory aura, migraine and, 201
Sensory changes, 90–93, 90f
Sensory loss
in elbow region, 323–324
in knee region, 448
Serious pathology
in lumbar region, 368
in wrist and hand examination, 336
Serratus anterior, strength testing of, 80f
Severe symptoms, in lumbar region, 369
Severity, of symptoms, 45b, 46, 158–160, 160b
Shared decision-making, 24–26, 25t–26t
Shingles, in thoracic region, 262t–264t
Short-leg gait, 412
Shoulder, examination of, 284–306
abnormal sensation in, 285
active physiological movements in, 287–289, 288f

Shoulder, examination of (*Continued*)
aggravating factors in, 286
areas relevant to the region being examined in, 285
biceps test and, 293
body chart in, 285–286
case study and, 303b–304b
completion of, 302
easing factors in, 286
glenohumeral joint instability and, 296–298
investigations in, 287
muscle tests and
control in, 298–299, 300f
strength in, 299
neurological examination and, 301
observation in, 287
pain in, quality of, 285
palpation in, 302
passive physiological movements in, 289–292
posterior shoulder tightness and, 289–292, 291f
past medical history in, 287
physical, 287–302
present condition in, history of, 286–287
referred symptoms to, from wrist and hand, 336
rotator cuff pathology tests and, 292–293
empty- and full-can tests, 292, 293f
external rotation lag sign as, 293, 294f
Gerber 'lift-off,', 292–293, 293f
rotator cuff-related shoulder pain in, 295–296
stage of the condition in, 286
subjective, 285–287
patient's perspective on, 285
serious pathology in, 285, 287b
superior labral anterior-posterior tests and, 293–295
active compression test, 294–295, 295f
biceps load tests I and II, 294, 295f
symptoms in
area of current, 285
behaviour of, 286
morning and evening, 286
Shoulder, examination of (*Continued*)
neurological, 286
night, 286
relationship of, 286
vascular, 286
trauma in, history of, 286
vascular assessment and, 301–302
Shoulder abduction test, 247
Shoulder girdle, in joint clearing tests, 77t
Shoulder impingement syndrome (SIS), 295
Shoulder instability, 296–298, 302b
apprehension test for, 298, 298f
load and shift test for, 297, 297f
posterior drawer test, 298, 298f
sulcus sign for, 297–298, 297f
Shoulder joint, in joint clearing tests, 77t
Shoulder symptom modification procedures (SSMPs), 289, 290f
Shoulder tests, 292
Shuttle walking test, 72
Side-flexion PPIVM, 212f
Sideways step down/landing test, 458
Signposting
in physical examination, 20
in remote consultations, 18
SIJ. *See* Sacroiliac joints
Single-leg squat, 448, 456
SIS. *See* Shoulder impingement syndrome
Skin colour, lumbar region and, 370
Skin moisture, localized increase of, 449
SLAP tests. *See* Superior labral anterior-posterior (SLAP) tests
SLR. *See* Straight-leg raise
Slump test, 110–111, 111f, 377
Small fibre testing, 93–96, 96f
Small talk, first impressions and, 8
SMART goals, 163, 163f
Smiling, in nonverbal behaviours, 9
Smooth pursuit neck torsion test, 204
SNAGs. *See* Sustained natural apophyseal glides
SNOOP mnemonic, yellow flag screening using, 206t
SOAP. *See* Subjective, objective, analysis and plan
Social history
for examination, in elbow region, 309
foot and ankle examination, 470–471
subjective examination and, 285
Social opportunity, 27
Socratic questions, 11, 11t
Soft tissues
of cervicothoracic region, 236
foot and ankle examination and, 475–476
hip region examination and, 412
knee region examination and, 437
observation of, 71
wrist and hand examination and, 339–340
Soleus, muscle length of, 448
Special tests, 67t
Specificity, in physical examination, 66
Speed of movement, in active physiological movements, 77
Speed's test, for bicipital tendinopathy, 293, 294f
Spinal cancer, red-flag screening for, 206t
Spinal cord compression, 367, 410, 473
Spinal fracture, red-flag screening for, 206t
Spinal manipulation, clinical prediction rules of,criteria for, 148t
Spinal masqueraders, 258, 262t–264t
Spinal spondylolysis, presence of, 158
Spine, lumbar region and, 364
Splenius capitis, 217
Spondylosis, in thoracic region, 262t–264t
Sports-related chronic groin pain, 419, 420t
Spurling's neck compression test, 247, 250f
Squeeze test
for foot and ankle, 481, 481f
for hip region, 419–420, 419f, 420t
SSMPs. *See* Shoulder symptom modification procedures
Stage of condition, 47–48
Stages-of-change model, 163, 164f, 164t

Stair climbing tests, 72
Stand-up test, 72, 321
Standard active testing, 73–74
Standing hip flexion test (Gillet test), for pelvis, 394, 394f
Stanmore Triangle, shoulder instability and, 297, 297f
Star excursion balance test (SEBT), 459, 459b, 484, 484f
STarT MSK Tool, 230, 259
Step-by-step approach, to subjective and physical examination, 1
Step down/single leg landing/load acceptance test, 457
Stereognosis, of hand, 349
Sternoclavicular joint, in joint clearing tests, 77t
Sternocleidomastoid (SCM), length testing of, 84f, 218
Sternocostal fibres, length testing of, 84f
Sternocostal joints, accessory movements in, 277t
Steroid therapy, 313, 369
Stiff shoulder, 296
Stiffness, in elbow region, 312
Straight-leg raise (SLR), 108, 109f, 377, 449
Stretch pattern, regular, 76
Stroke, 232–233
Sub-acromial pain syndrome (SAPS), 295
Subclinical stage, of cancer, 50
Subjective, objective, analysis and plan (SOAP), 150, 152b
Subjective examination, 34–64
  aggravating and easing factors in, 45–46
  aim of, 35–36
  body chart for, 37–44, 38f, 43f
    abnormal sensations in, 44
    area of current symptoms in, 37–38
    areas relevant to the region being examined in, 38
  of cervicothoracic region, 230–235
    assessment tools and patient reported outcome measures, 230
    patients' perspective, 230
  chronicity, risk factors for, 48, 48t
  clinical reasoning in, 35
Subjective examination (*Continued*)
  form of, using hypothesis categories, 59, 59f
  of elbow region, 309–314
  family history in, 56
  function of, impact on, 44–45
  of hip region, 408–411
  history of present condition in, 56
  of knee region, 431–435
  of lumbar region, 364–369
  pain in
    characteristics of, 39b
    definition of, 38–39
    dimensions of, 39f
    intensity, 39–41, 41f
    quality of, 39–44
    referred, 41–44, 42f, 44b
  past medical history in, 55
  patient's perspective in, 36–37
  of pelvis, 390–393
  physical examination, plan in, 56–58, 58f
  radiographs, medical imaging and tests in, 55
  screening/special questions for, 49–55, 49t–50t
    cancer in, 52
    cardiovascular disease in, 51–52
    cervical artery dysfunction in, 54
    diabetes mellitus in, 52
    drug therapy in, 55
    epilepsy in, 52
    general health in, 51
    human immunodeficiency virus, 52
    hypermobility spectrum disorder in, 54
    inflammatory arthritis in, 53
    neurological symptoms in, 53–54
    neuropathic pain symptoms in, 54
    osteoporosis in, 53
    respiratory disease in, 52
    thyroid disease in, 52
    tuberculosis in, 52
    weight loss in, 51
  of shoulder, 285–287
  stage of condition in, 47–48
  summary of, 37t
  symptoms in
    constant or intermittent, 44
    evening, 47
Subjective examination (*Continued*)
    morning, 47
    night, 47
    relationship of, 44
    severity and irritability, 46–47
    twenty-four-hour behaviour of, 47
  of thoracic region, 259–266
  of upper cervical region, 204–208
  of wrist and hand, 335–339
Suboccipital muscle group, 198f
Subscapularis
  strength testing of, 80f
  tendinopathy, Gerber 'lift-off' for, 292–293, 293f
Subtalar joint, 476–477
Sulcus sign, for shoulder instability, 297–298, 297f
Superior labral anterior-posterior (SLAP) tests, for shoulder region, 293–295
  active compression test, 294–295, 295f
  biceps load tests I and II, 294, 295f
Superior radioulnar joint, 308, 311
  accessory movements in, 326, 328f, 329t
  active physiological movements in, 316
  aggravating factors in, 310–311
Superior tibiofibular joint, accessory movements of, 450–451, 453t
Supine internal rotation in 90 degrees abduction, shoulder region and, 291, 291f
Supracondylar process syndrome, test for, 325
Suprascapular nerve, palpation of, 301
Supraspinatus
  full-thickness tears of, external rotation lag sign for, 293, 294f
  tear or tendinopathy of, empty- and full-can tests for, 292, 293f
Surgery, previous, lumbar region and, 368
Sustained movements, in active physiological movements, 77
Sustained natural apophyseal glides (SNAGs), 214, 215f
  in cervicothoracic region, 241, 244f
  headache, 215f
  upper cervical traction, 215f

Sustained single-leg stance, for hip region, 418, 418f
Swan-neck deformity of fingers, 339, 340f
Sway-back posture, 68, 69f
Sweater finger sign test, 349
Sweep test, 439–440
Swelling
  of elbow region
    observation of, 316
    sudden, 312
  of wrist and hand, tests for, 351
Symphysis pubis, 398
Symptom modification
  in elbow region, 317, 323
  in thoracic region, 268–271, 272f
  in wrist and hand examination, 340–341, 342f, 347f
Symptoms
  aggravating factors of, 45–46, 49t–50t
    in cervicothoracic region, 231
    in elbow region, 310–311
    in foot and ankle, 472
    in hip region, 408–409
    in knee region, 432, 437
    in lumbar region, 365
    in pelvis, 391
    in shoulder, 286
    in temporomandibular joint, 177
    in thoracic region, 260
    in upper cervical region, 205
    in wrist and hand, 336–337
  behaviour of, 37t
    in cervicothoracic region, 231–232
    in elbow region, 310–311
    in foot and ankle, 472
    in hip region, 408–409
    in knee region, 432–433
    in lumbar region, 365–367, 366t
    in shoulder, 286
    in temporomandibular joint, 177–178
    in thoracic region, 260–261
    in upper cervical region, 205
    in wrist and hand, 336–337
  constant or intermittent, 44, 158
    in cervicothoracic region, 231
    in elbow region, 310
Symptoms (*Continued*)
    in foot and ankle, 471
    in hip region, 408
    in temporomandibular joint, 177
    in thoracic region, 260
  evening, 47
  irritability of, 158–160, 160b
  morning, 47
  morning and evening, 47
    in cervicothoracic region, 232
    in elbow region, 311
    in foot and ankle, 472
    in hip region, 409
    in knee region, 432–433
    in lumbar region, 366–367
    in pelvis, 391–392
    in wrist and hand, 337
  neurological, 53–54
    in foot and ankle, 473
    in lumbar region, 367
    in shoulder, 286
    in thoracic region, 261
  neuropathic pain, 54
  night, 47
  relationship, 44
  relationship of, 44, 45b
    in cervicothoracic region, 231
    in elbow region, 310
    in foot and ankle, 472
    in hip region, 408
    in knee region, 432
    in lumbar region, 365
    in pelvis, 391
    in shoulder, 286
    in temporomandibular joint, 177
    in thoracic region, 260
    in upper cervical region, 204–205
    in wrist and hand, 336
  severity and irritability, 46–47
  severity of, 158–160
  twenty-four-hour behaviour of, 47
    in cervicothoracic region, 232
    in elbow region, 311
    in foot and ankle, 472
    in hip region, 409
    in knee region, 432–433
    in lumbar region, 366–367
    in pelvis, 391–392
Symptoms (*Continued*)
    in temporomandibular joint, 178
    in upper cervical region, 205
Systematic palpation, suggested approach to
  in elbow region, 326
  in wrist and hand, 351

T

Table-top relocation test, 321
Talar tilt, 480, 480f
Talocrural joint, 483
  anterior impingement sign of, 483, 483f
Talus, osteochondral defects affecting, 469
Tandem gait, 219
Tarsometatarsal joints, 484
TB. *See* Tuberculosis
Technology, concerns, in remote consultations, 19
Tectorial membrane, 198f
  distraction test for, 212f
TED questions, 10–11
Temperature sensation, 93
Temporal artery, palpation of, 188
Temporomandibular joint dysfunction (TMD), 174–176
  classification of, 175, 175t
  multidisciplinary team approach to, 189–191
    AROM, 193b
    diagnosis, 192b
    HPC, 192b
    impact on function, beliefs and expectations, 192b
    informal observation, 193b
    intraoral observation, 193b
    lifestyle/occupation/homelife, 192b
    outcome measures, 192b
    palpation, 193b
    planning the objective, 193b
    screening questions, 192b
    strength testing, 193b
  other nontemporomandibular joint causes of, 176
  relationship between the cervical spine, thoracic and, 175–176
  signs and symptoms of, 175

Temporomandibular joint (TMJ), 173–195
abnormal sensation in, 177
accessory movements in, 188, 189f, 189t
active physiological movements in, 182–185, 183f–185f, 185t
anatomy review of, 174
area of current symptoms in, 177
areas relevant to the region being examined in, 177
articular disc in, 174
bite test for, 189, 191f
bruxism and, 179
case study for, 192b–193b
cervical arterial dysfunction and, 179–180
clenching and, 179
clicking and, 178
clinical tests and, validity of, 189
completion of, 189
cranial nerve disorders and, 179
deflection of, 183
dental disorders and, 179
deviation of, 182
dynamic loading and distraction in, 189
easing factors in, 177–178
headaches and, 180
in joint clearing tests, 77t
miscellaneous test for, 188
muscle tests and, 186
endurance testing, 186
isometric, 186
muscle control, 186
muscle strength, 186, 187f
neurological tests for, 186–188
dermatomes, 186
integrity of nervous system, 186
myotomes, 186
neurodynamic tests, 186
reflex testing, 186
observation of, 181–182
formal, 181
informal, 181
of intraoral environment, 182, 182f
of muscle form, 182
of posture, 181, 181f
of soft tissues, 182
overpressures to, 184f
Temporomandibular joint (TMJ) (*Continued*)
pain in
intensity of, 177
myogenic, 179
quality of, 177
palpation of, 188, 188f
via external auditory meatus, 189, 191f
parafunctional habits in, 178, 178t
passive physiological movements in, 185–186
past medical history in, 180
physical examination of, plan of, 180–181
present condition for, history of, 180
subjective examination for, 176–181
body chart for, 176–177, 176f
patient's perspective in, 176
special questions and red-flag screening, 178–180
symptoms in
aggravating factors of, 177
behaviour of, 177–178
constant or intermittent, 177
ear, 180
morning and evening, 178
night, 178
trismus and, 179
Temporomandibular region, 173–195
Tenderness, of bone, 449
Tendinopathy, elbow
lateral, symptom modification for, 323, 324f
medial, 323
Tennis elbow, 309t
tests for, 322–323
Tenodesis action, of wrist and hand, 348
Tension-type headache (TTH), 200, 200t
Tensor fasciae latae, muscle length of, 448
Thenar eminence, muscle strength testing in, 347
Thessaly test, 446, 446f
Thigh, symptoms, referred from, knee region and, 438
Thigh thrust test, for pelvis, 396, 396f
Thompson's test, for Achilles tendon rupture, 481, 481f
Thoracic disc, 262t–264t
Thoracic outlet syndrome, test for, 249
Thoracic region, 257–283
abnormal sensation in, 260
active physiological movements in, 267–271, 269f–270f, 270t
differentiation and symptom modification for, 268–271, 271f–272f
aggravating factors in, 260
areas relevant to the region being examined in, 259
assessment tools and patient-reported outcome measures in, 259
body chart in, 259–260
case study in, 281b–282b
complaint in, history of, 265
completion of, 276–278
drug history in, 261
easing factors in, 260
general health in, 261
investigations, injections and imaging in, 261
miscellaneous tests and, 273–274
muscle testing and, 271, 273b
neurological integrity in, 271–273
neurological testing and, 271
observation in, 266–267, 267t
of aggravating functional activities or positions, 268
formal, 266–267
informal, 266
pain in, intensity of, 259–260
palpation in, 274
passive accessory intervertebral movements in, 274, 275f–276f, 277t, 278b
passive physiological intervertebral movements in, 271, 273f
past medical history in, 265
patient's perspective in, 259
pattern recognition and differential diagnosis in, 261, 262t–264t
physical, plan of, 265–274
presenting condition in, 265
in ribcage, 274–276, 276f
during respiration, 275–276, 277f

Thoracic region (*Continued*)
special/screening questions for, 261–265
state of the condition in, 261
subjective, 259–266
symptoms in
area of current, 259
behaviour of, 260–261
constant or intermittent, 260
morning and evening, 260–261
neurological, 261
night, 260
relationship of, 260
vascular, 261–265
thoracic spine and, 258–259
upper motor nerve lesions and, 273
vascular tests and, 274
Thoracic spine
in joint clearing tests, 77t
lumbar region and, 369
overpressures to, 269f–270f
overview of, 258–259
wrist and hand symptoms referred to, 336
Thoracic spine dysfunction, kinetic chain and, 258–259
Thoracic spine pain, 258
pattern recognition and differentiation for, 262t–264t, 265b
Thumb
accessory movements of, 352f, 355t–356t
in joint clearing tests, 77t
Thyroid disease, history of, 52
Thyroid dysfunction
in elbow region, 311
in wrist and hand examination, 337–338
Tibial nerve palpation, 422, 449
Tibial tubercle, enlarged, 437
Tibialis anterior, strength testing of, 80f
Tibialis posterior, 476
length testing of, 84f
muscle length of, 448
Tibiofemoral joint, accessory movements of, 450–451, 453t
Tinel test, 324
Tinel's sign, 245
at wrist, 350
Tissue resistance, 107
Tissue responses, healing and, 152–153
Tissue sources, physical impairments and, 154–155
TMD. *See* Temporomandibular joint dysfunction
TMJ. *See* Temporomandibular joint
Toe extension, 103f
Toe standing, 103f
Tongue scalloping, 182, 182f
Touch, role of, in physical examination, 22–23, 23b
Transverse ligament, 198f
Trapezius
length testing of, 84f, 218
strength testing of, 80f
Trauma
in ankle, 469
in elbow region, 309t, 312
history of, shoulder and, 286
in knee region, 433
in lumbar region, 369
to wrist and hand, 335
Treatment planning, of clinical reasoning, 160–166
Trendelenburg gait, 412
Trendelenburg sign, 412, 413f
Triangular fibrocartilaginous complex load test, 344–346, 348f
Triceps jerk, 105f
Trigger points, 126
active, referred pain in, 44
Trismus, temporomandibular joint and, 179
Trochanteric bursitis, 417
Trunk muscles, muscle control of, test of, 375
TTH. *See* Tension-type headache
Tuberculosis (TB), 309t
history of, 52
in thoracic region, 262t–264t
Twenty-four-hour behaviour of symptoms
in cervicothoracic region, 232
in elbow region, 311
in foot and ankle, 472
in hip region, 409
in knee region, 432–433
in lumbar region, 366–367
in pelvis, 391–392
in temporomandibular joint, 178
in upper cervical region, 205

U

UCI. *See* Upper cervical instability
UCS. *See* Upper cervical spine
Ulna, fracture of, 309t
Ulnar artery, Allen test for, 351
Ulnar drift, 339–340
Ulnar nerve
compression neuropathy tests, 324–325
compression of, 309t
test for, 350–351
of upper limb, 99f
upper-limb neurodynamic test for. *See* ULNT 3
ULNT 1, 111–120, 115f
ULNT 2a, 117, 118f
ULNT 2b, 117–120, 121f
ULNT 3, 120, 123f
ULNTs. *See* Upper limb neurodynamic tests
Ultrasound
of foot and ankle, 473–474
of wrist and hand, 338
Unstable surface (soft mat), 458
Upper cervical instability (UCI), innervation of, 197, 199f
Upper cervical region, 196–228
active physiological movements of, 208, 209f
differentiation tests, 208
anatomical overview of, 197–198
body chart for, 204–205
completion of examination for, 219–221
definition
C0-C1 (atlanto-occipital joint), 197
C1-C2 (atlantoaxial joint), 197
C2-3 facet joints, 197
muscle testing for, 214–218
isometric testing, 214–215
isotonic testing, 214
muscle length, 218
muscle strength, 214
neurological testing for, 208–211
nervous system, integrity of, 209
neurodynamic tests, 211
upper motor neurone lesion, pathological reflex testing for, 211
observation for, 208
palpation in, 211
nerve, 211

Upper cervical region (*Continued*)
passive accessory intervertebral movements of, 211–212, 213f, 214t
passive intervertebral examination for, 212f
physical examination for, 208–219
relationship of symptoms, 204–205
risk factors of, 207t
sensorimotor control, 215–216
subjective examination for, 204–208
patient's perspective, 204
special questions, 205
sustained natural apophyseal glides, 214, 215f
symptoms, behaviour of, 205
aggravating factors, 205
easing factors, 205
twenty-four-hour, 205
Upper cervical spine (UCS)
dizziness, 203
innervation of, 197
Upper limb
dermatomes of, 94f
median nerve of, 99f
nerves of, 98f
Upper limb neurodynamic tests (ULNTs), 111–120, 301
Upper motor neurone lesion, test for, 377

V

Valgus stress tests, 440–441, 441f
Valgus test, in elbow region, 315f, 318–319, 319f
VAs. *See* Vertebral arteries
Vascular assessment, for shoulder, 301–302
Vascular symptoms
in cervicothoracic region, 234, 234b
in shoulder, 286
in thoracic region, 261–265
Vascular tests
for foot and ankle, 482–483
for hip region, 421–422
for knee region, 449
for lumbar region, 378
for thoracic region, 274
Vastus intermedius
muscle strength of, 447–448
strength testing of, 80f
Vastus lateralis
muscle strength of, 447–448
strength testing of, 80f
Vastus medialis
muscle strength of, 447–448
strength testing of, 80f
Vastus medialis obliquus (VMO), 450
VDT. *See* Vibration disappearance threshold
Vertebral arteries (VAs), 198
dissection, pain presentation for, 207f
dysfunction, 207t
Vertebrobasilar insufficiency, 219
Vibration disappearance threshold (VDT), 92–93
Vibration sensation, 92–93
Visceral complaints, in thoracic region, 262t–264t
Visceral pain, 42
VISI. *See* Volar intercalated segment instability
Visual analogue scale, 41f
for recording pain intensity, 365
Visual aura, migraine and, 201
Volar intercalated segment instability (VISI), 341
Volkmann ischaemic contracture, 309t

W

WADs. *See* Whiplash-associated disorders
Walking tests, 72
Watson (scaphoid shift) test, 342, 347f
Weight-bearing joint, 308
Weight-bearing lunge test, 477, 479f
Weight loss, 51
lumbar region and, 368
Wells score, for suspected deep-vein thrombosis, 482–483
WHAT. *See* Wrist hyperflexion and abduction of the thumb
Whiplash-associated disorders (WADs), 203–204
Whiplash-related dizziness, 203–204
Wrist and hand, 334–362
behaviour of symptoms of, 336–337
aggravating factors in, 336–337
Wrist and hand (*Continued*)
easing factors in, 337
over time, 337
body charts of, 336, 336f
area of current symptoms in, 336
areas relevant to the region being examined, 336
constant or intermittent symptoms, 336
intensity of pain, 336
quality of symptoms, 336
relationship of symptoms, 336
case study on, 359b–360b
dysfunction of, 335, 335b
formal observation in, 339–340
muscle form, 339
posture, 339
soft tissues, 339–340
history in
past medical, 337–338
of present condition, 338, 338b
joint integrity tests for, 341–347
axial compression test (grind test), 346–347, 348f
ligamentous instability test for joints of thumb and fingers, 346
lunotriquetral ballottement (Reagan's) test in, 342–344
midcarpal shift test in, 344
triangular fibrocartilaginous complex load test in, 344–346, 348f
Watson (scaphoid shift) test in, 342, 347f
muscle tests for, 347–349
isometric muscle testing, 348–349
muscle length, 348
muscle strength, 347–348
other muscle/tendon tests, 349
neurological testing for, 349–351
compression neuropathy, testing for, 350–351
integrity of nervous system, 349–350
neurodynamic tests in, 350
observation in, 339–340
formal, 339–340
informal, 339
overview in, 335
physical examination for, 339–353

Wrist and hand (*Continued*)
accessory movements in, 351–353, 352f, 355t–357t, 357b
active physiological movements in, 340–341, 341t
completion of, 353–357
functional testing in, 340
joint integrity tests in, 341–347
muscle tests in, 347–349
observation in, 339–340
palpation, 351
passive physiological movements in, 341
planning of, 338–339
reassessment asterisks in, 353
special/screening questions on, 337
subjective examination for, 335–339

Wrist and hand (*Continued*)
behaviour of symptoms, 336–337
body chart in, 336, 336f
history of the present condition, 338, 338b
past medical history in, 337–338
patients' perspective on their experience, 335–336
planning physical examination in, 338–339
special/screening questions on, 337
symptom modification in, 340–341, 342f, 347f
vascular assessment for, 351
Allen test, 351
figure-of-eight measurement, 351

Wrist hyperflexion and abduction of the thumb (WHAT) test, 349, 350f
Wrist joint, in joint clearing tests, 77t

X

X-ray
for elbow region, 312
for knee region, 434
for lumbar region, 369, 369b
for scaphoid fractures, 338
for shoulder, 296

Y

Yellow flags, 48, 48t
Yergason's test, 293, 294f